POCKET ESSENTIALS OF
CLINICAL
MEDICINE

FOURTH EDITION

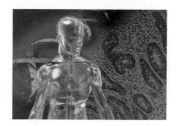

Pocket Essentials

Series Editors
Professor Parveen Kumar
Professor of Clinical Medical Education, Barts and the London, Queen Mary's School of Medicine and Dentistry, University of London, and Honorary Consultant Physician and Gastroenterologist, Barts and the London Hospitals NHS Trust and Homerton University Hospital NHS Foundation Trust, London, UK

and

Dr Michael Clark
Honorary Senior Lecturer, Barts and the London, Queen Mary's School of Medicine and Dentistry, University of London, UK

Commissioning Editor: Ellen Green
Development Editor: Hannah Kenner
Project Manager: Andrew Palfreyman
Design Direction: George Ajayi
Illustration Manager: Bruce Hogarth
Illustrator: Ethan Danielson, Richard Morris, Antbits

POCKET ESSENTIALS OF
CLINICAL
MEDICINE
FOURTH EDITION

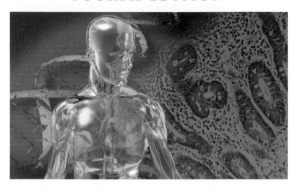

Anne Ballinger MD FRCP
Consultant Gastroenterologist and General Physician
Homerton University Hospital NHS Foundation Trust,
London, UK

Stephen Patchett MD FRCPI
Consultant Physician/Gastroenterologist,
Beaumont Hospital, Dublin, Ireland

Series Editors
Parveen Kumar and Michael Clark

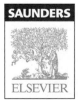

Edinburgh London New York Oxford Philadelphia
St Louis Sydney Toronto 2007

SAUNDERS
ELSEVIER

© 2008, Elsevier Limited. All rights reserved.

First edition 1995	Standard Edition ISBN 13: 978-0-7020-2830-4
Second edition 2000	Reprinted 2007
Third edition 2003	International Edition ISBN 13: 978-0-7020-2831-1
Fourth edition 2007	Reprinted 2007
	Book + CD of PDA version (pack)
	ISBN 13: 978-0-7020-2832-8
	CD of PDA version ISBN 13: 978-8-7020-2832-8

British Library Cataloguing in Publication Data
A catalogue record for this book is available from the British Library

Library of Congress Cataloging in Publication Data
A catalog record for this book is available from the Library of Congress

Note
Knowledge and best practice in this field are constantly changing. As new research and experience broaden our knowledge, changes in practice, treatment and drug therapy may become necessary or appropriate. Readers are advised to check the most current information provided (i) on procedures featured or (ii) by the manufacturer of each product to be administered, to verify the recommended dose or formula, the method and duration of administration, and contraindications. It is the responsibility of the practitioner, relying on their own experience and knowledge of the patient, to make diagnoses, to determine dosages and the best treatment for each individual patient, and to take all appropriate safety precautions. To the fullest extent of the law, neither the Publisher nor the Authors assume any liability for any injury and/or damage to persons or property arising out of or related to any use of the material contained in this book.

The Publisher

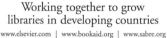

Series preface

Medical students and doctors in training are expected to travel to different hospitals and community health centres as part of their education. Many books are too large to carry around, but the information they contain is often vital for the basic understanding of disease processes.

The *Pocket Essentials* series is designed to provide portable, pocket-sized companions for students and junior doctors. They are most useful for clinical practice, whether in hospital or the community, and for exam revision.

The notable success of *Pocket Essentials of Clinical Medicine* over many editions is shown by its presence in the pockets of *all* healthcare professionals – nurses, pharmacists, physical and occupational therapists, to name a few – not simply medical students and doctors.

All the books in the series have the same helpful features:

- Succinct text
- Simple line drawings
- Emergency and other boxes
- Tables that summarize causes and clinical features of disease
- Exam questions and explanatory answers
- Dictionary of terms

They contain core material for quick revision, easy reference and practical management. The modern format makes them easy to read, providing an indispensable 'pocket essential.'

Parveen Kumar and **Michael Clark**
Series Editors

Series preface

Preface

Pocket Essentials of Clinical Medicine has been in print since 1995. With each edition we have continued the original concept of writing an easy-to-carry medical textbook based on its parent text, Kumar and Clark's *Clinical Medicine*. Like *Clinical Medicine*, we believe that an understanding of physiology, anatomy and pathophysiology is integral to learning about the clinical features and treatment of disease and we have continued to emphasize these aspects in the current edition. The fourth edition of *Pocket Essentials* has been thoroughly revised and updated, in line with changes in medicine and in the parent text.

We have continued to improve and expand the popular features associated with the *Pocket Essentials* series, such as emergency boxes, tables and diagnostic and treatment algorithms, while maintaining the core attribute of a succinct and highly portable text. We have updated the list of useful websites which was first introduced in the third edition. We have also added two new chapters: 'The special senses' and 'Therapeutics'. The special senses chapter – eyes and ENT – has been written in response to readers' suggestions for the parent text in that these are common conditions presenting to general practitioners and through Accident and Emergency. The therapeutics chapter describes those drugs commonly used in practice with their common or serious side-effects and contraindications; it is beyond the scope of this book to provide an exhaustive list to cover prescribing in all groups of patients. The Examination Questions have always been a popular feature of *Pocket Essentials* with enthusiastic reviews from our readers. We have updated this section in recognition of the increasing use of OSCEs, 'best of 5' and extended matching in examination scenarios.

Full colour throughout was first introduced in the third edition and we have made the most of this for the fourth edition with the addition of more colour pictures and diagrams. The use of colour also makes the text easier to navigate and to relate to the parent text, *Clinical Medicine* 6e, by using the same 'colour-coding' scheme for specific chapters. As with previous editions of *Pocket Essentials*, readers will find cross-referencing to *Clinical Medicine* 6e identified by the use of *K&C* 6e with the page number, thus making it easier to look up information in the larger book.

The third edition of *Pocket Essentials* was accompanied by an electronic product for use on hand-held computers or PDAs. This proved popular and we have extended this facility in the fourth edition with the addition of more medical calculators (▦ in the text) to the current version.

We would like to thank Mike Clark and Parveen Kumar for their support and assistance in the preparation of this fourth edition of *Pocket Essentials*, and to express our thanks to the contributors of the parent text, *Clinical Medicine*. Finally, without the continued help, support, hard work and keen eye of Hannah Kenner, Development Editor at Elsevier, this book would not have been completed in its present form.

Anne Ballinger and **Stephen Patchett**

Contents

Abbreviations

ACE	angiotensin-converting enzyme
ACTH	adrenocorticotrophic hormone
ADH	antidiuretic hormone
AF	atrial fibrillation
AIDS	acquired immunodeficiency syndrome
ALS	advanced life support
ANA	antinuclear antibodies
ANCA	antineutrophil cytoplasmic antibodies
ANF	antinuclear factor
ARDS	adult respiratory distress syndrome
AST	aspartate aminotransferase
AV	atrioventricular
AXR	abdominal X-ray
BCG	bacille Calmette–Guérin
BMI	body mass index
BP	blood pressure
CAL	chronic airflow limitation
CAPD	continuous ambulatory peritoneal dialysis
CCF	congestive cardiac failure
CCU	coronary care unit
CLL	chronic lymphatic leukaemia
CML	chronic myeloid leukaemia
CNS	central nervous system
CPR	cardiopulmonary resuscitation
CRP	C-reactive protein
CSF	cerebrospinal fluid
CT	computerized tomography
CVP	central venous pressure
CXR	chest X-ray
DIC	disseminated intravascular coagulation
DNA	deoxyribonucleic acid
DVT	deep venous thrombosis
ECG	electrocardiogram
EEG	electroencephalogram
ELISA	enzyme-linked immunosorbent assay
ERCP	endoscopic retrograde cholangiopancreatography

Abbreviations

ESR	erythrocyte sedimentation rate
FBC	full blood count
GABA	γ-aminobutyric acid
γ-GT	γ-glutamyltranspeptidase
GFR	glomerular filtration rate
GORD	gastro-oesophageal reflux disease
Hb	haemoglobin
5-HIAA	5-hydroxyindoleacetic acid
HIV	human immunodeficiency virus
HLA	human leucocyte antigen
Ig	immunoglobulin (e.g. IgM = immunoglobulin the M class)
i.m.	intramuscular
INR	international normalized ratio
iu/IU	international unit
i.v.	intravenous
IVP	intravenous pyelogram
JVP	jugular venous pressure
K&C	Kumar & Clark: *Clinical Medicine* 6e (Saunders 2005)
LP	lumbar puncture
LVF	left ventricular failure
MCV	mean corpuscular volume
ME	myalgic encephalomyelitis
MRI	magnetic resonance imaging
MRSA	methicillin-resistant *Staphylococcus aureus*
MSU	mid-stream urine
Na^+	concentration of sodium ions
nd	notifiable disease
NICE	National Institute for Health and Clinical Effectiveness
NSAIDs	non-steroidal anti-inflammatory drugs
P_aCO_2	partial pressure of carbon dioxide in arterial blood
P_aO_2	partial pressure of oxygen in arterial blood
PCR	polymerase chain reaction
PCV	packed cell volume
PPI	proton pump inhibitor
PR	per rectum (rectal instillation)
PT	prothrombin time
PTC	percutaneous transhepatic cholangiography
PTCA	percutaneous transluminal coronary angioplasty
PTTK	partial thromboplastin time with kaolin
QC	quick calculator in the PDA version

RAST	radioallergosorbent test
RCC	red cell count
RhF	rheumatoid factor
RIA	radioimmunoassay
RNA	ribonucleic acid
s.c.	subcutaneous
SLE	systemic lupus erythematosus
STI	sexually transmitted infection
SVC	superior vena cava
SVT	supraventricular tachycardia
TIA	transient ischaemic attack
TNM	tumour, node, metastasis classification
TPN	total parenteral nutrition
TRH	thyrotrophin-releasing hormone
TSH	thyroid-stimulating hormone
VDRL	Venereal Disease Research Laboratory (test for syphilis)
VF	ventricular fibrillation
VIP	vasoactive intestinal polypeptide
VT	ventricular tachycardia
WBC	white blood (cell) count
WCC	white cell count
WE	Wernicke's encephalopathy

Significant websites

General websites

http://gungadin.cs.brandeis.edu/~weiluo/main3.htm
Lists biomedical acronyms and their meanings

http://health.allrefer.com
Patient information site with medical encyclopaedia, information
on 1600 diseases and conditions and 2500 medical illustrations

http://www.bma.org
British Medical Association. A library, excellent ethics section
and healthcare information. More sections for members

http://www.cancerbacup.org.uk
Cancerbacup. Questions and answers for patients with all forms
of cancer

http://www.chi.nhs.uk/
Commission for Health Improvement

http://www.cochrane.org
The Cochrane Database. Regularly updated evidence-based
healthcare databases

http://www.dvla.gov.uk/at_a_glance/content.htm
UK Driver and Vehicle Licensing Agency. Up-to-date information
about fitness to drive and exclusions

http://www.emedicine.com
eMedicine features up-to-date, searchable, peer-reviewed
medical journals, on-line physician reference textbooks, and a
full-text article database. Also patient information leaflets

http://www.ncbi.nlm.nih.gov/PubMed
PubMed: Medline on the Web

http://www.nelh.nhs.uk/guidelinesfinder/
Details of UK national guidelines with links to Internet versions

http://www.nhsdirect.nhs.uk
Patient information site on numerous illnesses, operations, tests
and treatments

http://www.nice.org.uk
UK National Institute for Health and Clinical Effectiveness

http://www.nih.gov/health
US National Institutes of Health website (biomedical research, free)

http://www.sign.ac.uk
Scottish Intercollegiate Guidelines Network. Clinical guidelines on many subjects

Healthcare journals and magazines

http://www.bmj.com/index.shtml
British Medical Journal

http://www.doh.gov.uk/cmo/publications.htm
Chief Medical Officer's publications

http://www.jr2.ox.ac.uk/bandolier/
Bandolier (free abstracts and good links)

Medical societies and organizations

http://www.gmc-uk.org/
UK General Medical Council

1 Ethics and communication

http://www.bma.org.uk/ethics
British Medical Association ethics site

http://www.clinical-skills-net.org.uk
UK Clinical Skills Network

http://www.ethics-network.org.uk
UK Clinical Ethics Network

http://www.gmc-uk.org/
General Medical Council

http://www.nih.gov/sigs/bioethics/uk
National Institute of Health website – bioethics pages

http://www.nivel.nl/each
European Association for Communication in Healthcare

http://www.wma.net/e/policy.html
World Medical Association policy

2 Infectious diseases and tropical medicine

http://www.cdc.gov
Department of Health and Human Services Centers for Disease Control and Prevention (CDC). The CDC has a major role in public health efforts to prevent and control infectious and chronic diseases, injuries, workplace hazards, disabilities, and environmental health threats

http://www.doh.gov.uk/eaga/
Department of Health Expert Advisory Group on AIDS: information about post-exposure prophylaxis, guidelines for pre-test discussion on HIV testing and risks of transmission

http://www.hivatis.org/
Centers for Disease Control and Prevention: HIV/AIDS treatment/information service

http://www.idlinks.com
General starting point for infectious disease links

http://www.nfid.org/factsheets/
National Foundation for Infectious Disease, USA: fact sheets on infectious diseases

http://www.hpa.org.uk
Health Protection Agency website. Provides up-to-date information for medical practitioners on some infectious diseases and their prevention, particularly those that are new or where an epidemic is expected

http://www.phls.co.uk/
UK Public Health Laboratory Service: UK regional information on infections

http://www.who.int/en
The World Health Organization is the United Nations specialized agency for health. The website provides information and fact sheets on many infectious diseases, and much more

3 Gastroenterology and nutrition

http://www.ag.uiuc.edu/~food-lab/nat/
Free analysis of the nutrient content of food available to anyone (at University of Illinois, USA)

http://www.ama-assn.org/ama/pub/category/10931.html
American Medical Association – assessment and management of adult obesity

http://www.bsg.org.uk/
British Society of Gastroenterology. Regularly updated clinical practice guidelines for many common conditions

http://www.coeliac.co.uk
Coeliac disease

http://www.corecharity.org.uk
Provides information for patients and their families and friends about many gastrointestinal diseases

http://www.digestivedisorders.org.uk/leaflets/ibs.html
Irritable bowel syndrome

http://www.gastro.org
American Gastroenterology Association. Patient information
leaflets for various conditions

http://www.ific.org/
International Food Information Council (IFIC) – non-profit
organization providing access to health and nutrition resources
to improve communication of health and nutrition information to
consumers

http://www.nacc.org.uk
Provides information, support and services to patients with
inflammatory bowel disease

http://www.who.int/nutgrowthdb/
World Health Organization site, provides information on world-
wide nutritional issues, resources and research

4 Liver, biliary tract and pancreatic disease

http://www.britishlivertrust.org.uk
British Liver Trust. Information for patients and doctors,
including patient information leaflets in Hindi, Chinese and
Bengali

http://www.liverfoundation.org
Website of the American Liver Foundation. Patient information
leaflets for common liver conditions

http://www-micro.msb.le.ac.uk/335/Hepatitis.html
Viral hepatitis

http://www.pancreasfoundation.org
Patient information leaflets about pancreatitis and pancreatic
cancer

5 Diseases of the blood and haematological malignancies

http://www.bcshguidelines.com
The British Committee for Standards in Haematology. Guidelines
for medical practitioners on general haematology, thrombosis,
blood transfusion and haematological malignancies

http://www.blood.co.uk
UK National Blood Service. Lay person information site about
blood products, blood donation and transfusion

http://www.haemophilia.org.uk
For patients with haemophilia, von Willebrand's and related
disorders

http://www.hemophilia.org
US National Hemophilia Foundation

http://www.leukaemia.com/leukaemia-foundation
Leukaemia Foundation. Patient information about haematological
malignancies and current research. Information available in
languages other than English

www.sicklecellsociety.org
UK Sickle Cell Society. Care and information on sickle cell
anaemia (anemia) and other sickle cell disorders to healthcare
workers and patients

6 Rheumatology

http://www.arc.org.uk
Arthritis Research Campaign. Publications for medical
practitioners and patients with arthritis

http://www.nos.org.uk
National Osteoporosis Society. Recommendations and guidance
for medical practitioners and information for patients

http://www.rheumatology.org.uk
British Society for Rheumatology. Regularly updated clinical
guidelines for medical practitioners

http://www.rheumatology.org/publications/guidelines
American College of Rheumatology clinical practice guidelines

7 Water and electrolytes &

8 Renal disease

http://www.kidney.org
GFR calculator and clinical practice guidelines. Patient fact
sheets about renal disease. UK charity run by and for patients

http://www.nephronline.org
Management and guidance section for health professionals and
information for patients with renal disease

9 Cardiovascular disease

http://www.americanheart.org
American Heart Association. Patient information site

http://www.ecglibrary.com/ecghome.html
ECG tracings library

http://www.erc.edu
European Resuscitation Council. Latest guidelines on
resuscitation, as well as a full overview of the ERC educational
tools such as manuals, posters and slides

http://www.resus.org.uk
Resuscitation Council (UK). Adult advanced life support
resuscitation guidelines

10 Respiratory disease

http://www.brit-thoracic.org.uk
British Thoracic Society. Clinical practice guidelines and patient
information leaflets. Guidelines for the management of many
respiratory diseases including asthma. UK National Asthma
Campaign

http://www.goldcopd.org
The WHO Global Initiative for Chronic Obstructive Lung Disease
(GOLD). Clinical guidelines and patient information: diagnosis,
treatment and prevention of COPD

http://www.quitsmoking.com
The Quit Smoking Company

http://www.quitsmokinguk.com
Good site for those wanting to quit or to help patients to quit

http://www.thoracic.org
American Thoracic Society. Clinical practice guidelines and
patient education resource

11 Intensive care medicine

http://www.esicm.org
European Society for Intensive Care. Guidelines and
recommendations for medical practitioners

http://www.ics.ac.uk
Intensive Care Society (UK). Standards and guidelines for
medical practitioners and information for relatives and patients

http://www.survivingsepsis.org
Surviving Sepsis Campaign. Clinical guidelines and patient
information

12 Poisoning, drug and alcohol abuse

http://www.alcoholscreening.org
Patient information site for alcohol and health

http://www.doh.gov.uk/cmo/cmo0202.htm
Department of Health. Detailed information on CO poisoning

http://www.drinksafely.info
Patient-based website. Useful information about harmful effects
of alcohol and guidelines for safe drinking

http://www.spib.axl.co.uk
Toxbase. Database of UK National Poisons Information Service

http://www.toxnet.nlm.nih.gov
National Library of Medicine's Toxnet

http://www.who/int/ipcs
Contact details of all poisons centres world-wide

13 Endocrinology

http://www.endocrineweb.com
Website for thyroid, parathyroid and other endocrine disorders
for the education of patients and their families

http://www.niddk.nih.gov/health/endo/endo.htm
US National Institutes of Health, National Institute of Diabetes &
Digestive & Kidney Diseases

http://www.pituitary.org.uk
The Pituitary Foundation (UK). Information and support for those
living with pituitary disorders, including patients, their relatives,
friends and carers

14 Diabetes mellitus and other disorders of metabolism

http://www.diabetes.org
American Diabetes Association. Patient resource centre

http://www.diabetes.org.uk
Diabetes UK charity (formerly the British Diabetic Association).
Guidelines for healthcare professionals and patient resource
centre

http://www.jdf.org.uk
Juvenile Diabetes Foundation (UK)

http://www.sign.ac.uk/guidelines/index.html
Scottish Intercollegiate Guidelines Network. Guidelines on a
range of subjects including diabetes

15 The special senses

http://www.defeatingdeafness.org
Deafness Research UK. Patient information site for hearing and
information about conditions causing deafness

http://www.nei.nih.gov
National Eye Institute. Patient information about the eye and its
disorders

16 Neurology

http://www.epilepsy.org.uk
The British Epilepsy Association

http://www.gbs.org.uk
Guillain–Barré Syndrome Support Group. Past patients offer
visiting and counselling services

http://www.mssociety.org.uk
The Multiple Sclerosis Society

http://www.parkinsons.org.uk
Parkinson's Disease Society

http://www.stroke.org.uk
The Stroke Association (UK). Information resource for patients
and healthcare workers

http://www.theabn.org/public/patientcarer.php
Lists all the individual websites for patients and carers with
various neurological conditions

17 Dermatology

http://tray.dermatology.uiowa.edu/DermImag.htm
Dermatological image database (adult)

http://www.bad.org.uk
British Association of Dermatologists

http://www.eczema.org
UK National Eczema Society (atopic eczema)

http://www.paalliance.org
Psoriatic Arthropathy Alliance (psoriasis)

http://www.usc.edu/hsc/nml/e-resources/info/dermis.html
Dermatological image database (paediatric)

http://www.usc.edu/hsc/nml/index.html
Dermatology images (atlas)

19 Therapeutics

http://bnf.org
British National Formulary. Authoritative and practical
information on the selection and clinical use of drugs

http://www.dtb.org.uk/idtb
Drug and Therapeutics Bulletin. Independent reviews of medical
treatment. Registration is necessary for this website

Normal values

HAEMATOLOGY

Haemoglobin	
Male	13.5–17.7 g/dL
Female	11.5–16.5 g/dL
Mean corpuscular haemoglobin (MCH)	27–32 pg
Mean corpuscular haemoglobin concentration (MCHC)	32–36 g/dL
Mean corpuscular volume (MCV)	80–96 fL
Packed cell volume (PCV)	
Male	0.40–0.54 L/L
Female	0.37–0.47 L/L
White blood count (WBC)	$4–11 \times 10^9$/L
Basophil granulocytes	$<0.01–0.1 \times 10^9$/L
Eosinophil granulocytes	$0.04–0.4 \times 10^9$/L
Lymphocytes	$1.5–4.0 \times 10^9$/L
Monocytes	$0.2–0.8 \times 10^9$/L
Neutrophil granulocytes	$2.0–7.5 \times 10^9$/L
Platelet count	$150–400 \times 10^9$/L
Serum B_{12}	160–925 ng/L (150–675 pmol/L)
Serum folate	2.9–18 µg/L (3.6–63 nmol/L)
Red cell folate	149–640 µg/L
Red cell mass	
Male	25–35 mL/kg
Female	20–30 mL/kg
Reticulocyte count	0.5–2.5% of red cells ($50–100 \times 10^9$/L)
Erythrocyte sedimentation rate (ESR)	<20 mm in 1 hour

COAGULATION

Bleeding time (Ivy method)	3–9 min
Activated partial thromboplastin time (APTT)	23–31 s
Prothrombin time	12–16 s
International Normalized Ratio (INR)	1.0–1.3
D-dimer	<500 ng/mL

LIPIDS AND LIPOPROTEINS

Cholesterol	3.5–6.5 mmol/L (ideal <5.2 mmol/L)
HDL cholesterol	
Male	0.8–1.8 mmol/L
Female	1.0–2.3 mmol/L
LDL cholesterol	<4.0 mmol/L
Triglycerides	
Male	0.70–2.1 mmol/L
Female	0.50–1.70 mmol/L

BIOCHEMISTRY (SERUM/PLASMA)

Alanine aminotransferase (ALT)	5–40 U/L
Albumin	35–50 g/L
Alkaline phosphatase	39–117 U/L

Amylase	25–125 U/L
Aspartate aminotransferase (AST)	12–40 U/L
Bicarbonate	22–30 mmol/L
Bilirubin	<17 µmol/L (0.3–1.5 mg/dL)
Calcium	2.20–2.67 mmol/L (8.5–10.5 mg/dL)
Chloride	98–106 mmol/L
C-reactive protein	<10 mg/L
Creatinine	79–118 µmol/L (0.6–1.5 mg/dL)
Creatine kinase (CPK)	
Female	24–170 U/L
Male	24–195 U/L
CK-MB fraction	<25 U/L (<60% of total activity)
Ferritin	
Female	6–110 µg/L
Male	20–260 µg/L
Postmenopausal	12–230 µg/L
α-Fetoprotein	<10 kU/L
Glucose (fasting)	4.5–5.6 mmol/L (70–110 mg/dL)
γ-Glutamyl transpeptidase (γ-GT)	
Male	11–58 U/L
Female	7–32 U/L
Glycosylated (glycated) haemoglobin (HbA_{1c})	3.7–5.1%
Iron	13–32 µmol/L (50–150 µg/dL)
Iron-binding capacity (total) (TIBC)	42–80 µmol/L (250–410 µg/dL)
Magnesium	0.7–1.1 mmol/L
Osmolality	275–295 mOsm/kg
Phosphate	0.8–1.5 mmol/L
Potassium	3.5–5.0 mmol/L
Prostate-specific antigen (PSA)	≤4.0 µg/L
Protein (total)	62–77 g/L
Sodium	135–146 mmol/L
Urate	0.18–0.42 mmol/L (3.0–7.0 mg/dL)
Urea	2.5–6.7 mmol/L (8–25 mg/dL)

BLOOD GASES (ARTERIAL)

P_aCO_2	4.8–6.1 kPa (36–46 mmHg)
P_aO_2	10–13.3 kPa (75–100 mmHg)
$[H^+]$	35–45 nmol/L
pH	7.35–7.45
Bicarbonate	22–26 mmol/L

Ethics and communication 1

Ethical and moral issues are integrally involved with patient care, particularly with respect to controversial topics such as euthanasia, organ donation and genetic technology. A doctor with clinical responsibility for a patient has three corresponding duties of care:

- *Protect life and health.* Clinicians should practise medicine to a high standard and not cause unnecessary suffering or harm. Treatment should only be given when it is thought to be beneficial to that patient. Competent patients have the right to refuse treatment, but decisions not to provide life-sustaining treatment should only be taken with their informed consent on the basis of a clear explanation about the consequences of their refusal.
- *Respect autonomy.* Clinicians must respect the need to maintain the autonomy and self-determination of patients and thus recognize that the patient has the ability to reason, plan and make choices about the future. Wherever possible patients should remain responsible for themselves. Informed consent and confidentiality are fundamental parts of good medical practice and respect for human dignity. Medical information belongs to the patient and should not be disclosed to any other parties, including relatives, without the informed consent of the patient. However, the right to privacy does not entail the right to harm others in exercising it, and in certain circumstances clinicians must breach confidentiality, e.g. infectious patients who pose a threat to specific individuals through undisclosed risks. Breach of confidentiality in these circumstances is usually only done after informing the patient of the intent to do so.
- *Protect life and health and respect autonomy with fairness and justice.* All patients have the right to be treated equally regardless of race, fitness, social worth, class or any other arbitrary prejudice or favouritism.

Various regulatory bodies, common law and the Human Rights Act 1998 regulate medical practice and ensure that doctors take their duties of care seriously. The standards expected of healthcare professionals by their regulatory bodies (for example in the UK, the General Medical Council (GMC), the Royal College of Physicians, and British Medical Association) may at times be higher than the minimum required by law.

LEGALLY VALID CONSENT

It is a general legal and ethical principle that valid consent must be obtained before starting treatment or physical investigation, or providing personal care, for a patient. This principle reflects the right of patients to determine what happens to their own bodies. For instance, common law has established that touching a patient without valid consent may constitute the civil or criminal offence of battery. Furthermore, failure to obtain adequate consent may be a factor in a claim of negligence against the health professional involved, particularly if the patient suffers harm as a result of treatment.

The amount of information doctors provide to each patient will vary according to factors such as the nature and severity of the condition, the complexity of the treatment, the risks associated with the treatment or procedure and the patient's own wishes.

In the consent process enough information must be provided in order that the patient's decisions are informed. This should be in the form of a discussion with the patient and written information leaflets. For a patient who does not speak the native language this must be done with the aid of a health advocate. The type of information provided includes:

- The purpose of the investigation or treatment
- Details and uncertainties of the diagnosis
- Options for treatment including the option not to treat
- Explanation of the likely benefits and probabilities of success for each option
- Known possible side-effects: decide what information about risks a 'reasonable person' in the position of the patient would want before agreeing to treatment
- The name of the doctor who will have overall responsibility

- A reminder that the patient can change his or her mind at any time
- An opportunity to raise with patients the possibility of additional problems coming to light during the procedure, and discussion of possible action in this event.

Obtaining consent

For consent to be valid it must be given voluntarily after providing the patient with a reasonable amount of information about the risks of the proposed treatment or investigation. In addition, the patient must have the capacity to consent to the treatment in question, i.e. the patient must be able to comprehend and retain information about the treatment and use this information in the decision-making process. The clinician providing the treatment or investigation is responsible for ensuring that the patient has given valid consent before treatment begins. Consent may be verbal (e.g. for venepuncture) or written (e.g. always for a surgical procedure) depending on the proposed treatment or intervention. However, it should be remembered that a signed consent form is not legal or professional proof that proper informed consent has been obtained. The person obtaining consent should be the surgeon/physician who is doing the procedure or an assistant who is fully competent to carry out the procedure and therefore understands the potential complications. It is not acceptable for a junior doctor who does not perform and fully understand the procedure to obtain consent.

Special circumstances
Emergencies Treatment can only be given legally to adult patients without consent if they are temporarily or permanently incompetent to provide it and the treatment is necessary to save their life, or to prevent them from incurring serious and permanent injury.

Adults who lack capacity to consent In the case of adults who cannot give informed consent because of brain damage, the doctor must decide if the proposed treatment is in the best interests of the patient. The treatment should be discussed with the relatives but they should not be asked to provide consent. It must also be determined if the person has previously expressed any opinions regarding certain procedures, perhaps on the grounds of religious

3

or moral beliefs. This wish must be respected. It is only when the patient may die if an intervention is not made that this can be carried out without consent. However, if the patient had already expressed a clear opinion on this matter, the doctor cannot override this, whatever the consequences.

Children In the UK, the legal age of presumed competence to consent to treatment is 16 years. Below this age, those with parental responsibility are the legal proxies for their children and usually consent to treatment on their behalf. At any age, an attempt should be made to explain fully the procedures and potential outcomes to the child, even if the child is too young to be fully competent. Children under 16 years can give legally effective consent to medical treatment provided they have sufficient under-standing and intelligence.

Research procedures Doctors must ensure that patients asked to consider taking part in research are given written information presented in terms and in a form that they can understand. Patients must be aware that they are being asked to participate in a research project and that the results are not predictable. Adequate time must be given for reflection prior to the patient giving consent. Retention of human tissue for research or teaching requires written consent from the donor, or the next of kin of deceased patients or those who cannot speak for themselves.

Teaching It is necessary to obtain a patient's consent if a student or other observer would like to sit in during a consultation. The patient has the right to refuse without affecting the subsequent consultation. Consent must also be obtained if any additional procedure is to be carried out on an anaesthetized patient solely for the purposes of teaching. Consent must also be obtained if a video or audio recording is to be made of a procedure or consultation and subsequently used for teaching purposes.

HIV testing Doctors must obtain consent from patients before testing for HIV, except in rare circumstances such as in unconscious patients where testing would be in their immediate clinical interests, for example to help in making a diagnosis. In other circumstances, doctors must make sure that patients are given appropriate information about the implications of the test, including the advantages and disadvantages, and wherever possible allow patients appropriate time to consider and discuss them.

Advance directives Competent adults acting free from pressure and who understand the implications of their choice(s) can make an advance statement (sometimes known as a living will) about how they wish to be treated if they suffer loss of capacity. The advance statement may be a clear instruction refusing one or more medical procedures or a statement that specifies a degree of irreversible deterioration after which no life-sustaining treatment should be given. It is legally binding providing the patient criteria outlined above are fulfilled, the statement is clearly applicable to the current circumstances and there is no reason to believe that the patient has changed his or her mind.

COMMUNICATION

5

Communication is the way in which clinicians integrate clinical science with patient-centred, evidence-based shared healthcare. It is the process of exchanging information and ideas and also making a trusting relationship upon which the collaborative partnership between patients and their families and healthcare workers depends. Good communication improves health outcomes, including symptom resolution, reduction in adverse psychological outcomes, improved pain control and reduced patient anxiety. Failure of communication leads to poor delivery of information, lack of patient understanding and ultimately the patient feeling deserted and devalued. The majority of complaints against doctors are not based on failures of biomedical practice but on poor communication. Patients have identified qualities used by the doctor in the interview which lead to good relationships. Doctors who were considered to have communicated well:

- Orientated patients to the process of the visit, e.g. introductory comments: 'We are going to do this first and then go on to that'
- Used facilitative comments
- Asked patients their opinion
- Used active listening
- Used humour and laughter
- Conducted slightly longer visits (18 versus 15 minutes).

Ethics and communication

The medical interview

Clinicians must use their time to the greatest benefit of their patients. It is essential to find out not only the medical facts in detail but also what patients have experienced and what impact this experience has had upon them. There are three phases to an interview:

Opening The start of the interview will be helped by well-organized arrangements for appointments, reception and punctuality. The physician should come out of the room to greet the patient, establish eye contact and shake hands if appropriate. Clinicians should introduce themselves by telling patients their name, status and responsibility to the patient; a name badge will reinforce this information. The patient should sit beside the clinician and not on the far side of a desk.

Exploring and focusing In addition to obtaining a complete history, the clinician should also determine the impact of the problem on the patient's life, the patient's ideas and fears and the patient's attitude to similar problems in others. The clinician will obtain more information by starting with open questions and then guiding the history by using closed questions for further detail. An open question such as 'What has brought you to see me today?' allows the patient to speak freely and the clinician will obtain more information. A closed question such as 'What date exactly did the headache start?' will not allow patients to address all their concerns and they will not speak freely. During the interview a smile and eye contact from the physician will let the patient know that the doctor is listening attentively. Demonstrating empathy is a key skill in building the patient–clinician relationship and involves the patient's experiences being seen, heard and accepted with some feedback to demonstrate this. For instance, 'The last point made you look worried. Is there something more serious about that point you would like to tell me?' demonstrates that the patient's experiences have been seen. Patients are more likely to adhere to clinical advice if they get comprehensible information, if it makes sense of their problems, and if they can get easy access to more information if they need it. Patients must always be given information in a logical sequence, using simple language and avoiding medical terms, and if possible with the aid of simple diagrams and key words. It is useful to check that the patient understands before moving on to another point. Further aids for information such as medical support groups and reference web sites are always useful.

Closing Closing the interview may start with a brief summary of the patient's agenda and then of that of the clinician. The patient should be told the arrangements for further interviews and the commitment to informing other healthcare professionals involved with the patient. It is useful to make a written record in the patient's notes as to what the patient has been told and what has been understood. In some situations it is useful if the patient knows how to contact an appropriate team member as a safety net before the next interview. The interview is closed with an appropriate farewell and some words of encouragement.

Breaking bad news

Breaking bad news can be difficult, and the way that it is broken has a major psychological and physical effect upon patients. In these situations patients usually know more than anyone has guessed, welcome clear information and do not want to be drawn into a charade of deception which does not allow them to discuss their illness and the future. The clinician should begin the interview by finding out how much the patient knows and if anything new has developed since the last encounter. The clinician should give the patient a warning that the news is bad or more serious than initially thought, and then pause to allow the patient to think this over and only continue when the patient gives some lead to follow. The clinician should then give small chunks of information and ensure that the patient understands before moving on. Frequent pauses allow the patient to think. The interview should be stopped and resumed at a later date if necessary. The patient should be provided with some positive information and hope tempered with realism. The patient may ask for a time frame of events but it is often impossible to give an accurate time frame for a terminal disease. The importance of maintaining a good quality of life during this time must be stressed. The patient must be given the opportunity for other family members to meet with the clinician. The interview should close with a further interview date – preferably soon – a contact name as a safety net before the next interview and details regarding further sources of information.

Infectious diseases and tropical medicine 2 (K&C 6e p. 19)

Infection remains the main cause of morbidity and mortality in man, particularly in developing areas where it is associated with poverty and overcrowding. Although the prevalence of infectious disease has reduced in the developing world as a result of increasing prosperity, immunization and antibiotic availability, antibiotic-resistant strains of microorganisms and diseases such as human immunodeficiency virus (HIV) infection, variant Creutzfeldt–Jakob disease (vCJD) and severe acute respiratory syndrome (SARS) have emerged. Increasing global mobility has aided the spread of infectious disease with the result that more tropical diseases are now seen in the UK. In the elderly and immunocompromised the presentation of infectious disease may be atypical with few localizing signs and the normal physiological responses to infection (fever and sometimes neutrophilia) may be diminished or absent. A high index of suspicion is required in these populations.

The widespread use of antibiotics has led to bacterial resistance and changing patterns of disease. Methicillin-resistant *Staphylococcus aureus* (MRSA) is one such example. MRSA is a bacterium commonly found on the skin and/or in the noses of healthy people (they are 'colonized'). Infection is a result of MRSA spread (either from the same patient or between patients) from a site of colonization to a wound, burn or indwelling catheter where it causes clinical disease. The bacteria are resistant to multiple antibiotics, and infections are usually treated with vancomycin or teicoplanin. The risk of infection with MRSA is reduced by hospital staff washing their hands with antibacterial soap or alcohol hand scrub after contact with all patients, side-room isolation of colonized and infected patients (hospital staff wear disposable gowns and gloves before contact) and topical antibiotics for individuals colonized (identified by nasal and skin swabs) with MRSA.

In the UK some infectious diseases must be notified to the local Medical Officer for Environmental Health; these are indicated by the abbreviation nd where appropriate.

Common investigations in infectious disease

- **Blood tests**. Routine blood count, ESR and C-reactive protein, biochemical profile, urea and electrolytes are performed in the majority of cases.
- **Imaging**. X-ray, ultrasound, echocardiography, CT and MR scanning are used to identify and localize infections. Biopsy or aspiration of tissue for microbiological examination may also be facilitated by ultrasound or CT guidance.
- **Radionuclide scanning** after injection of indium- or technetium-labelled white cells (previously harvested from the patient) may occasionally help to localize infection. It is most effective when the peripheral white cell count is raised, and is of particular value in localizing occult abscesses.
- **Microscopy and culture** of blood, urine, cerebrospinal fluid and faeces should be performed as clinically indicated. Detection of a specific clostridial toxin is a more reliable test for diarrhoea caused by *Clostridium difficile* than culture of the organism itself.
- **Immunodiagnostic tests**. These either detect viral or bacterial antigen using a polyvalent antiserum or a monoclonal antibody, or they detect serological response to infection.

Pyrexia of unknown origin (*K&C* 6e p. 29)

Pyrexia (or fever) of unknown origin (PUO) is defined as a documented fever (> 38°C) lasting more than 2 weeks in which a clinical history (including travel, animal contact, sexual activity and intravenous drug use), repeated thorough physical examination and routine investigations have failed to reveal a cause. Occult infection remains the most common cause in adults. Collagen vascular disease, drug hypersensitivity and malignancy are other causes (Table 2.1).

Investigations

First-line investigations should be repeated as the results may have changed since the tests were first performed:

- Full blood count, including a differential white cell count (WCC) and blood film
- Erythrocyte sedimentation rate (ESR)

Table 2.1 Some causes of pyrexia of unknown origin

Infection (20–40%)
Pyogenic abscess: e.g. liver, pelvis, subphrenic
Tuberculosis
Infective endocarditis
Viruses: Epstein–Barr, cytomegalovirus
Primary HIV infection
Brucellosis
Lyme disease
Malaria

Malignant disease (10–30%)
Lymphoma
Leukaemia
Renal cell carcinoma
Hepatocellular carcinoma

Collagen vascular disease (15–20%)
Rheumatoid arthritis
Systemic lupus erythematosus
Wegener's granulomatosis
Giant cell arteritis
Adult Still's disease

Miscellaneous (10–25%)
Drug fever
Thyrotoxicosis
Inflammatory bowel disease
Sarcoidosis
Granulomatous hepatitis: e.g. tuberculosis, sarcoidosis
Factitious fever (switching thermometers, injection of pyogenic material)
Familial Mediterranean fever

- Serum urea and electrolytes, liver biochemistry and blood glucose
- Blood cultures – several sets from different sites at different times
- Microscopy and culture of urine, sputum and faeces
- Baseline serum for virology
- Chest X-ray
- Serum rheumatoid factor and antinuclear antibody.

Second-line investigations are performed in conditions that remain undiagnosed and when repeat physical examination is unhelpful.

- Abdominal imaging with ultrasound, CT or MRI to detect occult abscesses and malignancy
- Echocardiography for infective endocarditis
- Biopsy of liver and bone marrow; temporal artery biopsy (p. 763) should be considered in the elderly
- Determination of HIV status (after counselling)
- Radionuclide scanning.

Management

The treatment is of the underlying cause. Blind antibiotic therapy should not be given unless the patient is very unwell. In a few patients no diagnosis is reached after thorough investigation and in most of these the fever will resolve on follow-up.

Septicaemia (*K&C* 6e p. 74)

12

The term *bacteraemia* refers to the transient presence of organisms in the blood (generally without causing symptoms) as a result of local infection or penetrating injury. The term *septicaemia*, on the other hand, is usually reserved for the clinical picture that results from the systemic inflammatory response to infection. Inflammation is normally intended to be a local and contained response to infection. Activated polymorphonuclear leucocytes, macrophages and lymphocytes release inflammatory mediators including tumour necrosis factor, interleukin-1 (IL-1), platelet-activating factor, IL-6, IL-8, interferon and eicosanoids. In some cases, mediator release exceeds the boundaries of the local environment leading to a generalized response that affects normal tissues. This process is referred to as sepsis, and the clinical features include fever, tachycardia, an increase in respiratory rate and hypotension. Septicaemia has a high mortality without treatment, and demands immediate attention. The pathogenesis and management of septic shock is discussed on pages 552 and 556.

Aetiology

Overall, about 40% of cases are the result of Gram-positive organisms and 60% of Gram-negative ones. Fungi are much less common but should be considered, particularly in the immunocompromised. In the previously healthy adult, septicaemia may occur from a source of infection in the chest (e.g. with pneumonia), urinary tract (often Gram-negative rods) or biliary tree (commonly *Enterococcus faecalis, Escherichia coli*). Intravenous drug abusers may develop septicaemia as a result of *Staphylococcus aureus* and *Pseudomonas* sp. infection. Hospitalized patients are susceptible to infection from wounds, indwelling urinary catheters and intravenous cannulae.

Clinical features

Fever, rigors and hypotension are the cardinal features of severe septicaemia. Lethargy, headache and a minor change in conscious level may be preceding features. In elderly and immunocompromised patients the clinical features may be quite subtle and a high index of suspicion is needed.

Certain bacteria are associated with a particularly fulminating course:

- Staphylococci that produce an exotoxin called toxic shock syndrome toxin-1. The toxic shock syndrome is characterized by an abrupt onset of fever, rash, diarrhoea and shock. It is associated with the use of infected tampons in women but may occur in anyone, including children.
- Meningococci that produce the Waterhouse–Friderichsen syndrome. This is a rapidly fatal illness (without treatment), with a purpuric skin rash and shock. Adrenal haemorrhage (and hypoadrenalism) may or may not be present.

Investigations

In addition to blood count, serum electrolytes and liver biochemistry:

- Blood cultures
- Cultures from possible source: urine, abscess aspirate, sputum
- In some cases: chest radiography, abdominal ultrasonography and CT scan.

Management

Antibiotic therapy should be started immediately the diagnosis is suspected and after appropriate culture samples have been sent to the laboratory. The probable site of origin of sepsis will often be apparent, and knowledge of the likely microbial flora can be used to choose appropriate treatment. In cases where 'blind' antibiotic treatment is necessary, a reasonable combination would be intravenous gentamicin and piperacillin, or cefotaxime, with or without metronidazole for anaerobes. Therapy may subsequently be altered on the basis of culture and sensitivity results. Activated protein C is an endogenous protein that modulates the inflammatory cascade and has anti-inflammatory actions. Recombinant human activated protein C is added to full supportive treatment in patients with severe sepsis and multiorgan failure.

COMMON VIRAL INFECTIONS

Measles nd (*K&C* 6e p. 56)

Measles is caused by infection with an RNA paramyxovirus which is spread by droplets. With the introduction of aggressive immunization policies, the incidence has fallen in the West, but it remains common in developing countries, where it is associated with a high morbidity and mortality. One attack confers lifelong immunity.

Clinical features

The incubation period is 8–14 days. Two distinct phases of the disease can be recognized.

The infectious pre-eruptive and catarrhal stage There is fever, cough, rhinorrhoea, conjunctivitis and Koplik's spots in the mouth (small grey irregular lesions on an erythematous base, commonly on the inside of the cheek).

The non-infectious eruptive or exanthematous stage Characterized by the presence of a maculopapular rash which starts on the face and spreads to involve the whole body. The rash becomes confluent and blotchy.

Complications

These are uncommon in the healthy child but carry a high mortality in the malnourished or those with other diseases. They include gastroenteritis, pneumonia, otitis media, encephalitis, myocarditis and, rarely, subacute sclerosing panencephalitis. The latter is due to reactivation of persistent virus pre-pubertally. There is progressive mental deterioration and death.

Management

The diagnosis is usually clinical and treatment is symptomatic. Measles vaccine is given to children between 12 and 18 months of age, in combination with mumps and rubella vaccine (MMR) to prevent infection.

Mumps nd (*K&C* 6e p. 57)

Mumps is also caused by infection with a paramyxovirus, spread by droplets. The incubation period averages 18 days.

Clinical features

Mumps is predominantly an infection of school-aged children and young adults. There is fever, headache and malaise, followed by the development of parotid gland swelling. Less common features are orchitis, meningitis, pancreatitis, oophoritis, myocarditis and hepatitis.

15

Management

Diagnosis is usually clinical. In doubtful cases demonstration of a rise in serum antibody titres is necessary for diagnosis. Treatment is symptomatic. The disease is prevented by administration of a live attenuated mumps virus vaccine.

Rubella nd (*K&C* 6e p. 52)

Rubella ('German measles') is caused by an RNA virus and has a peak age of incidence of 15 years. The incubation period is 14–21 days. During the prodrome the patient complains of malaise, fever and lymphadenopathy (suboccipital, postauricular, posterior cervical nodes). A pinkish macular rash appears on the face and trunk after about 7 days and lasts for up to 3 days.

Diagnosis

The diagnosis may be suspected clinically and a definitive diagnosis is made by demonstrating a rising serum antibody titre in paired samples taken 2 weeks apart, or by the detection of rubella-specific IgM.

Management

Treatment is symptomatic. Complications are uncommon but include arthralgia, encephalitis and thrombocytopenia. Prevention is with a live vaccine (see Measles).

Congenital rubella syndrome (*K&C* 6e p. 52)

Maternal infection during pregnancy may affect the fetus, particularly if infection is acquired in the first trimester. Congenital rubella syndrome is characterized by the presence of fetal cardiac defects, eye lesions (particularly cataracts), microcephaly, mental handicap and deafness. There may also be persistent viral infection of the liver, lungs and heart, with hepatomegaly, pneumonitis and myocarditis. The teratogenic effects of rubella underlie the importance of preventing maternal infection with immunization.

16

Herpes viruses (*K&C* 6e p. 43)

Herpes simplex virus (HSV) infection (*K&C* 6e p. 43)
HSV-1 causes:

- Herpetic stomatitis with buccal ulceration, fever and local lymphadenopathy
- Herpetic whitlow: damage to the skin over a finger allows access of the virus, with the development of irritating vesicles
- Keratoconjunctivitis
- Encephalitis
- Systemic infection in immunocompromised patients.

HSV-2 is transmitted sexually and causes genital herpes, with painful genital ulceration, fever and lymphadenopathy. Anorectal infection may occur in male homosexuals. There may be systemic infection in the immunocompromised host, and in severe cases death may result from hepatitis and encephalitis. These divisions are not rigid, because HSV-1 can also give rise to genital herpes.

Recurrent HSV infection occurs when the virus lies dormant in ganglion cells and is reactivated by trauma, febrile illnesses and ultraviolet irradiation. This leads to recurrent labialis ('cold sores') or recurrent genital herpes.

Investigations

The diagnosis is often clinical but the virus may be cultured from lesions. Herpes simplex encephalitis is discussed on page 752.

Management

Aciclovir is used topically and systemically for both primary and recurrent infection of the skin and mucous membranes. Penciclovir is used topically as a cream for herpes labialis.

Herpes zoster (*K&C* 6e p. 45)
Varicella (chickenpox) (*K&C* 6e p. 45)   Primary infection with this virus causes chickenpox, which may produce a mild childhood illness, although this can be severe in adults and immunocompromised patients.

Clinical features

After an incubation period of 14–21 days there is a brief prodromal period of fever, headache and malaise. The rash, predominantly on the face, scalp and trunk, begins as macules and develops into papules and vesicles, which heal with crusting. Complications include pneumonia and central nervous system involvement.

Investigations

The diagnosis is usually clinical. Electron microscopy of vesicle fluid may reveal the virus.

Management

Healthy children require no treatment. Anyone over the age of 16 is given antiviral therapy with aciclovir because they are more at risk of severe disease. Because of the risk to both mother and fetus during pregnancy, pregnant women exposed to varicella zoster virus should receive prophylaxis with zoster-immune immunoglobulin (ZIG) and treatment with aciclovir if they develop chickenpox. Immuno-compromised patients are treated in a similar manner.

Herpes zoster (shingles) (*K&C* 6e pp. 45 & 1240)   After the primary infection, herpes zoster remains dormant in dorsal root ganglia and/or cranial nerve ganglia, and reactivation causes shingles.

Clinical features

Pain and tingling in a dermatomal distribution precede the rash by a few days. The rash consists of papules and vesicles in the same dermatome. The most common sites are the lower thoracic dermatomes and the ophthalmic division of the trigeminal nerve (p. 716).

Management

Treatment is with oral famciclovir given as early as possible. The main complication is postherpetic neuralgia, which can be severe and last for years. Treatment is with carbamazepine or phenytoin.

Infectious mononucleosis and Epstein–Barr virus infection (K&C 6e p. 47)

Infectious mononucleosis (glandular fever) is caused by the Epstein–Barr virus (EBV) and predominantly affects young adults. EBV is transmitted in saliva and by aerosol. EBV is also the major aetiological agent responsible for Burkitt's lymphoma, nasopharyngeal carcinoma, post-transplant lymphoma and the immunoblastic lymphoma of AIDS patients.

Clinical features

Many infections are asymptomatic. In symptomatic patients the main features are fever, headache, sore throat and a transient macular rash (more common following administration of amoxicillin given inappropriately for a sore throat). There may be palatal petechiae, cervical lymphadenopathy, splenomegaly and mild hepatitis. Rare complications include splenic rupture, myocarditis and meningitis.

Investigations

Atypical lymphocytes on a peripheral blood film strongly suggest infection. Detection of heterophile antibodies is the diagnostic test of choice. They react to antigens from phylogenetically unrelated species and agglutinate sheep red cells (the Paul–Bunnell reaction) and horse red blood cells (the 'Monospot test'). Measurement of EBV-specific antibodies may be necessary in the few patients with suspected

infectious mononucleosis and negative heterophile antibodies.

Management

Most cases require no treatment. Corticosteroids are given
if there is neurological involvement (encephalitis, meningitis)
or marked thrombocytopenia or haemolysis. Infection with
Toxoplasma gondii (*K&C* 6e pp. 103 & 137) or cytomegalovirus (*K&C* 6e p. 46) may produce a similar clinical picture
in immunocompetent adults.

BACTERIAL INFECTIONS

Most of the bacterial infections are discussed under the
relevant system, e.g. meningitis in the neurology chapter
and pneumonia in the respiratory chapter.

Lyme borreliosis (Lyme disease) (*K&C* 6e pp. 62 & 79)

19

Lyme disease is a multisystem inflammatory disease caused
by the spirochaete *Borrelia burgdorferi*. Infection is spread
from deer and other wild mammals by *Ixodes* ticks.

Clinical features

The clinical manifestations of Lyme disease are divided into
three phases. Not all stages need appear and, conversely,
clinical stages may overlap.

- Early localized disease includes erythema migrans (EM)
  and associated non-specific complaints of fever, malaise,
  headache or myalgia. EM usually occurs within 1 month
  of the tick bite, is usually asymptomatic and the rash
  expands over the course of several days with central
  clearing ('bull's eye' appearance).
- Early disseminated disease occurs days to months after
  the tick bite and consists of neurological (meningoencephalitis or polyneuropathy) or cardiac (myocarditis
  or conduction defects) problems.
- Late disease occurs months to years after the onset and
  consists of chronic and persistent neurological disease
  and/or arthritis.

Investigations

The diagnosis can be made on the basis of typical clinical
features in a patient living or visiting an endemic area.

Serology will show IgM antibodies in the first month and IgG antibodies late in the disease.

Management

Amoxicillin, doxycycline or cephalosporins are the treatments of choice in the early stages of disease. Intravenous benzylpenicillin should be given for later stages of disease. To prevent infection in tick-infested areas, repellants and protective clothing should be worn and ticks removed promptly from the site of a bite.

Leptospirosis (*K&C* 6e p. 77)

This zoonosis is caused by a Gram-negative organism, *Leptospira interrogans*, which is excreted in animal urine and enters the host through a skin abrasion or intact mucous membranes. Individuals who work with animals or take part in water sports which bring them into close contact with rodents (e.g. boating lakes, diving) are most at risk.

Clinical features

Following an incubation period of about 10 days, the initial leptospiraemic phase is characterized by fevers, headache, malaise and myalgia, followed by an immune phase, which is most commonly manifest by meningism. Most recover uneventfully at this stage. A small proportion go on to develop tender hepatosplenomegaly, jaundice, haemolytic anaemia, myocardial involvement and oliguric renal failure with microscopic haematuria (Weil's disease).

Investigations

Blood or CSF culture can identify the organisms in the first week of the disease. The organism may be detected in the urine during the second week.

Serology will show specific IgM antibodies by the end of the first week.

Management

Penicillin or erythromycin is most commonly used. The complications of the disease are treated appropriately.

SKIN AND SOFT TISSUE INFECTIONS

Infections of the skin and soft tissues beneath are common. The majority are caused by the Gram-positive cocci, *Staph. aureus* (part of the normal microflora of the skin) and *Streptococcus pyogenes*. Sometimes infection is introduced by an animal bite or a penetrating foreign body and in these cases more unusual organisms can be found.

Cellulitis is a superficial spreading infection involving subcutaneous tissue and is the most common skin infection leading to hospitalization. It falls into a continuum of skin infections that includes impetigo (superficial vesiculo-pustular infection in children; *K&C* 6e p. 1318), folliculitis (multiple erythematous lesions with a central pustule localized to the follicles; *K&C* 6e p. 1319) and carbuncles (abscesses in the subcutaneous tissue that drain via hair follicles; *K&C* 6e p. 1320). The last three infections are usually caused by *Staph. aureus*.

Cellulitis and erysipelas (*K&C* 6e p. 1319)

Cellulitis preferentially involves the lower extremities. Risk factors include lymphoedema, site of entry (leg ulcer, trauma, presence of tinea pedis – 'athlete's foot'), venous insufficiency, leg oedema and obesity. Beta-haemolytic streptococci and *Staph. aureus* are the common causative organisms. Erysipelas is a characteristic form of cellulitis that affects the superficial epidermis. In the majority of cases it is caused by group A beta-haemolytic streptococci.

Clinical features

The typical findings in cellulitis are erythema in the involved area, with poorly demarcated margins, swelling, warmth and tenderness. There may be a low-grade fever. In erysipelas the area is raised and erythematous and sharply demarcated from normal skin.

Diagnosis

The diagnosis is clinical. Patients should also be evaluated for risk factors for cellulitis such as tinea pedis, which may prevent recurrence if treated. In the majority of cases, culturing blood or skin aspirates does not reveal a pathogen. Deep venous thrombosis is the main differential diagnosis.

Treatment

Treatment is with intravenous benzylpenicillin and flucloxacillin, or single-agent clindamycin if penicillin allergic, with a switch to oral therapy when the skin signs have begun to subside. Antibiotics are continued for 10–14 days or longer if erythema persists.

Necrotizing fasciitis (*K&C* 6e p. 64)

This is a deep-seated infection of the subcutaneous tissue that results in progressive destruction of fascia and fat but may initially spare the skin. There is fulminant destruction of tissue and a high mortality. There is severe pain at the site of infection followed by spreading erythema, underlying crepitus and systemic toxicity.

There are two types:

- Type 1 is caused by a mixed infection with aerobic and anaerobic bacteria, and most commonly occurs after surgical procedures and in patients with diabetes and peripheral vascular disease.
- Type 2 is caused by group A streptococci and occurs in previously healthy patients after penetrating injury, childbirth or injection drug use.

Treatment is urgent surgical debridement and aggressive antibiotic treatment with benzylpenicillin and clindamycin ± metronidazole.

TROPICAL MEDICINE

Fever in the returned traveller (*K&C* 6e p. 28)

Fever is a common problem in people travelling between countries. Malaria is the single most common cause of fever in recent travellers from the tropics to the UK. Falciparum malaria has the potential to be rapidly fatal, and so evaluation of fever in this group of patients is often regarded as a medical emergency. Table 2.2 lists the causes of fever in travellers from the tropics; in about 25% of cases no specific cause is found. The most common causes are discussed in greater detail below.

Approach to diagnosis

An accurate history and physical examination will help formulate an appropriate differential diagnosis and guide

Table 2.2	Causes of fever after travel to the tropics
Malaria	
Viral hepatitis	
Febrile illness unrelated to foreign travel	80% of specific infections*
Dengue fever	
Enteric fever (typhoid and paratyphoid fevers)	
Gastroenteritis	
Rickettsia	
Leptospirosis	
Schistosomiasis	
Amoebic liver abscess	
Tuberculosis	
Acute HIV infection	
Others	

*Includes respiratory and urinary tract infection

Table 2.3 Typical incubation periods for tropical infections	
Incubation period	**Infection**
Short (< 10 days)	Arboviral infections (including dengue fever), enteric bacterial infections, paratyphoid, plague, typhus, haemorrhagic fevers
Medium (10–21 days)	Malaria (but may be much longer), typhoid fever (rarely 3–60 days) scrub typhus, Lassa fever, African trypanosomiasis, brucellosis, leptospirosis
Long (> 21 days)	Viral hepatitis, tuberculosis, HIV, schistosomiasis, amoebic liver abscess, visceral leishmaniasis, filariasis

initial investigations. In addition to a full medical history, an accurate travel history must be obtained:

- Countries visited, arrival and departure dates (for assessment of incubation period; Table 2.3).
- Travel in rural (where infection may be more common) or urban areas.
- Exposure to vectors: mosquitoes, ticks, flies and fresh water infested with snails containing schistosomes.

Tropical medicine

- Needle and blood exposure, e.g. blood transfusion or surgery, shared needles, acupuncture.
- Vaccination and prophylaxis: recent vaccination against yellow fever and hepatitis A and B is extremely effective; subsequent infection with these agents is very unlikely. Vaccination against typhoid is only partially effective, therefore infection is still a possibility. Malaria is always a possibility, even in those who have taken chemo-prophylaxis and used anti-mosquito precautions.
- History of unprotected sexual intercourse may suggest an acute HIV or hepatitis B seroconversion illness (p. 137).

Investigations

The initial work-up of a febrile patient who has travelled to the tropics is listed below. Additional studies depend upon exposure and other factors.

- Full blood count with differential white cell count, and thick and thin blood malaria films; repeat after 12–24 hours if initial films negative and malaria suspected
- Liver biochemistry – abnormal results found in many tropical infections
- Cultures of blood and stool
- Microscopy and culture of urine
- Chest X-ray
- 'Acute' serum for storage and subsequent antibody detection with paired convalescent serum at a later date.

Malaria nd (*K&C* 6e p. 95)

Malaria is a protozoan parasite widespread in the tropics and subtropics (Fig. 2.1). Each year 500 million people are affected, with a mortality rate of 0.2%. In endemic areas mortality is principally in children, and those who survive to adulthood acquire significant immunity. In hyperendemic areas an exaggerated immune response to repeated malarial infections leads to massive splenomegaly, anaemia and elevated IgM levels (tropical splenomegaly syndrome). Malaria parasites are scanty or absent in this syndrome and the disease responds to prolonged antimalarial treatment.

Aetiology

Travellers abroad are infected following the bite of an infected female mosquito of the genus *Anopheles*. Rarely

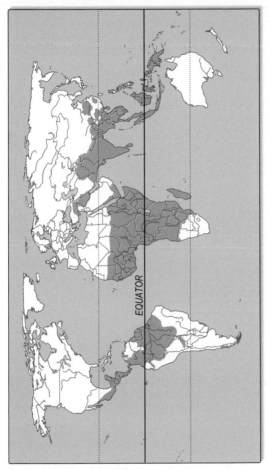

Fig. 2.1 **Malaria – geographical distribution.** (From Baird 2005, Copyright: © Massachusetts Medical Society. All rights reserved.)

the parasite is transmitted by importation of infected mosquitoes by air (airport malaria).

Four malaria parasites may infect humans; by far the most hazardous is *Plasmodium falciparum*, the symptoms of which can rapidly progress from an acute fever with rigors to severe multiorgan failure, coma and death. Once successfully treated this form does not relapse. The other malaria parasites, *P. vivax*, *P. ovale* and *P. malariae*, cause a more benign illness. However, *P. ovale* and *P. vivax* may relapse and *P. malariae* may run a chronic course over months or years.

Pathogenesis

The infective form of the parasite (sporozoites) passes through the skin and via the bloodstream to the liver. After a variable number of days they invade red blood cells and pass through further stages of development, which terminate with the rupture of the red cell. Rupture of red blood cells contributes to anaemia and releases pyrogens, causing fever. Red blood cells infected with *P. falciparum* adhere to the endothelium of small vessels and the consequent vascular occlusion causes severe organ damage, chiefly in the kidney, liver and brain. *P. ovale* and *P. vivax* may remain latent in the liver, and this is believed to be responsible for the relapses that may occur.

Clinical features

The incubation period varies:

- 10–14 days in *P. vivax*, *P. ovale* and *P. falciparum* infection
- 18 days to 6 weeks in *P. malariae* infection.

The onset of symptoms may be delayed in the partially immune or after prophylaxis. There is an abrupt onset of fever (> 40°C), tachycardia and rigors, followed by profuse sweating some hours later. This may be accompanied by anaemia and hepatosplenomegaly.

P. falciparum (Table 2.4) should be considered a medical emergency because patients may deteriorate rapidly. The following clinical forms are recognized and are more likely to occur when more than 1% of the red blood cells (RBC) are parasitized:

- *Cerebral malaria* is characterized by a high fever, convulsions, coma and eventually death. Hypoglycaemia, a complication of severe malaria, may present in a similar way and must be excluded.
- *Blackwater fever*, so called because of the production of dark brown-black urine (haemoglobinuria) resulting from severe intravascular haemolysis.

Table 2.4	Possible features of falciparum malaria
Central nervous system	Impaired consciousness and fits
Renal	Haemoglobinuria (Blackwater fever)
	Oliguria
	Uraemia (acute tubular necrosis)
Blood	Severe anaemia
	Disseminated intravascular coagulation
Respiratory	Acute respiratory distress syndrome/acute lung injury
Metabolic	Hypoglycaemia
	Metabolic acidosis
Gastrointestinal	Diarrhoea
	Jaundice
	Splenic rupture
Other	Hyperpyrexia
	Shock

27

Investigations

The conventional method for diagnosing malaria is light microscopy of a Giemsa-stained thick and thin blood smear. Thick smears are most useful for diagnosis of malaria and thin smears for quantification of the percentage of parasitized red cells and for species identification. Three to four smears should be taken over 48 hours before the diagnosis of malaria is ruled out. Antigen-detection methods for identifying malarial proteins and enzymes have been developed. Some are available as a rapid card or simple dipstick test from a finger-prick blood sample. They give a result in 10–15 minutes and are used in the field in developing countries. Other investigations include full blood count, serum urea and electrolytes, liver biochemistry and blood glucose.

Management

The acute treatment and eradication therapy of uncomplicated malaria is summarized in Table 2.5. Chloroquine resistance is now widespread, and chloroquine cannot be considered as treatment for *P. falciparum* in the UK. Antipyretics such as aspirin and paracetamol are given as necessary, and intravenous fluids may be required to combat dehydration and shock.

Table 2.5 Treatment of an acute uncomplicated attack of malaria	
Type of malaria	**Oral drug treatment**
P. vivax, P. ovale, P. malariae	Chloroquine: 600 mg followed by 300 mg 6 hours later and 300 mg daily for 2 days
P. falciparum	Quinine: 600 mg three times daily for 7 days followed by 3 tablets of Fansidar as a single dose or if Fansidar allergic or resistant (particularly areas of East Africa) give doxycycline 200 mg daily for 7 days
	Alternative therapy:
	Mefloquine: 25 mg/kg in 2 doses 8 hours apart
	Malarone (atovaquone 250 mg + proguanil 100 mg): 4 tablets daily for 3 days*
Eradication	
For *P. vivax, P. ovale*	Oral primaquine† 15 mg daily for 14 days

Chloroquine doses quoted are for the base drug;
Fansidar = pyramethamine/sulfadoxine
*Also used in the treatment of drug-resistant *P. falciparum* malaria
†Check for glucose-6-phosphate dehydrogenase deficiency first
(p. 206)

Severe falciparum malaria, indicated by the presence of any of the complications listed in Table 2.4 or if more than 2% of the RBCs are infected, constitutes a medical emergency, and optimal management may require admission to the ITU. Expert advice should be sought from a malaria reference centre. Quinine is given intravenously (20 mg/kg over 4 hours then 10 mg/kg over 4 hours every 8 hours until parasite count <1% and patient able to take oral quinine). In developing countries where facilities are not available for intravenous infusion, alternative routes are by intramuscular injection (chloroquine and quinine), nasogastric tube (chloroquine) or rectally (artemisinin). Intravenous glucose is given for hypoglycaemia and benzodiazepines for seizures. Early dialysis for acute renal failure should be commenced and positive-pressure ventilation for non-cardiogenic pulmonary oedema.

Prevention and control

Effective prevention of malaria includes the following elements.

- Awareness of risk
- Use of mechanical barriers such as insecticide-impregnated nets and mosquito repellents
- Chemoprophylaxis.

As a result of changing patterns of resistance, advice about chemoprophylaxis should be sought before leaving for a malaria-endemic area. Further details can be found in the *National Formulary* or from travel advice centres. Prophylaxis does not afford full protection. Drug regimens should be started at least 1 week before departure and continued without interruption for 4 weeks after return. The rationale for this advice is to ensure therapeutic drug levels before travelling and to enable unwanted effects to be dealt with before departure. The continued use of drugs after returning home will deal with infection contracted on the last day of exposure.

Chloroquine   300 mg weekly is recommended in travellers to chloroquine-sensitive areas. In areas of limited chloroquine resistance this is combined with proguanil 200 mg daily. This regimen has few side-effects and is safe in pregnancy.

Mefloquine   250 mg weekly is used in areas where falciparum malaria is highly resistant to chloroquine. With the now widespread geographic prevalence of chloroquine-resistant *P. falciparum*, mefloquine is for many travellers the mainstay of malarial chemoprophylaxis. An alternative is malarone (proguanil/atovaquone) or doxycycline.

Dengue fever (*K&C* 6e p. 54)

Dengue fever is caused by a flavivirus. It is found mainly in Asia, Africa, Central and South America where it is a common cause of fever and may be fatal. The virus is transmitted by the mosquito *Aedes aegypti*. After an incubation period of 5–6 days there is an abrupt onset of fever, headache, retro-orbital pain and severe myalgia, often with a skin rash. Some patients display a biphasic ('saddleback') fever curve with the second febrile phase lasting 1–2 days. Rare complications include shock and haemorrhagic manifestations, including purpura, epistaxis and melaena. Diagnosis is clinical and confirmed by acute and convalescent serum samples. Treatment is supportive.

Schistosomiasis (*K&C* 6e p. 112)

Schistosomiasis (also known as bilharzia) is virtually confined to travellers in Southern and sub-Saharan Africa especially those who undertake water sports in Lake Malawi. Acute symptoms are more common in non-immune individuals such as travellers. Parasite penetration through the skin may result in a localized pruritic papular rash ('swimmer's itch'). Parasite migration through the lungs and hepatic circulation 4–8 weeks after infection can be associated with fever, arthralgia and dry cough (Katayama fever). Chronic complications of schistosoma infection usually occur only in endemic areas where there is a high parasite load (Table 2.9).

Enteric fever (*K&C* 6e p. 85)

Typhoid fever and paratyphoid fever are caused by *Salmonella typhi* and *Salmonella paratyphi* (types A, B and C), respectively.

Typhoid fever nd (*K&C* 6e p. 85)

Humans are the only known reservoir of infection, and the spread is faecal–oral.

Clinical features

After an incubation period of 10–14 days there is an insidious onset of headache, dry cough and constipation, and a rising fever with relative bradycardia. In the second week of the illness an erythematous maculopapular rash that blanches on pressure and is referred to as 'rose spots' appears, chiefly on the upper abdomen and thorax, lasting for only 2–3 days. There is splenomegaly (75%), cervical lymphadenopathy and hepatomegaly (30%). Diarrhoea may develop. Complications, usually occurring in the third week, are pneumonia, meningitis, acute cholecystitis, osteomyelitis, intestinal perforation and haemorrhage. Recovery occurs in the fourth week.

Investigations

The diagnosis of enteric fever requires the culture of the causative microorganism from the patient. Organisms can be cultured from the blood, faeces and urine depending on the stage in the illness that individuals present for medical attention. In complicated cases or where the diagnosis remains in doubt, bone marrow cultures may be positive even after starting antibiotics.

Blood count   shows leucopenia.

Serologic tests   (Widal test) are of limited clinical utility.

Management

Treatment is with oral ciprofloxacin 750 mg twice daily for 7–14 days. Worldwide resistance is emerging to ciprofloxacin and an alternative is oral azithromycin 500 mg daily for 7 days. Infection is cleared when consecutive cultures of urine and faeces are negative. Some patients become chronic carriers, with the focus of infection in the gall bladder. Treatment is with amoxicillin and probenecid for 6 weeks. The most common method of prophylaxis for travellers is by intramuscular administration of a capsular polysaccharide vaccine.

Paratyphoid nd (*K&C* 6e p. 85)

Paratyphoid results in a milder illness that is otherwise clinically indistinguishable from typhoid fever. Treatment is with co-trimoxazole for 2 weeks.

Enterocolitis nd

Other *Salmonella* species (*S. choleraesuis* and *S. enteritidis*) cause a self-limiting infection presenting with diarrhoea and vomiting (Table 2.6) and are a cause of traveller's diarrhoea.

GASTROENTERITIS AND FOOD POISONING nd

Most causes of acute diarrhoea (lasting less than 14 days) with or without vomiting are due to a gastrointestinal infection with bacteria, virus or protozoa. Not all cases of gastroenteritis (*K&C* 6e p. 67) are food poisoning (*K&C* 6e p. 70), as the pathogens are not always food- or water-borne, e.g. *C. difficile* as a complication of antibiotic use.

Table 2.6 Pathogenic mechanisms of bacterial gastroenteritis where established

Pathogenesis	Mode of action	Clinical presentation	Examples
Mucosal adherence	Effacement of intestinal mucosa	Moderate watery diarrhoea	Entero-pathogenic *E. coli* (EPEC)
Mucosal invasion	Penetration and destruction of mucosa	Bloody diarrhoea	*Shigella* spp. *Campylo-bacter* spp. Enteroinvasive *E. coli* (EIEC)
Toxin production			
Enterotoxin	Fluid secretion without mucosal damage	Profuse watery diarrhoea	*Vibrio cholerae* *Salmonella* spp. *Campylo-bacter* spp. Enterotoxigenic *E. coli* (ETEC)
Neurotoxin	Preformed toxin	Variable diarrhoea and vomiting	*Bacillus cereus* *Staphylococcus aureus* producing enterotoxin B *Clostridium perfringens* type A
Cytotoxin	Damage to the mucosa	Bloody diarrhoea	*Salmonella* spp. *Campylo-bacter* spp. Enterohae-morrhagic *E. coli* (EHEC)

Individuals at increased risk of infection include infants and young children, the elderly, travellers (principally to developing countries), the immunocompromised and those with reduced gastric acid secretion. Viral gastroenteritis is a common cause of diarrhoea and vomiting in young children but is rarely seen in adults. Protozoal and helminthic gut infections are rare in the West but relatively common in developing countries.

Bacteria can cause diarrhoea in three different ways resulting in two broad clinical syndromes: watery diarrhoea and bloody diarrhoea, i.e. dysentery (Table 2.6).

The clinical features based on the principal presenting symptom associated with the causative organisms of food poisoning are summarized in Table 2.7. Listeriosis (infection with *Listeria monocytogenes*) is associated with contaminated coleslaw, non-pasteurized soft cheeses and other packaged chilled foods. The main feature of listeria infection is meningitis, occurring perinatally and in immunocompromised adults (see p. 751). Hepatitis A (p. 134) and *Toxoplasma gondii* (p. 19) are also acquired from infected foods and their major effects are extraintestinal.

Most infectious causes of diarrhoea are self-limiting. Routine stool examination for culture and microscopy for ova and parasites (three samples, since excretion is intermittent) and *C. difficile* toxin is not necessary other than in the following groups of patients: immunosuppressed, patients with inflammatory bowel disease (to distinguish a flare from infection), certain employees such as food handlers, bloody diarrhoea, persistent diarrhoea (> 7 days, possible *Giardia*, *Cryptosporidium*, *Cyclospora*), severe symptoms (fever, volume depletion) or recent antibiotic treatment or hospitalization. The management of patients with acute diarrhoea includes adequate hydration and antimotility agents such as loperamide (other than those with bloody diarrhoea or fever). Antibiotic therapy is not given in most cases since the illness is usually self-limited. Antibiotics are avoided in patients with suspected or proven enterohaemorrhagic *E. coli* infection as they may increase the risk of haemolytic uraemic syndrome. Empirical antibiotic therapy, e.g. ciprofloxacin and metronidazole, is given to patients with severe symptoms or bloody diarrhoea, pending the results of stool testing.

Traveller's diarrhoea (K&C 6e p. 70)

Acute gastrointestinal infection affects 30–50% of travellers from western countries to the developing world. Typically, abdominal cramps and diarrhoea begin 4–6 days after arrival and last 1–3 days. Less commonly, diarrhoea persists and may last for weeks.

Infection is most commonly due to enterotoxigenic *E. coli* (ETEC, Tables 2.7 and 2.8). To reduce the risk of infection,

33

Table 2.7 Major food-borne microbes by the principal presenting gastrointestinal symptom in immunocompetent adults nd

	Organism	Source/vehicles	Incubation period	Diagnosis	Recovery
Vomiting	Staph. aureus	Prepared food (e.g. sandwiches)	1–6 h	Diagnosis usually clinical for all organisms	<24 h
	Bacillus cereus	Rice, meat	1–6 h		2–3 days
	Norovirus (Norwalk-like virus)	Shellfish, prepared food	24–48 h		2–3 days
Watery diarrhoea	Clostridium perfringens	All by contaminated food and water	8–22 h	Stool testing by various methods is available for most organisms. ETEC and Clostridium perfringens usually require testing in reference laboratories	2–3 days
	Enterotoxigenic E. coli (ETEC)		6–24 h		1–5 days
	Enteric viruses		Variable		Variable
	Cryptosporidium parvum		5–28 days		7–14 days
	Cyclospora cayetanensis		7 days		Weeks to months
	Yersinia enterocolitica		1–9 days		1–22 days
	Vibrio cholerae		Hours – 6 days		2–3 days
Inflammatory diarrhoea Stools with mucus and blood	Campylobacter jejuni	Cattle and poultry – meat and milk	48–96 h	All detected on stool culture	3–5 days

Table 2.7 Major food-borne microbes by the principal presenting gastrointestinal symptom in immunocompetent adults nd —cont'd

	Organism	Source/vehicles	Incubation period	Diagnosis	Recovery
	Non-typhoidal salmonella	Cattle and poultry – eggs, meat	12–48 h		3–6 days, may be up to 2 weeks
	Enterohaerrorrhagic E. coli (usually serotype 0157:H7)*	Cattle – meat, milk	12–48 h		10–12 days
	Shigella spp.	Contaminated food and water	24–48 h		7–10 days
	Vibrio parahaemolyticus	Contaminated seafood	4–90 h		1–12 days
Non-gastrointestinal manifestations	Clostridium botulinum Paralysis due to neuromuscular blockade	Environment – bottled or canned food	18–24 h	Toxin in food or faeces	10–14 days
	Listeria monocytogenes Meningitis	Contaminated packaged chilled foods	Up to 6 weeks	CSF culture	Variable

*E. coli 0157:H7 also presents with the haemolytic uraemic syndrome (HUS) characterized by the triad of acute renal failure, haemolytic anaemia and thrombocytopenia. Patients who also have neurological symptoms are considered to have the related disorder thrombotic thrombocytopenic purpura (TTP)

Gastroenteritis and food poisoning nd

Table 2.8 Causes of traveller's diarrhoea

Bacteria – 70–90% of cases
Enterotoxigenic *Escherichia coli*
Shigella sp.
Salmonella sp.
Campylobacter jejuni
Aeromonas and *Plesimonas* spp.
Vibrio cholerae

Viruses – 10%
Rotavirus
Noroviruses (Norwalk-like virus)

Protozoa – < 5%
Giardia intestinalis
Entamoeba histolytica
Cryptosporidium parvum
Cyclospora cayetanensis

---

travellers are advised to drink bottled water, peel fruit before eating it and avoid salads because the ingredients may have been washed in contaminated water. Antibiotic prophylaxis, e.g. with ciprofloxacin, is not routinely recommended but is considered for patients with inflammatory bowel disease, immunosuppression and coexistent medical disease which would be compromised by dehydration, e.g. renal failure.

Treatment of traveller's diarrhoea is with rehydration, antibiotics, e.g. ciprofloxacin, for moderate to severe symptoms, and antidiarrhoeal agents, e.g. loperamide, for watery diarrhoea. Investigation, with microscopy and culture of three serial stool specimens, is usually only necessary for individuals with dysentery when invasive organisms are involved, or when diarrhoea persists in the returning traveller. In the latter case, this may reveal trophozoites (adult forms) or cysts of *Giardia intestinalis* or other parasites such as cryptosporidium. If stools are negative, empirical treatment for giardiasis with tinidazole 2 g as a single dose is given. Colonoscopy and biopsy are occasionally necessary in patients with persistent diarrhoea, particularly if an alternative diagnosis is considered, such as inflammatory bowel disease.

Amoebiasis nd (*K&C* 6e p. 104)

Amoebiasis is caused by infection of the human gastro-intestinal tract with the protozoal organism *Entamoeba histolytica*. Infection occurs world-wide, although much higher incidence rates are found in the tropics and sub-tropics. The modes of transmission are:

- Ingestion of cysts in contaminated food and water
- Person-to-person contact
- Sexual transmission among homosexual men.

Clinical features

Intestinal amoebiasis (amoebic dysentery) Invasion of the colonic epithelium by *E. histolytica* leads to tissue necrosis and ulceration. Ulceration may deepen and progress under the mucosa to form typical flask-like ulcers. The presentation varies from mild bloody diarrhoea to fulminating colitis, with the risk of toxic dilatation, perforation and peritonitis. In 10% of cases an amoeboma (inflammatory fibrotic mass) develops, commonly in the caecum or rectosigmoid region, which may bleed, cause obstruction, intussusception, or be mistaken for a carcinoma.

Amoebic liver abscess An amoebic liver abscess develops when organisms invade through the bowel serosa, enter the portal vein and pass into the liver. The abscess is usually single and in the right lobe of the liver. There is tender hepatomegaly, a high swinging fever and profound malaise. There may not be a history of colitis.

Investigations

Serology Amoebic fluorescent antibody test (FAT) is positive in 90% of patients with liver abscess and in 60–70% of patients with active colitis.

Colonic disease Microscopic examination of fresh stool or colonic exudate obtained at sigmoidoscopy shows the motile trophozoites, which contain red blood cells. *E. histolytica* must be distinguished by molecular techniques from the non-pathogenic *E. dispar* which appears identical.

Liver disease Liver abscesses should be considered when the serum alkaline phosphatase is elevated. Liver ultra-sonography or CT scan will confirm the presence of an abscess.

Differential diagnosis

Amoebic colitis must be differentiated from the other causes of bloody diarrhoea: inflammatory bowel disease, bacillary dysentery, *E. coli*, *Campylobacter* sp., salmonellae and, rarely, pseudomembranous colitis. Amoebic liver abscess must be differentiated from a pyogenic abscess and/or a hydatid cyst.

Management

Metronidazole is given for 5 days in amoebic colitis and a more prolonged course (10–14 days) in liver abscess. A large tense abscess may require percutaneous drainage under ultrasound guidance. After treatment of the invasive disease, the bowel should be cleared of parasites with a luminal amoebicide such as diloxanide furoate.

Control and prevention

Improved standards of personal hygiene and water supply are required. Travellers are advised to drink bottled water. Individual chemoprophylaxis is not advised because the risk of acquiring infection is low. There is no effective vaccine.

Shigellosis (bacillary dysentery) nd (*K&C* 6e p. 69)

Shigellosis is an acute self-limiting intestinal infection which occurs world-wide but is more common in tropical countries and in areas of poor hygiene. Transmission is by the faecal–oral route. The four *Shigella* species (*S. dysenteriae*, *S. flexneri*, *S. boydii* and *S. sonnei*) invade and damage the intestinal mucosa. Some strains of *S. dysenteriae* secrete a cytotoxin which results in diarrhoea.

Clinical features

After an incubation period of about 2 days there is an abrupt onset of fever, malaise, abdominal pain and watery diarrhoea, which may progress to bloody diarrhoea with mucus and tenesmus.

Investigations

The diagnosis is made on the basis of the stool culture.

Differential diagnosis

This is from other causes of bloody diarrhoea (see above). Sigmoidoscopic appearances may be the same as those in inflammatory bowel disease.

Management

The treatment of choice is ciprofloxacin 500 mg twice daily.

Cholera nd (*K&C* 6e p. 84)

Cholera is caused by the Gram-negative bacillus, *Vibrio cholerae*. Infection is common in tropical and subtropical countries in areas of poor hygiene. Infection is by the faecal–oral route, and spread is predominantly by ingestion of water contaminated with the faeces of infected humans. There is no identified animal reservoir.

Following attachment to and colonization of the small intestinal epithelium, *V. cholerae* produces its major virulence factor, cholera toxin. The B subunit of the toxin attaches to the enterocyte surface receptor, the ganglioside GM1; this allows migration of the A subunit into the cell to stimulate adenylate cyclase activity and increase cAMP levels. This produces massive secretion of isotonic fluid into the intestinal lumen. Cholera toxin also increases serotonin release from enterochromaffin cells in the gut, which contributes to the secretory activity and diarrhoea. Additional enterotoxins have been described in *V. cholerae* which may contribute to its pathogenic effect.

Clinical features

The incubation period varies from a few hours to 6 days. The illness varies from mild diarrhoea to profuse watery diarrhoea ('rice-water stools') resulting in dehydration, hypotension and death.

Investigations

The diagnosis is largely clinical. Fresh stool microscopy may show the motile vibrios.

Management

Management is aimed at effective rehydration, which is mainly oral but in severe cases intravenous fluids are given.

Gastroenteritis and food poisoning nd

Oral rehydration solutions (ORS) depend on the fact that there is a glucose-dependent sodium absorption mechanism not related to cAMP and thus unaffected by cholera toxin. The traditional World Health Organization ORS contains sodium (90 mmol/L) and glucose (111 mmol/L), along with potassium, chloride and citrate. New ORS solutions based on rice water may be more effective and are being evaluated.

Tetracycline for 3 days helps to eradicate the infection, decrease stool output and shorten the duration of the illness.

Prevention and control

Good hygiene and sanitation are the most effective measures for the reduction of infection. Oral cholera vaccines are under development.

Giardiasis (*K&C* 6e p. 105)

Giardia intestinalis is a flagellated protozoan that is found world-wide but is more common in tropical areas. It is a cause of traveller's diarrhoea and may cause prolonged symptoms (see later).

Clinical features

The clinical features are the result of damage to the small intestine, with subtotal villous atrophy in severe cases. There is diarrhoea, nausea, abdominal pain and distension, with malabsorption and steatorrhoea in some cases. Repeated infections can result in growth retardation in children.

Investigations

Treatment is often given based on clinical suspicion. If necessary, the diagnosis is made by finding cysts on stool examination or parasites in duodenal aspirates or biopsies.

Management

Metronidazole or tinidazole 2 g as a single dose daily for 3 days will cure most infections; some patients need two or three courses.

HELMINTHS (K&C 6e p. 106)

The helminths or worms that may infect man are of three classes (Table 2.9). In the UK only three species are commonly encountered: *Enterobius vermicularis*, *Ascaris lumbricoides* and *Taenia saginata*. Other species occur in tropical and sub-tropical countries and may be imported into the UK. A raised blood eosinophil count (eosinophilia) occurs at some stage in nearly all helminth infections.

SEXUALLY TRANSMITTED INFECTIONS (K&C 6e p. 117)

Sexually transmitted infections (STIs) remain endemic in all societies, and the range of diseases spread by sexual activity continues to increase. The three common presenting symptoms are:

41

- Urethral discharge (see below)
- Genital ulcers (see below)
- Vaginal discharge is caused by *Trichomonas vaginalis*, *Neisseria gonorrhoeae*, *Chlamydia trachomatis* and herpes simplex. Bacterial vaginosis is also characterized by a vaginal discharge but it is not clear to what extent this is a sexually transmitted infection. It occurs when the normal lactobacilli of the vagina are replaced by a mixed flora of *Gardnerella vaginalis* and anaerobes, resulting in an offensive discharge. Other causes of vaginal discharge are *Candida albicans*, retained tampon, chemical irritants, cervical polyps and neoplasia.

STIs predominantly seen in the tropics are chancroid, granuloma inguinale and lymphogranuloma venereum. They may present with genital ulceration and inguinal lymphadenopathy.

The aspects of management of all the STIs are:

- Accurate diagnosis and effective treatment
- Screening for other STIs (multiple STIs may coexist)
- Patient education
- Contact tracing: the patient's sexual partners must be traced so that they can be treated, thereby preventing the disease from spreading further
- Follow-up to ensure that infection is adequately treated.

Table 2.9 Summary of intestinal diseases caused by helminths (parasitic worms)

Helminth	Clinical manifestations	Diagnosis	Treatment of choice
Nematodes (roundworms)			
Small intestine *Strongyloides stercoralis*	Local dermatitis at site of skin penetration, diarrhoea, malabsorption, disseminated disease. Symptoms may continue for years as a result of autoinfection	Larvae in fresh stool. Detection of specific serum antibodies (serology)	Tiabendazole
Hookworm: *Ancylostoma duodenale*, *Necator americanus*	Local dermatitis at the site of skin penetration, nausea, epigastric pain, iron deficiency anaemia	Detection of eggs in faeces	Mebendazole
Roundworm: *Ascaris lumbricoides*	Often asymptomatic. Vomiting, abdominal discomfort, anorexia, intestinal obstruction. Pulmonary eosinophilia after migration to the lungs	Detection of eggs in faeces	Levamisole
Trichinella spiralis	Abdominal pain and diarrhoea. Larvae penetrate the bowel wall and invade striated muscle causing pain	Serology, muscle biopsy	Albendazole
Toxocara canis	Penetration of small intestine to lungs (bronchospasm), liver (hepatomegaly), heart, brain and eye	Serology	Albendazole

Table 2.9 Summary of intestinal diseases caused by helminths (parasitic worms)—cont'd

	Helminth	Clinical manifestations	Diagnosis	Treatment of choice
Large intestine	Whipworm: *Trichuris trichiura*	Often asymptomatic. Mucosal damage may result in bloody diarrhoea	Detection of eggs in faeces	Pyrantel pamoate
	Threadworm: *Enterobius vermicularis*	Pruritus ani	Apply adhesive tape to perineum and identify eggs	Mebendazole
Trematodes (flukes)				
Blood flukes	*Schistosoma* species	Snail vectors release cercariae which penetrate human skin (causing swimmer's itch) during swimming and paddling. Worms migrate to pelvic veins and bladder (*S. haematobium*) causing haematuria, hydronephrosis and renal failure. *S. mansoni* and *S. japonicum* migrate to the mesenteric veins and bowel causing bloody diarrhoea, intestinal strictures, hepatic fibrosis and portal hypertension	Detection of eggs in urine, stool or rectal biopsy. Serology	Praziquantel

Continued

Table 2.9 Summary of intestinal diseases caused by helminths (parasitic worms)—cont'd

	Helminth	Clinical manifestations	Diagnosis	Treatment of choice
Liver flukes	*Clonorchis sinensis* *Opisthorchis felineus* *and O. viverrini*	Cholangitis, biliary carcinoma	Detection of eggs on stool microscopy	Praziquantel
	Fasciola hepatica			Tiabendazole
Cestodes (tapeworms)				
	Taenia saginata	Beef tapeworm acquired by eating insufficiently cooked beef. Causes abdominal pain and malabsorption	Detection of eggs on stool microscopy	Praziquantel
	Taenia solium	Pork tapeworm from undercooked pork. Larvae penetrate the intestinal wall and cause disseminated disease involving skin, skeletal muscle and brain (fits, focal signs)	Serology, imaging of cysts in muscle and brain by X-ray, CT or MRI	Albendazole
	Echinococcus granulosus	Hydatid disease acquired by eating meat (from sheep, cattle) contaminated with ova excreted by dogs. Large cysts develop in liver, lung and brain. Anaphylactic reactions if cyst contents escape	Ultrasound, CT and MRI show the cysts and daughter cysts. Diagnosis by serology	Surgical excision and albendazole

Urethritis (*K&C* 6e p. 121)

Urethritis in men presents with urethral discharge and dysuria. It is often asymptomatic in women.

Gonorrhoea (*K&C* 6e p. 120)

The causative organism, *Neisseria gonorrhoeae* (gonococcus), is a Gram-negative intracellular diplococcus which infects epithelium, particularly of the urogenital tract, rectum, pharynx and conjunctivae.

Clinical features

The incubation period ranges from 2–14 days. In men the symptoms are purulent urethral discharge and dysuria. In homosexual men proctitis may produce anal pain, discharge and itch. Women may be asymptomatic or complain of vaginal discharge, dysuria and intermenstrual bleeding. Complications include salpingitis and Bartholin's abscess in women, epididymitis and prostatitis in men, and systemic spread with a rash and arthritis (p. 279). Infants born to infected mothers may develop ocular infections (ophthalmia neonatorum).

Diagnosis

Gram stain and culture of a swab taken from the urethra in men and the endocervix in women. Blood culture and microscopy of synovial fluid should be performed in cases of disseminated gonorrhoea. Nucleic acid amplification tests (NAATs) using urine specimens are non-invasive and highly sensitive, but may give false-positive results.

Management

Single-dose ciprofloxacin (500 mg by mouth) is the treatment of choice for uncomplicated anogenital infection in areas with a low prevalence of antibiotic resistance. Single-dose treatment with cefixime or ceftriaxone is used otherwise. Longer courses are required for complicated infections. Culture tests should be repeated at least 72 hours after treatment is complete.

Non-gonococcal urethritis (NGU) (*K&C* 6e p. 122)

The most common cause is infection with *Chlamydia trachomatis*, which in men presents with urethral discharge and dysuria. In women, infection may be asymptomatic and only found during investigations for infertility (secondary to salpingitis and fallopian tube blockage). The diagnosis of chlamydial urethritis is best made by nucleic acid amplification tests such as the polymerase chain reaction. The new urine-based diagnostic tests avoid the patient discomfort associated with urethral sampling. Treatment is with doxycycline or azithromycin (in pregnancy). Other causes of NGU are *Ureaplasma urealyticum*, *Bacteroides* sp. and *Mycoplasma* sp.

Genital ulcers (*K&C* 6e p. 118)

The infective causes of genital ulceration in the UK include syphilis, herpes simplex and herpes zoster. Non-infective causes are Behçet's disease, erythema multiforme major (p. 793), carcinoma and trauma.

Syphilis (*K&C* 6e p. 125)

The causative organism, *Treponema pallidum*, is a motile spirochaete which enters via a skin abrasion during close sexual contact. The organism may also pass transplacentally from mother to fetus.

Primary infection

After an incubation period of 10–90 days a papule develops at the site of infection. This ulcerates to become a painless, firm chancre which heals spontaneously within 2–3 weeks.

Secondary infection

This occurs 4–10 weeks after the appearance of the primary lesion. There may be one or more of the following features: fever, sore throat, arthralgia, generalized lymphadenopathy, widespread skin rash (except the face), superficial ulcers in the mouth (snail-track ulcers) and condylomata lata (warty perianal lesions). In most patients symptoms subside within 1 year.

Tertiary syphilis

This occurs after a latent period of 2 years or more. The characteristic lesion is a gumma (granulomatous lesion) occurring in the skin, bones, liver and testes. Cardiovascular syphilis is discussed on pages 459 and 482 and neurosyphilis on page 755.

Congenital syphilis

This usually becomes apparent between the second and sixth weeks after birth, early signs being nasal discharge, skin and mucous membrane lesions, and failure to thrive. Signs of late syphilis appear after 2 years of age, when there are also characteristic bone and teeth abnormalities as a result of earlier damage.

Diagnosis

- *Dark ground microscopy of fluid* taken from lesions shows organisms in primary and secondary disease. Serological tests may be negative in primary disease.
- *Serology.* The *T. pallidum* enzyme immunoassay (EIA) is the screening test of choice. A positive test is then confirmed with the *T. pallidum* haemagglutination assay (TPHA) and Venereal Disease Research Laboratory (VDRL) test. The VDRL test is detectable within 3–4 weeks of infection; it becomes negative in treated patients and in some untreated patients with late tertiary syphilis. Other diseases, e.g. autoimmune disease and malignancy, may give false-positive results. The *T. pallidum* EIA, TPHA and the fluorescent treponemal antibody test are positive in most patients with primary disease, and remain positive in spite of treatment. They do not distinguish between syphilis and other treponemes, e.g. yaws.

Management

Intramuscular procaine benzylpenicillin (procaine penicillin) for 10 days is given for primary and secondary syphilis. For tertiary syphilis, treatment is continued for 4 weeks. The Jarisch–Herxheimer reaction, characterized by malaise, fever and headache, occurs most commonly in secondary syphilis and is the result of release of TNF-α, IL-6 and IL-8 when organisms are killed by antibiotics.

HUMAN IMMUNODEFICIENCY VIRUS (HIV) AND AIDS

HIV is the cause of the acquired immune deficiency syndrome (AIDS). Estimates for 2002 are that 41 million people are infected with HIV world-wide with over 70% in sub-Saharan Africa. HIV is now the leading single cause of death in adults, causing 5 million deaths in 2003 with approximately 16 000 new infections occurring daily, the majority in young adults.

Epidemiology (K&C 6e p. 129)

Transmission is by:

- *Sexual intercourse.* World-wide, heterosexual intercourse accounts for the vast majority of infections. Homosexual transmission accounts for about two-thirds of infections in Europe, the USA and Australia.
- *Mother to child.* Transmission can occur in utero, although the majority of infections take place perinatally or via breast milk.
- *Contaminated blood, blood products and organ donations.* The risk is now minimal in developed countries since the introduction of screening blood products in 1985.
- *Contaminated needles.* This is a major route of transmission of HIV among intravenous drug addicts. Healthcare workers have a risk of approximately 0.3% following a single needle-stick injury with known HIV-infected blood.

HIV infection is not spread by ordinary social or household contact.

Pathogenesis of HIV infection (K&C 6e p. 130)

The virus consists of an outer envelope and an inner core. The core contains RNA and the enzyme reverse transcriptase, which allows viral RNA to be transcribed into DNA and then incorporated into the host cell genome (i.e. a retrovirus). The rapid emergence of viral quasispecies (closely related but genetically distinct variants) is due to the high mutation rate of reverse transcriptase and the high rate of viral turnover. This genetic diversification has implications for the evolution of viral variants with resistance to antiviral drugs.

HIV surface glycoprotein gp120 binds to the CD4 molecule on host lymphocytes. Other cells of the immune system bearing the CD4 receptor are also affected. The interaction between CD4 and HIV surface glycoprotein together with host chemokine co-receptors CCR5 and CXCR4 is responsible for HIV entry into cells and release of viral RNA. There is a progressive and severe depletion of infected CD4 helper lymphocytes which results in host susceptibility to infections with intracellular bacteria and mycobacteria. The coexisting antibody abnormalities predispose to infections with capsulated bacteria, e.g. *Strep. pneumoniae* and *H. influenzae*. The clinical illness associated with HIV infection is due to this immune dysfunction, and also to a direct effect of HIV on certain tissues.

Natural history of HIV infection (*K&C* 6e p. 132)

The typical pattern of HIV infection is shown in Figure 2.2. Throughout the course of HIV infection, viral load and immunodeficiency progress steadily, despite the absence of observed disease during the latency period.

   HIV infection is divided into the following stages:

■ *Category A* includes:
   – Primary HIV infection (also called acute HIV infection or acute seroconversion syndrome). Symptoms range from a mild glandular fever-like illness to an aseptic meningitis; severe symptoms are rare.
   – Clinical latent period with or without persistent generalized lymphadenopathy defined as nodes > 1 cm

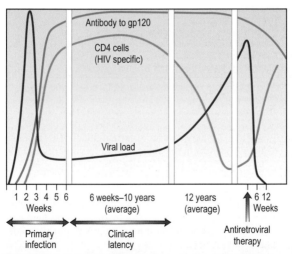

Fig. 2.2 Schematic representation of the course of HIV infection in vivo. The effect of antiretroviral therapy is also shown.

Table 2.10 AIDS-defining conditions*
Candidiasis of bronchi, trachea or lungs
Candidiasis, oesophageal
Cervical carcinoma, invasive
Coccidioidomycosis, disseminated or extrapulmonary
Cryptococcosis, extrapulmonary
Cryptosporidiosis, chronic intestinal (1-month duration)
Cytomegalovirus (CMV) disease (other than liver, spleen or nodes)
CMV retinitis (with loss of vision)
Encephalopathy (HIV-related)
Herpes simplex, chronic ulcers (1-month duration); or bronchitis, pneumonitis or oesophagitis
Histoplasmosis, disseminated or extrapulmonary
Isosporiasis; chronic intestinal (1-month duration)
Kaposi's sarcoma
Lymphoma, Burkitt's
Lymphoma, immunoblastic (or equivalent term)
Lymphoma (primary) of brain
Mycobacterium avium complex or *M. kansasii,* disseminated or extrapulmonary
Mycobacterium tuberculosis, any site
Mycobacterium, other species or unidentified species, disseminated or extrapulmonary
Pneumocystis carinii pneumonia
Pneumonia, recurrent
Progressive multifocal leucoencephalopathy
Salmonella septicaemia, recurrent
Toxoplasmosis of brain
Wasting syndrome, due to HIV

*USA definition also includes those with a CD4 count < 200 cells/μL (<200 cells/mm³)

in diameter at two or more extrainguinal sites for more than 3 months in the absence of causes other than HIV infection.

■ *Category B.* Early symptomatic HIV infection, which includes patients who do not have conditions specific to category A or C, e.g. persistent vaginal candidiasis, oral hairy leucoplakia, herpes zoster involving more than one dermatome, idiopathic thrombocytopenic purpura and pelvic inflammatory disease.

■ *Category C* includes patients with clinical conditions indicating that they have severe immunosuppression (AIDS; Table 2.10).

Table 2.11	Direct HIV effects
Neurological disease	AIDS dementia complex
	Sensory polyneuropathy
	Autonomic neuropathy causing diarrhoea and postural hypotension
	Aseptic meningitis
Eye	Retinal cotton wool spots – rarely troublesome
Mucocutaneous	Dry, itchy flaky skin
	Pruritic papular eruption
	Aphthous ulceration in the mouth
Haematological	Anaemia of chronic disease
	Neutropenia
	Autoimmune thrombocytopenia
Gastrointestinal	Anorexia leading to weight loss in advanced disease
	HIV enteropathy leading to diarrhoea and malabsorption
Renal	Renal impairment
	Nephrotic syndrome (due to focal glomerulosclerosis)
Respiratory	Chronic sinusitis and otitis media
	Lymphoid interstitial pneumonitis – lymphocytic infiltration of the lung, causing dyspnoea and a dry cough
Endocrine	Reduced adrenal function – infection may precipitate clear adrenal insufficiency
Cardiac	Myocarditis and cardiomyopathy

51

Effects of HIV infection

The clinical findings resulting from direct HIV infection are summarized in Table 2.11.

Conditions due to immunodeficiency (*K&C* 6e p. 135)

Immunodeficiency allows the development of opportunistic infections. These are diseases caused by organisms that are not usually considered pathogenic, unusual presentations of known pathogens, and the occurrence of tumours that have an oncogenic viral aetiology. Susceptibility increases as the patient becomes more immunosuppressed. When patients are profoundly immunocompromised (CD4 count < 100 cells/μL) disseminated infections with organisms of very low virulence such as *M. avium-intracellulare* and *Cryptosporidium* are able to establish themselves. The mortality and morbidity associated with HIV infection have declined dramatically since the introduction of highly active antiviral treatment (HAART). Similarly, long-term secondary chemoprophylaxis for previously life-threatening infections may not be necessary when HAART maintains the CD4 count above 200 cells/μL and the viral load is low.

Fungi (*K&C* 6e p. 136)

Pneumocystis carinii causes pneumonia (PCP) in severely immunocompromised patients (CD4 count < 200 cells/μL). There is an insidious onset of breathlessness, a non-productive cough, fever and malaise. Pneumothorax may complicate PCP. The chest X-ray may be normal or show bilateral perihilar interstitial infiltrates, which can progress to more diffuse shadowing. Definitive diagnosis is made by demonstrating the organisms in sputum by immuno-fluorescent staining. Specimens are obtained by sputum induced by nebulized hypertonic saline or, if non-diagnostic, bronchoscopy and bronchoalveolar lavage. Treatment is with intravenous co-trimoxazole, intravenous pentamidine or dapsone and trimethoprim for 21 days. Systemic cortico-steroids reduce mortality in severe cases (P_aO_2 < 9.5 kPa). Long-term prophylaxis, usually with oral co-trimoxazole, is required in patients whose CD4 count is below 200 cells/μL.

Cryptococcus most commonly causes meningitis in AIDS patients. There is an insidious onset of fever, nausea and headache, eventually with impaired consciousness and change in affect. Diagnosis is made by CSF microscopy (Indian ink staining shows the organisms directly), demonstration of cryptococcal antigen, and culture. CT scan is performed before lumbar puncture to exclude a space-occupying lesion. Treatment is with intravenous ampho-tericin B or fluconazole, and oral fluconazole continued long-term in the absence of HAART.

Candida infection (usually *Candida albicans*) presents as creamy plaques in the mouth, vulvovaginal region and oesophagus (producing dysphagia and retrosternal pain). Infection usually responds to treatment with fluconazole or itraconazole. Disseminated infection with *Aspergillus fumigatus* occurs in advanced HIV infection. The prognosis is poor, with amphotericin B being the mainstay of therapy.

Protozoal infections (*K&C* 6e p. 137)

Toxoplasma gondii most commonly causes encephalitis and cerebral abscess in AIDS patients. Clinical features include focal neurological signs, fits, fever, headache and possible confusion. Eye involvement with chorioretinitis may also be present. Diagnosis is made on the basis of positive toxoplasmosis serology and multiple ring-enhancing lesions on contrast-enhanced CT or MRI brain scan. Treatment is with pyrimethamine, sulfadiazine and folinic acid (leucovorin); lifelong maintenance may be required to prevent relapse. The differential diagnosis of multiple ring-enhancing CNS lesions in these patients includes lymphoma, mycobacterial (e.g. tuberculoma), bacterial (nocardia, streptococcus) or fungal (e.g. cryptococcoma) lesions.

Cryptosporidium parvum causes severe chronic watery diarrhoea and sclerosing cholangitis. Diagnosis is made by demonstrating cysts on stool microscopy or on small bowel biopsy specimens obtained at endoscopy. Treatment is symptomatic with antidiarrhoeal agents together with fluid, electrolyte and nutritional support.

Microsporidia infection (usually *Enterocytozoon bieneusi*) causes a diarrhoeal illness. Diagnosis is made by demonstrating spores in the stools. Treatment is with albendazole.

Viruses (*K&C* 6e p. 138)

Cytomegalovirus (CMV) causes:

■ Retinitis with floaters, loss of visual acuity and orbital pain, usually in a patient with CD4 count less than 100. The diagnosis is made on fundoscopy which shows a characteristic appearance of the retina with haemorrhages and exudate. Treatment is with intravenous ganciclovir or foscarnet, continued long term to prevent reactivation. Oral and topical forms of ganciclovir are available for maintenance treatment.

- Colitis, which presents with bloody diarrhoea and abdominal pain. Diagnosis is made by demonstrating characteristic 'cytomegalic cells' (large cells containing an intranuclear inclusion and sometimes intracytoplasmic inclusions) on light-microscopic examination of mucosal biopsy specimens. Treatment is with intravenous ganciclovir or foscarnet.
- Oesophageal ulceration, causing painful dysphagia.
- Less commonly, polyradiculopathy, encephalitis and pneumonitis.

Herpes simplex virus infection causes genital and oral ulceration, and systemic infection. Varicella zoster occurs at any stage of HIV infection, but may be more aggressive and longer lasting than in immunocompetent patients. Herpes-virus 8 is associated with Kaposi's sarcoma. Infection usually responds to aciclovir. Epstein–Barr virus (EBV) causes oral hairy leucoplakia, presenting as a pale, ridged lesion on the side of the tongue. Treatment is with aciclovir. Human papilloma virus (HPV) produces genital and plantar warts. HPV infection is associated with the more rapid development of squamous cell cancer of the cervix and anal cancer. Papovavirus causes progressive multifocal leucoencephalopathy, which presents with intellectual impairment and often hemiparesis and aphasia.

Hepatitis virus B and C (*K&C* 6e p. 138)

Because of the comparable routes of transmission of hepatitis viruses and HIV, co-infection is common, particularly in drug users and those infected by blood products. Hepatitis B does not seem to influence the natural history of HIV, though there is a reduced rate of clearance of the hepatitis B e antigen in co-infected patients and thus the risk of developing chronic infection is increased. Hepatitis C, on the other hand, is associated with a more rapid progression of HIV infection, and the progression of hepatitis C is more likely and more rapid.

Bacterial infection (*K&C* 6e p. 140)

This may present early in HIV infection, is often disseminated and frequently recurs. *Mycobacterium tuberculosis* (TB) can cause disease at all stages of HIV infection, but extrapulmonary TB is more common with advanced disease. *M. tuberculosis* infection usually responds well to standard treatment regimens, although the duration of therapy may be extended, especially in extrapulmonary infection. Treatment of TB in HIV co-infected patients presents specific challenges, particularly with regard to drug interactions and multidrug resistance, and requires input from a specialist physician.

Mycobacterium avium-intracellulare (MAI) (*K&C* 6e p. 141) occurs only in the later stages of HIV infection when patients are profoundly immunosuppressed (CD4 cell count $< 50/\mu L^3$). Clinical features include fever, anorexia, weight loss, diarrhoea and anaemia with bone marrow involvement. MAI is typically resistant to standard anti-tuberculous therapies. A combination of ethambutol, rifabutin and clarithromycin reduces the burden of organisms and provides symptomatic benefit. Other infections include *Strep. pneumoniae*, *H. influenzae*, staphylococcal skin infection and salmonella.

Neoplasia (*K&C* 6e p. 142)

The commonest tumours are Kaposi's sarcoma and non-Hodgkin's lymphoma. The incidence of all HIV-related malignancies has fallen since the introduction of HAART (see below).

- Kaposi's sarcoma is a vascular tumour which appears as red-purple, raised, well-circumscribed lesions on the skin, hard palate and conjunctivae, and in the gastro-intestinal tract. The lungs and lymph nodes may also be involved. Human herpesvirus 8 is implicated in the pathogenesis. Localized disease is treated with radio-therapy; systemic disease is treated with chemotherapy. Initiation of HAART may cause regression of lesions and prevent new ones emerging.
- Non-Hodgkin's lymphoma occurs in the brain, gut and lung.
- Squamous cell carcinoma of the cervix and anus is associated with HIV. Human papillomavirus may play a part in the pathogenesis.

Diagnosis and monitoring (*K&C* 6e p. 142)

Testing for HIV infection must only be undertaken with informed consent, and the patient should receive advice from a trained counsellor about the implications of a positive test (e.g. difficulties in obtaining life insurance, mortgages).

HIV infection is diagnosed by the following tests:

- Serum IgG antibodies against envelope components (gp120 and its subunits) may not appear for up to 3 months after infection. They are the most commonly used marker of HIV infection.
- Measurement of HIV RNA (viral load) in plasma.
- Measurement of viral p24 antigen (p24ag) in plasma if RNA assay is unavailable. Antigen disappears 8–10 weeks after exposure.

Following a diagnosis of HIV infection, the numbers of circulating CD4 lymphocytes are measured 3-monthly; patients with counts below 200 cells/μL are at greatest risk of HIV-related pathology (normal CD4 count in a healthy adult is > 500/μL). Plasma levels of HIV RNA ('viral load', measured in copies of RNA per mL) are a measure of viral replication. The viral load is the best indicator of long-term prognosis, and levels fall with effective antiretroviral medication.

The diagnosis of AIDS is made when an HIV-positive patient develops one or more of a defined list of opportunistic infections, malignancies or HIV-associated illnesses (Table 2.10) in the absence of other causes of immunosuppression, e.g. leukaemia, immunosuppressive drugs.

Management (*K&C* 6e p. 143)

Management involves treatment with antiretroviral drugs, social and psychological care, prevention of opportunistic infections and prevention of transmission of HIV. Although HIV infection cannot be cured, the advent of highly active antiretroviral therapy (HAART) has transformed HIV into a chronic controllable condition. The aims of treatment are to maintain physical and mental health, to avoid transmission of the virus, and to provide appropriate palliative support as needed. Table 2.12 lists the antiretroviral drugs currently available.

Treatment regimens for HIV infection are complicated and require a long-term commitment to high levels of adherence. A combination of clinical assessment and laboratory marker data, including viral load and CD4 counts, together with individual circumstances, should guide therapeutic decision-making.

Table 2.12 Antiretroviral drugs

Class of drug	Mechanism of action	Drug	Side-effects
Reverse transcriptase inhibitors			
Nucleoside analogues	Bind to viral DNA and inhibit reverse transcriptase, also act as DNA chain terminators	Abacavir Didanosine Lamivudine Stavudine Zalcitabine Zidovudine	Nausea, mitochondrial dysfunction, lactic acidosis and polyneuropathy may occur with any of these drugs. In addition, pancreatitis with didanosine, myelosuppression with lamivudine and zidovudine, myelopathy with zidovudine
Non-nucleoside reverse transcriptase inhibitors	Bind directly to, and inhibit reverse transcriptase	Efavirenz Nevirapine	Rash and Stevens–Johnson syndrome. Hepatic toxicity with nevirapine, CNS effects with efavirenz
Nucleotide analogues	Competitive reverse transcriptase inhibitors	Tenofovir (available in Europe on named-patient basis only)	
Protease inhibitors	Act competitively on HIV aspartyl protease enzyme which is	Amprenavir Indinavir Nelfinavir Ritonavir Saquinavir	Nausea, diarrhoea, abnormalities of fat distribution, raised plasma lipids, hyper-glycaemia, abnormal liver biochemistry/

Continued

Table 2.12	Antiretroviral drugs—cont'd		
Class of drug	Mechanism of action	Drug	Side-effects
	involved in pro-duction of func-tional viral proteins and enzymes		hepatotoxicity. Perioral para-esthesia with amprenavir and ritonavir
Fusion inhibitors	Inhibits fusion of HIV with target cell	Enfurvitide	Reactions at subcutaneous injections sites

In the UK, the current recommendations for initiation of treatment are shown in Table 2.13.

Treatment is initiated with a combination of drugs started simultaneously. The preferred regimen is two nucleoside reverse transcriptase inhibitors in combination with either a non-nucleoside reverse transcriptase inhibitor, a protease inhibitor, or with abacavir as a third drug. The goal is to achieve a viral load of less than 50 copies/mL within 3–6 months of therapy. Patients may need to change therapy because of virological failure or side-effects.

Prevention and control

- The risk of HIV transmission (p. 48) following a needle-stick injury involving contaminated blood is reduced by about 80% with post-exposure prophylaxis using a combination of zidovudine, lamivudine and indinavir for 4 weeks. Prophylaxis should be started as soon as possible after exposure.
- Pregnant HIV-positive women should receive antiviral therapy to reduce the risk of vertical transmission. Mothers with a high viral load might further reduce the risk to the baby if they deliver by elective caesarean section. They should be advised against breast-feeding.
- The use of condoms reduces sexual transmission of HIV.

Table 2.13 UK recommendations for starting antiretroviral therapy

Clinical presentation	Laboratory markers	Treatment recommendation
Symptomatic HIV infection, AIDS	Any CD4 count or viral load	Treat
Established, asymptomatic infection	CD4 < 200, any viral load	Treat
	CD4 201–350	Consider treatment based on viral load, rate of CD4 decline, coexisting clinical conditions, patient preference
	CD4 > 350	Defer treatment
Primary HIV infection		Treatment only recommended in a clinical trial or for severe symptoms

59

■ Advise drug addicts not to share needles; some areas provide free sterile needles.

Prognosis

The rate of progression among patients infected with HIV varies greatly. The average life expectancy for an HIV-infected patient in the absence of treatment is approximately 10 years. The mean survival following a CD4 count of 200 cells/μL is about 3 years. The introduction of HAART has resulted in a dramatic decrease in mortality and opportunistic infections in patients with HIV.

Gastroenterology and nutrition 3

GASTROENTEROLOGY

SYMPTOMS OF GASTROINTESTINAL DISEASE

Abdominal pain

Acute abdominal pain is discussed on page 115.

Dysphagia

Dysphagia is difficulty in swallowing. The causes are listed in Table 3.1.

Table 3.1 **Causes of dysphagia**

Intrinsic lesion
Benign (peptic) stricture
Malignant stricture
Foreign body
Oesophageal ring or web
Pharyngeal pouch

Neuromuscular disorders
Bulbar palsy
Pharyngeal disorders
Myasthenia gravis

Motility disorders
Achalasia
Scleroderma
Diffuse oesophageal spasm
Presbyoesophagus (oesophagus of old age)
Diabetes mellitus
Chagas' disease

Extrinsic pressure
Goitre
Mediastinal glands
Enlarged left atrium in mitral valve disease

Heartburn

Heartburn is a retrosternal burning discomfort which spreads up towards the throat and is a common symptom of acid reflux (p. 69). The pain can sometimes be difficult to distinguish from the pain of ischaemic heart disease, although a careful history will usually differentiate between the two (pp. 69 and 396).

Dyspepsia

Dyspepsia describes a range of symptoms referable to the upper gastrointestinal tract, e.g. nausea, heartburn, acidity, pain or distension. Patients are more likely to use the term 'indigestion' for these symptoms. Dyspepsia is a common symptom, and the most common cause is functional dyspepsia (p. 114) also referred to as non-ulcer dyspepsia. Other patients will have a peptic ulcer, gastro-oesophageal reflux disease or rarely a gastro-oesophageal cancer. The investigation and management are discussed on page 80.

Flatulence

Flatulence describes excessive wind, presenting as belching, abdominal distension and the passage of flatus per rectum. It is rarely indicative of serious underlying disease.

Vomiting

Vomiting occurs as a result of stimulation of the vomiting centres in the lateral reticular formation of the medulla. This may result from stimulation of the chemoreceptor trigger zones in the floor of the fourth ventricle or from vagal afferents from the gut. It is associated with many gastrointestinal conditions, but nausea and vomiting without abdominal pain are frequently non-gastrointestinal in origin. Non-gastrointestinal causes of vomiting include CNS disease (e.g. raised intracranial pressure, migraine), drugs especially chemotherapeutic agents, metabolic conditions (e.g. uraemia, diabetic ketoacidosis) and pregnancy. Persistent nausea and vomiting without any other symptoms is often functional in origin (p. 114).

Constipation

Constipation is difficult to define because there is considerable individual variation, but it is usually taken to mean infrequent passage of stool (< twice weekly) or the difficult passage of hard stools.

Diarrhoea

Diarrhoea implies the passage of increased amounts of loose stool (stool weight >200g/24h) (p. 110). This must be differentiated from the frequent passage of small amounts of stool (which patients often refer to as diarrhoea), which is commonly seen in functional bowel disorders. Investigation and management are discussed on page 112.

Steatorrhoea

Steatorrhoea is the passage of pale bulky stools that contain fat (> 18 mmol/24 h) and indicates fat malabsorption as a result of small bowel, pancreatic or biliary disease. The stools often float because of increased air content and are difficult to flush away.

INVESTIGATION OF GASTROINTESTINAL DISEASE (*K&C* p. 268)

Endoscopy

Endoscopic investigation of the gastrointestinal tract is usually performed as an outpatient procedure. The investigations require an explanation to the patient and written informed consent.

Oesophagogastroduodenoscopy

Oesophagogastroduodenoscopy is often referred to as OGD, gastroscopy, or upper endoscopy. A flexible endoscope is passed by mouth into the oesophagus, stomach and duodenum following the administration of local anaesthetic spray to the pharynx. Light sedation with intravenous midazolam may also be used. Patients should fast for 6 hours prior to the procedure and be warned not to drive for 24 hours if sedation is given. The procedure is useful for the investigation of dyspepsia, dysphagia, weight loss and iron deficiency anaemia. Duodenal biopsies can be obtained to establish a diagnosis of coeliac disease, and therapeutic options include arresting upper GI bleeding, oesophageal dilatation of peptic strictures, and stent insertion for palliation of oesophageal malignancy.

Sigmoidoscopy

This can be performed with a rigid instrument allowing examination of the rectum and distal sigmoid, or with a flexible instrument allowing examination of the left colon. Bowel preparation is achieved with one or two phosphate enemas, and sedation is rarely required.

Colonoscopy

This allows endoscopic examination of the entire colon and terminal ileum. Full bowel preparation on the day before the examination is achieved with oral sodium picosulfate or polyethylene glycol. Sedation is usually required and patients should be warned not to drive for 24 hours following the procedure. It is useful for the investigation of patients with altered bowel habit, rectal bleeding, abdominal pain or a strong family history of bowel cancer. Therapeutic options include removal of polyps (polypectomy) or diathermy of bleeding lesions such as angiodysplasia. Bowel perforation and bleeding following polypectomy are uncommon complications of the procedure.

Radiology and imaging

Plain X-rays

Plain chest and abdominal X-rays are usually used in the investigation of the acute abdomen. They may show free gas with a perforated viscus, dilated loops of bowel with intestinal obstruction and colonic dilatation in a patient with toxic megacolon in ulcerative colitis. Calcification in the pancreas (just to the left of L1) indicates chronic pancreatitis, and faecal loading is seen with constipation.

Barium examination

Ingestion of barium followed by X-rays allows examination of the oesophagus (barium swallow), stomach and duodenum (barium meal) and small intestine (barium follow-through). For examination of the colon (barium enema), barium and air are inserted per rectum and the patient is rotated until barium reaches the caecum.

Computed tomography (CT scan)

CT scanning (p. 952) is frequently used in the investigation of gastrointestinal disease, particularly in the staging of intra-abdominal malignancy and in the investigation and assessment of the acute abdomen. CT colonoscopy (virtual colonoscopy) uses spiral CT images and sophisticated software to generate a computer-simulated intraluminal view of the air-filled colon. The technique requires full bowel preparation as with conventional colonoscopy and air distension of the colon. The images obtained can visualize colonic polyps and cancer. The indications are evolving and currently it is mainly used where conventional colonoscopy cannot be performed because of patient intolerance or technical difficulties.

Ultrasound

Transabdominal ultrasound is useful for visualization of the liver, gall bladder and biliary tree, and kidneys. It is commonly used for investigation of abnormal liver blood tests, hepatomegaly and for characterization of abdominal masses. High-resolution ultrasound is also used in the diagnosis of patients with suspected appendicitis and diverticulitis, and to identify associated complications such as perforation and abscess formation. It is also used for the detection of bowel wall thickening and for determining the extent of involved segments in Crohn's disease, but is not disease specific.

Endoscopic ultrasound (EUS) is an endoscopic technique that utilizes an endoscope with an ultrasound probe at its tip. This allows more accurate visualization of the walls of the upper and lower gastrointestinal tract and nearby organs such as the pancreas and gall bladder. It is commonly used for tumour and nodal staging of oesophageal, gastric or pancreatic cancer or for non-invasive imaging of the biliary tree.

Endoanal ultrasonography involves the passage of a transducer into the rectum. It is used to assess the anal sphincters, particularly in patients with faecal incontinence.

Magnetic resonance imaging (MRI)

MRI (p. 959) is particularly used to image the pelvis and is used in the assessment of patients with perianal Crohn's disease and in the staging of rectal cancer. The magnetic field of an MR imaging system may cause movement of a ferromagnetic object within the body. Thus MRI may be contraindicated in patients with pacemakers, prosthetic heart valves and intraorbital metallic foreign bodies. In these cases the procedure should be discussed with the responsible radiologist in advance.

Positron emission tomography (PET) scanning

PET scanning (p. 961) is used with other imaging modalities such as CT scan in the investigation of suspected malignancy and for detection of metastases in known malignancy.

Oesophageal pH monitoring and manometry

Insertion of a pH probe into the lower oesophagus via the nose allows continual monitoring of acid reflux over 24 hours. Data are captured on a small device worn on a belt, and transferred to a computer at the end of the 24-hour period. The frequency and duration of reflux episodes are then calculated automatically This test is usually performed to confirm GORD prior to surgery or in difficult diagnostic cases. Oesophageal manometry involves the passage of a small tube containing several pressure transducers into the oesophagus via the nose. The patient is then asked to take a swallow allowing oesophageal peristalsis and pressure to be assessed. Manometry may be used in the investigation of patients with dysphagia particularly to establish the diagnosis of suspected achalasia or oesophageal spasm, or for detecting oesophageal motor abnormalities in patients with systemic disease, e.g. systemic sclerosis.

Wireless video endoscopy (video capsule endoscopy)

This is a non-invasive technique designed primarily to provide imaging of the small intestine, an anatomical site that has proved difficult to visualize with endoscopy. After an overnight fast the video capsule is swallowed and images are recorded by sensors and a recorder worn on an abdominal belt. The indications for its use are still being established.

THE MOUTH

Problems in the mouth are common and often trivial, although they can cause severe symptoms.

Mouth ulcers (*K&C* 6e p. 271)

Non-infective
- Recurrent aphthous ulceration is the most common cause of mouth ulcers and affects at least 20% of the population; in most cases the aetiology is unknown. The history is of recurrent self-limiting episodes of painful oral ulcers (rarely on the palate). Topical corticosteroids

are used for symptomatic relief but they have no effect on the natural history. In a few cases ulcers are associated with trauma or gastrointestinal and systemic diseases, e.g. anaemia, inflammatory bowel disease, coeliac disease, Behçet's disease, Reiter's disease, systemic lupus erythematosus, pemphigus, pemphigoid, and fixed drug reactions.

■ Squamous cell carcinoma presents as an indolent ulcer, usually on the lateral borders of the tongue or floor of the mouth. Aetiological factors include tobacco (smoking and chewing) and alcohol. Treatment is with surgery, radiotherapy or a combination of both.

Infective

Many infections can affect the mouth, though the most common are viral and include:

■ Herpes simplex virus type 1
■ Coxsackie A virus
■ Herpes zoster virus.

Oral white patches

Oral white patches are associated with smoking, *Candida* infection, lichen planus, trauma and syphilis. Leucoplakia is the term used to describe oral white patches or plaques for which no local cause can be found (i.e. a diagnosis of exclusion). Leucoplakia is occasionally a premalignant lesion and thus oral white patches must be biopsied to exclude malignancy. Hairy leucoplakia is an Epstein–Barr-related white patch on the side of the tongue, which is almost pathognomonic of HIV infection; it is not premalignant.

Atrophic glossitis

A smooth sore tongue with loss of filiform papillae may occur in patients with iron, vitamin B_{12} or folate deficiency.

Geographical tongue

This affects 1–2% of the population and describes discrete areas of depapillation on the dorsum of the tongue. This may be asymptomatic or produce a sore tongue. The aetiology is unknown and there is no specific treatment.

Periodontal disorders

Gum bleeding is most commonly caused by gingivitis, an inflammatory condition of the gums associated with dental plaque. Bleeding may also be associated with generalized conditions such as bleeding disorders and leukaemia. Acute ulcerative gingivitis (Vincent's infection) is characterized by the development of crater-like ulcers, with bleeding, involving the interdental papillae, followed by lateral spread along the gingival margins. It is thought to be the result of spirochaetal infection occurring in the malnourished and immunocompromised. Treatment is with oral metronidazole and good oral hygiene.

Salivary gland disorders (*K&C* 6e p. 273)

Xerostomia (mouth dryness) may be caused by anxiety, drugs such as tricyclic antidepressants, Sjögren's syndrome and dehydration.

Infection (parotitis) may be viral, i.e. mumps virus, or bacterial (staphylococci or streptococci).

Sarcoidosis produces enlargement of the parotid glands and, if combined with lacrimal gland enlargement, is known as the Mikulicz syndrome.

Calculus formation usually occurs in the duct of the submandibular gland, and causes painful swelling of the gland before or during mastication.

Tumours most commonly affect the parotid gland and are usually benign, e.g. pleomorphic adenoma. Treatment is with surgical resection. Involvement of the VIIth cranial nerve raises the suspicion of malignancy.

THE OESOPHAGUS

The main oesophageal symptoms are dysphagia, heartburn and painful swallowing (odynophagia):

- Dysphagia is usually investigated with a barium swallow, followed by gastroscopy where appropriate. The causes are listed in Table 3.1. The commonest causes are peptic or malignant strictures and bulbar palsies. Typically, mechanical narrowing of the oesophagus, particularly in oesophageal malignancy, produces progressive dysphagia, initially for solids and eventually for liquids. Motor disorders, e.g. achalasia and scleroderma, produce dysphagia for both solids and liquids together.
- Heartburn is a retrosternal or epigastric burning sensation produced by the reflux of gastric acid into the oesophagus. The pain may radiate up to the throat and be confused with chest pain of cardiac origin. It is often aggravated by bending or lying down.

- Painful swallowing occurs with infections of the oesophagus (herpes simplex virus, *Candida*) or in gastro-oesophageal reflux disease, particularly with alcohol and hot liquids.

Gastro-oesophageal reflux disease (GORD) (*K&C* 6e p. 275)

Reflux of gastric contents into the oesophagus is a normal event and clinical symptoms occur only when there is prolonged contact of gastric contents with the oesophageal mucosa.

Pathophysiology

The lower oesophageal sphincter (LOS) tone is reduced, and there are frequent transient LOS relaxations. There is increased mucosal sensitivity to gastric acid and reduced oesophageal clearance of acid. Delayed gastric emptying and prolonged postprandial and nocturnal reflux also contribute. Mechanical or functional aberrations associated with a hiatus hernia may contribute to GORD in some patients, but patients may also have reflux in the absence of a hiatus hernia. Other predisposing factors in GORD include obesity, pregnancy, systemic sclerosis and certain drugs (e.g. nirates, tricyclics).

Clinical features

Heartburn (p. 62) is the major symptom of GORD. The burning is aggravated by bending, stooping and lying down, and may be relieved by antacids. There may be pain on drinking hot drinks. Cough and nocturnal asthma can occur from aspiration of gastric contents into the lungs. Symptoms do not correlate well with the severity of oesophagitis.

Investigations

The diagnosis is clinical and investigation is not usually required in patients without 'alarm' symptoms (weight loss, dysphagia, anaemia).

Gastroscopy is the investigation of choice and may show oesophagitis (mucosal erythema, erosions and ulceration). The mucosa can, however, be normal in patients with symptoms of reflux.

Barium swallow may show an ulcerated lower oeso-phagus and demonstrate a hiatus hernia if present.

24-Hour intraluminal pH monitoring (p. 66) is usually reserved for the confirmation of GORD prior to surgery or in difficult diagnostic cases.

Management

Conservative measures with weight loss, a reduction in alcohol intake, cessation of smoking and simple antacids are often sufficient for mild symptoms.

- *Alginate-containing antacids* are usually first-line treatments; they prevent reflux by forming a 'foam raft' on gastric contents.
- H_2-*receptor antagonists* (e.g. ranitidine) improve the symptoms of heartburn.
- *Prokinetic agents*, such as metoclopramide and dom-peridone, are occasionally helpful.
- *Proton pump inhibitors* (PPIs) (e.g. omeprazole, esome-prazole, lansoprazole, pantoprazole) inhibit gastric hydrogen/potassium-ATPase and block the luminal secretion of gastric acid. They are potent acid blockers and the drugs of choice for all but mild cases. Given the propensity of reflux symptoms to relapse, maintenance acid-suppressive therapy is often necessary. In these cases the aim is to reduce to the minimum dose necessary to control symptoms ('step-down approach').
- *Endoscopic therapy.* Endoscopic gastroplasty (sutures are placed endoscopically in the lower oesophagus), the Stretta procedure (radiofrequency energy is delivered to the LOS to induce fibrosis), and endoscopic injection of submucosal polymers to bolster the LOS are being increasingly employed in patients dependent on PPIs.
- *Surgery* may be necessary for the few patients who continue to have symptoms in spite of full medical therapy, or in young people whose symptoms return rapidly on stopping treatment. The fundus of the stomach is sutured around the lower oesophagus to produce an antireflux valve (Nissen fundoplication). This procedure is now usually performed laparoscopically.

Complications

Oesophageal stricture formation is the major complication of reflux and presents with intermittent dysphagia. It is treated with endoscopic dilatation. Long-standing acid reflux may cause metaplasia from squamous to columnar epithelium in the lower oesophagus, a change known as Barrett's oesophagus. The diagnosis is made at endoscopy when the pale glossy squamous epithelium is replaced by red-coloured columnar epithelium. Barrett's oesophagus is premalignant for adenocarcinoma of the oesophagus and patients with this condition should undergo regular endoscopic surveillance with multiple biopsies to look for dysplasia or carcinoma.

Achalasia (*K&C* 6e p. 277)

Achalasia is a disease of unknown aetiology, characterized by aperistalsis and non-propulsive tertiary contractions in the body of the oesophagus, and the failure of relaxation of the lower oesophageal sphincter (LOS) on initiation of swallowing.

Pathology

There is a decrease in ganglionic cells in the nerve plexus of the oesophageal wall and degeneration in the vagus nerve.

Clinical features

The disease can present at any age but is rare in childhood. There is usually a long history of dysphagia for both liquids and solids, which may be associated with regurgitation. Severe retrosternal chest pain may occur, particularly in younger patients.

Investigations

- Barium swallow often shows dilatation of the oesophagus, lack of peristalsis, a gradually tapering lower end (beak deformity) and asynchronous contractions of the oesophagus.
- Gastroscopy may be necessary to exclude oesophageal cancer, which can produce similar symptoms and X-ray appearance.
- Oesophageal manometry demonstrates aperistalsis and failure of LOS relaxation.
- Chest X-ray may show a dilated oesophagus with a fluid level behind the heart. The fundal gas shadow is not present.

Management

There is no cure for achalasia and the goal of treatment is relief of patient symptoms and improved oesophageal emptying. The two most effective treatment options are endoscopic graded pneumatic balloon dilatation of the LOS and surgical division of the sphincter (Heller's cardio-myotomy). For patients who are at high risk for these techniques, endoscopic injection of the LOS with botulinum toxin (Botox) or pharmacological treatment with calcium-channel blockers may be acceptable alternatives. Both relax the LOS, Botox by inhibiting the release of acetylcholine from cholinergic nerve terminals in the myenteric plexus and so reducing smooth muscle contraction and LOS tone. GORD is a complication of all treatments, particularly surgery.

Complications

There is a slight increase in the incidence of squamous carcinoma of the oesophagus. The risk is not reduced by endoscopic or surgical treatment.

Systemic sclerosis (K&C 6e p. 278)

There is oesophageal involvement in over 90% of patients with systemic sclerosis. The smooth muscle layer is replaced by fibrous tissue. The LOS pressure is reduced, thereby permitting reflux. Patients may be asymptomatic or complain of reflux and dysphagia. Dysphagia is caused by stricture formation complicating reflux. Treatment is as for reflux and stricture formation.

Diffuse oesophageal spasm (K&C 6e p. 278)

This is a severe form of abnormal oesophageal motility which most commonly presents in middle age, and can produce chest pain and dysphagia. A 'corkscrew' appearance may be seen on barium swallow. 'Nutcracker oesophagus' is a variant characterized by high-amplitude peristaltic waves in the oesophagus. Treatment of these disorders is difficult, but calcium-channel blockers, e.g. oral nifedipine, may be helpful. Treatment of GORD may help.

Hiatus hernia (K&C 6e p. 274)

A hiatus hernia refers to herniation of a part of the stomach through the oesophageal hiatus of the diaphragm. There are two main forms:

- *Sliding.* This accounts for more than 95% of cases. The gastro-oesophageal junction slides through the hiatus and lies above the diaphragm. On its own, a sliding hiatus hernia is not responsible for symptoms unless there is associated reflux.
- *Para-oesophageal hernias* are uncommon. The gastric fundus rolls up through the hiatus alongside the oesophagus, the gastro-oesophageal junction remaining below the diaphragm. These never regress and pose a serious risk of complications including gastric volvulus (rotation and strangulation of the stomach), bleeding and respiratory complications. They should be treated surgically.

Malignant oesophageal tumours (*K&C* 6e p. 279)

Pathology

- Squamous cell, usually of the middle third of the oesophagus
- Adenocarcinoma of the lower third of the oesophagus.

73

Epidemiology

Squamous carcinoma The incidence is 5–10 per 100 000 in the UK, although it varies greatly throughout the world, being particularly high in China and parts of Africa and Iran. It is most common in the 60- to 70-year age group. It is associated with heavy alcohol intake, heavy smoking and a high intake of salted fish and pickled vegetables. Other predisposing factors include achalasia and coeliac disease.

Adenocarcinoma This arises from the columnar-lined epithelium of the lower oesophagus (Barrett's oesophagus) which results from long-standing reflux.

Clinical features

Symptoms include progressive dysphagia (initially for solids and later for liquids), weight loss, and chest pain, which may be due to bolus food impaction or local infiltration. Physical signs are usually absent.

Investigations

- Gastroscopy and biopsy of the tumour is the initial investigation to make the diagnosis. A barium swallow will show the strictured area but biopsies cannot be taken.

■ CT scan of the chest and abdomen, MRI and endoscopic ultrasonography of the oesophagus are helpful in staging the lesion to decide the most appropriate treatment.

Management

In many patients, only symptomatic treatment to relieve the dysphagia is possible. This is usually performed endoscopically, and options include:

■ Insertion of an expanding metal stent to keep the oesophagus open
■ Laser to photocoagulate the tumour
■ Alcohol injections into the tumour to cause local necrosis.

Surgical resection may be carried out in a few patients when staging has shown that the tumour has not infiltrated outside of the oesophageal wall. The combination of chemotherapy and radiotherapy prior to surgery (neo-adjuvant chemotherapy) may increase survival. Radiation alone is sometimes employed with limited success in both squamous cell carcinoma and adenocarcinoma.

Prognosis

The prognosis overall is poor (9% 5-year survival) as most patients can only be treated palliatively.

Benign oesophageal tumours (*K&C* 6e p. 281)

See page 82 (GIST tumours).

Oesophageal perforation (*K&C* 6e p. 279)

The commonest cause of oesophageal perforation is iatrogenic and occurs after endoscopic dilatation of oesophageal strictures (usually malignant) or achalasia. It may also occur after forceful vomiting (Boerhaave's syndrome), when there is also usually severe chest pain and collapse. On examination there may be fever, hypotension and surgical emphysema. Diagnosis is by chest X-ray, which may be normal or show air in the mediastinum and neck, and a pleural effusion. A gastrografin swallow (not barium) will confirm the diagnosis. Treatment is with intra-venous antibiotics, nil by mouth and intravenous fluids. Surgical repair is needed for patients with large tears or who fail to settle with conservative management.

THE STOMACH AND DUODENUM

Gastropathy and gastritis (K&C 6e p 287)

Gastropathy is the term used when there is injury to the gastric mucosa associated with epithelial cell damage and regeneration. There is little or no accompanying inflammation. *Gastritis* is inflammation of the gastric mucosa. This distinction has caused considerable confusion, since gastritis is often used to describe endoscopic or radiological characteristics of the gastric mucosa rather than specific histological findings.

Gastropathy

The commonest cause of gastropathy is mucosal damage associated with the use of aspirin or other non-steroidal anti-inflammatory drugs (NSAIDs). These drugs deplete mucosal prostaglandins, by inhibiting the cyclo-oxygenase pathway, which leads to mucosal damage (p. 848). Other causes include infections, e.g. cytomegalovirus and herpes simplex virus, and alcohol in high concentrations. Gastric erosions can also be seen after severe stress (stress ulcer), burns (Curling's ulcer), and in renal and liver disease. Common symptoms include indigestion, vomiting and haemorrhage, although these correlate poorly with endoscopic and pathological findings. Erosions (superficial breaks in the mucosa < 3 mm) and subepithelial haemorrhage are most commonly seen at endoscopy. Treatment is with a proton pump inhibitor with removal of the offending cause if possible. Prophylaxis is also given to prevent future damage in patients who continue to take aspirin or NSAIDs.

Gastritis

The commonest cause of gastritis is *Helicobacter pylori* infection (p. 76). Other causes are autoimmune gastritis (the cause of pernicious anaemia associated with antibodies to gastric parietal cells and intrinsic factor), viruses and duodenogastric reflux. Gastritis is a histological diagnosis and is usually discovered incidentally when a gastric mucosal biopsy is taken for histology at endoscopy. It is classified as acute or chronic. Acute inflammation is associated with neutrophilic infiltration, while chronic inflammation is characterized by mononuclear cells, chiefly lymphocytes, plasma cells and macrophages. Gastritis is usually asymptomatic; whether *H. pylori* gastritis itself produces functional dyspepsia is controversial (p. 114). At endoscopy the mucosa may appear reddened or normal. No specific treatment is required although eradication treatment for *H. pylori* is often given.

Helicobacter pylori and the upper gastrointestinal tract (*K&C* 6e p. 283)

Helicobacter pylori is a Gram-negative urease-producing spiral-shaped bacterium found predominantly in the gastric antrum and in areas of gastric metaplasia in the duodenum. It is closely associated with chronic active gastritis, peptic ulcer disease, gastric cancer and gastric B cell lymphoma (p. 82). However, most patients with the infection are asymptomatic. Some strains of *H. pylori* (CagA-positive strains) are particularly associated with gastroduodenal disease.

Epidemiology

The incidence of *H. pylori* infection is higher in the older age groups and associated with lower socio-economic status. Most cases of infection probably occur in childhood, and transmission is most likely via the oral–oral or faecal–oral routes.

Clinicopathological features

H. pylori infection produces a gastritis mainly in the antrum of the stomach. In some individuals gastritis can involve the body of the stomach, leading to atrophic gastritis and in some cases intestinal metaplasia, which is a premalignant condition.

Investigations

Invasive tests (endoscopy and biopsy of the gastric antrum)
- Rapid urease test (CLO test) is the test of first choice on an antral biopsy. A biopsy which contains *H. pylori* when added to a urea-containing solution breaks down urea to release ammonia and produces a pH-dependent colour change in the indicator present.
- Histology with direct visualization of the organism.
- Gram stain and culture. This is not a routine method of testing.

Non-invasive tests

■ Urea breath test. ^{13}C (or ^{14}C) labelled urea is given by mouth; the detection of ^{13}C in expired air indicates infection with urease-producing *H. pylori*. The breath test is particularly useful to confirm eradication of the organism after appropriate treatment.
■ Serological tests detect IgG antibodies to *H. pylori*. They are used to diagnose infection but are not useful for confirming eradication because patients may have antibodies for years after eradication of the organism.
■ Stool tests. A specific immunoassay for qualitative detection of *H. pylori* is available with a sensitivity and specificity of greater than 90%.

Management

Eradication of *H. pylori* is indicated for all patients with proven peptic ulcer disease, atrophic gastritis, patients who are first-degree relatives of patients with gastric cancer and in patients with gastric lymphoma (p. 82). Recurrence is very uncommon in those in whom the infection is successfully eradicated. Several treatment regimens are available, although proton-pump inhibitor (PPI)-based triple therapy regimens are favoured, e.g.

■ PPI (e.g. omeprazole 20 mg) plus metronidazole 400 mg and clarithromycin 500 mg all twice daily for 1 week
■ PPI (e.g. omeprazole 20 mg) plus amoxicillin 1 g and clarithromycin 500 mg all twice daily for 1 week.

Peptic ulcer disease (*K&C* 6e p. 285)

A peptic ulcer is an ulcer of the mucosa in or adjacent to an acid-bearing area. Most occur in the stomach or proximal duodenum.

Epidemiology

Duodenal ulcers are three to four times more common than gastric ulcers and occur in 15% of the population at some time. They are more common in men than in women (4:1) and both are more common in elderly people. There is a significant geographical variation.

Table 3.2   Proposed pathogenic mechanisms of *H. pylori*
Increased gastric acid secretion due to:
increased fasting and meal-stimulated serum gastrin
increased parietal cell mass
decreased somatostatin (D) cells in the antrum
Increased pepsinogen-1
Disruption of mucous protective layer
Production of virulence factors:
vacuolating toxin (Vac A)
cytotoxic associated protein (CagA)
urease
adherence factors

Aetiology

The precise mechanism of how peptic ulceration occurs is unclear, though infection with *H. pylori* plays a central role. Potential pathogenic mechanisms are listed in Table 3.2. Genetic factors may have a role to play. Aspirin and NSAIDs are also a cause of gastric ulceration, though less commonly duodenal ulcers. Peptic ulceration is also seen in hyperparathyroidism and the Zollinger–Ellison syndrome (p. 182).

Clinical features

Epigastric pain is the most common presenting symptom. This is typically relieved by antacids but has a variable relationship to food. Duodenal ulcer pain, however, often occurs when the subject is hungry and classically occurs at night. Other symptoms, such as nausea, heartburn and flatulence, may occur. Occasionally ulcers may present with the complications of perforation or painless upper gastrointestinal haemorrhage.

Investigations

Patients less than 55 years with ulcer-type symptoms should undergo screening for *H. pylori* infection by either serology, breath test or stool test; upper gastrointestinal endoscopy is not usually necessary (see Management of dyspepsia, p. 80). Older patients should undergo endoscopy particularly to rule out a gastric cancer. In patients found to have a gastric ulcer at endoscopy, multiple biopsies from the centre and edge of the ulcer must be taken, because it is often impossible to distinguish by naked eye a benign from malignant gastric ulcer. A barium meal is useful if gastric outlet obstruction is suspected.

Management

Ulcers associated with *H. pylori* Treatment regimens (p. 77) that successfully eradicate *H. pylori* from the gastric antrum result in ulcer healing rates of over 90% and prevent recurrence unless reinfection occurs, which is unusual. There is normally no need to continue antisecretory treatment (with a proton pump inhibitor or H_2-receptor antagonist) unless the ulcer is complicated by haemorrhage or perforation. This approach to treatment is indicated in all patients with *H. pylori*-associated peptic disease.

***H. pylori*-negative peptic ulcers** Most *H. pylori*-negative peptic ulcers are associated with aspirin and NSAID ingestion. Treatment involves the use of acid-suppressing drugs and stopping the NSAID if at all possible. PPIs (p. 70) heal most ulcers and are the drugs of choice. After ulcer healing NSAIDs can only be continued with ulcer prophy-laxis (such as with a PPI or misoprostil (a prostaglandin agonist)) or therapy is switched to a selective COX-2 inhibitor (p. 850).

Follow-up endoscopy plus biopsy should be performed for all gastric ulcers to demonstrate healing and exclude malignancy (initial biopsies may be false negatives).

Surgery With the introduction of modern drugs, surgery is rarely performed for peptic ulceration but is reserved for the treatment of complications: recurrent haemorrhage, perforation and outflow obstruction.

Complications

Perforation is uncommon. Duodenal ulcers perforate more commonly than gastric ulcers, usually into the peritoneal cavity. Management is surgical, with closure of the perforation and drainage of the abdomen. *H. pylori* should subsequently be eradicated. Conservative treatment with intravenous fluids and antibiotics may be indicated in elderly or very ill patients.

Gastric outlet obstruction   This is now rare following ulcer disease, and carcinoma is the commonest cause. Outflow obstruction occurs because of surrounding oedema or scarring following healing. Copious projectile vomiting is the main symptom, and a succussion splash may be detectable clinically. Metabolic alkalosis may develop as a result of loss of acid. In patients with peptic ulcer disease the oedema will usually settle with conservative management with nasogastric suction, replacement of fluids and electrolytes and proton pump inhibitors. Surgery is now rarely required.

Haemorrhage   See page 82.

Management of dyspepsia (*K&C* 6e p. 288)

Significant gastrointestinal pathology is uncommon in most young people with dyspepsia. Furthermore, the close association of *H. pylori* with peptic ulcer disease has led most practitioners to agree that investigation with endoscopy is unnecessary in all patients with dyspepsia. Older patients (> 55 years) with persistent dyspepsia should be investigated with a gastroscopy or a barium meal to rule out gastro-oesophageal malignancy, as should all patients with 'alarm symptoms' such as dysphagia, weight loss, vomiting or gastrointestinal bleeding. In other patients *H. pylori* status should be assessed by a non-invasive method and, if positive, eradication therapy instituted. Further investigation can then be reserved for those who remain symptomatic or who are *H. pylori*-negative on initial testing.

Malignant gastric tumours (*K&C* 6e p. 288)

Epidemiology

Gastric cancer is the sixth most common fatal cancer in the UK. The incidence increases with age and is more common in men. The frequency varies throughout the world, being more common in Japan and Chile, and relatively less common in the USA. Although the incidence overall is decreasing world-wide, proximal gastric cancers are increasing in frequency.

Aetiology

This is unknown; *H. pylori* infection is implicated, causing chronic gastritis which in some individuals leads to atrophic gastritis and intestinal metaplasia, a premalignant pathological change. Other risk factors include advanced age, male gender, cigarette smoking, diets low in fruits and vegetables or high in salted, smoked or preserved foods, pernicious anaemia, and family history of gastric cancer.

Pathology

Tumours most commonly occur in the antrum and are almost always adenocarcinomas. They may be localized ulcerated lesions with rolled edges (intestinal type), or more diffuse with extensive submucosal spread, giving the picture of linitus plastica (diffuse type).

Clinical features

Pain similar to peptic ulcer pain is the most common symptom. With more advanced disease, nausea, anorexia and weight loss are common. Vomiting with outflow obstruction occurs if the tumour is near the pylorus, or dysphagia can occur with lesions in the cardia. Almost 50% have a palpable epigastric mass, and a lymph node is sometimes felt in the supraclavicular fossa (Virchow's node). In patients with advanced disease there may be evidence of metastatic spread to the peritoneum and liver, with ascites and hepatomegaly. Skin manifestations of malignancy, such as dermatomyositis and acanthosis nigricans, are occasionally associated.

Investigations

Gastroscopy and biopsy is the initial investigation of choice. CT, MRI and endoscopic ultrasonography are useful in staging the tumour and guiding operability.

Management

Surgery is the best form of treatment if the tumour is operable. Adjuvant (postoperative) chemoradiotherapy should be considered for more advanced tumours. Palliative chemotherapy is sometimes used for unresectable lesions, with a modest improvement in survival.

Prognosis

The overall survival is poor (10% 5-year survival). Those patients undergoing curative operations, however, have a

5-year survival of 50%. In Japan, where the incidence of the disease is high and there is an active screening programme, earlier diagnosis and an aggressive surgical approach have resulted in a 5-year survival of 90%.

Other gastric tumours

Gastrointestinal stromal cell tumours (GIST) occur most commonly in the oesophagus and stomach. They were previously considered to be benign but it is now clear that on prolonged follow-up, many have malignant potential. They are usually asymptomatic and discovered incidentally when an upper GI endoscopy is performed for dyspepsia. They can ulcerate and bleed. Gastric lymphoma (non-Hodgkin's B type) presents similarly to gastric carcinoma. Treatment is usually with chemotherapy and radiotherapy. Gastric lymphomas in mucosa-associated lymphoid tissue are caused by *H. pylori* and some can be treated by eradication of *H. pylori* only.

Gastric polyps are uncommon and usually regenerative. Adenomatous polyps can occur but are rare.

GASTROINTESTINAL BLEEDING

Acute upper gastrointestinal bleeding (*K&C* 6e p. 291)

Haematemesis is the vomiting of blood. Melaena is the passage of black tarry stools, which is the result of altered blood from the upper intestine (50 mL or more is required to produce melaena).

Aetiology

Peptic ulceration is the most common cause of upper gastrointestinal bleeding (Fig. 3.1). Relative incidences vary according to patient population. Aspirin and NSAIDs may be responsible for bleeding from both duodenal and gastric ulcers, particularly in elderly people. Corticosteroids have been implicated, but in the usual therapeutic dosage they probably have no relationship to gastrointestinal bleeding.

Management

A large-bore (16-gauge) intravenous cannula should be placed in a peripheral vein and blood taken for full blood count, liver biochemistry, urea and electrolytes, clotting

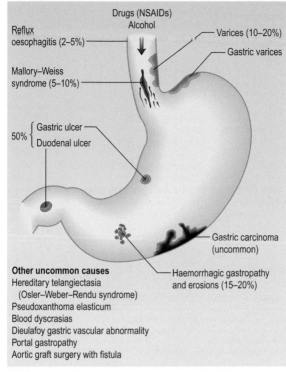

Drugs (NSAIDs)
Alcohol

Reflux oesophagitis (2–5%)

Varices (10–20%)

Gastric varices

Mallory–Weiss syndrome (5–10%)

50% { Gastric ulcer
Duodenal ulcer }

Gastric carcinoma (uncommon)

Other uncommon causes
Hereditary telangiectasia
  (Osler–Weber–Rendu syndrome)
Pseudoxanthoma elasticum
Blood dyscrasias
Dieulafoy gastric vascular abnormality
Portal gastropathy
Aortic graft surgery with fistula

Haemorrhagic gastropathy and erosions (15–20%)

Fig. 3.1 **Causes of upper gastrointestinal haemorrhage.**

screen and 'group and save'; cross-match at least 4 units of blood if there is evidence of a large bleed (blood pressure < 100 mmHg, pulse > 100 beats per min, cool or cold extremities with slow capillary refill, Hb < 10 g/dL). The 'Rockall' Score (Table 3.3, 📟 QC 3.1) is a mortality risk assessment score for patients admitted with non-variceal upper gastrointestinal bleeding. It is simple to use and helps to identify those at highest risk of dying and needing active intervention. It also identifies those for safe, early hospital discharge (pre-endoscopy score 0, post-endoscopy ≤ 2).

Gastrointestinal bleeding

Table 3.3 Rockall Score for upper gastrointestinal haemorrhage

		Score
Age	< 60 years	0
	60–79 years	1
	> 80 years	2
Shock	None	0
	Pulse > 100 + Systolic BP > 100	1
	Systolic BP < 100	2
Co-morbidity	None	0
	Cardiac failure, IHD or any major co-morbidity	2
	Renal/liver failure or disseminated malignancy	3
PRE-ENDOSCOPY ROCKALL SCORE (max. 7)		
Endoscopic diagnosis	Mallory–Weiss tear, no lesion seen, and no SRH	0
	All other diagnoses	1
	Malignancy of upper GI tract	2
	Major SRH	
	None or dark spot only	0
	Blood in upper GI tract, adherent clot, visible or spurting vessel	2
FINAL ROCKALL SCORE (max. score 11)		

SRH, stigmata of recent haemorrhage
Low-risk patients (post-endoscopy score ≤ 2), < 5% risk rebleeding, 0% risk of death
High-risk patients (post-endoscopy score 5–11), 11–41% risk of death

84

Resuscitate In many patients no specific treatment is required, bleeding stops spontaneously and the patient remains well compensated. In patients with large bleeds or clinical signs of shock, urgent transfusion, ideally with whole blood, is required (p. 217). Monitoring pulse rate and venous pressure will guide transfusion requirements.

Determine site of bleeding This may be evident from the history, e.g. bleeding from a peptic ulcer is suggested by a history of aspirin or NSAID ingestion or previous peptic ulceration. Mallory–Weiss syndrome (haematemesis from a tear in the oesophagus) is suggested by a history of vomiting preceding the haematemesis. After resuscitation, endoscopy should be performed as soon as possible, and preferably within 24 hours. More urgent endoscopy may be indicated if varices are strongly suspected from the history and examination (i.e. signs of chronic liver disease). Endoscopy can detect the site of haemorrhage in 80% or more of cases.

Specific management A stepwise approach to the management of upper gastrointestinal bleeding is illustrated in Emergency Box 3.1.

At endoscopy varices should be treated with sclerotherapy or banding (p. 150). Ulcers that are actively bleeding or demonstrate stigmata of recent bleeding (a visible vessel or overlying clot) should be treated by one or more of three methods: injection of dilute epinephrine (adrenaline),

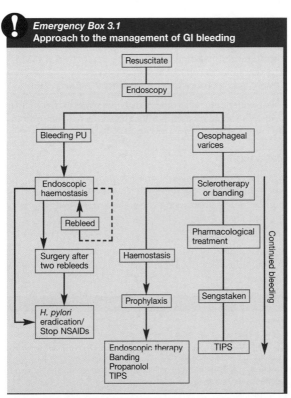

> **Emergency Box 3.1**
> **Approach to the management of GI bleeding**

TIPS, transjugular intrahepatic portosystemic shunt; PU, peptic ulcer
Bleeding oesophageal varices are discussed on page 150.

coagulation of the vessel with the heater or bipolar probe, or application of mechanical clips (endoclips) to the vessel. Mallory–Weiss tears usually stop bleeding spontaneously. In general, young patients with peptic ulcer bleeding who are otherwise fit and haemodynamically stable and who at endoscopy have no stigmata of recent haemorrhage can be discharged from hospital within 24 hours (post-endoscopy Rockall Score < 2). Intravenous proton pump inhibitors (omeprazole 80 mg bolus i.v. and then 8 mg per hour by infusion for 72 hours) are given following endoscopic therapy in acute peptic ulcer bleeding; they reduce re-bleeding rates and transfusion requirements. Surgery is required for persistent or recurrent bleeding from ulcers.

Prognosis

The mortality increases with increasing Rockall Score, and overall mortality rate is 5–10%.

Lower gastrointestinal bleeding (K&C 6e p. 293)

Massive bleeding is rare and usually the result of diverticular disease or ischaemic colitis. Minor bleeds from haemorrhoids are common. The causes are listed in Table 3.4.

Management

With large bleeds, resuscitation with intravenous fluids/ whole blood may be required. The site of bleeding must then be determined using the following investigations as appropriate:

- Rectal examination, e.g. carcinoma
- Proctoscopy, e.g. haemorrhoids
- Sigmoidoscopy, e.g. inflammatory bowel disease

Table 3.4 **Causes of lower GI bleeding**

Haemorrhoids
Anal fissure
Colon cancer
Colitis: ulcerative colitis, Crohn's, infective, ischaemic
Angiodysplasia (abnormal collections of blood vessels)
Diverticular disease
Polyps
Meckel's diverticulum

- Barium enema – any mucosal lesion
- Colonoscopy – diagnosis and removal of polyps
- Angiography – vascular abnormality, e.g. angiodysplasia.

Specific management Lesions should be treated as appropriate.

Chronic gastrointestinal bleeding

Chronic gastrointestinal bleeding usually presents with iron deficiency anaemia. Blood loss producing anaemia in all men, and in women after the menopause, is always the result of bleeding from the gastrointestinal tract and requires investigation. The causes of chronic blood loss are those that cause acute bleeding (see Fig. 3.1 and Table 3.4). However, oesophageal varices, duodenal ulcers and diverticular disease very rarely bleed chronically. Malabsorption (most frequently from coeliac disease), previous gastrectomy and, rarely, poor dietary intake are also causes of iron deficiency anaemia and thus will present similarly to anaemia as a result of chronic blood loss.

Investigations

The initial investigation is a 'top and tail', performed at the same endoscopic session, i.e. gastroscopy and colonoscopy; a distal duodenal biopsy is taken at endoscopy to look for coeliac disease as the cause of iron deficiency.

Further investigations, usually in the order listed, are only warranted in anaemia not responding to iron treatment or where there is visible blood loss:

- Small bowel barium follow-through (usually only helpful if there are symptoms to suggest Crohn's disease)
- Small bowel enteroscopy and/or wireless capsule endoscopy
- Coeliac axis and mesenteric angiography
- Technetium-labelled red cell scan.

Management

The cause of the bleeding is treated and oral iron (p. 188) is given to treat the anaemia.

THE SMALL INTESTINE

The small intestine has a number of functions, many of which are concerned with the digestion and absorption of

Table 3.5 Disorders of the small intestine causing malabsorption

Coeliac disease
Crohn's disease
Dermatitis herpetiformis
Tropical sprue
Small bowel bacterial overgrowth
Intestinal resection
Whipple's disease
Radiation enteritis
Parasite infection, e.g. *Giardia intestinalis*

nutrients. Nutrients are absorbed throughout the small intestine, with the exception of vitamin B_{12} and bile salts, which have specific receptors in the terminal ileum (*K&C* 6e p. 295).

The presenting features of small bowel disease are diarrhoea, steatorrhoea (p. 63), abdominal pain or discomfort, and weight loss, which is the result of accompanying anorexia. The two most common causes of small bowel disease in developed countries are coeliac disease and Crohn's disease. In many small bowel diseases malabsorption of specific substances occurs, but these deficiencies do not dominate the clinical picture. An example is Crohn's disease, in which malabsorption of vitamin B_{12} can be demonstrated, but this is not usually a clinical problem. The major disorders of the small intestine that cause malabsorption are shown in Table 3.5.

Coeliac disease (gluten-sensitive enteropathy) (*K&C* 6e p. 301)

Coeliac disease is a condition in which there is an abnormal jejunal mucosa that improves morphologically when the patient is treated with a gluten-free diet and relapses when gluten is reintroduced. Gluten is contained in wheat, rye and barley. Pure oats are not harmful.

Epidemiology

World-wide distribution, but it is rare in African people and more common in Ireland (incidence 1 in 100; 1 in 300 in UK).

Aetiology

The toxic portion of gluten is the peptide α-gliadin. The exact mechanism by which gluten causes damage to the intestinal mucosa is not known. The strong association with the haplotypes HLA-A1, -B8, -DR3, -DR7 and -DQ2 suggests an immunological origin. It is thought that gluten-sensitive T lymphocytes recognize gluten-derived peptide epitopes when presented in association with DQ2. Upon activation, these gluten-sensitive T cells develop a Th1/Th0-type inflammatory response which produces the observed mucosal damage. The enzyme tissue transglutaminase (tTG) modifies gluten and this increases its stimulating effect on gluten-sensitive T cells.

Pathology

There are absent or stunted small intestinal villi with elongation of crypts (subtotal villous atrophy). There is a chronic inflammatory cell infiltrate in the lamina propria, with an increase in intraepithelial cell lymphocytes.

Clinical features

Coeliac disease can present at any age but there are two peaks in incidence: in infancy, after weaning on to gluten-containing foods, and in adults at 30–40 years. It often presents with non-specific symptoms of tiredness and malaise, or symptoms of small intestinal disease (see above).

Physical signs are usually few and non-specific, and related to anaemia and nutritional deficiency. There is an increased incidence of atopy and autoimmune disease.

Investigations

Distal duodenal biopsies are obtained endoscopically. The mucosa shows the histological features described above. Other causes of villous atrophy (Table 3.6) are rare in adults in the western world.

Serum antibodies Endomysial (EMA) and tissue transglutaminase (tTG) antibodies have a very high sensitivity and specificity for coeliac disease and can also be used to screen patients who have non-specific symptoms or an associated autoimmune condition such as type I diabetes mellitus. Antigliadin and antireticulin antibodies are less

Table 3.6 Causes of villous atrophy in adults
Coeliac disease
Dermatitis herpetiformis
Giardiasis
Malnutrition
Ischaemia
Lymphoma
Whipple's disease
Tropical sprue

commonly used now owing to lower sensitivity and specificity.

Blood count   A mild anaemia is present in 50% of cases. There is almost always folate deficiency, commonly iron deficiency and, rarely, vitamin B_{12} deficiency.

Radiology   Small bowel follow-through may show a dilated bowel with thickened folds.

Bone densitometry   (DEXA scan, p. 257) should be performed in all patients because of the increased risk of osteoporosis in these patients.

Management

Treatment is with a gluten-free diet, which should be continued lifelong, and nutritional supplements if there are vitamin deficiencies. Definitive diagnosis is confirmed when symptoms resolve subsequently with a gluten-free diet. A demonstration of normalized histology following a gluten-free diet is no longer required for a definitive diagnosis of coeliac disease.

Complications

There is an increased incidence of malignancy, particularly intestinal lymphoma, small bowel and oesophageal cancer. The incidence may be reduced by a gluten-free diet.

Dermatitis herpetiformis (*K&C* 6e pp. 303 & 1348)

Dermatitis herpetiformis is an itchy, symmetrical eruption of vesicles and crusts over the extensor surfaces of the body, with deposition of granular immunoglobulin (Ig) A at the dermoepidermal junction of the skin including areas not involved with the rash. Most patients also have a gluten-sensitive enteropathy, which is usually asymptomatic. The skin condition responds to dapsone, but both the gut and the skin will improve on a gluten-free diet.

Tropical sprue (*K&C* 6e p. 303)

Tropical sprue is a progressive small intestinal disorder presenting with malabsorption which occurs in residents or visitors to a tropical area where the disease is endemic (Asia, some Caribbean islands, Puerto Rico, parts of South America).

Aetiology

The aetiology is unknown but the disease occurs in epidemics and improves with antibiotics, suggesting an infectious aetiology.

Clinical features

The disease may present many years after patients have been in the tropics. There is diarrhoea, anorexia and abdominal distension. Nutritional deficiencies develop over a variable period of time.

Investigations

Malabsorption should be demonstrated, particularly of fat and vitamin B_{12}. The intestinal mucosa shows partial villous atrophy affecting the whole small bowel. Infective causes of diarrhoea, particularly *Giardia intestinalis*, should be excluded.

Management

Treatment is with a combination of folic acid and tetracycline, which may be required for up to 6 months. Nutritional deficiencies must also be corrected.

Bacterial overgrowth (*K&C* 6e p. 304)

The upper small intestine is almost sterile. Bacterial over-growth may occur when there is stasis of intestinal contents as a result of abnormal motility, e.g. systemic sclerosis, or a structural abnormality, e.g. previous small bowel surgery or a diverticulum.

The small intestine

Clinical features

There may be diarrhoea and/or steatorrhoea caused by the deconjugation of bile salts by bacteria. Vitamin B_{12} deficiency, resulting from its metabolism by bacteria, can also occur.

Diagnosis

Breath tests   The hydrogen or ^{14}C breath tests are the investigations of choice. These depend on the ability of the organisms to metabolize either glucose or labelled bile salts, given by mouth, with the production of either hydrogen (from glucose) or $^{14}CO_2$ (from bile salts), which are then absorbed and can be measured in the exhaled air.

Proximal small intestinal aspirates   Proximal small intestinal aspirates (obtained endoscopically) will reveal high numbers of coliforms and *Bacteroides* sp. on culture.

In clinical practice, a therapeutic trial of antibiotics in the appropriate clinical setting is often employed.

Management

If possible, the underlying cause should be corrected. This may not be possible and rotating courses of antibiotics are then necessary, such as tetracycline and metronidazole.

Whipple's disease (*K&C* 6e p. 305)

Whipple's disease is a rare systemic disease which almost always involves the small intestine and is due to infection with the bacterium *Tropheryma whipplei*. Common clinical features include steatorrhoea, abdominal pain, fever, lymphadenopathy, arthritis and neurological involvement. Small bowel biopsy shows periodic acid–Schiff (PAS)-positive macrophages. On electron microscopy the macrophages are seen to contain the causative bacteria. Treatment is with co-trimoxazole for 6 months.

Intestinal resection (*K&C* 6e p. 304)

The effects of small intestinal resection depend on the extent and the area involved. Resection of the terminal ileum leads to malabsorption of:

■ Vitamin B_{12}, leading to megaloblastic anaemia

■ Bile salts, which overflow into the colon and interfere with salt and water absorption, producing diarrhoea. Bile salts in the colon also increase oxalate absorption, which may result in renal oxalate stones (p. 362).

If there is extensive resection, increased hepatic bile salt synthesis cannot compensate for faecal loss and there is steatorrhoea secondary to bile salt deficiency. After massive intestinal resection there is severe loss of water and electrolytes, with malnutrition.

Miscellaneous small intestinal conditions
(*K&C* 6e p. 306)

Tuberculosis (TB) (*K&C* 6e pp. 306 & 344)

This results from reactivation of the primary disease caused by *Mycobacterium tuberculosis* (p. 523), and in the UK is most commonly seen in Asian immigrants. The ileocaecal valve is the most common site affected.

Clinical features

There is abdominal pain, diarrhoea, anorexia, weight loss and fever. A mass may be palpable. The symptoms, signs and radiology (see below) can be similar to those of Crohn's disease, and TB must always be considered in the differential diagnosis of Asians presenting with apparent Crohn's disease.

Diagnosis

Imaging The chest X-ray will show evidence of pulmonary tuberculosis in 50% of cases. The small bowel follow-through may show features similar to those of Crohn's disease (p. 99). Abdominal ultrasonography shows mesenteric thickening and lymphadenopathy.

Endoscopy Colonoscopy with terminal ileal biopsies is usually performed. It is not always possible to obtain bacteriological confirmation on tissue culture, and treatment is started if there is a high degree of suspicion.

Surgery Laparoscopy or laparotomy is rarely needed for diagnosis.

Management

Treatment is similar to that for pulmonary tuberculosis (p. 527) although 1 year's treatment is required.

Protein-losing enteropathy (*K&C* 6e p. 306)

This involves increased protein loss across an abnormal intestinal mucosa. If there is inadequate hepatic synthesis of albumin to compensate for the intestinal loss, patients develop hypoalbuminaemia and oedema. Causes include Crohn's disease, Ménétrièr's disease (thickening and enlargement of gastric folds), coeliac disease and lymphatic disorders, e.g. lymphangiectasia.

Meckel's diverticulum (*K&C* 6e p. 306)

This is a congenital abnormality affecting 2–3% of the population. A diverticulum projects from the wall of the ileum approximately 60 cm from the ileocaecal valve. About 50% will contain gastric mucosa which secretes acid, and peptic ulceration may occur, with complications of bleeding or perforation. Diverticula may also become inflamed and present similarly to appendicitis. Treatment is surgical removal.

Chronic intestinal ischaemia (*K&C* 6e p. 307)

This is rare and results from atheromatous occlusion of mesenteric vessels in elderly people. The characteristic symptom is abdominal pain occurring after food. Diagnosis is made using angiography.

Malignant small intestinal tumours (*K&C* 6e p. 308)

These are rare and present with abdominal pain, diarrhoea, anorexia and anaemia. Carcinoid tumours have additional clinical features, described below.

Carcinoid tumours (*K&C* 6e p. 309)

Pathology

These originate from enterochromaffin cells (serotonin producing) of the intestine. The most common sites are the appendix, terminal ileum and rectum. *Carcinoid syndrome* is the term applied to the symptoms that arise as a result of products synthesized and released into the circulation by the tumour. These mediators include serotonin (5-hydroxytryptamine, or 5-HT), kinins, histamine and prostaglandins. The liver normally inactivates these mediators.

Clinical features of the carcinoid syndrome

Patients with gastrointestinal carcinoid tumours have the carcinoid syndrome only if they have liver metastases because tumour products are able to drain directly into the hepatic vein (without being metabolized) and then into the systemic circulation, where they produce a variety of effects resulting in the carcinoid syndrome: flushing, wheezing, diarrhoea and abdominal pain, and right-sided cardiac valvular fibrosis causing stenosis and regurgitation.

Investigations

A high level of 5-hydroxyindoleacetic acid (5-HIAA), the breakdown product of serotonin, is found in the urine in the carcinoid syndrome. A liver ultrasound confirms the presence of secondary deposits.

Management

Treatment of the carcinoid syndrome is symptomatic and aimed at:

- Inhibition of tumour products with the somatostatin analogue, octreotide, or with 5-HT antagonists, e.g. cyproheptadine
- Reducing tumour mass through surgical resection, hepatic artery embolization, radiofrequency ablation or chemotherapy.

Adenocarcinoma (*K&C* 6e p. 308)

Adenocarcinoma accounts for 50% of malignant small bowel tumours; there is an increased incidence in coeliac disease and Crohn's disease.

Lymphoma (*K&C* 6e p. 308)

Non-Hodgkin's lymphoma constitutes 15% of malignant small bowel tumours and may be B cell or T cell in origin. The latter occur with increased frequency in coeliac disease.

Benign small bowel tumours (*K&C* 6e p. 309)

- The Peutz–Jegher syndrome is an autosomal dominant condition with mucocutaneous pigmentation (circumoral, hands and feet) and hamartomatous gastrointestinal polyps. Polyps may occur anywhere in the gastrointestinal

tract, but are most common in the small bowel. They may bleed or cause intussusception, and may undergo malignant change.
- Adenomas, leiomyomas and lipomas are rare. They are usually asymptomatic and discovered incidentally.
- Familial adenomatous polyposis (p. 107).

INFLAMMATORY BOWEL DISEASE (K&C 6e p. 309)

Two main forms are recognized: Crohn's disease, which affects any part of the gastrointestinal tract, and ulcerative colitis (UC), which affects the large bowel only.

Epidemiology

Inflammatory bowel disease (IBD) is more common in the western world, occurring at any age but most commonly between the ages of 20 and 40 years. Both sexes are affected. In western populations the prevalence of UC is approximately 1 in 1000 and of Crohn's disease 1 in 1500.

Aetiology

It is probable that environmental factors operate in a genetically predisposed individual. It is proposed that disruption of the intestinal epithelial integrity allows bacteria and luminal antigens to trigger an immune response. In the genetically predisposed individual, there is an exaggerated immune response. In Crohn's disease, the T cell immune response is T helper cell 1 (Th1) dominant as manifested by increased production of the pro-inflammatory cytokines, interferon-γ and tumour necrosis factor-α (TNF-α) and reduced production of the anti-inflammatory cytokines, interleukin-4 (IL-4) and IL-10. In contrast, in UC there is a Th2-dominant response with increased production of IL-5. There is also activation of other cells (neutrophils, mast cells and eosinophils) which leads to increased production of a wide variety of inflammatory mediators, all of which can lead to cell damage.

Environmental
- *Infective agents.* Measles virus and *Mycobacterium paratuberculosis* have been put forward as possible causes of Crohn's disease, but a causal relationship has not been established.

- *Smoking.* Crohn's disease is more common in smokers and UC less common. In Crohn's disease smoking doubles the risk of postoperative recurrence.

Genetic There is a familial tendency in both UC and Crohn's disease; twin studies suggest a stronger genetic influence in Crohn's disease than in UC. Mutations within the *NOD2/CARD15* gene present on chromosome 16 confer susceptibility to Crohn's disease. Having one copy of the risk alleles confers a two- to fourfold risk for developing Crohn's disease, whereas having both alleles increases the risk 20- to 40-fold. This is likely to be one of many genes that contribute to the Crohn's phenotype. The wild-type NOD2 protein regulates macrophage activation in response to bacterial lipopolysaccharides, and it is not known how mutations lead to sustained activation of inflammatory pathways in Crohn's disease. There is an increased incidence of HLA-B27 in inflammatory bowel disease with ankylosing spondylitis.

Pathology

UC and Crohn's disease have differences at both macroscopic and microscopic levels, and immunologically (Table 3.7).

Clinical features

Crohn's disease is a progressive chronic disease with symptomatology depending on the region(s) of involved bowel; the commonest site is ileocaecal (in 40% of patients). The main feature in patients with small bowel disease is abdominal pain, usually with weight loss. Less commonly, terminal ileal disease presents as an acute abdomen with right iliac fossa pain mimicking appendicitis. Colonic disease presents with diarrhoea, bleeding and pain related to defecation. In perianal disease there are anal tags, fissures, fistulae and abscess formation.

UC presents with diarrhoea, often containing blood and mucus. The clinical course may be one of persistent diarrhoea, relapses and remissions, or severe fulminant colitis (Table 3.8).

Patients with IBD may have one or more extraintestinal manifestations, and these are listed in Table 3.9.

Table 3.7 Differences between Crohn's disease and ulcerative colitis

	Crohn's disease	Ulcerative colitis
Macroscopic	Affects any part of the gut from mouth to anus	Affects only the colon
	Begins in the rectum and extends proximally in varying degrees	Oral and perianal disease
	Discontinuous involvement ('skip lesions')	Continuous involvement
	Deep ulcers and fissures in the mucosa: 'cobblestone appearance'	Red mucosa which bleeds easily
		Ulcers and pseudopolyps (regenerating mucosa) in severe disease
Histology/ immunology	Transmural inflammation	Mucosal inflammation
	Granulomata may be present	No granulomata but goblet cell depletion and crypt abscesses
	Dominant Th1 response	Dominant Th2 response

Table 3.8 Definition of a severe attack of ulcerative colitis

Bloody diarrhoea	> 6/day
With one of:	
Fever	> 37.5°C
Tachycardia	> 90/min
ESR	> 30 mm/h
Anaemia	Hb < 10 g/dL
Serum albumin	< 30 g/L

Investigations

The purpose of investigations is to define the nature of the disease and the extent and severity of bowel involvement.

Table 3.9 Non-gastrointestinal manifestations of inflammatory bowel disease

Eyes	Uveitis, episcleritis, conjunctivitis
Joints	Small joint arthritis*, monoarticular arthritis (knees and ankles), ankylosing spondylitis*, sacroileitis
Skin	Erythema nodosum, pyoderma gangrenosum (necrotizing ulceration of the skin, commonly on the lower legs)
Liver*†	Fatty change, primary sclerosing cholangitis, chronic hepatitis, cirrhosis
Calculi*	Increased incidence of gall bladder and renal calculi
Venous thrombosis	
Vasculitis	(Rare)
Amyloidosis	(Rare)

*These manifestations are not related to disease activity
†Biochemical abnormalities are common; clinically overt disease is uncommon

Blood count Anaemia is common and is usually the normochromic, normocytic anaemia of chronic disease, although iron deficiency anaemia may occur. The platelet count, ESR and C-reactive protein are often raised in acute Crohn's disease, and the serum albumin may be low in severe disease.

Endoscopy Rigid or flexible sigmoidoscopy will establish the diagnosis of UC and, less commonly, Crohn's disease. A rectal biopsy can be taken for histological examination to determine the nature of the inflammation. Colonoscopy allows the exact extent and severity of colonic and terminal ileal inflammation to be determined, and biopsies to be taken. The role of capsule endoscopy is at present unclear.

Other investigations In Crohn's disease a small bowel follow-through often shows an asymmetrical alteration in the mucosal pattern, with deep ulceration and areas of narrowing (string sign) commonly confined to the ileum. Skip lesions may be seen. Ultrasonography and CT scanning are particularly helpful in delineating abscesses, and will show thickened bowel in involved areas. MRI is useful in perianal disease.

Table 3.10 Summary of treatments used in inflammatory bowel disease

Remission induction	Maintenance of remission
5-ASA	5-ASA (in UC)
Corticosteroids	Azathioprine/6-mercaptopurine
Liquid enteral nutrition	Methotrexate
Metronidazole	Infliximab
Methotrexate	
Ciclosporin	
Infliximab (anti-TNF-α antibody)	

5-ASA, aminosalicyclic acid

A plain X-ray should be performed in all patients admitted to hospital. This helps to assess extent of colonic involvement and will identify toxic dilatation of the colon.

White cell scanning is a safe, non-invasive investigation, but lacks specificity.

Differential diagnosis

Crohn's disease must be differentiated from other causes of chronic diarrhoea, malabsorption and malnutrition. In children it is a cause of short stature. Other causes of terminal ileitis are TB and *Yersinia enterocolitica* infection (causing an acute illness). IBD affecting the colon must be differentiated from other causes of colitis: infection (p. 33), ischaemia and microscopic colitis (p. 103).

Management (Table 3.10)

Medical Patients with Crohn's disease who smoke should be advised to stop, as this will decrease the number of relapses and reduce postoperative recurrence. The precise mechanisms responsible for the clinical efficacy of many of these treatments is not known. In general they have many anti-inflammatory and immunosuppressive properties combined with an antibacterial action in some cases (e.g. metronidazole).

■ 5-Aminosalicylic acid (5-ASA) tablets (mesalazine, olsalazine, balsalazide) will induce a remission in mild attacks of UC and in colonic Crohn's disease. In lower

Management

> ! **Emergency Box 3.2**
> **Management of acute severe colitis**
>
> **Admit to hospital**
> - Joint inpatient management between gastroenterologist and colorectal surgeon
>
> **Investigations**
> - Full blood count, C-reactive protein
> - Liver biochemistry and serum albumin
> - Serum urea and electrolytes
> - Blood cultures (Gram-negative sepsis occurs)
> - Plain abdominal X-ray looking for toxic dilatation (diameter, colon > 5 cm), mucosal islands, and/or perforation
> - Stool cultures (×3) to exclude coincidental infection
>
> **Treatment**
> - Intravenous steroids: hydrocortisone 100 mg 6-hourly
> - Correct electrolyte and fluid imbalance
> - Consider i.v. ciclosporin (2 mg/kg over 24 h) in patients not responding to steroids
> - Low-molecular-weight heparin to prevent venous thrombosis

doses they are useful as a maintenance treatment to reduce the number of relapses. 5-ASA preparations can also be administered as an enema or suppository to treat proctosigmoiditis (i.e. inflammation of the rectum and sigmoid colon).

- Corticosteroids: oral steroids (e.g. prednisolone 40 mg daily) are used to treat acute attacks, and the dose is tailed off by 5 mg weekly as symptoms improve. In severe attacks intravenous steroids are necessary (Emergency Box 3.2). Proctosigmoiditis can be treated locally with steroid enemas or suppositories. Budesonide is a poorly absorbed corticosteroid with limited bioavailability and extensive first-pass metabolism that has therapeutic benefit with reduced systemic toxicity in ileocaecal Crohn's disease.

- Azathioprine or its metabolite 6-mercaptopurine is used in patients with Crohn's disease and UC who continue to have frequent relapses despite taking an adequate dose of 5-ASAs. The major side-effects are bone marrow suppression (neutropenia, thrombocytopenia and anaemia), acute pancreatitis and allergic reactions. Monitoring of the full blood count must be performed weekly for the first 4 weeks of treatment and 3-monthly thereafter to look for evidence of bone marrow suppression, although this can occur unpredictably.

- Liquid enteral nutrition with an elemental (liquid preparation of amino acids, glucose and fatty acids) or polymeric diet will induce a remission in active Crohn's disease. The exact mode of action is not known. These diets are unpalatable and may have to be given via a nasogastric tube.
- Metronidazole is useful in severe perianal Crohn's disease as a result of both its antibacterial and immuno-suppressive action.
- Methotrexate is used in the minority of patients with active Crohn's disease that is resistant to conventional treatment with steroids. The long-term efficacy of this treatment is not known.
- Ciclosporin is useful in patients with severe acute UC who fail to improve after treatment with intravenous steroids. The management of severe colitis is summarized in Emergency Box 3.2. Management should be in conjunction with the appropriate surgical team because patients not responding to medical therapy will need to undergo colectomy.
- Infliximab is a chimeric anti-TNF monoclonal antibody which is given as a single infusion. It produces clinical improvement in 60% of patients with steroid-resistant Crohn's disease and is also useful in patients with fistulating disease. Further infusions may be given at 8-weekly intervals to maintain remission, though the optimal duration of treatment is unclear at present.

Surgery Surgery is indicated for:
- Failure of medical therapy
- Complications (Table 3.11)
- Failure to grow in children.

Table 3.11   Complications of inflammatory bowel disease
Toxic dilatation of the colon + perforation
Stricture formation*
Abscess formation (Crohn's disease)
Fistulae and fissures (Crohn's)*
Colon cancer

*Surgical intervention only necessary if symptomatic and not responding to medical treatment

In Crohn's disease, resections are kept to a minimum as recurrence is almost inevitable in the remaining bowel. In some patients with small bowel disease, strictures can be widened (strictuloplasty) without resection.

The surgical options in UC are:

- Colectomy with ileoanal anastomosis, in which the terminal ileum is used to form a reservoir (a 'pouch'), and the patient is continent with a few bowel motions per day. The pouch may become inflamed ('pouchitis'), leading to bloody diarrhoea which is treated initially with metronidazole.
- Panproctocolectomy with ileostomy (the whole colon and rectum are removed and the ileum brought out on to the abdominal wall as a stoma).

Cancer in inflammatory bowel disease

Patients with extensive UC of more than 10 years' duration are at an increased risk of colorectal cancer (cumulative risk 12% after 25 years). Patients with long-standing Crohn's colitis are also at risk, although less so than with UC. These patients are usually offered surveillance colonoscopy with multiple colonic biopsies (to look for dysplasia) at intervals of 1–3 years. Since the risk of cancer increases with duration of disease, testing should be done more frequently as time goes on. A history of primary sclerosing cholangitis adds significantly to the already high risk of dysplasia and colorectal cancer in patients with ulcerative colitis, and these patients should be tested annually. Colectomy is recommended if high-grade dysplasia is discovered.

Prognosis

Both diseases are characterized by relapses and remissions. Almost all patients with Crohn's disease have a significant relapse over a 20-year period. The prognosis of UC is variable. Only 10% of patients with proctitis develop more extensive disease, but with severe fulminant disease there is a risk of colonic perforation and death.

Microscopic colitis

Microscopic colitis is an inflammatory condition of the colon in which the colonic mucosa appears normal under endoscopic and radiological examination, but histological examination reveals specific features. Microscopic colitis is two separate but related diseases, collagenous colitis (CC) and lymphocytic colitis (LC). The two are similar in presentation and natural history, but differ in histological appearance. In both conditions, the colonic mucosa's lamina propria is inflamed and has increased intraepithelial lymphocytes. In CC, but not in LC, there is marked thickening of the subepithelial collagen layer. Presentation is with chronic watery non-bloody diarrhoea, most commonly in middle-aged to elderly patients. Treatment is symptomatic initially with antidiarrhoeal drugs such as loperamide. 5-ASA drugs (p. 100) and steroids are used in more resistant cases.

THE COLON AND RECTUM

Diverticular disease (*K&C* 6e p. 324)

Pouches of mucosa extrude through the muscular wall through weakened areas near blood vessels to form diverticula. The term diverticulosis means the presence of diverticula. Diverticulitis implies inflammation, which occurs when faeces obstruct the neck of the diverticulum. Diverticula are common, affecting 50% of the population over 50 years of age.

Aetiology

The precise cause of diverticular disease is unknown, although it appears to be related to the low-fibre diet eaten in western populations. It is thought that insufficient dietary fibre leads to increased intracolonic pressure, which causes herniation of the mucosa at sites of weakness.

Clinical features

It is asymptomatic in 90% and usually discovered incidentally when a barium enema or colonoscopy is performed for other reasons. Symptoms are the result of bleeding or acute diverticulitis (left iliac fossa pain, fever, nausea, vomiting). Complications include abscess formation, perforation, haemorrhage, fistula formation and intestinal obstruction. Acute diverticulitis is diagnosed by CT scan or in some cases by ultrasound.

Table 3.12 Causes of constipation
Irritable bowel syndrome
Idiopathic slow transit
Pelvic floor dyssynergia
Intestinal obstruction, e.g. by colon cancer
Intestinal pseudo-obstruction
Painful anal conditions
Drugs, e.g. opiates, aluminium antacids, antimuscarinics
Hypothyroidism
Hypercalcaemia
Spinal cord lesion
Depression
Immobility
Hirschsprung's disease

Management

Acute attacks are treated with antibiotics (ciprofloxacin and metronidazole). Surgery is indicated rarely for complications and for frequent attacks of diverticulitis.

Constipation (Table 3.12) (*K&C* 6e p. 320)

This is a very common problem in the general population, and often requires no more than dietary advice and reassurance. It is particularly common in elderly people, in whom it is often associated with immobility and poor diet, and in young women in whom it may be associated with slow colonic transit or postpartum pelvic floor abnormalities. In many patients it is part of the irritable bowel syndrome (p. 114). Colorectal cancer should always be excluded in middle-aged and elderly people.

Management

A high-fibre diet and bulking agents should be the first line of treatment. Long-term laxatives (e.g. magnesium sulphate) should only be used in severe cases.

Faecal Incontinence (*K&C* 6e p. 323)

This is defined as recurrent uncontrolled passage of faecal material. Continence depends on a number of factors including mental function, stool volume and consistency, structural and functional integrity of the anal sphincters, puborectalis muscle, pudendal nerve function, rectal distensibility and anorectal sensation. Faecal impaction is a common cause of faecal incontinence in the elderly. Anal sphincter tears or trauma to the pudendal nerve can occur after childbirth or anal surgery (e.g. for haemorrhoids). Impaired rectal sensation occurs with diabetes mellitus, multiple sclerosis, dementia and spinal cord injuries. A detailed history and examination with digital rectal examination will help diagnose and exclude most common causes. Specific investigations include sigmoidoscopy to exclude mucosal disease, imaging of the anal sphincters (by anal endosonography, or MRI), anorectal manometry (to assess anal sphincter pressures), and sensory testing by rectal balloon distension to assess rectal sensation and compliance. Treatment depends on the cause.

Miscellaneous conditions

Megacolon (K&C 6e p. 322)

This term describes a number of conditions in which the colon is dilated. The most common cause is chronic constipation. Other causes are Chagas' disease and Hirschsprung's disease (congenital aganglionic segment in the rectum). Treatment is with laxatives, although Hirschsprung's disease responds to surgical resection.

Ischaemic colitis (K&C 6e p. 323)

This usually presents in the older age groups, with abdominal pain and rectal bleeding, and occasionally shock. Sigmoidoscopy is often normal apart from blood. Treatment is symptomatic, although surgery may be required for gangrene, perforation or stricture formation.

Colon polyps and the polyposis syndromes (K&C 6e p. 326)

A polyp is an elevation above the mucosal surface. They may be single or multiple, are usually asymptomatic and 70–80% of colonic polyps are adenomas. Colonic polyps are classified as neoplastic (adenomas and carcinomas), non-neoplastic or hamartomatous. Non-neoplastic polyps are usually hyperplastic polyps composed of normal cellular components with no dysplasia and with no malignant potential. They may be indistinguishable from adenomas at endoscopy. Inflammatory polyps (also non-neoplastic) occur on a background of inflammatory bowel disease and represent healing regenerating mucosa.

In the polyposis syndromes hundreds of polyps may be present.

Hamartomatous polyps   Hamartomas are benign tumours composed of an overgrowth of mature cells and tissues that normally occur in the affected part, in this case the colon. They may be one of two types:

- *Juvenile polyps.* These are dominantly inherited polyps which occur in children and teenagers, and present early with diarrhoea, bleeding or intussusception.
- *Peutz–Jeghers polyps* (p. 95).

Adenomatous polyps   are tumours of benign neoplastic epithelium. They are common, occurring in about 10% of the population. The aetiology is unknown, although genetic and environmental factors have been implicated. They rarely produce symptoms, although large polyps can bleed and cause anaemia, and villous adenomas can occasionally present with diarrhoea and hypokalaemia. Adenomatous polyps carry a malignant risk which increases with polyp size. Treatment is by endoscopic removal.

Familial adenomatous polyposis (FAP)   is an autosomal dominantly inherited condition in which individuals usually develop hundreds of adenomatous polyps throughout the gastrointestinal tract at an early age, resulting inevitably in colon cancer unless the large bowel is removed. FAP arises from germline mutations of the *APC* gene (adenomatous polyposis coli) located on chromosome 5. Gene testing is offered to unaffected members of FAP families to establish whether or not they carry the gene. Many of these patients have congenital hypertrophy of the retinal pigment epithelium (CHRPE) and this, along with genetic analysis, facilitates screening of young patients. Carriers of the gene are counselled and offered prophylactic colectomy in young adulthood. After colectomy these patients remain at risk of small bowel cancer, particularly of the duodenum, and surveillance gastroscopy is recommended.

Colorectal cancer (*K&C* 6e p. 328)

Most colorectal cancers occur sporadically. In 5–10% of patients they occur in patients with hereditary non-polyposis colorectal cancer (HNPCC) (see p. 110) or FAP. Colorectal cancer may also occur on a background of long-standing UC or colonic Crohn's disease.

Sporadic colorectal cancer

Epidemiology

This is the second most common cause of cancer death in the UK, and the incidence increases with age: most patients are over 50 years. Colon cancer is rare in Africa and Asia, largely because of environmental differences. A diet high in meat and animal fat and low in fibre is thought to be an important aetiological factor. In the West, the lifetime risk is 1 in 50, increasing to 1 in 17 in those with one affected first-degree relative.

Inheritance

Multiple molecular genetic abnormalities are now thought to be involved in the development of sporadic colon cancer. These include the activation of tumour-promoting genes or oncogenes (K-*ras*, c-*myc*) and the inactivation of tumour suppressor genes (*MCC*, *DCC*, *p53*). The risk of a tumour developing increases with increasing number of genetic abnormalities.

Pathology

It is likely that most carcinomas (other than on a back-ground of IBD) start as a benign adenoma, the so-called 'adenoma–carcinoma' sequence. Spread is by direct invasion through the bowel wall, with later invasion of blood vessels and lymphatics and spread to the liver. The mortality of colorectal cancer is directly related to the stage at presentation, and the stage is classified according to the modified Dukes' (Table 3.13) or TNM (tumour, node, metastases) classification. Synchronous (i.e. more than one tumour) tumours are present in 2% of cases.

Table 3.13	Modified Dukes' grading of colon cancer
Dukes' A	Tumour confined to the bowel wall
Dukes' B	Tumour extending through the bowel wall
Dukes' C	Regional lymph nodes involved
Dukes' D	Distant metastases

Clinical features

Most tumours are in the left side of the colon. They cause rectal bleeding and stenosis, with symptoms of increasing intestinal obstruction such as an alteration in bowel habit and colicky abdominal pain. Carcinoma of the caecum and ascending colon often presents with iron deficiency anaemia or a right iliac fossa mass. Clinical examination is usually unhelpful, although a mass may be palpable trans-abdominally or in the rectum. Hepatomegaly may be present with liver metastases.

Investigation

Examination of the colon is performed with a double-contrast barium enema or colonoscopy. A full blood count may show anaemia, and abnormal serum liver biochemistry suggests the presence of liver secondaries. Faecal occult blood tests are used in population screening studies but are not of value diagnostically.

Management (*K&C* 6e p. 330)

109

Treatment is surgical, with tumour resection and end-to-end anastomosis of bowel if possible. Adjuvant chemotherapy with 5-fluorouracil and leucovorin increases survival in Dukes' grade C (TNM stage III) cases, and in some cases with Dukes' B cancer. Preoperative radiotherapy improves survival in some patients with rectal cancer, and radiotherapy can also offer effective palliation in patients with locally advanced disease. Patients with up to two or three liver metastases confined to one lobe of the liver may be offered hepatic resection. Patients with unresectable metastatic disease are commonly offered chemotherapy in the form of 5-fluorouracil and leucovorin in combination with irinotecan or oxplatinin, which increases median survival and improves quality of life.

Prognosis

The overall 5-year survival rate is 40%, but is over 95% in tumours confined to the bowel wall (Dukes' grade A).

Screening

High-risk individuals (i.e. patients from HNPCC families or with a first-degree relative developing colon cancer < 50 years) should be offered screening colonoscopy. Mass

> *Table 3.14* Modified Amsterdam criteria for diagnosis of HNPCC
>
> ■ Three or more relatives with histologically verified HNPCC-associated cancer (colorectal, endometrium, small bowel, ureter or renal pelvis), one of whom is a first-degree relative of the other and in whom FAP has been excluded
>
> ■ Families with colorectal cancer involving at least two generations
>
> ■ One or more cancers were diagnosed before the age of 50

population screening of the over-50s with faecal occult blood tests (with colonoscopy when positive) or sigmoidoscopy has been shown to reduce the mortality from colon cancer, but this strategy has not yet been widely adopted because of the cost implications and the relatively poor uptake by healthy individuals.

Hereditary non-polyposis colorectal cancer (HNPCC) (*K&C* 6e p. 328)

HNPCC has an autosomal dominant mode of transmission with incomplete penetrance. It results from a mutation in one of six DNA mismatch repair genes which in turn leads to widespread genomic instability. Mutations in two of these, *hMLH1* and *hMSH2* account for > 95% of HNPCC families. These patients have an increased risk of developing tumours at an early age, and more often develop right-sided tumours. Many of these patients also have an increased incidence of gynaecological, urinary tract, biliary and other malignancies. Diagnostic criteria (Amsterdam criteria) to help identify those with HNPCC, based on family history have been devised (Table 3.14). A detailed family history should always be taken in any patient presenting with cancer.

DIARRHOEA (*K&C* 6e p. 331)

True diarrhoea is defined as an increase in stool weight to more than 200 g in 24 hours. Acute diarrhoea is usually due to infection or dietary indiscretion; chronic diarrhoea is defined as diarrhoea persisting for more than 14 days. Diarrhoea must be differentiated from the frequent passage of small amounts of stool (usually functional). Symptoms suggestive of an organic cause of diarrhoea as opposed to functional include nocturnal diarrhoea, bloody stools and weight loss. The next step in the assessment of diarrhoea is to distinguish malabsorptive from colonic/inflammatory forms of diarrhoea. Colonic, inflammatory and secretory (see below) causes of diarrhoea typically present with liquid loose stools with blood or mucous discharge. Malabsorption is often accompanied by steatorrhoea (p. 63). In occasional cases where differentiation between organic and functional bowel disease is difficult it may be necessary to measure stool weight by a 3-day stool collection as a hospital inpatient. Occasionally diarrhoea is factitious due to surreptitious laxative ingestion, or the patient deliberately dilutes the faeces by adding water or urine.

There are three main mechanisms: osmotic, secretory, motility related.

Osmotic diarrhoea

This occurs when there are large quantities of non-absorbed hypertonic substances in the bowel lumen. The diarrhoea stops when the patient stops eating or the malabsorptive substance is discontinued. The causes of osmotic diarrhoea are as follows:

- Ingestion of non-absorbable substance, e.g. a laxative such as magnesium sulphate
- Generalized malabsorption so that high concentrations of solute (e.g. glucose) remain in the lumen
- Specific malabsorptive defect, e.g. disaccharidase deficiency.

Secretory diarrhoea

Secretory diarrhoea results from the net secretion of fluid and electrolytes into the bowel lumen, and continues when the patient fasts. The causes are:

- Inflammation, e.g. ulcerative colitis, Crohn's disease
- Infection, e.g. shigella, salmonella
- Enterotoxins, e.g. from E. coli, cholera toxin
- Hormone-secreting tumours, e.g. VIPoma (p. 182)
- Bile salts (in the colon) following ileal disease or resection; also in idiopathic bile acid malabsorption
- Fatty acids (in the colon) following ileal resection
- Some laxatives.

Motility related

Abnormal motility often produces frequency rather than true diarrhoea. Causes are thyrotoxicosis, diabetic autonomic neuropathy and post-vagotomy.

Investigation

Acute diarrhoea lasting a few days is the result of dietary indiscretion or an infection. Investigation is not needed and treatment is symptomatic to maintain hydration. Chronic diarrhoea always requires investigation. Figure 3.2 outlines an approach to the investigation of a patient with chronic diarrhoea. Laxative abuse, usually seen in young females, must be excluded as a cause of chronic diarrhoea. Patients taking anthraquinone purgatives, e.g. Senokot, develop pigmentation of the colonic mucosa (melanosis coli) which may be seen at sigmoidoscopy. Other laxatives may be detected in the stool or urine.

Diarrhoea is a common problem in patients with AIDS, resulting either from a specific AIDS enteropathy or from an infection (cryptosporidia, microsporidia, cytomegalovirus infection).

FUNCTIONAL BOWEL DISORDERS (K&C 6e p. 335)

This is a large group of gastrointestinal disorders that are termed 'functional' because symptoms occur in the absence of any demonstrable abnormalities in the digestion and absorption of nutrients, fluid and electrolytes and no structural abnormality can be identified in the gastro-intestinal tract. Functional bowel disorders are extremely common world-wide, accounting for up to 80% of patients seen in the gastroenterology clinic. Rather than a diagnosis of exclusion after normal investigations (as the definition would suggest), this is frequently a positive diagnosis made in a patient with symptoms suggestive of a functional gastrointestinal disorder (Table 3.15). It is estimated that only 25% of persons with this condition seek medical care for it, and studies suggest that those who seek care are more likely to have behavioural and psychiatric problems than those who do not seek care. Altered bowel motility, visceral hypersensitivity (they have a lower pain threshold when tested with balloon distension of the rectum), psychosocial factors, an imbalance in neurotransmitters, and gastro-

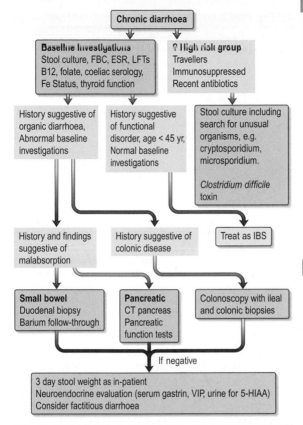

VIP = Vasoactive intestinal polypeptide; 5-HIAA = 5-hydroxyindole acetic acid

Fig. 3.2 **Approach to the investigation of chronic diarrhoea.** IBS, irritable bowel syndrome; VIP, vasoactive intestinal polypeptide.

intestinal infection have all been proposed as playing a part in the development of functional bowel disorders. Low-dose antidepressant treatment is frequently used for these disorders if initial symptom-based treatments do not prove beneficial.

Functional bowel disorders

> **Table 3.15   Chronic gastrointestinal symptoms suggestive of a functional gastrointestinal disorder**
>
> Nausea alone
> Vomiting alone
> Belching
> Chest pain unrelated to exercise
> Postprandial fullness
> Abdominal bloating
> Abdominal discomfort/pain (right or left iliac fossa)
> Passage of mucus per rectum
> Frequency of bowel actions with urgency first thing in the morning

Common functional gastrointestinal disorders are:

■ *Functional oesophageal disorders* occur in the absence of dysphagia, heartburn or other oesophageal disorder. They include globus (a sensation of a lump in the throat), effortless regurgitation of recently ingested food, and chest pain. Sometimes these symptoms will respond to high-dose acid suppression.

■ *Functional dyspepsia.* Common symptoms include indigestion, wind, nausea, early satiety and heartburn. Symptoms are sometimes very similar to peptic ulceration. Investigation is frequently unnecessary in younger people (< 55 years) but endoscopy is usually required in older people or in those with 'alarm symptoms' (see p. 80). Management is mainly by reassurance. Antacids and H_2-receptor antagonists are rarely of benefit. Eradication of *H. pylori* is often practised but there is little evidence that this improves symptoms. The prokinetic agents metoclopramide and domperidone are sometimes helpful, particularly in those with fullness and bloating.

■ *Irritable bowel syndrome (IBS).* Crampy abdominal pain relieved by defecation or the passage of wind, altered bowel habit, a sensation of incomplete evacuation, abdominal bloating and distension are common symptoms. Symptoms are more common in women than men, and the history is usually prolonged. Characteristically the patient looks healthy. Examination is usually normal, although sigmoidoscopy and air insufflation may reproduce the pain. If frequency of defecation is a feature, a rectal biopsy should be performed to exclude inflammatory bowel disease. Investigation depends on the individual patient. Young patients with classic symptoms do not require investigation. New symptoms in an elderly patient should prompt a search for underlying disease. Management is reassurance, with a discussion of lifestyle and diet. A high-fibre diet and antispasmodics, e.g. mebeverine, are useful in some patients. Other treatments, such as antidepressants, biofeedback and hypnotherapy, may be tried.

THE ACUTE ABDOMEN (K&C 6e p. 340)

This section deals with acute abdominal conditions that cause patients to be hospitalized within a few hours of the onset of their pain. Most are admitted under the care of the surgical team, and some will need a laparotomy. Medical conditions that may present as an acute abdomen include diabetic ketoacidosis, myocardial infarction and pneumonia. The irritable bowel syndrome may also present with acute severe abdominal pain.

History

A detailed history, which should include gynaecological symptoms, will often point to the cause of the pain.

- Acute abdominal pain may be intermittent or continuous. Intermittent (colicky) pain describes pain that occurs for a short period (usually a few minutes) and is interspersed with pain-free periods lasting a few minutes or up to half an hour. This is characteristic of mechanical obstruction of a hollow viscus, e.g. ureteric calculus or bowel obstruction (Table 3.16). Additional symptoms of bowel obstruction, which may or may not be present, are abdominal distension, vomiting and absolute constipation

Table 3.16 Causes of mechanical intestinal obstruction	
Constriction from the outside	Bowel entrapped in a hernia
	Adhesions
	Volvulus, particularly of the sigmoid
Disease of the bowel wall	Crohn's disease
	Carcinoma
	Diverticular disease
Intraluminal obstruction	Foreign body
	Gallstones

(i.e. failure to pass flatus or stool). Biliary pain (previously called biliary colic) resulting from obstruction of the gall bladder or bile duct is not colicky but usually a constant upper abdominal pain.

Continuous pain is relentless with no periods of complete relief. It occurs in many abdominal conditions.

■ The onset of pain may be sudden or gradual. Sudden onset suggests perforation of a viscus (e.g. duodenal ulcer), rupture of an organ (e.g. aortic aneurysm) or torsion (e.g. ovarian cyst). The pain of acute pancreatitis often begins suddenly.
■ The site of the pain must be noted. In general, upper abdominal pain is produced by pathology of either the upper abdominal viscera – e.g. acute cholecystitis, acute pancreatitis – or the stomach and duodenum. The pain of small bowel obstruction is often in the centre of the abdomen. A common cause of acute right iliac fossa pain is acute appendicitis.
■ Radiation of pain to the back suggests acute pancreatitis, rupture of an aortic aneurysm or renal tract disease.

Examination

A general physical examination should be made and the following points noted:

■ The presence of shock (pale, cool peripheries, tachycardia, hypotension) suggests rupture of an organ, e.g. aortic aneurysm, ruptured ectopic pregnancy. It may also occur in the later stages of generalized peritonitis resulting from bowel perforation (see below).
■ Fever is common in acute inflammatory conditions.
■ Peritonitis and bowel obstruction produce specific signs on abdominal examination.

The signs of peritonitis are tenderness, guarding and rigidity on palpation. Guarding is an involuntary contraction of the abdominal muscles when the abdomen is palpated. Peritonitis may be localized or generalized (see below). Bowel sounds are absent with generalized peritonitis.

Mechanical bowel obstruction produces distension and active 'tinkling' bowel sounds. A strangulated hernia may produce obstruction, and the hernial orifices must always be examined.

In most cases a rectal and pelvic examination should be performed.

Investigations

- Blood tests. The white cell count may be raised in inflammatory conditions. The serum amylase may be raised in any acute abdomen, but levels greater than five times normal indicate acute pancreatitis.
- Imaging. An erect chest X-ray may show air under the diaphragm with a perforated viscus. A plain abdominal X-ray shows dilated loops of bowel and fluid levels in obstruction. Ultrasound examination is useful in the diagnosis of acute cholecystitis, appendicitis and gynaecological conditions.
- Surgery. Laparoscopy or laparotomy may be required, depending on the diagnosis.

Acute appendicitis (K&C 6e p. 342)

Acute appendicitis occurs when the lumen of the appendix becomes obstructed by a faecolith.

Epidemiology

It affects all age groups but is rare in the very young and very old.

Clinical features

The typical clinical presentation is the onset of central abdominal pain which then becomes localized to the right iliac fossa (RIF), accompanied by anorexia and sometimes vomiting and diarrhoea. The patient is pyrexial, with tenderness and guarding in the RIF.

Investigations

In many cases the diagnosis is clinical. There is a raised white cell count and ultrasonography may show an inflamed appendix. CT is also used to make the diagnosis.

Differential diagnosis

Conditions that mimic acute appendicitis include non-specific mesenteric lymphadenitis, terminal ileitis due to Crohn's disease or *Yersinia* infection, acute salpingitis in women, inflamed Meckel's diverticulum and functional bowel diseases.

Management

The treatment is surgical, with removal of the appendix either by open surgery or laparoscopically.

Complications

These arise from gangrene and perforation, leading to localized abscess formation or generalized peritonitis.

Acute peritonitis (*K&C* 6e p. 342)

Localized peritonitis occurs with all acute inflammatory conditions of the gastrointestinal tract, and management depends on the underlying condition, e.g. acute appendicitis, acute cholecystitis.

Generalized peritonitis occurs as a result of rupture of an abdominal viscus, e.g. perforated duodenal ulcer, perforated appendix. There is a sudden onset of abdominal pain which rapidly becomes generalized. The patient is shocked and lies still, as movement exacerbates the pain. A plain abdominal X-ray shows air under the diaphragm; serum amylase must be checked to exclude acute pancreatitis.

Intestinal obstruction (*K&C* 6e p. 343)

Intestinal obstruction is either mechanical or functional.

Mechanical (Table 3.16)   The bowel above the level of the obstruction is dilated, with increased secretion of fluid into the lumen. The patient complains of colicky abdominal pain, associated with vomiting and absolute constipation. On examination there is distension and 'tinkling' bowel sounds. Small bowel obstruction may settle with conservative management (i.e. nasogastric suction and intravenous fluids to maintain hydration). Large bowel obstruction is treated surgically.

Functional   This occurs with a paralytic ileus, which is often seen in the postoperative stage of peritonitis or of major abdominal surgery, or in association with opiate treatment (acute colonic pseudo-obstruction, Ogilvie's syndrome). It also occurs when the nerves or muscles of the intestine are damaged, causing intestinal pseudo-obstruction.

Unlike mechanical obstruction, pain is often not present and bowel sounds may be decreased. Gas is seen throughout the bowel on a plain abdominal X-ray. Management is conservative.

THE PERITONEUM (K&C 6e p. 344)

The peritoneal cavity is a closed sac lined by mesothelium. It contains a little fluid to allow the abdominal contents to move freely. Conditions which affect the peritoneum are listed below.

- Infective (peritonitis)
  - secondary to gut disease, e.g. appendicitis, perforation
  - chronic peritoneal dialysis
  - spontaneous (associated with ascites)
  - tuberculous
- Neoplasia
  - secondary deposits, e.g. from ovary
  - primary mesothelioma
- Vasculitis: connective tissue disease.

119

NUTRITION

Dietary requirements (K&C 6e p. 229)

Food is necessary to provide the body with energy. The average daily requirement (Table 3.17) of a middle-aged adult female in the UK is 8100 kJ (1940 kcal), and for a man is 10 600 kJ (2550 kcal). This is made up of 50% carbohydrate, 35% fat and 15% protein, plus or minus 5% alcohol. Energy requirements increase during periods of rapid growth, such as adolescence, pregnancy and lactation, and with sepsis.

Table 3.17 Protein, energy and water requirement of normal and hypercatabolic adults

Metabolic state	Nutritional requirements	
	Normal	Hypercatabolic
Protein (g/kg)	1	2–3
Nitrogen (g/kg)	0.17	0.3–0.45
Energy (kcal/kg)	25–30	35–50
Water (mL/kg)	30–35	30–35

Bodyweight is maintained at a 'set point' by a precise balance of energy intake and total energy expenditure (the sum of the resting metabolic rate, activity energy expenditure and the thermic effect of food eaten). Weight gain is almost always due solely to an increase in energy intake which exceeds the total energy expenditure. Occasionally weight gain is due to a decrease in energy expenditure, e.g. hypothyroidism, or to fluid retention, e.g. heart failure or ascites. On the other hand, weight loss associated with cancer and chronic diseases is due to a reduction in energy intake secondary to a loss of appetite (anorexia). In a few conditions, such as sepsis and severe trauma, there is an increase in energy requirements (hypercatabolic or hyper-metabolic) which will result in a negative energy balance if there is no compensatory increase in energy intake.

A balanced diet also requires sufficient amounts of minerals and vitamins. In the western world vitamin deficiency is rare except in specific groups, e.g. alcoholics and patients with small bowel disease, who may have multiple vitamin deficiencies, and patients with liver and biliary tract disease who are susceptible to deficiency of the fat-soluble vitamins (A, D, E, K). Deficiencies of the B vitamins, riboflavin and biotin, are rare in all patient groups and are not discussed further. Dietary deficiency of vitamin B_6 (pyridoxine, pyridoxal and pyridoxamine) is also extremely rare, but drugs (e.g. isoniazid and penicillamine) that interact with pyridoxal phosphate may cause B_6 deficiency and a polyneuropathy. Vitamin B_{12} and folate deficiency are discussed on pages 189 and 192 and vitamin D deficiency on page 304.

NUTRITIONAL SUPPORT (*K&C* 6e p. 257)

Patients should be screened for nutritional status on admission to hospital and during their hospital stay. Current recommendations suggest that:

- Patients should be asked simple questions about recent weight loss, their usual weight and whether they have been eating less than usual.
- Their weight and height should be recorded and body mass index (BMI) calculated (weight [kg]/height [m]^2, QC3.2). The acceptable range of BMI is 20–25 kg/m^2 for men and 19–24 kg/m^2 for women.

Some form of nutritional supplementation is required in those patients who cannot eat, should not eat, will not eat or cannot eat enough. It is necessary to provide nutritional support for:

■ All severely malnourished patients on admission to hospital: severe malnutrition is indicated by a BMI of less than 15
■ Moderately malnourished patients (BMI 15–19) who, because of their physical illness, are not expected to eat for 3–5 days
■ Normally nourished patients not expected to eat for 7–10 days.

Enteral nutrition is cheaper, more physiological and has fewer complications than parenteral (intravenous) nutrition, and should be used if the gastrointestinal tract is functioning normally. With both enteral and parenteral nutrition a complete feeding regimen consisting of fat, carbohydrates, protein, vitamins, minerals and trace elements can be provided to provide the nutritional requirements of the individual (Table 3.17). Ideally a multidisciplinary nutrition support team should supervise the provision of artificial nutritional support.

Enteral nutrition (K&C 6e p. 258)

Foods can be given by:

■ Mouth
■ Fine-bore nasogastric tube for short-term enteral nutrition
■ Percutaneous endoscopic gastrostomy (PEG): this is useful for patients who need feeding for longer than 2 weeks
■ Percutaneous jejunostomy where a tube is inserted directly into the jejunum either endoscopically or at laparotomy.

A polymeric diet with whole protein, carbohydrate and fat is usually used; sometimes an elemental diet composed of amino acids, glucose and fatty acids is used for patients with Crohn's disease (p. 102).

Total parenteral nutrition (TPN) (K&C 6e p. 259)

Parenteral nutrition may be given via a feeding catheter placed in a peripheral vein or a silicone catheter placed in

Nutritional support

Table 3.18 Complications of total parenteral nutrition
Catheter related: sepsis, thrombosis, embolism and pneumothorax
Metabolic, e.g. hyperglycaemia, hypercalcaemia
Electrolyte disturbances
Liver dysfunction

the subclavian vein. Central catheters must only be placed by experienced clinicians under strict aseptic conditions in a sterile environment. The risk of introducing infection is reduced if these catheters are only used for feeding purposes, and not the administration of drugs or blood. Peripheral feeding lines usually only last for about 5 days and are reserved for when feeding is necessary for a short period. Central lines may last for months to years. Complications of TPN are given in Table 3.18.

Monitoring of artificial nutrition

Patients receiving nutritional support should be weighed twice weekly: they require regular clinical examination to check for evidence of fluid overload or depletion. Patients receiving nutritional support in hospital initially require daily measurements of urea and electrolytes and blood glucose. More frequent measurement of blood glucose with BM Stix is indicated in patients beginning TPN. Liver biochemistry, calcium and phosphate are measured twice weekly. Serum magnesium, zinc and nitrogen balance (see below) are measured weekly. The frequency of biochemical monitoring is adjusted according to the patient's clinical and metabolic status.

It is necessary to give 40–50 g of protein per 24 hours to maintain nitrogen balance, which represents the balance between protein breakdown and synthesis. The aim of any regimen is to achieve a positive nitrogen balance, which can usually be obtained by giving 3–5 g of nitrogen in excess of output. The amount of protein required to maintain nitrogen balance in a particular individual can be calculated from the amount of urinary nitrogen loss, using the formula:

$$N_2 \text{ loss (g/24 h)} = \text{Urinary urea (mmol/24 h)} \times 0.028 + 2$$

Urinary nitrogen $\times$ 6.25 = grams of protein required (most proteins contain about 16% nitrogen).

Most patients require about 12 g of nitrogen per 24 hours, but hypercatabolic patients require more, about 15 g/day.

Refeeding syndrome

The refeeding syndrome occurs within the first few days of refeeding by the oral, enteral or parenteral route. It is under-recognized and can be fatal. It involves a shift from the use of fat as an energy source during starvation to the use of carbohydrate as an energy source during refeeding. With the introduction of artificial nutrition and carbohydrate by any source, insulin release is augmented and there is rapid intracellular passage of phosphate, magnesium and potassium resulting in hypophosphataemia, hypomagnesaemia (p. 326), and hypokalaemia (p. 322). Phosphate is an integral part of cellular machinery. Deficiency results in widespread organ dysfunction (muscle weakness, rhabdomyolysis, cardiac failure, immune suppression, haemolytic anaemia, thrombocytopenia, coma, hallucinations, fits). Thiamine deficiency can be precipitated. Patients at risk of refeeding are underweight (e.g. anorexia nervosa, chronic alcoholism) or those with recent rapid weight loss (5% within preceding month), including patients after treatment for morbid obesity. These at-risk patients should receive Pabrinex (1 pair twice daily for 5–7 days beginning before feeding), and begin feeding at 25–50% of estimated calorie requirements, increasing by 100 calories per day. Serum phosphate, magnesium, calcium, potassium, urea and creatinine, bodyweight and evidence of fluid overload should be checked daily for the first week, and electrolyte deficiencies corrected as necessary.

123

DISORDERS OF BODYWEIGHT

Obesity (K&C 6e p. 252)

Obesity, defined as an excess of body fat contributing to co-morbidity, is a common problem in developed countries and is becoming more common in developing countries. A BMI of 25 kg/m^2 or greater is a standard commonly used to define obesity. Obesity is associated with an increased prevalence of ischaemic heart disease, hypertension, diabetes mellitus, hyperlipidaemia, obstructive sleep apnoea, fatty liver and gallstones. Weight reduction can be achieved with a reduction in calorie intake and an increase in physical activity, although in practice this is difficult to achieve. Drug treatment such as orlistat, an inhibitor of pancreatic lipase and hence fat digestion, is sometimes used in the severely obese patient. Surgical treatments for obesity such as gastric banding or intestinal bypass are used in patients resistant to other treatments.

Anorexia nervosa (*K&C* 6e p. 1310)

Anorexia nervosa is a psychological illness, predominantly affecting young females and characterized by marked weight loss (BMI < 17.5 kg/m^2), intense fear of gaining weight, a distorted body image and amenorrhoea. Patients with anorexia nervosa control their body weight by a process of semi-starvation and/or self-induced vomiting (bulimia) and may develop consequences of undernutrition. Treatment is difficult and usually undertaken in a specialist eating disorders unit.

Liver, biliary tract and pancreatic disease 4

The pancreas secretes the hormones insulin and glucagon (both regulate blood sugar) in addition to pancreatic enzymes involved in the digestion of fat, carbohydrate and protein in the small intestine (*K&C* 6e p. 406). The main functions of the liver (*K&C* 6e p. 349) are:

- Control of synthesis and metabolism of carbohydrate, lipids, protein (including most plasma proteins and coagulation factors) and drugs. The liver manufactures most of the body's cholesterol; the rest comes from food. Cholesterol is used to make bile salts and is also needed to make certain hormones, including oestrogen, testosterone, and the adrenal hormones. The liver is the major site for converting excess carbohydrates and proteins into fatty acids and triglycerides, which are then exported and stored in adipose tissue. Sugars are also stored in the liver as glycogen and then broken down and released into the bloodstream as glucose when needed.
- The metabolism and excretion of bilirubin and bile acids (necessary for digestion and absorption of dietary fat).

In most western countries alcohol and hepatitis C are the major causes of liver disease. Elsewhere, infection with hepatitis B virus is a common cause but the incidence is decreasing with vaccination.

SYMPTOMS OF LIVER DISEASE

Acute liver disease, e.g. viral hepatitis, may be asymptomatic or it presents with generalized symptoms of lethargy, anorexia and malaise in the early stages, with jaundice developing later (p. 129).

Chronic liver disease may also be asymptomatic and discovered from an incidental finding of abnormal liver biochemistry. Some patients with chronic liver disease may present at a late stage with complications of cirrhosis, causing:

- Ascites with abdominal swelling and discomfort (p. 152)
- Haematemesis and melaena due to bleeding oesophageal varices (p. 151)
- Confusion and drowsiness due to hepatic encephalopathy (p. 154).

Patients presenting in this way are often extremely unwell and a detailed history may not be obtained. However, physical examination will often reveal the signs of chronic liver disease (p. 141) and thus point to liver disease as the cause of the presenting illness.

Pruritus (itching) occurs in cholestatic jaundice from any cause (p. 131), but is particularly common in primary biliary cirrhosis, when it may be the only symptom (without jaundice) at presentation. Pruritus may occur in association with other systemic diseases (e.g. hyperthyroidism, polycythaemia, renal failure, malignant disease) and skin diseases (e.g. scabies, eczema), but in these cases there are usually additional symptoms or signs that suggest the diagnosis.

INTERPRETING LIVER BIOCHEMISTRY AND LIVER FUNCTION TESTS (K&C 6e p. 352)

A routine blood sample sent to the laboratory for liver biochemistry will be processed by an automated multi-channel analyser to produce serum levels of bilirubin, aminotransferases, alkaline phosphatase, γ-glutamyl transpeptidase (γ-GT) and total proteins. These tests are often referred to as 'liver function tests' (LFTs) but this term is misleading as they do not accurately reflect how well the liver is functioning. These tests are best referred to as liver blood tests or liver biochemistry. Liver synthetic function is determined by measuring the serum albumin and the prothrombin time (clotting factors are synthesized in the liver), which are reduced and increased respectively with impaired liver function. Hypoalbuminaemia may also occur with chronic inflammatory disease, sepsis and the nephrotic syndrome (p. 351). A prolonged prothrombin time may also occur as a result of vitamin K deficiency in biliary obstruction (low concentration of intestinal bile salts results in poor absorption of vitamin K); however, unlike in liver disease, clotting is corrected by giving 10 mg of vitamin K intravenously.

■ *Bilirubin* (normal range < 17 µmol/L, 1.00 mg/dL) is the breakdown product of haem metabolism (see p. 130). An isolated rise in serum bilirubin with otherwise normal liver biochemistry is likely to be due to an inherited defect in bilirubin metabolism (usually Gilbert's disease), haemolysis or ineffective erythropoiesis (premature death of the red cell in the bone marrow). Hyper-bilirubinaemia caused by hepatobiliary disease is almost always accompanied by other abnormalities of liver biochemistry; very high levels occur most frequently in biliary tract obstruction. Serial measurements are useful in following the progress of some diseases, e.g. primary biliary cirrhosis, or the response to treatment, e.g. after placement of a stent in cancer of the head of the pancreas.

■ *Aminotransferases.* These enzymes are present in hepatocytes and leak into the blood with liver cell damage. Very high levels may occur with acute hepatitis (20–50 times normal). Aspartate aminotransferase (AST, normal range 10–40 U/L) is also present in heart and skeletal muscle, and raised serum concentrations are seen with myocardial infarction and skeletal muscle damage. Alanine amino-transferase (ALT, normal range 5–40 U/L) is more specific to the liver than AST.

■ *Alkaline phosphatase* (normal range 25–115 U/L) is situated in the canalicular and sinusoidal membranes of the liver. Raised serum alkaline phosphatase concentrations are seen in cholestasis from any cause, whether intra- or extrahepatic disease. Circulating alkaline phosphatase is also derived from the placenta and bone, and raised serum levels occur in pregnancy, Paget's disease, osteomalacia, growing children, and bony meta-stases. In these cases differentiation from cholestasis is made by the absence of a rise in serum γ-glutamyl trans-peptidase (γ-GT) (see below). The placenta secretes its own alkaline phosphatase isoenzyme and the serum level is raised in pregnancy.

■ γ-Glutamyl transpeptidase (normal range: male < 50 U/L, female < 32 U/L) is a liver microsomal enzyme which may be induced by alcohol and enzyme-inducing drugs, e.g. phenytoin. A raised serum concentration is a useful screen for alcohol abuse. In cholestasis the γ-GT rises in parallel with the serum alkaline phosphatase because it has a similar pathway of excretion.

Approach to the asymptomatic person with abnormal liver biochemistry

The widespread routine testing of liver biochemistry has led to identification of abnormal liver blood tests in asymptomatic people. The pattern of abnormalities often provides a clue to the underlying disorder. A predominant elevation of serum aminotransferases indicates hepatocellular injury. Elevation of the serum bilirubin and alkaline phosphatase in excess of aminotransferases indicates a cholestatic disorder such as primary biliary cirrhosis, primary sclerosing cholangitis or extrahepatic bile duct obstruction. An isolated rise in bilirubin is most likely to be due to Gilbert's disease. A careful history (alcohol consumption, exposure to hepatotoxic drugs, risk factors for chronic liver disease), physical examination (particularly features of chronic liver disease) and simple laboratory tests to look for viral hepatitis (B and C), metabolic (haemochromatosis, Wilson's disease, α_1-antitrypsin deficiency) and autoimmune liver disease (Table 4.4) are the usual first steps in patients with a persistent elevation of serum aminotransferases.

OTHER INVESTIGATIONS IN LIVER AND BILIARY DISEASE (K&C 6e p. 354)

Endoscopic retrograde cholangiopancreatography (ERCP) is an endoscopic procedure performed under intravenous sedation. The pancreatic and bile ducts are imaged after the injection of radiographic contrast medium via the ampulla of Vater. Stones in the ducts can be removed and stents placed to relieve obstruction caused by strictures. Complications of ERCP include bleeding (after cutting of the sphincter to aid bile duct cannulation or stone removal), acute pancreatitis, perforation and cholangitis.

Magnetic resonance cholangiopancreatography (MRCP) is a radiological technique that produces images of the pancreaticobiliary ducts that are similar in appearance to those obtained by invasive radiographic methods, such as ERCP. It is a non-invasive test and does not require the administration of any exogenous contrast materials. It is used to confirm a diagnosis prior to ERCP and is useful in patients with allergies to iodine-based contrast materials.

Percutaneous transhepatic cholangiopancreatography (PTC) involves injection of contrast into the biliary system via a percutaneously placed needle inserted into an intrahepatic duct. It is performed in patients with biliary dilatation in whom ERCP has failed or is not possible.

Liver biopsy for histological examination is usually performed via a percutaneous approach under local anaesthesia. Contraindications include an uncooperative patient, a prolonged prothrombin time (by more than 3–5 s), platelet count $< 50 \times 10^9/L$, extrahepatic cholestasis and suspected haemangioma.

JAUNDICE (*K&C* 6e p. 358)

Jaundice (icterus) is a yellow discoloration of the sclerae and skin as a result of a raised serum bilirubin, and is usually detectable clinically when the bilirubin is greater than 50 μmol/L (3 mg/dL).

Bilirubin is derived predominantly from the breakdown of haemoglobin in the spleen, and is carried in the blood bound to albumin. Unconjugated bilirubin is conjugated in the liver by glucuronyl transferase to bilirubin glucuronide, and this is excreted into the small intestine in bile. In the terminal ileum conjugated bilirubin is converted to urobilinogen and excreted in the faeces (as stercobilinogen) or reabsorbed and excreted by the kidneys (Fig. 4 1).

The usual division of jaundice into prehepatic, hepatocellular and obstructive is an oversimplification, because in hepatocellular jaundice there is invariably cholestasis, and the clinical problem is whether the cholestasis is intrahepatic or extrahepatic. Jaundice is therefore considered under the following headings:

- Haemolytic jaundice (prehepatic)
- Congenital hyperbilirubinaemias
- Cholestatic jaundice.

Haemolytic jaundice

Increased breakdown of red cells leads to increased production of bilirubin, which usually results in mild jaundice only, as the liver can usually handle the increased bilirubin derived from haemolysis. The unconjugated bilirubin is not water soluble and therefore does not pass into the urine,

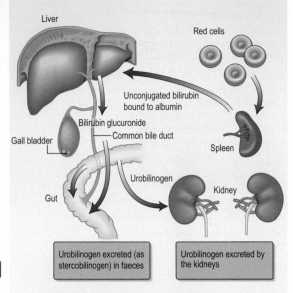

Fig. 4.1   Pathways in bilirubin metabolism.

unlike the conjugated hyperbilirubinaemia of cholestatic jaundice. The urinary urobilinogen is increased. The causes are those of haemolytic anaemia (p. 197), with the clinical features dependent on the cause. Investigations show features of haemolysis (p. 198), with raised serum unconjugated bilirubin and normal alkaline phosphatase and transferases.

Congenital hyperbilirubinaemia (K&C 6e p. 358)

The most common is Gilbert's syndrome, which affects 2–7% of the population. It is asymptomatic and is usually picked up as an incidental finding of a slightly raised serum bilirubin (17–102 μmol/L). Mutations in the gene coding for UDP-glucuronyl transferase lead to reduced enzyme activity and reduced conjugation of bilirubin with glucuronic acid. The diagnosis is based on the findings of unconjugated

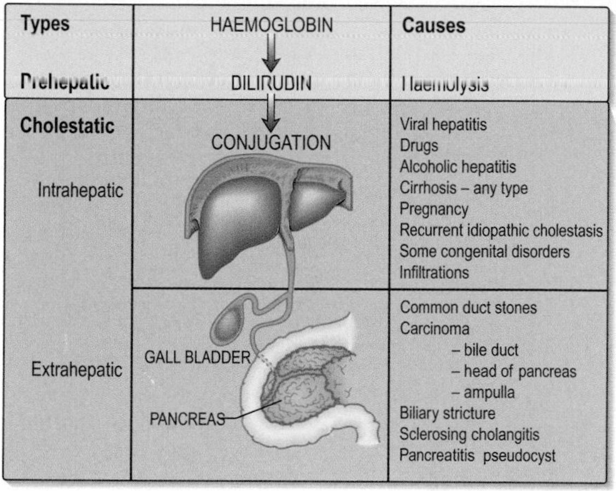

Fig. 4.2 Causes of jaundice.

hyperbilirubinaemia with otherwise normal liver bio-chemistry, normal full blood count, smear and reticulocyte count (thus excluding haemolysis) and absence of signs of liver disease. The patient should be reassured that no further investigation or treatment is necessary.

The other congenital abnormalities of bilirubin metabolism (Crigler–Najjar, Dubin–Johnson, and Rotor syndromes) are rare.

Cholestatic jaundice

This can be divided into the following (Fig. 4.2):

- Intrahepatic cholestasis, caused by hepatocellular swelling in parenchymal liver disease or abnormalities at a cellular level of bile excretion
- Extrahepatic cholestasis resulting from obstruction of bile flow at any point distal to the bile canaliculi.

Investigations

An outline of the approach to the investigation of jaundice is shown in Figure 4.3.

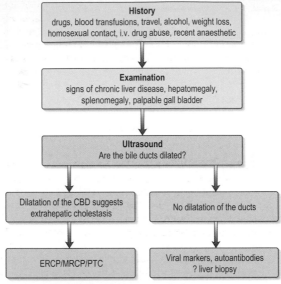

History
drugs, blood transfusions, travel, alcohol, weight loss,
homosexual contact, i.v. drug abuse, recent anaesthetic

Examination
signs of chronic liver disease, hepatomegaly,
splenomegaly, palpable gall bladder

Ultrasound
Are the bile ducts dilated?

Dilatation of the CBD suggests
extrahepatic cholestasis

No dilatation of the ducts

ERCP/MRCP/PTC

Viral markers, autoantibodies
? liver biopsy

ERCP = endoscopic retrograde cholangiopancreatography
MRCP = magnetic resonance cholangiopancreatography
PTC = percutaneous transhepatic cholangiogram

Fig. 4.3 **Approach to the investigation of cholestatic
jaundice.** The order of investigation is influenced by the age of
the patient and hence the likely cause of jaundice. A young
person is most likely to have intrinsic liver disease, e.g. viral
hepatitis, and it may be more appropriate to organize tests to
exclude these conditions before proceeding to ultrasound. See
page 134 for clinical features.

- Serum liver biochemistry will confirm the jaundice. The
  AST tends to be high early in the course of hepatitis, with
  a smaller rise in alkaline phosphatase. Conversely, in
  extrahepatic obstruction the alkaline phosphatase is
  elevated, with a smaller rise in the AST.
- Ultrasound examination will show dilated bile ducts in
  extrahepatic cholestasis and identify the level of
  obstruction.
- Serum viral markers for hepatitis A or hepatitis B may be
  present in acute viral hepatitis. Antibodies to hepatitis C
  virus develop late in the course of acute infection.

■ Other tests. Cholestasis impairs the absorption of fat-soluble vitamins. Malabsorption of vitamin K often results in a prolonged prothrombin time, which is reversed by intravenous administration of vitamin K. Impairment of liver synthetic function in advanced liver disease also results in a prolonged prothrombin time and a low serum albumin. Serum autoantibodies are present in autoimmune liver disease (see later).

HEPATITIS

The pathological features of hepatitis are liver cell necrosis and inflammatory cell infiltration. Clinically the liver may be enlarged and tender, jaundice may be evident, and laboratory evidence of hepatocellular damage is invariably found in the form of elevated serum transferase levels. Hepatitis is divided into acute and chronic types (Table 4.1) on the basis of clinical and pathological criteria. Acute hepatitis is most commonly caused by one of the hepatitis viruses. Acute hepatitis is usually self-limiting with a return to normal structure and function. Occasionally there is

Table 4.1 The causes of acute and chronic hepatitis	
Acute	**Chronic**
Viruses	Viruses
Hepatitis A, B ± D, C, and E	Hepatitis B ± D, and C
Epstein–Barr virus	
Cytomegalovirus	
Non-viral infections	Autoimmune hepatitis
Leptospira icterohaemorrhagica	
Toxoplasma gondii	
Coxiella burnetii (Q fever)	
Alcohol	Alcohol
Drugs	Drugs
Anti-TB, e.g. isoniazid	Methyldopa
Non-steroidal anti-inflammatory drugs	Nitrofurantoin
Halogenated anaesthetics	
Paracetamol poisoning	
Others	Metabolic disorders
Pregnancy	Wilson's disease
Poisons, e.g. carbon tetrachloride	α_1-Antitrypsin deficiency
Wilson's disease	

progression to massive liver cell necrosis, which may result in death. Raised serum ALT is the best indicator of acute hepatic injury but does not reflect disease severity (prothrombin time and bilirubin are required for this). Several characteristic laboratory abnormalities occur in patients with alcoholic hepatitis including serum AST/ALT ratio > 2 (rarely seen in other forms of liver disease), only a moderate rise in the transaminases (< 500 IU/L) and very high serum concentrations of bilirubin and γ-GT.

Chronic hepatitis due to any cause is defined as sustained inflammatory disease of the liver lasting for more than 6 months.

Viral hepatitis nd

The most common causes of viral hepatitis are hepatitis A, B and C. Hepatitis D and E are infrequent causes in the UK. Features of these viruses are summarized in Table 4.2. All cases of viral hepatitis must be notified to the appropriate public health authority. This allows contacts to be traced and provides data on disease incidence.

Hepatitis A nd (K&C 6e p. 362)

Epidemiology

Hepatitis A is the most common type of acute viral hepatitis. It occurs world-wide and affects particularly children and young adults. Spread is faecal–oral and arises from the ingestion of contaminated food (e.g. shellfish, clams) or water. The virus is excreted in the faeces of infected individuals for about 2 weeks before, and 7 days after, the onset of the illness. It is most infectious just before the onset of the jaundice.

Clinical features

Hepatitis A virus (HAV) infection varies from subclinical to fulminant hepatitis. The incubation period averages 30 days, after which the illness in symptomatic patients begins with non-specific prodromal symptoms of nausea, vomiting, diarrhoea, malaise, abdominal discomfort and mild fever. After 1 or 2 weeks some patients become jaundiced with dark urine and pale stools and the prodromal symptoms improve. There is moderate hepatomegaly and the spleen is palpable in 10% of cases. Occasionally lymphadenopathy

Table 4.2 Some features of the hepatitis viruses

	A	B	C	Hepatitis D	E
Virus	RNA	DNA	RNA	RNA	RNA
Transmission	Faecal–oral	Parenteral Sexual Vertical	Parenteral	Parenteral	Faecal–oral
Incubation	Short (2–7 weeks)	Long (1–5 months)	Long	Intermediate	Short
Chronicity	No	Yes	Yes	Yes (only with B)	No
Mortality rate (%) in acute infection	< 0.5	< 1	< 1		1–2 (20% in pregnancy)

and a skin rash are present. The illness is self-limiting and usually over in 3–6 weeks. Rarely there is fulminant hepatitis (p. 144), coma and death.

Investigations

- Liver biochemistry shows a raised serum AST and ALT and raised bilirubin when jaundice develops.
- The blood count may show a leucopenia with relative lymphocytosis and a high ESR.
- Acute HAV infection is diagnosed by IgM anti-HAV in the serum; the presence of IgG anti-HAV indicates past infection.

Management

No specific treatment is required. Hospital admission is not usually necessary and avoidance of alcohol advised only when the patient is ill.

Prophylaxis

Active immunization with an inactivated strain of the virus is recommended for the following groups:

- Travellers to areas of high prevalence (Africa, Asia, South America, Eastern Europe, the Middle East)
- Patients with chronic liver disease in whom the disease is more severe
- Homosexuals, people with haemophilia and persons who have occupational risk for exposure.

Control of hepatitis also depends on good hygiene. Travellers to high-risk areas should drink only boiled or bottled water and avoid risky foods.

Passive immunization with immunoglobulin is given to close contacts of confirmed cases of hepatitis A to prevent infection.

Hepatitis B nd (*K&C* 6e p. 364)

Epidemiology

Hepatitis B virus (HBV) is present world-wide and is particularly prevalent in parts of Africa, the Middle and Far East. It is spread through the intravenous route (infected blood products, contaminated needles of intravenous drug abusers and tattooists) and through sexual intercourse, particularly in male homosexuals. Vertical transmission from mother to child during parturition is the most common means of transmission world-wide. Hepatitis B is becoming rare in countries such as Taiwan where universal vaccination is performed. This approach has not been adopted in the UK.

Viral structure

The whole virus is the Dane particle (Fig. 4.4), which consists of an inner core and an outer surface coat, the hepatitis B surface antigen (HBsAg). The inner core contains double-stranded DNA, DNA polymerase/reverse transcriptase, the core antigen (HBcAg) and e antigen (HBeAg). HBeAg is produced in excess during active viral replication, and its detection in the serum indicates a high degree of infectivity. Mutations in all regions of the HBV genome have been found in patients with chronic HBV infection. HBV mutations can potentially modulate the severity of liver disease by altering the level of HBV replication or the expression of immunogenic epitopes (the site against which T cells respond). Some variants such as that produced by the precore stop codon mutation, do not make HBeAg but the virus can continue to replicate with the presence of HBV DNA in the serum and elevated liver enzymes. HBV DNA must therefore always be measured in an HbsAg-positive patient to determine the level of viral replication.

Acute infection   *HBitanGgen just shows prevrous exposue.*

Acute infection with HBV may be asymptomatic or produce symptoms and signs similar to those seen in hepatitis A. Occasionally it is associated with a rash or polyarthritis affecting the small joints. The sequence of events following acute infection is depicted in Figure 4.5.

Investigation is generally the same as for hepatitis A. The viral markers for HBV are shown in Figure 4.5. If HBsAg is present, a full viral profile is performed. There is no specific therapy for *acute* HBV infection and management is supportive.

Most patients recover completely. This is marked by the disappearance of HBsAg from the serum, the development of antibodies to surface antigen (anti-HBs) and immunity to subsequent infection (Fig. 4.5). One per cent of patients with acute hepatitis develop fulminant liver failure.

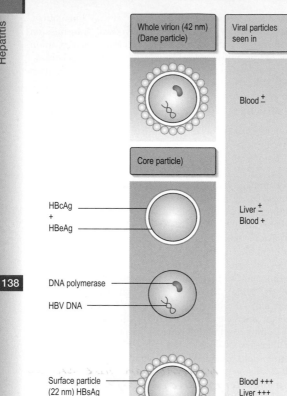

Fig. 4.4   **Hepatitis B virus: the antigenic components.**

A minority of patients do not clear HBsAg from the serum and become chronic carriers. The risk of developing chronic HBV infection is inversely related to age at the time of infection. Ninety per cent of infants infected at birth will

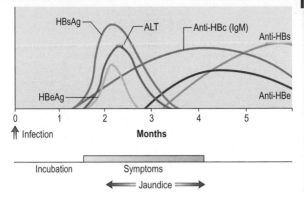

- **HBsAg**
  is found in acute hepatitis and persists in chronic carriers

- **HBsAg with HBeAg**
  is present in acute hepatitis
  its presence in chronic HBV infection is correlated with increased
  infectivity and development of chronic liver disease

- **HBsAg with anti-HBe**
  occurs in recovery from acute infection. In chronic infection it
  indicates decreased infectivity

- **Anti-HBs appears late and indicates immunity**

- **HBV DNA suggests continued viral replication**

Fig. 4.5 **Time course of the events and serological
changes seen following infection with hepatitis B virus.**

become chronically infected with HBV, but only about 5%
of adults (Fig. 4.6).

Chronic HBV carriers

The persistence of HBsAg in the serum for more than
6 months after acute infection defines the carrier status.
Carriers who, in addition, have HBeAg or viral DNA in the
serum (i.e. have active viral replication) are highly infectious
and are at greatest risk of developing chronic hepatitis (see
below) and cirrhosis, with the attendant increased risk of
hepatocellular carcinoma. Patients in this group with
abnormal liver biochemistry should be considered for
treatment (see below). Patients with only HBsAg (low
replication) and antibodies to eAg (anti-HBeAg) are usually

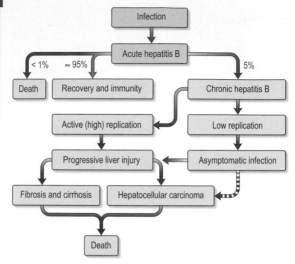

N.B. Acute HBV infection may also be subclinical and present later as chronic liver disease

Fig. 4.6 **The natural history of hepatitis B infection in adults.**

asymptomatic with normal liver biochemistry, and are of relatively low infective risk. Treatment is not indicated for this group of patients but they should have annual assessment of hepatitis B serology and liver biochemistry, since some will develop progressive disease and require treatment.

Chronic hepatitis (*K&C* 6e p. 370)

Approximately 3–5% of patients with acute viral hepatitis B progress to chronic hepatitis. The condition may be asymptomatic, or present with established liver disease and the signs of chronic liver disease on physical examination (see Fig. 4.7). Serum liver biochemistry, particularly the transferases, is usually abnormal. Liver biopsy and histological examination will show the severity of the disease varying from mild inflammatory changes to established cirrhosis.

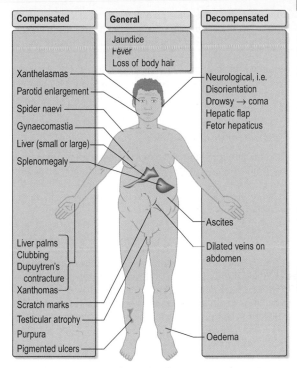

Compensated	General	Decompensated
	Jaundice Fever Loss of body hair	

Xanthelasmas

Parotid enlargement

Spider naevi

Gynaecomastia

Liver (small or large)

Splenomegaly

Liver palms
Clubbing
Dupuytren's
 contracture
Xanthomas

Scratch marks

Testicular atrophy

Purpura

Pigmented ulcers

Neurological, i.e.
Disorientation
Drowsy → coma
Hepatic flap
Fetor hepaticus

Ascites

Dilated veins on
abdomen

Oedema

Fig. 4.7 Physical signs in chronic liver disease.

Treatment of chronic hepatitis B

Treatment is indicated for patients with HBsAg and HBV DNA in the serum with abnormal serum aminotransferases and chronic hepatitis on liver biopsy. Most of these patients will also have HBeAg in the serum unless they have a mutant virus (see above). The aim of treatment is to eliminate HBeAg and HBV DNA from the serum and reduce inflammatory necrosis of the hepatocyte; this is accomplished in 25–40% of patients.

There are three antiviral agents for the treatment of chronic hepatitis B: pegylated alpha-interferon (IFN), lamivudine and adefovir. IFN is administered by subcutaneous injection weekly for 16–24 weeks. Side-effects include flu-like symptoms, depression and neutropenia. Lamivudine and adefovir are administered orally for at least 1 year. They are generally well tolerated but the durability of response is less than with IFN. Long-term therapy with lamivudine is associated with development of drug-resistant mutants with reappearance of HBV DNA in the serum.

Prophylaxis (*K&C* 6e p. 366)

The avoidance of high-risk factors (needle sharing, prostitutes and multiple male homosexual partners) and counselling patients who are potentially infective are important aspects of prevention. Active immunization with a recombinant yeast vaccine is universal in most developed countries. In the UK it is only recommended for those at increased risk, e.g. healthcare workers, homosexuals, intravenous drug abusers and haemodialysis patients. The immunity that develops after active immunization lasts for over 10 years. Combined prophylaxis (i.e. active immunization and passive immunization with specific antihepatitis B immunoglobulin) is given to non-immune individuals after high-risk exposure, e.g. a needle-stick injury from a carrier, newborn babies of HBsAg-positive mothers and HBV-negative sexual partners of HBsAg-positive patients.

Hepatitis D (delta or δ agent) nd (*K&C* 6e p. 367)

Hepatitis D virus (HDV) is an incomplete RNA virus enclosed in a shell of HBsAg. It is unable to replicate on its own, but is activated by the presence of HBV. It can affect all risk groups for HBV infection, but is seen particularly in intravenous drug abusers. HDV infection can occur as a co-infection with HBV or as a superinfection in an already HBsAg-positive patient, and thus presents as an illness indistinguishable from acute HBV infection or as a flare-up of previously quiescent chronic HBV infection. Diagnosis is by finding IgM anti-D in the serum.

Hepatitis C nd (*K&C* 6e p. 367)

Epidemiology

Hepatitis C virus (HCV) is an RNA virus. It is present world-wide, but is more common in southern Europe,

Africa and Egypt. The virus is transmitted by blood and blood products. In about 20% of patients the exact mode of infection is not known. There are six genotypes of hepatitis C (types 1–6) of which type 1 is the most common in Europe and the US.

Clinical features

Acute infection is usually mild, with jaundice developing in less than 10% of cases. Most patients infected with HCV go on to develop chronic liver disease and will not be diagnosed until they present, years later, with elevated serum aminotransferase levels found on routine biochemistry (e.g. at health checks) or with symptoms and signs of chronic liver disease and cirrhosis (Fig. 4.7). Patients with cirrhosis secondary to chronic HCV are at increased risk for the development of hepatocellular carcinoma. Extrahepatic manifestations of chronic HCV infection include arthritis, glomerulonephritis associated with cryoglobulinaemia, and porphyria cutanea tarda.

Diagnosis

This is made by finding HCV antibody in the serum. Antibodies may take 6 weeks to appear after acute infection, and thus an early negative result does not exclude acute HCV infection. Patients with antibodies to hepatitis C should undergo further tests to look for the presence of HCV RNA in the serum. A positive result indicates ongoing infection, and a liver biopsy is usually then performed to assess the histological activity of disease and to detect the presence or absence of fibrosis and cirrhosis.

Management

Treatment of HCV is with pegylated IFN-α and ribavirin, both of which inhibit viral replication. The addition of polyethylene glycol (PEG) to IFN prolongs its half-life leading to sustained plasma levels, fewer side-effects and better efficacy than standard IFN. The aim of treatment is sustained viral clearance, i.e. the absence of HCV RNA in the serum 6 months after treatment. Patients with genotypes 2 and 3 are treated for 24 weeks, with 80% sustained response rates. Patients with other genotypes are treated for 48 weeks (40–50% sustained response).

Table 4.3	Grading of hepatic encephalopathy
Grade I	Daytime somnolence, asterixis (flapping tremor of outstretched hands)
Grade II	Confusion, disorientation, agitation and impaired coordination
Grade III	Increasing drowsiness, stupor, no communication possible
Grade IV	Coma, increased rigidity, extensor plantar response

Hepatitis E nd (K&C 6e p. 368)

This is due to an RNA virus which causes enteral (epidemic or water-borne) hepatitis similar to hepatitis A, particularly in developing countries. There is no chronic carrier state and it does not progress to chronic liver disease, but the mortality rate from fulminant hepatic failure is about 1–2%, rising to 20% in pregnant women.

Fulminant hepatic failure (K&C 6e p. 368)

Fulminant hepatic failure is defined as hepatic failure with encephalopathy developing in less than 2 weeks in a patient with a previously normal liver, or in patients with an acute exacerbation of underlying liver disease. It is an infrequent complication of acute hepatitis (from any cause) and occurs as a result of massive liver cell necrosis. In the UK, viral hepatitis and paracetamol overdose are the most common causes. Presentation is with hepatic encephalopathy of varying severity (Table 4.3), accompanied by severe jaundice and a marked coagulopathy. The complications include cerebral oedema, hypoglycaemia, severe bacterial and fungal infections, hypotension and renal failure (hepatorenal syndrome). Fulminant hepatic failure should be managed with supportive treatment in a specialist liver unit. Emergency liver transplantation has become a useful treatment, depending on the cause, for the very severe cases (grade IV encephalopathy), of which 80% might otherwise die.

Autoimmune hepatitis (K&C 6e p. 373)

Autoimmune hepatitis is usually a progressive liver disease which is often associated with other autoimmune diseases, e.g. pernicious anaemia, thyroiditis. It is most common in young and middle-aged women but can occur in any age in either sex.

Aetiology

The aetiology is unknown but the disease is characterized by immunological abnormalities including hypergammaglobulinaemia with the most pronounced rise in IgG levels, the presence of circulating autoantibodies and interface hepatitis with portal plasma cell infiltration on liver biopsy.

Clinical features

The onset is often insidious, with anorexia, malaise, nausea and fatigue. Twenty-five per cent present as an acute hepatitis, with rapidly progressive liver disease. The signs of chronic liver disease are often present, with palmar erythema, spider naevae, hepatosplenomegaly and jaundice. Features of other autoimmune diseases may be present.

Investigations

Circulating autoantibodies (antinuclear, smooth muscle, soluble liver antigen, liver/kidney microsomal antibodies) are the hallmarks of the disease. There is hypergammaglobulinaemia (particularly IgG), and the serum bilirubin and aminotransferases are elevated. Liver biopsy will show the non-specific changes of chronic hepatitis, with interface hepatitis and often cirrhosis.

Treatment

Prednisolone 30 mg daily is given for 2–3 weeks. A subsequent reduction in the dose depends on clinical response, but maintenance doses of 10–15 mg are usually required. Azathioprine should be added as a steroid-sparing agent and is usually continued lifelong.

Prognosis

Steroid and azathioprine therapy induce remission in over 80% of cases. The length of treatment is lifelong in most cases with a 5-year survival rate of 90%.

Cirrhosis is a histological diagnosis. It is a diffuse process that results from necrosis of liver cells followed by fibrosis and nodule formation. The end result is impairment of liver cell function and gross distortion of the liver architecture, leading to portal hypertension.

Aetiology

The causes of cirrhosis are shown in Table 4.4. Alcohol is the most common cause in the western world, but viral hepatitis is the most common cause world-wide.

Pathology

Histologically two types of cirrhosis have been described: micronodular and macronodular.

- Micronodular cirrhosis is characterized by uniform, small nodules up to 3 mm in diameter. This type is often caused by alcohol damage.
- In macronodular cirrhosis large nodules up to several centimetres in diameter are present. This type is often seen following hepatitis B infection.
- There is also a mixed picture, with both small and large nodules.

Clinical features

These are secondary to portal hypertension and liver cell failure (Fig. 4.7). Cirrhosis with the complications of encephalopathy, ascites or variceal haemorrhage is designated decompensated cirrhosis. Cirrhosis without any of these complications is termed compensated cirrhosis.

Investigations

These are performed to assess the severity of liver disease, identify the aetiology and screen for complications.

Severity
- Liver biochemistry may be normal. In most cases there is at least a slight elevation of the serum alkaline phosphatase and aminotransferase.
- Liver function. Serum albumin and prothrombin time are the best indicators of liver function, both reflecting reduced hepatic synthesis.

Table 4.4 Causes of chronic liver disease and cirrhosis

Cause	Non-invasive markers of aetiology
Common	
Alcohol	History of excess alcohol
Chronic hepatitis B	HBsAg ± HBeAg/DNA in serum
Chronic hepatitis C	HCV antibodies and HCV RNA in serum
Others	
Haemochromatosis	Family history, ↑ serum ferritin + transferrin saturation
Non-alcoholic fatty liver disease	Features of the metabolic syndrome, hyperechoic liver on ultrasound
Primary biliary cirrhosis	Presence of serum antimitochondrial antibodies
Sclerosing cholangitis: primary (PSC) and secondary	Most PSC patients have IBD and serum pANCA (p. 948), multifocal stricturing and dilatation of bile ducts on cholangiography (either MRCP or ERCP)
Autoimmune hepatitis	Circulating autoantibodies (p. 145), hypergammaglobulinaemia
Cystic fibrosis	Presence of extrahepatic manifestations of CF (p. 506)
Budd–Chiari syndrome	Presence of known risk factors (p. 165), caudate lobe hypertrophy, abnormal flow in major hepatic veins on US
Wilson's disease	Young age, ↓ serum caeruloplasmin and total copper, ↑ 24-h urinary copper excretion, Kayser–Fleischer rings
α_1-Antitrypsin (AAT) deficiency	Young age, associated emphysema, ↓ serum AAT
Drugs, e.g. methotrexate	Drug history

IBD, inflammatory bowel disease

- Serum electrolytes. A low sodium concentration indicates severe liver disease secondary to either impaired free water clearance or excess diuretic therapy.
- Serum α fetoprotein (AFP). This is usually undetectable after fetal life, but raised levels may occur in chronic liver disease. It is measured principally to screen for the complication of hepatocellular carcinoma (HCC). The normal range is 10–20 ng/mL, and a level of greater than 400 ng/mL is usually regarded as diagnostic of HCC.

Aetiology

The cause of cirrhosis can usually be determined by the history combined with laboratory investigations (Table 4.4). A liver biopsy is performed to confirm the severity and type of liver disease.

Further investigations

Oesophageal varices are sought with endoscopy. An ultrasound is useful for detection of hepatocellular carcinoma, and to assess the patency of the portal and hepatic veins (p. 164).

Management

Cirrhosis is irreversible and frequently progresses. Management is that of the complications seen in decompensated cirrhosis as they arise. Correcting the underlying cause, e.g. venesection for haemochromatosis, abstinence from alcohol for alcoholic cirrhosis, may halt the progression of liver disease. Screening for hepatocellular carcinoma (measurement of serum AFP and ultrasonography every 6 months) is performed to identify tumours at an early stage. Liver transplantation should be considered in patients with end-stage cirrhosis. Patients should also be offered influenza immunization.

Prognosis

This is variable and depends on the aetiology and the presence of complications. The severity and prognosis of liver disease can be graded according to five variables: encephalopathy, ascites, prothrombin time, serum bilirubin and albumin (Child's grading, or modifications thereof). Overall the 5-year survival rate is approximately 50%.

Complications

The complications of cirrhosis are shown in Table 4.5.

Portal hypertension (K&C 6e p. 378)

The portal vein carries blood from the gut and spleen to the liver, and accounts for 75% of hepatic vascular inflow (25% is via the hepatic artery). Blood vessels enter the liver via the hilum (porta hepatis) and blood passes into the hepatic

Table 4.5	Complications of cirrhosis

Portal hypertension and variceal haemorrhage
Ascites
Infected ascites (spontaneous bacterial peritonitis)
Portosystemic encephalopathy
Acute renal failure (hepatorenal syndrome)
Hepatocellular carcinoma (HCC)
Malnutrition
Osteoporosis

Table 4.6	Causes of portal hypertension
Prehepatic	Portal vein thrombosis
Intrahepatic	Cirrhosis
	Alcoholic hepatitis
	Idiopathic non-cirrhotic portal hypertension
	Schistosomiasis
Posthepatic	Budd–Chiari syndrome
	Veno-occlusive disease
	Right heart failure – rare
	Constrictive pericarditis

sinusoids via the portal tracts and leaves the liver through the hepatic veins to join the inferior vena cava. The normal portal pressure is 8–10 mmHg. The inflow of portal blood to the liver can be partially or completely obstructed at a number of sites, leading to high pressure proximal to the obstruction and the diversion of blood into portosystemic collaterals. The most important site for collateral formation is at the gastro-oesophageal junction (varices), where they are superficial and liable to rupture, causing massive gastrointestinal haemorrhage.

The main sites of obstruction are:

- Prehepatic, caused by blockage of the portal vein before the liver
- Intrahepatic, resulting from distortion of the liver architecture
- Posthepatic, as a result of obstruction of the hepatic veins.

Aetiology

The causes of portal hypertension are outlined in Table 4.6. The most common cause is cirrhosis.

Cirrhosis

Clinical features

The characteristic clinical manifestations of portal hypertension are:

- Gastrointestinal bleeding from oesophageal or less commonly gastric varices
- Ascites
- Hepatic encephalopathy.

Variceal haemorrhage (*K&C* 6e p. 379)

Only 30% of patients with varices ever bleed from them, and bleeding is most common in those with large varices. Bleeding is often massive and mortality is as high as 50%.

Management

The general management of GI bleeding is discussed on page 82.

Acute bleeding Patients should be resuscitated and undergo urgent gastroscopy to confirm the diagnosis and exclude bleeding from other sites.

- Endoscopic therapy is the treatment of choice for active variceal haemorrhage and will stop bleeding in 80% of cases bleeding from oesophageal varices. Two forms are available: sclerotherapy or variceal band ligation. Sclerotherapy involves injection of a sclerosant solution (e.g. ethanolamine) into the varices. Variceal band ligation is similar to haemorrhoidal banding and involves placing small elastic bands around the varices.
- Pharmacological treatment is used for emergency control of bleeding whilst waiting for endoscopy and in combination with endoscopic techniques. Terlipressin is a synthetic analogue of vasopressin that restricts portal inflow by splanchnic arterial constriction. It is given by intravenous bolus injection (2 mg 6-hourly) and is contraindicated in patients with ischaemic heart disease. Octreotide (a somatostatin analogue, 50 µg i.v. stat followed by 50 µg hourly by intravenous infusion) lowers portal pressure by a similar mechanism to terlipressin but is less effective.
- Balloon tamponade with a Sengstaken–Blakemore tube is used if bleeding continues (p. 813). It can have serious complications, such as aspiration pneumonia, oesophageal

rupture and mucosal ulceration. To reduce complications, the airway should be protected, and the tube left in situ for no longer than 12 hours

- TIPS (transjugular intrahepatic portosystemic shunting) is used when there is a second rebleed after treatment. A metal stent is passed over a guidewire in the internal jugular vein. The stent is then pushed into the liver substance, under radiological guidance, to form a shunt between the portal and hepatic veins, thus lowering portal pressure.
- Surgery (oesophageal transection and ligation of varices) is occasionally necessary if bleeding continues in spite of all the above measures.
- Additional treatment. Patients require high-dependency/ ITU nursing. Bacterial infection is common after upper gastrointestinal bleeding in cirrhotic patients and all patients should have antibiotic prophylaxis with ciprofloxacin (500 mg twice daily for 7 days). Lactulose should be given to prevent portosystemic encephalopathy, and sucralfate to reduce oesophageal ulceration, a complication of endoscopic therapy.

Prophylaxis Following an episode of variceal bleeding there is a high risk of recurrence (60–80% over a 2-year period), and therefore treatment is given to prevent further bleeds (secondary prophylaxis). The main options are:

- Oral propranolol, which decreases portal pressure, but some patients are intolerant of treatment because of side-effects. Propranolol is also given to patients with varices who have never bled (primary prophylaxis).
- Repeated courses of variceal banding at 2-weekly intervals until the varices are obliterated.
- TIPS or occasionally a surgical portosystemic shunt (portal vein to vena cava – or splenorenal) which is performed if endoscopic or medical therapy fails. Liver transplantation should always be considered when there is poor liver function.

Ascites (*K&C* 6e p. 381)

This is the presence of fluid in the peritoneal cavity and is a common complication of cirrhosis of the liver.

Aetiology

In cirrhosis, peripheral arterial vasodilatation (mediated by nitric oxide and other vasodilators) leads to a reduction in effective blood volume, with activation of the sympathetic nervous system and renin–angiotensin system, thus promoting renal salt and water retention. The formation of oedema is encouraged by hypoalbuminaemia and mainly localized to the peritoneal cavity as a result of the portal hypertension.

Clinical features

There is fullness in the flanks, with shifting dullness. Tense ascites is uncomfortable and may produce respiratory distress. A pleural effusion (usually right-sided) and peripheral oedema may be present.

Investigations

A diagnostic aspiration (paracentesis, p. 812) of 10–20 mL of fluid should be carried out in all patients, and the following performed:

- Cell count. A neutrophil count > 250 cells/mm^3 indicates underlying (usually spontaneous) bacterial peritonitis
- Gram stain and culture for bacteria and acid-fast bacilli
- Protein. An ascitic protein of 11 g/L or more below the serum albumin level suggests a transudate; a value of < 11 g/L suggests an exudate
- Cytology for malignant cells
- Amylase to exclude pancreatic ascites.

The causes of ascites are listed in Table 4.7; the commonest cause is cirrhosis.

Table 4.7 Causes of ascites	
Transudate	**Exudate**
Cirrhosis	Malignancy
Constrictive pericarditis	Infection, e.g. pyogenic, tuberculous
Cardiac failure	Pancreatitis
Hypoalbuminaemia, e.g. nephrotic syndrome	Budd–Chiari syndrome
Meig's syndrome*	Myxoedema
	Lymphatic obstruction (chylous ascites)

*Meig's syndrome is the combination of an ovarian tumour, ascites and hydrothorax

Management

Treatment of ascites depends on the cause. The management of ascites due to portal hypertension is described below. In other cases, ascites will improve with treatment of the underlying condition.

Diuretics The management of ascites resulting from cirrhosis is based on a stepwise approach, starting with dietary sodium restriction (60 mmol/day) and oral spironolactone 100 mg daily, increasing gradually to 400 mg daily if necessary. Furosemide (frusemide) 20–40 mg daily is added if the response is poor and increased gradually to 160 mg if necessary. The rate of fluid loss is best assessed by changes in bodyweight. The aim of diuretic therapy is to produce weight loss of about 0.5 kg/day, because the maximum rate of transfer of fluid from the ascitic to the vascular compartment is only about 700 mL/day. Too rapid a diuresis causes volume depletion and hypokalaemia, and precipitates encephalopathy. In combination with dietary sodium restriction this medical approach is effective in over 90% of patients.

Paracentesis This is used in patients with tense ascites or who are resistant to standard medical therapy. All the ascites can be removed over several hours, providing rapid symptom relief and reduced hospital stay compared to treatment with diuretics. The major danger of this approach is the production of hypovolaemia because the ascites reaccumulates at the expense of the circulating volume. This is largely overcome by the intravenous infusion of albumin (8 g per litre removed) administered immediately after paracentesis.

Transjugular intrahepatic portosystemic shunt (TIPS, p. 151) is occasionally used for resistant ascites.

Complications

Spontaneous bacterial peritonitis (SBP) occurs in 8% of cirrhotic patients with ascites and has a mortality rate of 25%. The most common infecting organism is *Escherichia coli*. Clinical features may be minimal, but include abdominal pain and fever. Diagnosis is made on the ascitic fluid white cell count, and Gram stain and culture (p. 152). Empirical therapy, e.g. intravenous cefotaxime 2 g 8-hourly, should be

Cirrhosis

started in patients with an ascitic fluid neutrophil count of ≥ 250 cells/mm^3 rather than waiting for the results of culture. Recurrence is common and is reduced by antibiotic prophylaxis with oral norfloxacin. SBP is also an indication for referral to a liver transplant centre.

Portosystemic encephalopathy (K&C 6e p. 383)

The term 'portosystemic encephalopathy' (PSE) refers to a chronic neuropsychiatric syndrome which occurs with advanced hepatocellular disease, either chronic (cirrhosis) or acute (fulminant hepatic failure). It is also seen in patients following TIPS.

Pathophysiology

The mechanisms are unclear but are believed to involve 'toxic' substances, normally detoxified by the liver, bypassing the liver via the collaterals and gaining access to the brain. A putative toxin is ammonia produced from the breakdown of dietary protein by gut bacteria. In chronic liver disease there is an acute-on-chronic course, with acute episodes precipitated by a number of possible factors (Table 4.8).

Clinical features

The earliest features are lethargy, mild confusion, anorexia and a reversal of the sleep pattern, with the patient sleeping during the day and restless at night. Later there is disorientation, a decreased conscious level and eventually coma (see Table 4.3). The signs are fetor hepaticus (a sweet

154

Table 4.8 Factors precipitating portosystemic encephalopathy

Gastrointestinal haemorrhage (i.e. a high protein load)
Infection
Fluid and electrolyte disturbance (spontaneous or
    diuretic-induced)
Sedative drugs, e.g. opiates, diazepam
Development of a hepatoma
Portosystemic shunt operations and TIPS
Constipation
High dietary protein

smell to the breath), a flapping tremor of the outstretched hand (asterixis), inability to draw a five-pointed star (constructional apraxia) and a prolonged trail-making test (the ability to join numbers and letters within a certain time). Serial attempts are easily compared and used to monitor patient progress.

Differential diagnosis

None of the manifestations of hepatic encephalopathy are specific to this disorder. Alternative diagnoses such as other metabolic or toxic encephalopathies or intracranial mass lesions may present similarly and should be considered.

Investigations

The diagnosis is clinical. An EEG (showing δ waves) and visual evoked potentials may aid diagnosis in difficult cases.

Management

The aims of management are to identify and treat any precipitating factors (Table 4.8) and to minimize the absorption of nitrogenous material, particularly ammonia, from the gut. This is achieved by the following:

- Laxatives. Oral lactulose (10–30 mL three times daily) is an osmotic purgative that reduces colonic pH and increases transit. It may be given via a nasogastric tube if the patient is comatose. The dose should be titrated to result in 2–4 soft stools daily.
- Antibiotics are given to reduce the number of bowel organisms and hence production of ammonia. Rifaximin is mainly unabsorbed and well tolerated. Oral metronidazole (200 mg four times daily) is also used.
- Maintenance of nutrition with adequate calories. Protein is initially restricted but increased after 48 hours as encephalopathy improves.

Prognosis

The prognosis is that of the underlying liver disease.

Hepatorenal syndrome (K&C 6e pp. 384 & 665)

This is the development of acute renal failure in a patient who usually has advanced liver disease, either cirrhosis or alcoholic hepatitis. Splanchnic vasodilatation results in a fall in systemic vascular resistance and severe vasoconstriction of the renal circulation with markedly reduced renal perfusion. The diagnosis is made on the basis of oliguria, a rising serum creatinine (over days to weeks), a low urine sodium (< 10 mmol/L), absence of other causes of renal failure, and lack of improvement after volume expansion (if necessary) and withdrawal of diuretics. The prognosis is poor, and renal failure will often only respond to an improvement in liver function. Albumin infusion and terlipressin have been used with some success.

TYPES OF CHRONIC LIVER DISEASE AND CIRRHOSIS

Alcoholic

This is discussed in the section on alcoholic liver disease (p. 163).

Hereditary haemochromatosis (*K&C* 6e p. 386)

Hereditary haemochromatosis (HH) is a common autosomal recessive disorder with a prevalence in the Caucasian population of 1 in 400, with approximately 10% of the population being carriers. It is characterized by excess iron deposition in various organs, leading to eventual fibrosis and functional organ failure.

Aetiology

HH is characterized by inappropriately increased iron absorption from the upper small intestine. The clinical manifestations are related to excessive iron deposition in various parenchymal organs, notably the liver, pancreas, joints, heart, pituitary gland and skin. HH is due to a mutation in the gene *HFE* on the short arm of chromosome 6. The normal HFE protein is expressed in the small intestine and plays a role in the regulation of iron absorption. Two missense mutations of the *HFE* gene account for most patients with HH – one resulting in a change of cysteine at position 282 for tyrosine (known as the C282Y mutation). The second is a change of histidine at position 63 to aspartate (known as the H63D mutation). HLA-A3, -B7 and -B14 occur with increased frequency compared to the general population.

Table 4.9 Clinical presentation of haemochromatosis
Health screening (often symptomatic) Abnormal liver biochemistry Abnormal iron studies Familial and/or population screening
Symptomatic disease Lethargy Arthralgia Loss of libido Hepatomegaly Diabetes mellitus Congestive cardiac failure Cardiac dysrhythmias Increased skin pigmentation

Clinical features

Most patients are currently diagnosed when elevated serum iron or ferritin levels are noted on routine biochemistry, or screening is performed because a relative is diagnosed with HH. Presentation may also be with symptoms and signs of iron loading in parenchymal organs (Table 4.9). There is a reduced incidence of overt disease in women, presumably because of iron lost in blood during menstruation.

Investigations

- Serum liver biochemistry is often normal even with cirrhosis.
- Serum iron is elevated and total iron-binding capacity (TIBC) reduced. The transferrin saturation (serum iron/ TIBC) is > 60% (normal < 33%).
- Serum ferritin reflects iron stores and is usually greatly elevated (often > 500 µg/L).
- Genotyping (by PCR reaction using whole blood samples) for mutation analysis of the *HFE* gene is performed in patients with elevated ferritin and transferrin saturation.
- Patients with abnormal iron studies and mutations of the *HFE* gene are treated by phlebotomy without the need for biopsy. Liver biopsy to document the degree of fibrosis is performed in patients who are predicted to

have significant hepatic injury (abnormal liver bio-chemistry or serum ferritin > 1000 µg/L) and to measure hepatic iron content if the diagnosis is in doubt.

Causes of secondary iron overload, such as multiple transfusions, must be excluded. In addition, in alcoholic liver disease hepatic iron stores may increase. The precise reason is unknown, but the hepatic iron concentration does not reach the very high levels seen in haemochromatosis.

Management

The aim of treatment is to remove excess tissue iron and render the patient iron deficient (ferritin < 50 µg/L) while maintaining a haemoglobin of greater than 11 g/dL. This is best achieved by venesection: 500 mL of blood (containing 250 mg of iron) are removed twice-weekly, and this may need to be continued for up to 2 years. Three or four venesections per year are then required life-long to prevent the reaccumulation of iron. Surveillance (p. 167) for HCC is performed in patients with cirrhosis.

Genotyping to detect *HFE* mutations and iron studies should be performed on first-degree relatives of affected individuals.

Prognosis

The major complication is the development of hepato-cellular carcinoma in patients with cirrhosis. This can be prevented by venesection before cirrhosis develops, and life expectancy is then much the same as for the normal population.

Primary biliary cirrhosis (*K&C* 6e p. 385)

Primary biliary cirrhosis (PBC) is a chronic disorder in which there is progressive destruction of intrahepatic bile ducts causing cholestasis, eventually leading to cirrhosis.

Epidemiology

It affects predominantly women in the age range 40–50 years.

Aetiology

The cause of PBC is unknown but most data suggest that it is due to an inherited abnormality of immunoregulation, leading to immune-mediated damage to bile duct epithelial cells. It is thought that disease expression results from an environmental trigger, possibly infective, in a genetically susceptible individual. Antimitochondrial antibodies (AMAs) are present in almost all (> 95%) patients, but their role in the pathogenesis of this disorder is unclear.

Clinical features

Pruritus, with or without jaundice, is the single most common presenting complaint. In advanced disease there is, in addition, hepatosplenomegaly and xanthelasma (PBC is a cause of secondary hypercholesterolaemia). Asymptomatic patients may be discovered on routine examination or screening to have hepatomegaly, a raised serum alkaline phosphatase or autoantibodies. Patients with advanced disease may have steatorrhoea and malabsorption of fat-soluble vitamins owing to decreased biliary secretion of bile acids and the resulting low concentrations of bile acids in the small intestine. Autoimmune disorders, e.g. Sjögren's syndrome, scleroderma and rheumatoid arthritis, occur with increased frequency.

Investigations

- Liver biochemistry may show only a raised serum alkaline phosphatase, often very high (> 1000 U/L).
- Serum AMAs are found in more than 95% of patients and a titre of 1 : 160 or greater makes the diagnosis very likely. M2 antibody is specific. Other non-specific antibodies, e.g. antinuclear factor, may also be present.
- Serum IgM may be high.
- Liver biopsy shows loss of bile ducts, lymphocyte infiltration of the portal tracts, granuloma formation and, at a later stage, fibrosis and eventually cirrhosis.
- An ultrasound scan is sometimes performed in the jaundiced patient to exclude extrahepatic biliary obstruction.

Management

Ursodeoxycholic acid (ursodiol, 10–15 mg/kg by mouth) is a naturally occurring dihydroxy bile acid. It improves biochemistry, though it is unclear whether prognosis is altered. The mechanism of benefit of ursodiol in PBC is incompletely understood. Pruritus may be helped by colestyramine, and malabsorption of fat-soluble vitamins (A, D, K) is treated by supplementation. Liver transplantation is indicated for patients with advanced disease (bilirubin > 100 µmol/L).

Prognosis

Asymptomatic patients may show a near-normal life expectancy. In symptomatic patients with jaundice there is a steady downhill course, with death in approximately 5 years without transplantation.

Secondary biliary cirrhosis (K&C 6e p. 386)

Cirrhosis can result from prolonged (for months) large duct biliary obstruction. Causes include bile duct strictures, common bile duct stones and sclerosing cholangitis. Ultrasound examination followed by MRCP is performed to outline the ducts. ERCP may then be necessary to treat the cause, e.g. stone removal.

Wilson's disease (hepatolenticular degeneration) (K&C 6e p. 387)

This is a rare, recessively inherited disorder in which there is failure of biliary excretion of copper, resulting in accumulation of copper and deposition in the liver, basal ganglia of the brain and the cornea. Although this is a rare disease it is potentially treatable and therefore all young patients with liver disease must be screened for this condition.

Clinical features

Children usually present with hepatic problems ranging from fulminant hepatic failure to cirrhosis. Young adults have more neurological problems, which start with a mild tremor and speech problems and progress to involuntary movements and eventual dementia. A specific sign is the Kayser–Fleischer ring, which is caused by copper deposition in Descemet's membrane in the cornea. It appears as a greenish-brown pigment at the periphery of the cornea, best seen with a slit-lamp. Additional features are haemolytic anaemia and renal tubular defects.

Investigations

The diagnosis is usually made by demonstrating the following:

- Total serum copper and caeruloplasmin (the copper-carrying protein) are usually low but can be normal
- Urinary copper is usually increased on a 24-hour collection
- Increased hepatic copper concentration in a liver biopsy specimen.

Management

Lifelong treatment with penicillamine is effective in chelating copper, which is then excreted in the urine. Liver transplantation may be offered to those with end-stage liver disease. First-degree relatives are screened by slit-lamp examination of the eye, serum caeruloplasmin measurements and, where possible, genotype testing based on the findings in the index patient. Asymptomatic homozygotes should be treated.

α_1-Antitrypsin deficiency (K&C 6e p. 388)

This is a rare cause of cirrhosis. Mutations in the α_1-antitrypsin (α_1-AT) gene on chromosome 14 lead to reduced production of α_1-AT, which normally inhibits the proteolytic enzyme elastase. The genetic variants of α_1-AT are characterized by their electrophoretic mobilities as medium (M), slow (S) or very slow (Z). The normal genotype is PiMM, the homozygote for Z is PiZZ and the heterozygotes are PiMZ and PiSZ. S and Z variants are caused by single amino acid substitutions in the polypeptide chain that favours the formation of polymers which are retained within hepatocytes as inclusion bodies, leading to hepatocellular damage. In the lung, deficiency of α_1-AT leads to proteolytic lung damage and predisposes to emphysema.

Clinical features

The majority of patients with clinical disease are homozygous with a PiZZ phenotype. They have very low circulating levels of α_1-AT, associated with chronic liver disease and pulmonary emphysema (especially in smokers). The risk of liver disease is much smaller in heterozygotes, e.g. PiSZ or PiMZ.

Investigations

The serum α_1-AT is low. Liver biopsy demonstrates cirrhosis and α_1-AT-containing globules in the hepatocytes.

Management

There is no specific treatment. Patients should be advised to stop smoking.

Non-alcoholic fatty liver disease (NAFLD) (*K&C* 6e p. 374)

In this condition the liver biopsy findings show changes indistinguishable from those ascribed to alcohol excess but they occur in the absence of heavy drinking. When there is inflammation as well as fatty change the condition is called non-alcoholic steatohepatitis (NASH). Fatty liver is frequently associated with obesity, type II diabetes mellitus, hypertension and hyperlipidaemia (the metabolic syndrome). The exact pathogenesis is not known but it is thought that insulin resistance is a key mechanism leading to fatty liver and then a 'second hit' or oxidative injury is required to manifest the inflammatory component or steatohepatitis.

Clinical features

Most patients with NAFLD are asymptomatic and the most common presentation is mild elevations of transaminases discovered on routine laboratory testing. Hepatomegaly is a frequent finding on clinical examination.

Investigations

Ultrasonography often shows a hyperechoic texture or bright liver because of diffuse fatty infiltration. Similarly CT and MRI can show fatty liver but the findings are non-specific and these investigations do not show the degree of inflammation or fibrosis. Other causes of chronic liver disease should be excluded (Table 4.4). Liver biopsy allows staging the disease but when this should be performed is unclear. Most would biopsy if the ALT is persistently over twice normal.

Management

There is no proven effective therapy for NASH and management centres on treatment of risk factors such as obesity (see above). Transplantation may be needed for end-stage disease.

Alcohol and the liver (K&C 6e p. 389)

Alcohol is the most common cause of chronic liver disease in the western world. Alcoholic liver disease occurs more commonly in men, usually in the fourth and fifth decades, although subjects can present in their 20s with advanced disease. Although alcohol acts as a hepatotoxin, the exact mechanism leading to hepatitis and cirrhosis is unknown. As only 10–20% of people who drink excessively develop cirrhosis, genetic predisposition and immunological mechanisms have been proposed.

There are three major pathological lesions and clinical illnesses associated with excessive alcohol intake.

Alcoholic fatty liver

This is the most common biopsy finding in alcoholic individuals. Metabolism of alcohol within the liver produces fat, which accumulates within the hepatocyte (steatosis). Symptoms are usually absent, and on examination there may be hepatomegaly. Laboratory tests are often normal, although an elevated mean corpuscular volume (MCV) often indicates heavy drinking. The γ-GT level is usually elevated. The fat disappears on cessation of alcohol intake but with continued drinking may progress to fibrosis and cirrhosis.

Alcoholic hepatitis

There is necrosis of the liver cells and infiltration of polymorphonuclear leucocytes, with accumulation of dense cytoplasmic material called a Mallory body in the hepatocytes. It may progress to cirrhosis, particularly with continued alcohol consumption. Presentation encompasses a broad spectrum of patients, from those who are asymptomatic to those who are very ill with hepatic failure. Investigations show a leucocytosis with elevated bilirubin and transferases. However, the AST and ALT are usually less than 500IU/L and higher values suggest hepatitis due to another cause (p. 133). The albumin may be low and prothrombin time prolonged. Treatment is supportive and

163

adequate nutritional intake must be maintained. Cortico-steroids are of benefit in severe disease.

Alcoholic cirrhosis

This represents the final stage of liver disease from alcohol abuse. There is destruction and fibrosis, with regenerating nodules producing a classic micronodular cirrhosis. Patients may be asymptomatic, although they often present with one of the complications of cirrhosis and there are usually signs of chronic liver disease. Investigation is as for cirrhosis in general. Management is directed at the complications of cirrhosis, and patients are advised to stop drinking for life. Abstinence from alcohol improves the 5-year survival rate.

LIVER TRANSPLANTATION (*K&C* 6e p. 376)

Liver transplantation should be considered for acute or chronic liver failure of any cause. Careful selection of patients is crucial. Psychological assessment and education of patients and their families is essential before trans-plantation. In adults primary biliary cirrhosis is a common indication and, in these patients where the natural history is well defined, transplantation is offered when the serum bilirubin reaches 100 µmol/L. Absolute contraindications to transplantation are active sepsis outside the liver and biliary tree, malignancy outside the liver, liver metastases and if the patient is not psychologically committed. With rare exceptions, patients over 65 years are not transplanted. Graft rejection is reduced by immunosuppression with a ciclosporin- or tacrolimus-(FK506)-based regimen. Early complications include haemorrhage, sepsis and acute rejection (< 6 weeks), which is reversible with intensive immunosuppression. Late complications include recurrence of disease (hepatitis B and C) and chronic rejection, which is not reversible and requires retransplantation. The out-come of liver transplantation is good, with an overall 5-year survival rate of 70–85%.

BUDD–CHIARI SYNDROME (*K&C* 6e p. 390)

Budd–Chiari syndrome is caused by occlusion of the hepatic vein, thereby obstructing venous outflow from the liver. The resulting venous stasis and congestion within the liver leads to hypoxic damage and necrosis of hepatocytes.

Aetiology

Myeloproliferative disorders (polycythaemia vera, essential thrombocythaemia) and the accompanying hypercoagulable state are the commonest cause of Budd–Chiari syndrome. Malignancy, oral contraceptives, pregnancy and the inherited thrombophilias are also associated with venous thrombosis and occlusion of the hepatic vein. The cause is unknown in 20% of cases.

Clinical features

Clinical manifestations depend on the extent and rapidity of the hepatic vein occlusion and whether a venous collateral circulation has developed. Right upper quadrant pain, hepatomegaly, jaundice and ascites are typical features. Acute disease may also present with fulminant hepatic failure. Cirrhosis may develop in the chronically congested liver resulting in portal hypertension and the development of varices and other features of portal hypertension (p. 150).

Investigations

Doppler ultrasound is the initial investigation of choice. This will show abnormal flow in the major hepatic veins or inferior vena cava and thickening, tortuosity, and dilatation of the walls of the hepatic veins. Non-specific findings include hepatomegaly, splenomegaly, ascites and caudate lobe hypertrophy. CT scan or MRI may demonstrate abnormalities of the hepatic veins if the ultrasound is normal and clinical suspicion is high.

Treatment

The goals of therapy are threefold:
- To restore hepatic venous drainage. This is usually only feasible in the acute situation and includes thrombolysis, angioplasty and stent insertion, or TIPS.
- Treatment of complications related to ascites and portal hypertension (p. 150).
- Detection of underlying hypercoagulable disorder and prevention of further clot formation.

LIVER ABSCESS (K&C 6e p. 391)

Liver abscesses are pyogenic, amoebic or hydatid (p. 44).

Aetiology

The cause of pyogenic liver abscess is often unknown, although biliary sepsis or portal pyaemia from intra-abdominal sepsis may be responsible. Other causes include trauma, bacteraemia or direct extension from, for example, a perinephric abscess. The organism found most commonly is *Escherichia coli. Streptococcus milleri* and anaerobic organisms such as *Bacteroides* are often seen. An amoebic abscess results from spread of the organism *Entamoeba histolytica* from the bowel to the liver via the portal venous system.

Clinical features

There are non-specific symptoms of fever, lethargy, weight loss and abdominal pain. The liver may be enlarged and tender and there may be consolidation or an effusion in the right side of the chest. Patients with amoebic abscess often do not give a history of dysentery.

Investigations

■ Laboratory abnormalities reflect the non-specific findings of infection including anaemia, raised ESR and low albumin. Serum alkaline phosphatase and bilirubin may be high.
■ An ultrasound will show single or multiple rounded lesions that are hypoechoic in relation to the surrounding liver. CT scan will show the abscesses as non-enhancing cavities with a surrounding rim of inflammation that enhances in relation to the rest of the liver.
■ Serological tests for amoebae, e.g. complement-fixation test or enzyme-linked immunosorbent assay (ELISA), are almost always positive with amoebic abscess.

Management

Patients with clinical and radiological features suggesting amoebic liver abscess can be treated with metronidazole (800 mg three times daily by mouth for 10 days) without the need for aspiration of the abscess. These are patients who are migrants from and travellers to endemic countries and who have a single abscess in the right lobe of the liver. Patients with a presumed pyogenic abscess should have percutaneous aspiration under radiological control and usually placement of a pigtail catheter for continued drainage. Initial antibiotic therapy (intravenous metronidazole and cefuroxime) may be subsequently altered depending on the organisms obtained from aspiration.

JAUNDICE IN PREGNANCY (K&C 6e p. 393)

Viral hepatitis is the single most common cause of jaundice in pregnancy. Three types of liver disease are specific to pregnancy: acute fatty liver of pregnancy (a severe fulminating illness with jaundice, vomiting and hepatic coma); recurrent intrahepatic cholestasis (presenting with jaundice and pruritus); and haemolysis (occasionally producing jaundice), which occurs in pre-eclamptic toxaemia. The three conditions present most commonly in the third trimester and resolve with delivery of the baby.

LIVER TUMOURS (K&C 6e p. 394)

The most common malignant liver tumours are metastatic, particularly those from the gastrointestinal tract, breast or bronchus. Primary liver tumours may be either benign or malignant.

Hepatocellular carcinoma (hepatoma)

Hepatocellular carcinoma (HCC) is one of the most common cancers world-wide, although it is uncommon in the West. The differences in geographical distribution of HCC are probably due to regional variations in exposure to hepatitis B and C virus, and environmental pathogens.

Aetiology

HCC usually develops on a background of cirrhosis particularly due to viral hepatitis. Other suggested aetiological factors include aflatoxin (a metabolite of a fungus found in groundnuts), androgenic steroids and, possibly the contraceptive pill.

Clinical features

Weight loss, anorexia, fever, ascites and abdominal pain occur. The rapid development of these features in a patient with cirrhosis is suggestive of HCC. Because of surveillance, by measurement of serum α-fetoprotein and liver ultrasound, asymptomatic HCC is being found increasingly in asymptomatic patients with known cirrhosis. A focal lesion in the liver in a patient with cirrhosis is highly likely to be HCC.

Investigations

- Serum α-fetoprotein may be raised but is normal in at least a third of patients.
- Ultrasound or CT scanning shows large filling defects in 90% of cases.
- MRI or angiography is useful in cases where there is diagnostic doubt.
- Biopsy is only performed when there is diagnostic doubt, as there is a risk of tumour seeding in the percutaneous needle biopsy tract. For instance, in a patient with cirrhosis and a liver mass greater than 2 cm in diameter, the lesion is almost certainly HCC and biopsy is not indicated.

Management

Surgical resection or liver transplantation is occasionally possible. Percutaneous ablative therapies using ethanol injection or high-frequency ultrasound probes will produce necrosis of the tumour. Transarterial chemoembolization involves the injection of a chemotherapeutic agent and lipiodol into the hepatic artery. It is used in the treatment of large unresectable tumours. Chemotherapy given intravenously has a very limited role.

Prognosis

Overall, the median survival is only 6–20 months.

Benign liver tumours

The most common are haemangiomas, usually found incidentally on a liver ultrasound or CT scan. They require no treatment. Hepatic adenomas are less common and associated with use of oral contraceptives. Resection is required if there are symptoms (e.g. pain, intraperitoneal bleeding).

GALLSTONES (K&C 6e p. 398)

Gallstones are present in 10–20% of the population. They are most common in women, and the prevalence increases with age.

Pathophysiology

Gallstones are of two types:

- *Cholesterol gallstones* are composed mainly of cholesterol, and account for 80% of all gallstones in the western world. Cholesterol is held in solution by the detergent action of bile salts and phospholipids, with which it forms micelles and vesicles. Cholesterol gallstones only form in bile which has an excess of cholesterol, either because there is a relative deficiency of bile salts and phospholipids or a relative excess of cholesterol (supersaturated or lithogenic bile). The formation of cholesterol crystals and gallstones in lithogenic bile is promoted by factors that favour nucleation, such as mucus and calcium. Gallstone formation is further promoted by reduced gallbladder motility and stasis. The mechanism of cholesterol gallstone formation in patients with risk factors (Table 4.10) is frequently multifactorial (cholesterol supersaturation, nucleation factors and reduced gallbladder motility).
- *Pigment stones*, consisting of bilirubin polymers and calcium bilirubinate. They are seen in patients with

169

Table 4.10 Risk factors for cholesterol gallstones

Increased age
Gender (F > M)
Family history
Multiparity
Obesity
Rapid weight loss
Diet (high in animal fat)
Ileal disease or resection
Diabetes mellitus
Drugs (HRT, oral contraceptives, octreotide, ceftriaxone)
Acromegaly treated with octreotide
Liver cirrhosis

HRT, hormone replacement therapy

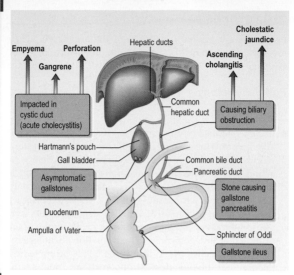

Fig. 4.8 **The complications of gallstones.**

chronic haemolysis, e.g. hereditary spherocytosis and sickle cell disease, in which bilirubin production is increased, and also in cirrhosis. Pigment stones may also form in the bile ducts after cholecystectomy and with duct strictures.

Clinical presentation

Most gallstones never cause symptoms, and cholecystectomy is not indicated in asymptomatic cases. The complications are summarized in Figure 4.8.

Biliary pain (*K&C* 6e p. 399)

Biliary pain (colic) is the term used for the pain associated with the temporary obstruction of the cystic or common bile duct (CBD) by a stone.

Clinical features

There are recurrent episodes of severe constant pain in the upper abdomen, which subsides after several hours. The pain may radiate to the right shoulder and right sub-scapular region and is often associated with vomiting. Examination is usually normal.

Investigations

The diagnosis is usually made on the basis of a typical history and an ultrasound showing gallstones. Increases of serum alkaline phosphatase and bilirubin during an attack support the diagnosis of biliary pain. The absence of inflammatory features (fever, white cell count and local peritonism) differentiates this from acute cholecystitis.

Management

The treatment is analgesia and elective cholecystectomy. Abnormal liver biochemistry or a dilated CBD, or stone in the CBD on ultrasonography, is an indication for pre-operative MRCP and/or ERCP.

Acute cholecystitis (K&C 6e p. 399)

Acute cholecystitis follows the impaction of a stone in the cystic duct or neck of the gall bladder. Very occasionally acute cholecystitis may occur without stones (acalculous cholecystitis).

Clinical features

The initial clinical features are similar to those of biliary colic. However, over a number of hours there is progression to severe pain localized in the right upper quadrant, which is associated with a fever and tenderness and muscle guarding on examination. The tenderness is worse on inspiration (Murphy's sign). Complications include an empyema (pus) and perforation with peritonitis. The diagnosis of acute cholecystitis is usually straightforward. The differential diagnosis includes acute pancreatitis, perforated peptic ulcer, intrahepatic abscess and basal pneumonia.

Investigations

- White cell count shows a leucocytosis.
- Serum liver biochemistry may be mildly abnormal.
- Radiology. The diagnosis is made by ultrasonography showing gallstones and a distended gall bladder with a

thickened wall. There is focal tenderness directly over the visualized gall bladder (sonographic Murphy's sign).

Management

The initial treatment is conservative, with nil by mouth, intravenous fluids, pain relief and intravenous antibiotics, e.g. cefotaxime. Cholecystectomy is usually performed within 48 hours of the acute attack, and always if complications (see above) develop.

Chronic cholecystitis (K&C 6e p. 404)

Chronic inflammation of the gall bladder is often found in association with gallstones. There is no evidence that this produces any symptoms, and cholecystectomy is not indicated. Chronic right hypochondrial pain and fatty food intolerance are likely to be functional in origin and gallstones an incidental finding.

Acute cholangitis (K&C 6e p. 401)

Cholangitis is an infection of the biliary tree; bacterial infection is the commonest and may be polymicrobial. Human bile is normally sterile. However, it can become infected with microorganisms from the gut if its flow is impeded by biliary obstruction. Common bile duct stones (choledocholithiasis) are the commonest cause of acute cholangitis. Other causes are benign biliary strictures following biliary surgery or associated with chronic pancreatitis, primary sclerosing cholangitis, HIV cholangiopathy (p. 174) and in patients with biliary stents. Bile duct obstruction due to cancer of the head of pancreas or bile duct (cholangiocarcinoma) can also cause cholangitis and this is more likely after ERCP. In the Far East, parts of Eastern Europe and the Mediterranean, biliary parasites can cause blockage and cholangitis.

Clinical features

The classic description of cholangitis with fever, jaundice and right upper quadrant pain (Charcot's triad) is not always present, although most patients have fever often with rigors. Jaundice is cholestatic in type, and therefore the urine is dark, the stools pale and the skin may itch. Elderly patients may present with non-specific symptoms such as confusion and malaise.

Investigations

- White cell count shows a leucocytosis.
- Blood cultures are positive (*E. coli, E. faecalis*, sometimes anaerobes) in about 30% of patients.
- Liver biochemistry shows a cholestatic picture with a raised serum bilirubin and alkaline phosphatase.
- Ultrasound shows a dilated common bile duct and may show the cause of the obstruction.
- Abdominal CT scan can further assess the site and cause of obstruction.
- ERCP is the definitive investigation and will also allow biliary drainage (see below). It will show the site of obstruction and the cause, and bile can be sampled for culture and cytology (if a malignant cause is suspected).

Management

Treatment of acute cholangitis includes resuscitation and volume replacement in shocked patients, pain relief, treatment of infection with appropriate intravenous antibiotics and relief of obstruction by biliary drainage. A suitable antibiotic regimen is a third-generation cephalosporin, e.g. cefotaxime (ciprofloxacin if allergic), plus metronidazole. An alternative regimen is amoxicillin, gentamycin (with appropriate monitoring) and metronidazole. In endemic areas primary parasite infection must also be treated.

Biliary drainage and/or clearance is usually achieved at ERCP with or without sphincterotomy. The urgency of this procedure depends on the clinical condition of the patient and the initial response to antibiotics. Stones can be removed from the CBD, a stent can be placed in the biliary tree if stones cannot be removed or to relieve obstruction in patients with a cancer of the head of pancreas or CBD. Antibiotics are continued after biliary drainage until symptom resolution, usually 7–10 days.

Common bile duct stones (choledocholithiasis)

CBD stones may also be asymptomatic with no features of cholangitis and present with abnormal liver biochemistry, usually with a cholestatic picture. Ultrasound will usually show gallbladder stones and may show the obstructed CBD containing a stone. Endoscopic ultrasound is more sensitive than transabdominal ultrasonography and is sometimes performed if there is a high index of suspicion and the latter is negative. MRCP is an alternative non-invasive technique for imaging the biliary system.

Management of gall bladder stones (K&C 6e p. 400)

Cholecystectomy is the treatment of choice for symptomatic gallstones, and is now almost always done laparoscopically. Non-surgical treatment of gallstones by dissolution therapy or lithotripsy is occasionally performed in patients who are not fit for or refuse cholecystectomy.

PRIMARY SCLEROSING CHOLANGITIS (K&C 6e p. 404)

Primary sclerosing cholangitis (PSC) is a chronic cholestatic liver disease characterized by a progressive obliterating fibrosis of the intra- and extrahepatic ducts. Episodes of ascending cholangitis and jaundice are common. PSC is a progressive disease, ultimately leading to liver cirrhosis and associated decompensation. Cholangiocarcinoma (bile duct cancer) occurs in up to 20% of patients. It is of unknown cause; 75% or more cases have ulcerative colitis which may be asymptomatic. Eighty per cent of patients have myeloperoxidase ANCA antibodies (p. 948), liver biopsy shows fibrosis around the bile ducts (onion skin lesion) and ERCP shows multiple strictures. Extrahepatic strictures may be amenable to dilatation. Treatment is limited to management of the general complications of the disease, such as pruritus, fat malabsorption and complications arising from chronic liver disease. No specific treatment has been shown to retard the rate of disease progression and the only option is eventual liver transplantation. Patients with AIDS can develop sclerosing cholangitis which is believed to be infectious in origin.

PANCREATITIS

The classification of pancreatitis is difficult because of the inability to separate acute and chronic forms clearly. By definition, acute pancreatitis, which can occur as isolated or recurrent attacks, is distinguished from chronic pancreatitis in that the process occurs on the background of a previously normal pancreas and the pancreas returns

Table 4.11 Causes of pancreatitis	
Acute	**Chronic**
Gallstones*	Alcohol*
Alcohol*	Idiopathic
Idiopathic (unknown cause)	Protein–energy malnutrition
Metabolic: hypercalcaemia, hyperlipidaemia	Hereditary
	Cystic fibrosis
Iatrogenic: post-surgical, post-ERCP	Autoimmune
Drugs: e.g. azathioprine, corticosteroids	

ERCP, endoscopic retrograde cholangiopancreatography
*Commonest causes in the western world

functionally and structurally to normal after the episode. The causes are shown in Table 4.11.

Acute pancreatitis (*K&C* 6e p. 409)

This is an acute condition presenting with abdominal pain and raised pancreatic enzymes in the blood or urine, resulting from inflammatory disease of the pancreas.

Pathogenesis

The exact pathophysiology is not well understood. Whatever the initiating event, there is acinar cell injury and release of activated proteases into the pancreatic interstitium. Disruption of acinar cells promotes migration of inflammatory cells from the microcirculation into the interstitium. Release of a variety of mediators and cytokines leads to a local inflammatory response, and sometimes a systemic inflammatory response that can result in single or multiple organ failure.

Clinical features

Epigastric or upper abdominal pain radiating through to the back is the cardinal symptom. There is often nausea and vomiting, and in severe cases multiorgan failure may develop. On examination there is epigastric tenderness, guarding and rigidity. Ecchymoses around the umbilicus (Cullen's sign) or in the flanks (Grey Turner's sign) indicate severe necrotizing pancreatitis.

Diagnosis

- *Blood tests.* A raised serum amylase, in conjunction with an appropriate history and clinical signs, strongly suggests a diagnosis of acute pancreatitis. Normal levels occur if the patient presents late when urinary amylase or serum lipase levels may still be raised. Serum amylase may also be moderately raised in other abdominal conditions, such as acute cholecystitis and perforated duodenal ulcer, although very high amylase levels (> 3 times normal) strongly suggest pancreatitis. Full blood count, CRP, urea and electrolytes, liver biochemistry, plasma calcium, and arterial blood gases are also measured as a guide to the severity of pancreatitis (Table 4.12).
- *Radiology.* An erect chest X-ray is performed to exclude perforated peptic ulcer as the cause of the pain and raised amylase. Abdominal ultrasound is performed as a screening test to look for gallstones as a cause of pancreatitis and may show swelling of the inflamed pancreas. Contrast-enhanced spiral CT scanning or MRI is performed in all but the mildest attack of pancreatitis to look for evidence of pancreatic necrosis (shown by non-enhancement of pancreatic parenchyma and indicating a severe attack) and peripancreatic fluid collections.

Management

Most attacks of pancreatitis are mild without systemic complications and associated only with interstitial inflammation; these patients usually recover within 5–7 days. In contrast, severe pancreatitis is associated with failure of one or more organ systems, such as renal or respiratory failure, and impaired coagulation with disseminated intravascular coagulation. These severe attacks are usually associated with pancreatic necrosis, which is identified on CT scanning as focal areas of reduced tissue perfusion. Several scoring systems have been developed in order to predict those patients with severe pancreatitis. The Glasgow scoring system is based on an initial admission score and subsequent repeat tests over 48 hours (Table 4.12). The acute physiology and chronic health evaluation score (APACHE) may be a more accurate predictor of disease severity and can be updated continuously but is more cumbersome to use.

Table 4.12 Glasgow scoring system for the initial prediction of severity in acute pancreatitis

Age	> 55 years
White blood cell count	$> 15 \times 10^9$/L
Glucose	> 10 mmol/L
Urea	> 16 mmol/L
P_aO_2	< 60 mmHg
Calcium	< 2 mmol/L
Albumin	< 32 g/L
Lactate dehydrogenase	600 units/L
Aspartate/alanine aminotransferase	> 100 units/L

Predicted severe pancreatitis ≥ 3 positive criteria on initial admission and repeat tests over 48 hours

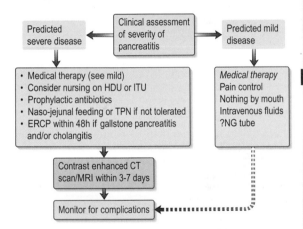

Fig. 4.9 The management of acute pancreatitis.

The management of acute pancreatitis is summarized in Figure 4.9. Patients with biliary pancreatitis and evidence of cholangitis or progressive jaundice (both of which suggest a stone impacted in the common bile duct) may require urgent ERCP and stone removal.

■ *Prophylactic antibiotics.* Broad-spectrum antibiotics, e.g. cefuroxime or aztreonam, reduce the risk of infected necrosis and are given from the outset.

177

- *Analgesia requirements.* Pethidine and tramadol are the drugs of choice, usually administered by a patient-control system. Morphine is avoided because it increases sphincter of Oddi pressure and may aggravate pancreatitis.
- *Feeding.* In patients with a severe episode of pancreatitis there is little likelihood of oral nutrition for a number of weeks. Nutrition is provided via a nasojejunal tube, and usually feeding is well tolerated and can maintain adequate nutritional input. The nasojejunal position of the feeding tube placed endoscopically overcomes the frequent problem of gastric paresis and there is less likelihood of pancreatic stimulation than with gastric placement.
- *Surgery.* Surgical treatment is sometimes required for very severe necrotizing pancreatitis, particularly if it is infected, or if complications such as pancreatic abscesses or pseudocysts occur.

Complications

Acute complications include hyperglycaemia, hypocalcaemia, renal failure and shock.

Prognosis

The mortality rate varies from 1% in mild cases to 50% in severe cases. Patients who recover may have recurrent attacks, depending on the aetiology.

Chronic pancreatitis (*K&C* 6e p. 411)

Chronic pancreatitis is defined as continuing inflammatory disease of the pancreas, characterized by irreversible morphological change and/or permanent impairment of function. Chronic calcifying pancreatitis is the commonest form in most developed countries, and is usually caused by alcohol. The disease is not reversible but it is possible to arrest the disease process, if the patient stops drinking alcohol.

Clinical features

There is central abdominal pain which is located in the epigastrium and characteristically radiates to the back. The pain may be intermittent or constant, and exacerbations are precipitated by an alcoholic binge. The abdominal pain is accompanied by severe weight loss as a result of anorexia, and may be difficult to distinguish from the pain of pancreatic cancer.

Diabetes may develop and steatorrhoea (p. 63) occurs when the secretion of pancreatic lipase is reduced by 90%. Occasionally the patient presents with biliary obstruction, jaundice and cholangitis. The differential diagnosis is from pancreatic carcinoma, which may also develop on a background of chronic pancreatitis. Carcinoma should be considered when there is a short history and localized ductular abnormalities on imaging.

Investigations

The diagnosis of chronic pancreatitis is made by radiological techniques which demonstrate structural changes in the gland, and metabolic studies which demonstrate functional abnormalities.

- *Radiology.* A plain abdominal X-ray will show pancreatic calcification in some cases. Ultrasonography and CT scanning may show a dilated pancreatic duct and demonstrate irregular consistency and outline of the gland. ERCP demonstrates dilatation of the pancreatic duct, with stenotic segments. MRCP and endoscopic ultrasound are sometimes used if the diagnosis is not confirmed with other imaging tests.

- *Functional assessment.* This relies upon measuring decreased concentrations of the products of synthetic compounds, e.g. fluorescein dilaurate (pancreolauryl) or N-benzoyl-L-tryosyl-p-amino benzoic acid (NBT-PABA), that appear in the stool, urine or blood after intraluminal hydrolysis and gut absorption. The pancreolauryl test for example involves the ingestion of fluorescein dilaurate, which is hydrolysed by pancreatic esterases to release fluorescein. Fluorescein is rapidly absorbed, conjugated in the liver and excreted in the urine. The various stages of the test require 3 days to perform and prolonged urine collection. Nevertheless, the test is simple, easily reproducible and has a high negative predictive value for pancreatic exocrine insufficiency. A faecal elastase level will be abnormal in patients with moderate to severe disease. The serum amylase is of no use in the diagnosis of chronic pancreatitis, but may be raised during an acute episode of pain. A raised blood sugar indicates diabetes mellitus.

Treatment

The patient should be advised to stop drinking alcohol. The pain may require opiates for control, with the attendant risk of addiction. Surgical resection combined with drainage of the pancreatic duct into the small bowel (pancreatico-jejunostomy) is of value for severe disease with intractable pain. Pancreatic strictures or stones are sometimes amenable to endoscopic treatment with ERCP. Pancreatic supplements are useful for those with steatorrhoea and may reduce the frequency of attacks of pain in those with recurrent symptoms. Diabetes requires appropriate treatment with diet, oral hypoglycaemics or insulin.

CARCINOMA OF THE PANCREAS (K&C 6e p. 414)

Epidemiology

Pancreatic cancer is the fifth most common cause of cancer death in the western world. Men are affected more commonly than women, and the incidence increases with age (peak in the seventh decade).

Aetiology

The aetiology is unknown but smoking, alcohol, coffee and dietary fat ingestion have all been implicated.

Clinical features

Cancer affecting the head of the pancreas presents with painless jaundice as a result of obstruction of the common duct, and weight loss. Examination may reveal jaundice and a distended palpable gall bladder (Courvoisier's law: if in a case of painless jaundice the gall bladder is palpable, the cause will not be gallstones). In gallstone disease chronic inflammation and fibrosis prevent distension of the gall bladder.

Cancer of the body or tail presents with abdominal pain, weight loss and anorexia.

Diabetes may occur and there is an increased risk of thrombophlebitis.

Investigations

The diagnosis is made with ultrasonography and/or CT. Duodenoscopy and ERCP may detect tumour in the head of the pancreas or at the ampulla. Endoscopic ultrasound is used for staging and in difficult cases for diagnosis.

Management

Surgical resection offers the only hope of cure but few patients have resectable disease at diagnosis. Tumour adherence or invasion into adjacent structures, particularly major blood vessels (locally advanced disease), makes complete resection difficult, and these patients are treated with combined chemotherapy and radiotherapy. 5-Fluorouracil and gemcitabine have been shown to improve survival in advanced disease and have also demonstrated survival benefit as an adjuvant therapy to pancreatic resection. Palliative treatment is often necessary for patients with unresectable pancreatic cancer to relieve obstructive jaundice (usually by endoscopic placement of a stent across the obstructed distal common bile duct), gastric outflow obstruction, and pain.

Prognosis

Overall, the prognosis is appalling. For the few patients who have had surgical resection with curative intent the 3-year survival is 30–40%. The median survival for treated patients with locally advanced disease is 8–12 months and for patients with metastatic disease 3–6 months.

NEUROENDOCRINE TUMOURS (K&C 6e p. 416)

These tumours arise in the pancreas from APUD (amine precursor uptake and decarboxylation) cells, and are sometimes called APUDomas. They usually secrete one hormone that produces the clinical effect, although other hormones are often also synthesized. Circulating hormone concentrations can be measured and high levels provide the diagnosis. Most neuroendocrine tumours express large numbers of somatostatin receptors. Intravenous injection of ^{111}In-labelled octreotide is therefore taken up readily by these tumours, and this test is the investigation of choice to localize the tumour and demonstrate the presence of metastases in patients suspected of having a neuro-endocrine tumour. Endoscopic ultrasonography is also used in some patients to localize the tumour.

Gastrinomas (Zollinger–Ellison syndrome)

Gastrinomas arise from the G cells of the pancreas and secrete large amounts of gastrin. This stimulates maximal gastric acid secretion, resulting in the development of peptic ulcers, which are often multiple, large and may be resistant to conventional treatment. Diarrhoea may also occur as a result of inhibition of digestive enzymes at low pH in the intestine. High-dose proton pump inhibitors are used to suppress symptoms but surgical resection is the only curative treatment.

VIPomas

These rare tumours produce vasoactive intestinal polypeptide (VIP), which stimulates intestinal water and electrolyte secretion, causing severe watery diarrhoea, hypokalaemia and dehydration. Treatment is with surgical resection or octreotide.

Glucagonomas

Glucagonomas arise from the α-cells of the pancreas and produce pancreatic glucagon. Patients present with diabetes mellitus and a unique necrolytic migratory erythematous rash.

Diseases of the blood and haematological malignancies 5

INTRODUCTION

Blood consists of red cells, white cells, platelets, and plasma in which the other components are suspended. Plasma is the liquid component of blood which contains soluble fibrinogen. Serum is what remains after the formation of the fibrin clot.

Haemopoiesis is the formation of blood cells (*K&C* 6e p. 419). The bone marrow is the only source of blood cells during normal childhood and adult life. Pluripotential stem cells, under the influence of a number of haemopoietic growth factors, give rise to lymphoid and myeloid stem cells. The former gives rise to T and B cells. The myeloid stem cell gives rise to CFU-GEMM (colony-forming unit, committed to the production of granulocytes, erythroid cells, monocytes and megakaryocytes). The growth factor erythropoietin controls the production of red blood cells. Reticulocytes are young red cells recently released from the bone marrow and still contain RNA. Reticulocytes normally represent 0.5–2.0% of total circulating red blood cells. The reticulocyte count gives a guide to the erythroid activity in the bone marrow and increases with haemorrhage, haemolysis and after treatment with specific haematinics in deficiency states.

ANAEMIA (*K&C* 6e p. 423)

Introduction

The principal physiological function of haemoglobin (Hb) is to carry and deliver oxygen to the tissues from the lungs. Hb is a tetramer consisting of two pairs of globin polypeptide chains: one pair of alpha chains and one pair of non-alpha chains. A haem group, consisting of a single molecule of protoporphyrin IX bound to a single ferrous ion (Fe^{2+}) is linked covalently at a specific site to each globin chain. Oxygenation and deoxygenation of haemoglobin occur at the haem iron (*K&C* 6e p. 423).

Table 5.1 Normal values for adult peripheral blood		
	Men	**Women**
Hb (g/dL)	13.5–17.7	11.5–16.5
PCV (haematocrit, L/L)	0.42–0.53	0.36–0.45
RCC (10^{12}/L)	4.5–6.0	3.9–5.1
MCV (fL)	80–96	
MCH (pg)	27–32	
MCHC (g/dL)	32–36	
WCC (10^9/L)	4.0–11.0	
Platelets (10^9/L)	150–400	
ESR (mm/h)	< 20	
Reticulocytes (% of total RCC)	0.2–2.0	

ESR, erythrocyte sedimentation rate; Hb, haemoglobin; MCH, mean corpuscular haemoglobin; MCHC, mean corpuscular haemoglobin concentration; MCV, mean corpuscular volume of red cells; PCV, packed cell volume; RCC, red cell count; WCC, white cell count

Anaemia is present when there is a decrease in the level of Hb in the blood below the reference range for the age and sex of the individual. Reduction of Hb is usually accompanied by a fall in red cell count (RCC) and packed cell volume (PCV, haematocrit), although an increase in plasma volume (as with massive splenomegaly) may cause anaemia with a normal RCC and PCV ('dilutional anaemia'). The normal values for these indices are given in Table 5.1, all of which are measured using automated cell counters as part of a routine full blood count (FBC).

Clinical features

Symptoms depend on the severity and speed of onset of anaemia. A very slowly falling level of Hb allows for haemodynamic compensation and enhancement of the oxygen-carrying capacity of the blood, and thus patients with anaemia may be asymptomatic. In general, elderly people tolerate anaemia less well than young people. The symptoms are non-specific and include fatigue, faintness and breathlessness. Angina pectoris and intermittent claudication may occur in those with coexistent atheromatous arterial disease. On examination the skin and mucous membranes are pale; there may be a tachycardia and a systolic flow murmur. Cardiac failure may occur in elderly people or those with compromised cardiac function.

Table 5.2 Classification of the anaemias based on the MCV

Microcytic	Normocytic	Macrocytic
Small red cells, MCV < 80 fL	Normal-sized red cells, normal MCV	Large red cells, MCV > 96 fL
Iron deficiency	Acute blood loss	Megaloblastic
Anaemia of chronic disease	Anaemia of chronic disease	Vitamin B_{12} deficiency
Thalassaemia	Aplastic anaemia	Folate deficiency
Sideroblastic anaemia	Combined deficiency, e.g. iron and folate	Normoblastic
	Haemolytic anaemia	Myelodysplasia
	Endocrine disorders, e.g. hypo-thyroidism	Haemolysis
		Other defects of DNA synthesis, e.g. chemotherapy

Classification of anaemia (Table 5.2)

The causes of anaemia are classified according to the measurement of red blood cell size. The normal red blood cell has a volume of 80–96 femtoliters (fL). Automatic cell counters provide a value for the mean of the red blood cell volume based on counting millions of cells (the mean corpuscular volume, MCV). This classification is useful because the type of anaemia then indicates the underlying causes and necessary investigations. Irrespective of the cause, most patients with chronic anaemia do not require blood transfusion and the appropriate management, unless severely anaemic, is treatment of the underlying cause.

Microcytic anaemia

Microcytosis usually reflects a decreased Hb content within the red blood cell and is then often associated with a reduction in the mean corpuscular haemoglobin (MCH) and mean corpuscular haemoglobin concentration (MCHC) producing a hypochromic appearance on the blood film. The causes of microcytic anaemia are listed in Table 5.2: α- or β-thalassaemia minor (p. 201) is associated with a microcytosis usually in the absence of anaemia.

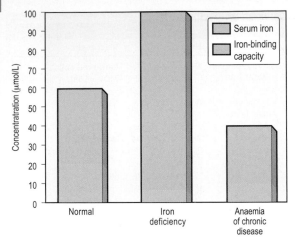

Fig. 5.1 **Serum iron and total iron-binding capacity (transferrin) in normal subjects, iron deficiency anaemia and anaemia of chronic disease.**

Iron deficiency

Iron is necessary for the formation of haem, and iron deficiency is the most common cause of anaemia worldwide. Absorption of dietary iron occurs primarily in the duodenum at a rate of about 1–2 mg per day, which represents about 10% of dietary iron. Factors that promote intestinal absorption include gastric acid, iron deficiency and increased erythropoietic activity. Iron is transported in the plasma bound to the protein transferrin, which is synthesized in the liver and normally about one-third saturated with iron (Fig. 5.1). Most of the body's iron content is incorporated into haemoglobin in developing erythroid precursors and mature red cells. Most of the remaining body iron is stored as ferritin and haemosiderin in hepatocytes, skeletal muscle and reticuloendothelial macrophages. A fixed amount of iron, about 1 mg each day, is lost in sloughed skin and mucosal cells through sweat, urine and faeces. In women there is an additional loss during menses, and premenopausal women may often border on iron deficiency.

Causes of iron deficiency

- Blood loss
- Decreased absorption in small bowel disease or after gastrectomy
- Increased demands, e.g. during growth and pregnancy
- Poor intake; this is rare in developed countries.

Most iron deficiency is due to blood loss, usually from the uterus or gastrointestinal tract. On a world-wide basis hookworm is a common cause of intestinal blood loss and iron deficiency. In women of childbearing age, menstrual blood loss, pregnancy and breast-feeding contribute to iron deficiency.

Clinical features

Symptoms and signs are the result of anaemia (see earlier) and of decreased epithelial cell iron, which causes brittle hair and nails, atrophic glossitis and angular stomatitis. The Paterson–Brown–Kelly syndrome (pharyngeal webs causing dysphagia) and koilonychia (spoon-shaped nails) are rarely seen.

Investigations

- Blood count shows a low Hb with a low MCV.
- Blood film. The red cells are microcytic and hypochromic, with anisocytosis (variation in size) and poikilocytosis (variation in shape).
- Serum ferritin reflects iron stores and is low.
- Serum iron is low and the total iron-binding capacity (TIBC) is high, resulting in a transferrin saturation (serum iron divided by TIBC) < 19% (Fig. 5.1).
- Serum soluble transferrin receptor: the number of transferrin receptors increases in iron deficiency.
- Bone marrow examination is only necessary in complicated cases, and shows erythroid hyperplasia and absence of iron.

Iron deficiency is almost always the result of chronic, often occult, gastrointestinal blood loss in men and in post-menopausal women, and further investigation of the gastrointestinal tract is required to determine the cause of the blood loss (see p. 87). Iron deficiency anaemia in premenopausal women is usually the result of menstrual blood loss. The only investigation necessary is serology for coeliac disease, and endoscopic investigation if there are intestinal symptoms or a family history of colorectal cancer (two first-degree relatives or one < 45 years of age).

Differential diagnosis

This is from other causes of a microcytic/hypochromic anaemia (see Table 5.2).

Management

■ Find and treat the underlying cause.
■ Oral iron, e.g. ferrous sulphate 200 mg three times daily, is given for about 6 months to correct the anaemia and replace iron stores. A response to iron treatment is characterized by an increase in the reticulocyte count followed by an increase in Hb at a rate of about 1 g/dL every week until the Hb concentration is normal.
■ Parenteral iron is rarely necessary and used only when patients are intolerant or there is a poor response to oral iron, e.g. severe malabsorption.

Anaemia of chronic disease (*K&C* 6e p. 429)

This occurs in patients with a variety of chronic diseases, including chronic renal failure, chronic inflammatory diseases such as Crohn's disease and polymyalgia rheumatica, and chronic infections such as tuberculosis and infective endocarditis. Anaemia of chronic disease presents with a normochromic, normocytic or microcytic anaemia. Characteristic laboratory findings include low serum iron levels, low serum iron-binding capacity (Fig. 5.1) and increased or normal serum ferritin. The anaemia of chronic disease is the result of decreased release of iron from bone marrow to developing erythroblasts, inadequate erythropoietin response to the anaemia, and decreased red cell survival. Treatment is of the underlying cause.

Sideroblastic anaemia (*K&C* 6e p. 429)

Sideroblastic anaemia is a rare disorder of haem synthesis characterized by a refractory anaemia with hypochromic cells in the peripheral blood and ring sideroblasts in the bone marrow. Ring sideroblasts are erythroblasts with iron deposited in mitochondria and reflect impaired utilization of iron delivered to the developing erythroblast. It may be inherited or acquired (secondary to myelodysplasia, alcohol, lead or isoniazid, or idiopathic). Treatment is to withdraw the causative agents. Some cases respond to pyridoxine (vitamin B_6). In many cases anaemia is transfusion dependent and iron overload becomes a problem.

Macrocytic anaemia

Macrocytosis is a rise in mean cell volume of the red cells above the normal range. Macrocytic anaemia can be divided into megaloblastic and non-megaloblastic types, depending on the bone marrow findings. In practice, macrocytosis is usually investigated without performing a bone marrow examination. The initial investigation is measurement of serum B_{12} and red cell folate.

Megaloblastic anaemia (*K&C* 6e p. 430)

Megaloblastic anaemia is characterized by the presence in the bone marrow of developing red blood cells with delayed nuclear maturation relative to that of the cytoplasm (*megaloblasts*). The underlying mechanism is defective DNA synthesis, which may also affect the white cells (causing hypersegmented neutrophil nuclei with six lobes, and sometimes leucopenia) and platelets (causing thrombocytopenia). The most common cause (see Table 5.2) of megaloblastic anaemia is deficiency of vitamin B_{12} or folate, which are both necessary to synthesize DNA.

Vitamin B_{12} deficiency

Animal products (meat and dairy products) provide the only dietary source of vitamin B_{12} for humans. The daily requirement is $1 \mu g$, which is easily supplied by a balanced western diet (containing $5–30 \mu g$ daily). Vitamin B_{12} is liberated from protein complexes in food by gastric acid and pepsin and binds to a vitamin B_{12}-binding protein 'R' binder derived from saliva. Free B_{12} is then released by pancreatic enzymes and becomes bound to intrinsic factor, which, along with H^+ ions, is secreted from gastric parietal cells. This complex is delivered to the terminal ileum, where vitamin B_{12} is absorbed and transported to the tissues by the carrier protein transcobalamin II. Vitamin B_{12} is stored in the liver, where there is sufficient supply for 2 or more years. About 1% of an oral dose of B_{12} is absorbed 'passively' without the need for intrinsic factor, mainly through the duodenum and ileum. The causes of vitamin B_{12} deficiency are listed in Table 5.3.

Table 5.3 Vitamin B_{12} deficiency – causes
Low dietary intake
Vegans
Impaired absorption
Stomach
Pernicious anaemia
Gastrectomy
Small bowel
Ileal disease or resection, e.g. Crohn's disease
Coeliac disease
Tropical sprue
Bacterial overgrowth
Congenital transcobalamin II deficiency (rare)

Pernicious anaemia

Pernicious anaemia (PA) is an autoimmune condition in which there is atrophy of the gastric mucosa with failure of intrinsic factor production and consequent vitamin B_{12} malabsorption. It is the most common cause of vitamin B_{12} deficiency in adults in western countries.

Epidemiology

This is a disease of elderly people (1–2% over the age of 60 years affected); most cases are undiagnosed. It is more common in women and in people with fair hair and blue eyes. There is an association with other autoimmune diseases, particularly thyroid disease and vitiligo.

Pathology

There is glandular atrophy of the gastric mucosa causing absent acid and intrinsic factor secretion.

Clinical features

The onset of PA is insidious, with progressively increasing symptoms of anaemia. There may be glossitis (a red sore tongue), angular stomatitis and mild jaundice. Neurological features can occur with very low levels of serum B_{12} and include a polyneuropathy caused by symmetrical damage to the peripheral nerves and posterior and lateral columns of the spinal cord (subacute combined degeneration of the cord). The latter presents with progressive weakness, ataxia and eventually paraplegia if untreated. Dementia and visual disturbances due to optic atrophy may also occur. There is a higher incidence of gastric carcinoma with PA (1–3%) than in the general population.

Investigations

- Blood count and film. There is a macrocytic anaemia (MCV often > 110 fL) with hypersegmented neutrophil nuclei and, in severe cases, leucopenia and thrombocytopenia.
- Serum vitamin B_{12} is low, frequently < 50 ng/L (normal > 160 ng/L).
- Red cell folate may be reduced because vitamin B_{12} is necessary to convert serum folate to the active intracellular form.
- Serum autoantibodies. Parietal cell antibodies are present in 90% and antibodies to intrinsic factor in 50%.
- Serum bilirubin may be raised as a result of excess breakdown of haemoglobin, owing to ineffective erythropoiesis in the bone marrow.
- In most cases, the cause is apparent from the history and autoantibody screen. A small bowel barium follow-through (to look at the terminal ileum) and distal duodenal biopsies (to look for coeliac disease) may be necessary in some patients.
- Bone marrow examination shows a hypercellular bone marrow with megaloblastic changes. This is not necessary in straightforward cases.

Differential diagnosis

Vitamin B_{12} deficiency must be differentiated from other causes of megaloblastic anaemia, principally folate deficiency, but this is usually clear from the blood levels of these two vitamins. Pernicious anaemia should be distinguished from other causes of vitamin B_{12} deficiency (Table 5.3).

Management

Traditionally, treatment is with intramuscular hydroxocobalamin (vitamin B_{12}). Injections (1 mg) are given twice weekly for 3 weeks to replenish body stores, and then

Table 5.4	Causes of folate deficiency
Poor intake	Old age, poverty, alcohol excess (also impaired utilization), anorexia
Malabsorption	Coeliac disease, Crohn's disease, tropical sprue
Excess utilization	Physiological: pregnancy, lactation, prematurity
	Pathological: chronic haemolytic anaemia, malignant and inflammatory diseases, renal dialysis
Drugs	Phenytoin, trimethoprim, sulfasalazine, methotrexate

3-monthly injections continued for life. Oral B_{12} (150 mg per day) is given to treat dietary deficiency.

Folate deficiency

Folate is found in green vegetables and offal, and absorbed in the upper small intestine. The daily requirement for folate is 100–200 µg and a normal mixed diet contains 200–300 µg. Body stores are sufficient for about 4 months, but folate deficiency may develop much more rapidly in patients who have a poor intake and excess utilization of folate, for example patients in intensive care. The causes of folate deficiency are shown in Table 5.4. The main cause is poor intake, which may occur alone or in combination with excessive utilization or malabsorption.

Clinical features

Symptoms and signs are the result of anaemia.

Investigations

Red cell folate is low (normal range 160–640 µg/mL) and is a more accurate guide to tissue folate than serum folate, which is also usually low (normal range 4.0–18 µg/L). If the history does not suggest dietary deficiency as the cause, further investigations such as a jejunal biopsy should be performed to look for small bowel disease.

Management

The underlying cause must be treated and folate deficiency corrected by giving oral folic acid 5 mg daily for 4 months, higher daily doses may be necessary with malabsorption. In megaloblastic anaemia of undetermined cause, folic acid alone must not be given, as this will aggravate the neuropathy of vitamin B_{12} deficiency. Prophylactic folic acid is given to patients with chronic haemolysis (5 mg weekly) and pregnant women.

Prevention of neural tube defects with folic acid To prevent first occurrence of neural tube defects, women who are planning a pregnancy should be advised to take folate supplements (at least $400 \, \mu g/day$) before conception and during the first 12 weeks of pregnancy. Larger doses (5 mg daily) are recommended for mothers who already have an infant with a neural tube defect.

Differential diagnosis of megaloblastic anaemias

A raised MCV with macrocytosis on the peripheral blood film can occur with a normoblastic rather than a megaloblastic bone marrow (Table 5.5). The most common cause of macrocytosis in the UK is alcohol excess. The exact mechanism for the large red cells in each of these conditions is uncertain, but in some it is thought to be due to altered or excessive lipid deposition on red cell membranes.

Table 5.5 Causes of macrocytosis other than megaloblastic anaemia

Physiological
Pregnancy
Newborn

Pathological
Alcohol excess
Liver disease
Reticulocytosis
Hypothyroidism
Haematological disorders
Myelodysplastic syndrome (a frequent cause in the elderly)
Sideroblastic anaemia
Aplastic anaemia
Drugs: hydroxycarbamide (hydroxyurea) and azathioprine
Cold agglutinins

Anaemia

Anaemia caused by marrow failure (aplastic anaemia) (*K&C* 6e p. 435)

Aplastic anaemia is defined as pancytopenia (deficiency of all cell elements of the blood) with *hypocellularity* (aplasia) of the bone marrow. It is an uncommon but serious condition which may be inherited but is more commonly acquired.

Aetiology

A list of the main causes of pancytopenia and aplasia is given in Table 5.6. Aplastic anaemia can be induced by a variety of disorders. However, immune mechanisms with local lymphocyte activation and release of interferon-γ leading to apoptotic cell death of bone marrow stem cells is thought to be a final common pathway. Many drugs have been associated with the development of aplastic anaemia, and this occurs as a predictable dose-related effect (e.g. chemotherapeutic agents) or as an idiosyncratic reaction (e.g. chloramphenicol).

Table 5.6 Causes of pancytopenia

Hypocellular bone marrow	Cellular bone marrow
Congenital	Megaloblastic anaemia
Idiopathic acquired (50% of cases)	Bone marrow infiltration or replacement
Cytotoxic drugs and radiation	Lymphoma
Idiosyncratic drug reaction	Acute leukaemia
Chloramphenicol	Myeloma
Gold	Secondary carcinoma
NSAIDs	Myelofibrosis
Chemicals: benzene, insecticides	Myelodysplastic syndrome
Infections	Hypersplenism
Parvovirus B19	
HIV	
Epstein–Barr	
Viral hepatitis	
Immune disorders	
Systemic lupus erythematosus	
Graft-versus-host	
Miscellaneous	
Paroxysmal nocturnal haemoglobinuria	
Overwhelming sepsis	

Clinical features

Symptoms are the result of the deficiency of red blood cells, white blood cells and platelets, and include anaemia, increased susceptibility to infection, and bleeding. Physical findings include bruising, bleeding gums and epistaxis. Mouth infections are common.

Investigations

- Blood count shows pancytopenia with low or absent reticulocytes.
- Bone marrow examination shows a hypocellular marrow with increased fat spaces.

Differential diagnosis

This is from other causes of pancytopenia (Table 5.6). A bone marrow trephine biopsy is essential for assessment of the bone marrow cellularity.

Management

Treatment includes withdrawal of the offending agent, supportive care and some form of definitive therapy (see below). Blood and platelet transfusions are used cautiously in patients who are candidates for bone marrow transplantation to avoid sensitization. Patients with severe neutropenia (absolute neutrophil count < 500 cells/μL) are at risk of serious infections. The responsible pathogens are usually bacteria but can also be fungal (e.g. candida and aspergillosis) and viral (herpes virus). Fever in a neutropenic patient is a medical emergency. The assessment and management are summarized in Emergency Box 5.1.

The course of aplastic anaemia is very variable, ranging from a rapid spontaneous remission to a persistent, increasingly severe pancytopenia, which may lead to death through haemorrhage or infection. Bad prognostic features are the following:

- A peripheral blood neutrophil count $< 0.5 \times 10^9/L$
- A peripheral blood platelet count $< 20 \times 10^9/L$
- A reticulocyte count of $< 40 \times 10^9/L$ (0.1% of total circulating red blood cells).

In those patients who do not undergo spontaneous recovery the options for treatment are as follows:

> **Emergency Box 5.1**
> **Assessment and treatment of the febrile neutropenic patient**
>
> **Definition**
> Single temperature > 38°C or temperature > 37.5°C for 1 hour
>
> **Assessment**
> Careful review of symptoms
> Detailed physical examination including mucous membranes, oropharynx, surgical sites and intravenous lines
>
> **Investigations**
> Full blood count and differential white cell count
> Urea and electrolytes
> Liver biochemistry
> Chest X-ray
> Microscopy and cultures of:
>   Blood from peripheral blood and intravenous lines
>   Sputum
>   Urine
>   Stool if diarrhoea
> Consider further imaging if localizing signs, e.g. CT scan of abdomen and pelvis
>
> **Antibiotics**
> Seek expert help from microbiologist and oncologist
> Start empirical antibiotic treatment, e.g. tazocin and aminoglycoside, to cover Gram-negative organisms and *Pseudomonas*
> Add vancomycin if clinical deterioration, fever persists or suspected MRSA infection
> Subsequent treatment is adjusted on the basis of cultured organisms and clinical progress.

- Bone marrow transplantation (BMT) from a histo-compatible sibling donor is the treatment of choice for patients under 40 years of age.
- Immunosuppressive therapy with antilymphocyte globulin, ciclosporin and corticosteroids is used for patients over the age of 40 years in whom BMT is not indicated because of the high risk of graft-versus-host disease.

HAEMOLYTIC ANAEMIA (K&C 6e p. 436)

Haemolytic anaemia results from increased destruction of red cells with a reduction of the circulating life-span

Table 5.7 Causes of haemolytic anaemia

Inherited	Acquired

Red cell membrane defect
  Hereditary spherocytosis
  Hereditary elliptocytosis
	Immune
	  Autoimmune haemolytic
	    anaemia
	  Haemolytic transfusion
	    reactions
	  Drug-induced

Haemoglobin abnormalities
  Thalassaemia
  Sickle cell disease
	Non-immune
	  Paroxysmal nocturnal
	    haemoglobinuria
	  Microangiopathic haemolytic
	    anaemia
	  March haemoglobinuria

Red cell metabolic defects
  Glucose-6-phosphate
    dehydrogenase
    deficiency
  Pyruvate kinase
    deficiency
	Miscellaneous
	  Infections (e.g. malaria)
	  Drugs/chemicals
	  Hypersplenism

(normally 120 days). Red cell destruction may be extra-vascular (within the reticuloendothelial system) or intra-vascular (within the blood vessels). The causes of haemolytic anaemia in adults are listed in Table 5.7.

In most haemolytic conditions, red cell destruction is extravascular, and cells are removed from the circulation by macrophages in the reticuloendothelial system, particularly the spleen.

When red cells are broken down within the circulation, haemoglobin appears in the plasma as the oxidized form, methaemoglobin, which dissociates into ferrihaem and globin. Binding of ferrihaem to albumin forms *methaem-albumin* and this can be detected in the plasma (Schumm's test). Free haemoglobin binds to plasma *haptoglobins*; the haemoglobin–haptoglobin is rapidly removed by the liver, leading to a reduction in plasma haptoglobin. Haemoglobin that is unbound to haptoglobin is filtered by the glomerulus and appears in the urine as *haemoglobinuria*. Some Hb is broken down in the renal tubular cells and appears as *haemosiderin* in the urine. Figure 5.2 shows an approach to investigating the patient with suspected haemolytic anaemia.

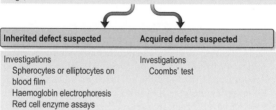

Evidence for haemolysis	
Increased red cell breakdown	**Increased red cell production**

• Increased unconjugated serum bilirubin
• Increased serum lactate dehydrogenase (released from haemolysed RBC)
• Spherocytes on the blood film
• With intravascular haemolysis
  – increased free plasma Hb
  – haemosiderinuria
  – very low or absent plasma haptoglobins
  – presence of methaemalbumin (positive Schumm's test)
	• Increased MCV (as a result of increased reticulocytes)
	• Increased reticulocyte count
	• Erythroid hyperplasia on the bone marrow

History	Examination
e.g. family history, systemic illness, drugs, race	e.g. jaundice, hepatosplenomegaly

Inherited defect suspected	Acquired defect suspected

Investigations
  Spherocytes or elliptocytes on blood film
  Haemoglobin electrophoresis
  Red cell enzyme assays
	Investigations
	  Coombs' test

Fig. 5.2 **An algorithm for investigation of suspected haemolytic anaemia.**

INHERITED HAEMOLYTIC ANAEMIAS

Inherited haemolytic anaemias are due to defects in one or more components of the mature red blood cell:

■ Cell membrane
■ Haemoglobin
■ Metabolic machinery of the red blood cell.

Membrane defects

Hereditary spherocytosis (*K&C* 6e p. 438)
Hereditary spherocytosis is the most common inherited

198

haemolytic anaemia in northern Europeans, and is inherited in an autosomal dominant manner. It is the result of a defect in the red cell membrane of which the commonest cause is a deficiency of the structural membrane protein *spectrin*. Red cells become spherical in shape, are more rigid and less deformable than normal red cells, and are thus destroyed prematurely in the spleen.

Clinical features

Hereditary spherocytosis may present with jaundice or be asymptomatic. Patients may develop anaemia, splenomegaly and leg ulcers. As in many haemolytic anaemias, the course of the disease may be interrupted by aplastic, haemolytic and megaloblastic crises. Aplastic anaemia usually occurs after infections, particularly with parvovirus B19, whereas megaloblastic anaemia is the result of folate depletion caused by hyperactivity of the bone marrow. Chronic haemolysis may lead to the development of pigment gallstones.

Investigations

- Blood count demonstrates reticulocytosis and anaemia, which is usually mild.
- The blood film shows spherocytes (also seen in auto-immune haemolytic anaemia) and reticulocytes.

The diagnosis is made by demonstration of increased red cell osmotic fragility when placed in hypotonic solutions.

Management

Splenectomy should be performed in all but the mildest of cases. This is usually postponed until after childhood, to minimize the risk of overwhelming pneumococcal infection. Patients undergoing splenectomy should receive appropriate prophylaxis against infection (p. 217).

Hereditary elliptocytosis

Hereditary elliptocytosis is similar to spherocytosis but the red cells are elliptical in shape. It is milder clinically and usually does not require treatment.

Haemoglobin abnormalities *(K&C 6e p. 439)*

Normal adult Hb is made up of haem and two polypeptide globin chains, α and β. The haemoglobinopathies can be

Table 5.8	Types of haemoglobin		
	Haemoglobin	Structure	Comment
Normal	A	$\alpha_2\beta_2$	97% of adult haemoglobin
	A_{1C}	$\alpha_2\beta_2$	$\leq 5\%$ of HbA (glycosylated Hb)
	A_2	$\alpha_2\delta_2$	2% of adult Hb; elevated in β-thalassaemia
	F	$\alpha_2\gamma_2$	Normal Hb in fetus from 3rd to 9th month; increased in β-thalassaemia
Abnormal chain production	H	β_4	Found in α-thalassaemia
	Barts	γ_4	Found in homozygous α-thalassaemia, biologically useless
Abnormal chain structure	S	$\alpha_2\beta_2$	Substitution of valine for glutamic acid in position 6 of the β chain
	C	$\alpha_2\beta_2$	Substitution of lysine for glutamic acid in position 6 of the β chain

classified into two subgroups: *abnormal chain production* or *abnormal chain structure* of the polypeptide chains (Table 5.8).

Thalassaemia (*K&C* 6e p. 440)

In normal Hb there is a balance (1 : 1) in the production of α and β chains. The thalassaemias are a group of disorders arising from one or multiple gene defects, resulting in a reduced rate of production of one or more globin chains. The imbalanced globin chain production leads to precipitation of globin chains within red cells or precursors. This results in cell damage, death of red cell precursors in the bone marrow (ineffective erythropoiesis), and haemolysis. The thalassaemias affect people throughout the world.

There are two main types:

- α-Thalassaemia: reduced α chain synthesis
- β-Thalassaemia: reduced β chain synthesis.

β-Thalassaemia In homozygous β-thalassaemia there is little or no β chain production, resulting in excess α chains. These combine with whatever δ and γ chains are produced, leading to increased Hb A$_2$ and Hb F. There are three main clinical forms of β-thalassaemia:

- β-*Thalassaemia minor (trait)*. This is the asymptomatic heterozygous carrier state. Anaemia is mild or absent, with a low MCV and MCH. Iron stores and serum ferritin levels are normal.
- β-*Thalassaemia intermedia*. This includes patients with moderate anaemia (Hb 7–10 g/dL) that does not require regular blood transfusions. Splenomegaly, bone deformities, recurrent leg ulcers and gallstones are other features. This may be caused by a combination of homozygous β- and α-thalassaemias.
- β-*Thalassaemia major (homozygous β-thalassaemia)*. This presents in the first year of life with severe anaemia (*Cooley's anaemia*), failure to thrive and recurrent infections. Hypertrophy of the ineffective bone marrow leads to bony abnormalities: the thalassaemic facies, with an enlarged maxilla and prominent frontal and parietal bones. Resumption of haemopoiesis in the spleen and liver (extramedullary haemopoiesis), the chief sites of red cell production in fetal life, leads to hepatosplenomegaly.

Investigations

In homozygous disease, blood count and film show a hypochromic/microcytic anaemia, raised reticulocyte count and nucleated red cells in the peripheral circulation.

The diagnosis is made by haemoglobin electrophoresis, which shows an increase in Hb F and absent or markedly reduced Hb Λ.

Management

In homozygous patients, the mainstay of treatment is blood transfusion, aiming to keep the haemoglobin above

10 g/dL, thus suppressing ineffective erythropoiesis, preventing bony abnormalities and allowing normal development. Iron overload caused by repeated blood transfusions may lead to damage to endocrine glands, liver, pancreas and heart, with death in the second decade from cardiac failure. Treatment with the iron-chelating agent desferrioxamine decreases iron loading. Ascorbic acid 200 mg daily is given, along with desferrioxamine, as it increases the urinary excretion of iron in response to desferrioxamine. Bone marrow transplantation has been used in some cases of thalassaemia.

α-Thalassaemia The clinical manifestations of this disorder vary from a mild anaemia with microcytosis to a severe condition incompatible with life. There are four α-globin genes per cell. The manifestations depend on whether one, two, three or all four of the genes are deleted, and thus whether α chain synthesis is partial or completely absent. In the most severe form, where there is complete absence of α-globin (Hb Barts), infants are stillborn (hydrops fetalis).

Antenatal diagnosis of haemoglobin abnormalities

It is possible to identify a fetus with severe haemoglobin abnormalities by DNA analysis of chorionic villus samples taken in the first trimester, or by testing umbilical cord blood in the second trimester. Abortion is offered if the fetus is found to be affected. This examination is appropriate if the mother is found to have a haemoglobin defect during antenatal testing and if, on subsequent screening, her partner is also affected.

Sickle cell disease (*K&C* 6e p. 442)

Sickle cell disease is a family of haemoglobin disorders in which the sickle β-globin gene is inherited. The gene for sickle haemoglobin (haemoglobin S) results in the substitution of the amino acid valine for glutamine normally present in position 6 of the β chain of haemoglobin. In the homozygous state (*sickle cell anaemia*) both genes are abnormal (Hb SS), whereas in the heterozygous state (*sickle cell trait*, Hb AS) only one chromosome carries the abnormal gene. Inheritance of the HbS gene from one parent and HbC from the other parent gives rises to Hb SC disease, which tends to run a milder clinical course than sickle cell disease but with more thromboses.

The sickle β gene is spread widely throughout Africa (25% carry the gene), the Middle East and Mediterranean countries. One of the main factors in this distribution is that patients with sickle cell trait have a relative resistance to malaria, so are more likely to survive, breed and pass on their genes.

In the deoxygenated state Hb S molecules link to form chains, and this process results in increased rigidity of the red cells, causing the classic sickle appearance. Sickling results in premature destruction of red cells (haemolysis) and obstruction of the microcirculation (vaso-occlusion), leading to tissue infarction. As the production of Hb F is normal, the disease is usually not manifest until Hb F decreases to adult levels at about 6 months of age.

Clinical features

In the heterozygous state, Hb AS (sickle cell trait), there are usually no symptoms unless the patient is exposed to extreme hypoxia, e.g. very poor anaesthesia.

Symptoms of the homozygous state, Hb SS (sickle cell anaemia), are due to vaso-occlusion and haemolysis.

Vaso-occlusion Avascular necrosis of bone marrow results in the bone pain crisis, which may be precipitated by hypoxia, dehydration or infection. In adults, bone pain most commonly affects the juxta-articular parts of the long bones, the ribs, spine and pelvis. In early childhood the small bones of the hands and feet are affected (dactylitis), which may result in shortened deformed bones. Most patients with a painful crisis are managed in the community, but hospital admission is necessary when the pain is not controlled by non-opiate analgesia such as paracetamol and non-steroidal anti-inflammatory drugs, or if there are complications listed in Table 5.9. The management of a painful sickle crisis is summarized in Emergency Box 5.2. Other complications of vaso-occlusion include splenic atrophy (resulting in susceptibility to infection with pneumococcus, *Salmonella* species and haemophilus), cerebral infarction (causing fits and hemiplegia) and retinal ischaemia (which may precipitate proliferative sickle retinopathy and visual loss).

Table 5.9 **Complications of sickle cell disease requiring inpatient management**

Pain uncontrolled by non-opiate analgesia
Swollen painful joints
Central nervous system deficit
Acute sickle chest syndrome or pneumonia
Mesenteric sickling and bowel ischaemia
Splenic or hepatic sequestration
Cholecystitis
Renal papillary necrosis resulting in colic or severe haematuria
Hyphema (a layer of red cells in anterior chamber of eye) or
    retinal detachment

Emergency Box 5.2
Management of a painful sickle cell crisis in hospital

● **Analgesia**
 ⇒ diclofenac 1 mg/kg every 8 hours orally
 ⇒ morphine 10–40 μg/kg/h by intravenous or subcutaneous
   infusion if no response to diclofenac.
   Side-effects of morphine include nausea, respiratory
   depression and hypotension.

● **Oxygen**, 60% by face mask if arterial oxygen saturation
 < 95%.

● **Rehydrate** with intravenous fluids.

● **Immediate investigations:**
 – full blood count and reticulocyte count
 – urea and electrolytes
 – blood cultures
 – urine microscopy and culture
 – oxygen saturation by pulse oximetry
 – chest X-ray
 – arterial blood gases (if oxygen saturation < 90% breathing
   air, chest X-ray shadowing or respiratory symptoms).

● Search for and treat any source of infection.

● Check Hb and reticulocyte count at least once daily.

● Examine daily: the respiratory system for the acute chest
 syndrome, and the abdomen for increase in liver or spleen
 size which may indicate a sequestration crisis.

Haemolysis Symptoms vary from mild anaemia to severe haemolysis. Chronic haemolysis is associated with increased formation of pigment gallstones. Most patients with sickle cell anaemia have a steady-state Hb of 6–8 g/dL with a high reticulocyte count (10–20%). Most patients do not have symptoms of anaemia because tissue oxygen delivery is normal owing to a hyperdynamic circulation and the lower oxygen affinity of Hb S, which releases oxygen to the tissues more easily than normal Hb. A rapid fall in the Hb may be due to:

- Aplastic crisis. This is often due to parvovirus B19 infection, which destroys erythrocyte precursors
- Acute sequestration crisis. The liver and spleen become engorged with red cells, leading to a fall in Hb and rapid enlargement of these organs
- Haemolysis due to drugs or infection.

Other complications of sickle cell disease include renal papillary necrosis and chronic renal failure, leg ulcers, and the acute chest syndrome. The latter is the commonest cause of death of adults with sickle cell disease. It is a medical emergency and characterized by fever, cough, dyspnoea and pulmonary infiltrates on the chest X-ray. It is caused by infection, fat embolism from necrotic bone marrow or pulmonary infarction due to sequestration of sickle cells. Sequestration of red cells within the corpora cavernosa causes priapism (prolonged erections) and eventual impotence.

Investigations

- Blood count. In sickle cell disease there is a low haemoglobin (6–8 g/dL) with a high reticulocyte count. Patients with sickle cell trait are not anaemic.
- Blood film shows sickled erythrocytes.

Diagnosis is made with Hb electrophoresis showing 80–90% Hb SS and absent Hb A. In addition, sickling can be induced in vitro with sodium metabisulphite.

Treatment and screening

Asymptomatic anaemia requires no treatment. Folic acid is given to patients with severe haemolysis, and to women before conception and during pregnancy. The risk of pneumococcal infection is reduced by prophylaxis with pneumococcal vaccine and daily oral penicillin. Routine vaccination against *Haemophilus influenzae* is given to all children in the UK. Exchange transfusions may be used to reduce the frequency of crises, or as prophylaxis in pregnancy or before surgery.

Hydroxycarbamide (hydroxyurea) raises the concentration of fetal Hb and ameliorates the clinical course, but concerns remain over its myelosuppressive side-effects. Bone marrow transplantation from an HLA-matched sibling has been used in some patients with severe disease.

People from areas with a high prevalence of sickle cell disease should be screened before general anaesthesia, and before or during pregnancy.

Prognosis

The median survival is 40–50 years.

Metabolic red cell disorders (*K&C* 6e p. 445)

A number of red cell enzyme deficiencies may produce haemolytic anaemia, the most common of which is glucose-6-phosphate dehydrogenase (G6PD) deficiency.

Glucose-6-phosphate dehydrogenase deficiency

G6PD is a vital enzyme in the hexose monophosphate shunt, which maintains glutathione in the reduced state. Glutathione protects against oxidant injury in the red cell. G6PD deficiency is a common heterogeneous X-linked trait found predominantly in African, Mediterranean and Middle Eastern populations.

G6PD deficiency causes neonatal jaundice, chronic haemolytic anaemia, and acute haemolysis precipitated by the ingestion of fava beans and oxidizing drugs such as quinine, sulphonamides and nitrofurantoin. Diagnosis is by direct measurement of enzyme levels in the red cell. Treatment is the avoidance of precipitating factors, and transfusion if necessary.

ACQUIRED HAEMOLYTIC ANAEMIA

Autoimmune haemolytic anaemia (*K&C* 6e p.448)

Acquired haemolytic anaemia is due to immunological destruction of red blood cells mediated by autoantibodies

Table 5.10 Features of autoimmune haemolytic anaemia

	Warm antibody	Cold antibody
Temperature at which antibody attaches best to red cell	37°C	Lower than 37°C
Type of antibodies	IgG	IgM
Direct Coombs' test	Strongly positive	Positive
Cause of primary condition	Idiopathic	Idiopathic
Cause of secondary condition	Autoimmune disorders, e.g. SLE Lymphomas Drugs, e.g. methyldopa	Infections *Mycoplasma* sp. Infectious mononucleosis Viruses Lymphomas Paroxysmal cold haemoglobinuria (rare)

207

directed against antigens on the patient's red blood cells. Autoimmune haemolytic anaemia is classified according to whether the antibody reacts best at body temperature (*warm antibodies*) or at lower temperatures (*cold antibodies*) (Table 5.10). IgG or IgM antibodies attach to the red cell, resulting in extravascular haemolysis through sequestration in the spleen, or in intravascular haemolysis through activation of complement. The autoimmune haemolytic anaemias are diagnosed on the basis of a positive direct antiglobulin test (direct Coombs' test, Fig. 5.3).

Warm antibody haemolysis

Clinical features

This anaemia occurs at all ages in both sexes, with a variable clinical picture ranging from mild haemolysis to life-threatening anaemia. About 50% are associated with other autoimmune disorders or lymphoma.

Investigation

There is evidence of haemolysis (p. 198) and the direct Coombs' test is positive (Fig. 5.3). A Coombs' test is a test

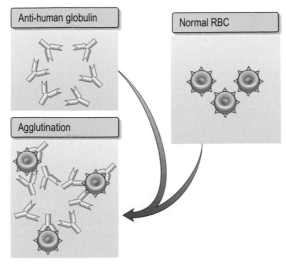

Direct antiglobulin test

Patient's cells sensitized in vivo
e.g. autoimmune haemolytic anaemia,
    haemolytic transfusion reaction,
    HDN,
    drug-induced immune haemolytic
     anaemia

Anti-human globulin

Normal RBC

Agglutination

Fig. 5.3 **Antiglobulin (Coombs' test).** The red blood cells of the patient are washed free of adherent proteins and reacted with antiserum or monoclonal antibodies against various immunoglobulins and complement. The anti-human globulin forms bridges between the sensitized cells causing visible agglutinations. The direct test detects patients' cells sensitized in vivo. HDN, haemolytic disease of newborn; RBC, red blood cell.

for antibodies or complement (another protein/enzyme that works with antibodies) attached to the surface of red blood cells. The red blood cells of the patient are reacted with antiserum or monoclonal antibodies prepared against the various immunoglobulins and the third component of complement (C3d). If either or both of these are present on the red cell surface, agglutination of red cells will be detected.

Management

High-dose steroids (e.g. prednisolone 1 mg/kg daily) induce remission in 80% of cases. Splenectomy is useful in those failing to respond to steroids. Occasionally, immuno-suppressive drugs such as azathioprine and cyclophosphamide are beneficial.

Cold antibody haemolysis

Clinical features

IgM antibodies (cold agglutinins) attach to red cells in the cold peripheral parts of the body and cause agglutination and complement-mediated intravascular haemolysis. Infection with mycoplasma or Epstein–Barr virus may lead to increased synthesis of cold agglutinins (normally produced in insignificant amounts) and produce transient haemolysis. A chronic idiopathic form occurs in elderly people, with recurrent haemolysis and peripheral cyanosis.

Investigation

There is evidence of haemolysis, and the direct Coombs' test is positive. Examination of a peripheral blood film at room temperature shows red cell agglutination.

Management

This does not usually require treatment other than for the underlying condition and avoiding exposure to cold.

Drug-induced haemolysis

Two types of mechanisms have been identified:

- In the commonest form, the drug may associate with structures on the red cell membrane and thus be part of the antigen in a haptenic reaction. There is severe complement-mediated intravascular haemolysis which resolves quickly after drug withdrawal.
- The drug may induce a subtle alteration of one component of the red cell membrane, rendering it antigenic. There is extravascular haemolysis and a protracted clinical course.

The mechanisms for drug-induced haemolytic anaemia probably also apply to drug-induced thrombocytopenia and neutropenia.

Non-immune haemolytic anaemia

Paroxysmal nocturnal haemoglobinuria (*K&C* 6e p. 452)

The pathogenic defect in paroxysmal nocturnal haemoglobinuria (PNH) is an inability to produce the glycosyl-phosphatidylinositol (GPI) anchor which tethers several proteins to the cell membrane. Deficiency of two of these proteins, CD59 and decay-accelerating factor, renders the red cell exquisitely sensitive to the haemolytic action of complement. The clinical manifestations of this rare disease are related to abnormalities in haemopoietic function including intravascular haemolysis, venous thrombosis and bone marrow aplasia. Progression to myelodysplasia and acute leukaemia can also occur. PNH should be considered in any patient with chronic or episodic haemolysis. Diagnosis is made by demonstrating deficiency of the GPI-anchored proteins on haematopoietic cells by flow cytometry. There is no specific treatment for PNH and management is supportive. Bone marrow transplantation has been successful in selected patients.

Mechanical haemolytic anaemia (*K&C* 6e p. 453)

Red cells may be injured by physical trauma in the circulation. Examples of this form of haemolysis include the following:

- Leaking prosthetic heart valves: damage to red cells in their passage through the heart
- March haemoglobinuria: damage to red cells in the feet from prolonged marching
- Microangiopathic haemolysis: fragmentation of red cells in abnormal microcirculation caused by malignant hypertension, haemolytic uraemic syndrome or disseminated intravascular coagulation.

MYELOPROLIFERATIVE AND MYELODYSPLASTIC DISORDERS

Myeloproliferative and myelodysplastic syndromes are both clonal haemopoietic stem cell disorders which arise from a single abnormal multipotential cell in the bone marrow. Both have the potential to transform into acute leukaemia. *Myelodysplastic syndromes* are characterized by ineffective erythropoiesis and peripheral blood cytopenias (see p. 194). *Myeloproliferative disorders* are characterized by the overproduction of one or more cell lines (myeloid, erythroid or megakaryocyte), and comprise chronic myeloid leukaemia (CML), polycythaemia vera, essential thrombocythaemia and myelofibrosis. These disorders differ from the acute leukaemias (also clonal proliferation of a single cell line), where the cells also do not differentiate normally but where there is progressive accumulation of immature cells.

Polycythaemia

Polycythaemia is defined as an increase in Hb, packed cell volume (PCV) and red cell count (RCC). These measurements are all concentrations and are therefore directly dependent upon plasma volume as well as red blood cell mass. The production of red cells by the bone marrow is normally regulated by the hormone erythropoietin, which is produced in the kidney. The stimulus for erythropoietin production is tissue hypoxia. *Absolute polycythaemia* (Fig. 5.4) is therefore the result of an appropriate increase in erythropoietin secondary to hypoxia, an inappropriate increase in erythropoietin resulting from abnormal production by certain tumours, or escape by marrow stem cells from erythropoietin control (polycythaemia vera). Absolute polycythaemia must be differentiated from *apparent poly-*

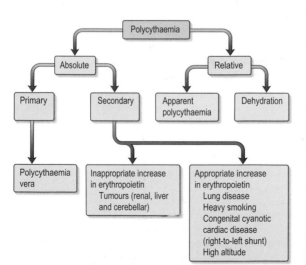

Fig. 5.4 **The causes of polycythaemia.**

Myeloproliferative and myelodysplastic disorders

cythaemia (Gaisböck's syndrome), where PCV is normal but plasma volume is decreased. Apparent polycythaemia usually affects middle-aged obese men and is associated with smoking, increased alcohol intake and hypertension. The causes of polycythaemia are shown in Figure 5.4. The most common cause is hypoxia secondary to cardiopulmonary disease. Apparent polycythaemia is uncommon.

Primary polycythaemia: polycythaemia vera (*K&C* 6e p. 453)

Clinical features

Polycythaemia vera, like the other myeloproliferative disorders, occurs principally in middle-aged and elderly people. It is characterized by an excessive proliferation of erythroid, myeloid and megakaryocytic progenitor cells due to a failure of apoptosis. Symptoms and signs are the result of hypervolaemia and hyperviscosity. Typical symptoms include headache, dizziness, tinnitus, visual disturbance, angina pectoris, intermittent claudication, pruritus and venous thrombosis. Physical signs include a plethoric complexion and hepatosplenomegaly as a result of extramedullary haemopoiesis. Splenomegaly, if present, reliably distinguishes primary polycythaemia from the other polycythaemias. There is an increased risk of haemorrhage as a result of friable haemostatic plugs, and gout caused by increased cell turnover and uric acid production.

Investigations

- Blood count shows a high Hb and PCV. The WCC is raised in 70% and the platelet count in 50% of patients; such abnormalities are rarely present in polycythaemia from other causes.
- Red cell volume, measured with ^{51}Cr-labelled red cells, is increased.
- Plasma volume, measured using ^{131}I-labelled albumin dilution, is normal or increased (compare with relative polycythaemia).
- Bone marrow shows erythroid hyperplasia with increased numbers of megakaryocytes.

Differential diagnosis

This is from secondary and relative polycythaemia. An abdominal ultrasound, arterial P_{O_2} and carboxyhaemoglobin (increased in heavy smokers) and measurement of serum erythropoietin may be necessary to differentiate. Erythropoietin is low or normal in polycythaemia vera, and usually high in secondary polycythaemia.

Management

There is no cure, and treatment is given to maintain a normal blood count and to prevent the complications of the disease, particularly thrombosis and haemorrhage.

- Venesection to maintain PCV < 0.45 L/L. Regular venesection (e.g. 3-monthly) may be all that is needed in many patients.
- Chemotherapy. Hydroxycarbamide (hydroxyurea) and busulfan are particularly useful to reduce the platelet count.
- Radioactive phosphorus (^{32}P) is sometimes used in patients over 70 years of age. Its use is restricted in younger patients because of the increased incidence of leukaemic conversion in patients treated with ^{32}P.
- Allopurinol is given to decrease uric acid levels.

213

Prognosis

Median survival in untreated patients is 1–2 years and may be increased to approximately 14 years with treatment. Thirty per cent will develop myelofibrosis and 5% acute leukaemia. The risk of acute myeloid leukaemia is marginally increased by treatment with busulfan or ^{32}P.

Secondary polycythaemia (*K&C* 6e p. 454)
Secondary polycythaemia presents with similar clinical features to primary polycythaemia, although the white cell and platelet counts are normal and the spleen is not enlarged. In patients with tumours the primary disease must be treated to lower the level of erythropoietin. In hypoxic patients, oxygen therapy (p. 500) may reduce the Hb, and a small-volume phlebotomy (400 mL) may help those with severe symptoms. Smokers should be advised to stop.

Primary (essential) thrombocythaemia (*K&C* 6e p. 455)

Essential thrombocythaemia is characterized by very high platelet counts (usually $> 1000 \times 10^9$/L). Platelet size and function are abnormal, and presentation may be with

Table 5.11 Differential diagnosis of a raised platelet count

Reactive thrombocytosis
    Connective tissue disorders
    Chronic infections
    Inflammatory bowel disease
    Malignancy
    Haemorrhage
    Surgery
    Splenectomy and functional hyposplenism

Primary thrombocythaemia
Primary polycythaemia
Myelofibrosis
Myelodysplasia

bleeding or thrombosis. Busulfan, hydroxycarbamide (hydroxyurea) or α-interferon are used to reduce platelet production. Differential diagnosis is from secondary causes of a raised platelet count and other myeloproliferative disorders (Table 5.11).

Primary myelofibrosis (myelosclerosis) (*K&C* 6e p. 455)

Myelofibrosis is characterized by haemopoietic stem-cell proliferation associated with marrow fibrosis (abnormal megakaryocyte precursors release fibroblast-stimulating factors such as platelet-derived growth factor).

Clinical features

There are constitutional symptoms of fever, weight loss and lethargy. Bleeding occurs in the thrombocytopenic patient. There is hepatomegaly and massive splenomegaly caused by extramedullary haemopoiesis.

Investigations

- Blood count shows anaemia. The white cell and platelet counts are high initially, but fall with disease progression as a result of marrow fibrosis.

- Blood film examination shows a leucoerythroblastic picture (immature red cells caused by marrow infiltration) and 'teardrop'-shaped red cells.
- Bone marrow is usually unobtainable by aspiration ('dry tap'); trephine biopsy shows increased fibrosis.
- The Philadelphia chromosome is absent; this helps to distinguish myelofibrosis from most cases of CML which may present similarly.

Management

- Supportive treatment including transfusions for anaemia and allopurinol to decrease serum uric acid levels.
- Hydroxycarbamide (hydroxyurea) or busulfan are used to reduce the raised white cell and platelet count.
- Splenic irradiation may be useful to reduce a large painful spleen.
- Splenectomy is performed if the spleen is very large and painful and the transfusion requirements are high.

Prognosis

The median survival is 3 years. Transformation to acute myeloid leukaemia occurs in 10–20%.

Myelodysplasia (*K&C* 6e p. 455)

Myelodysplasia is a group of acquired bone marrow disorders caused by a defect in stem cells. There is progressive bone marrow failure, which tends to evolve into acute myeloid leukaemia. The myelodysplastic syndromes are predominantly diseases of the elderly, and are increasingly being diagnosed when a routine full blood count shows an unexplained macrocytosis, anaemia, thrombocytopenia or neutropenia. The diagnosis is made on the basis of characteristic blood film and bone marrow appearances. The paradox of peripheral pancytopenia and a hypercellular bone marrow reflects premature cell loss by apoptosis.

For most elderly patients with symptomatic disease, treatment is supportive, with red cell and platelet transfusions. Allogeneic bone marrow transplantation offers the hope of cure in the minority of patients who are under the age of 50 years. Overall median survival is 20 months.

E SPLEEN (K&C 6e p. 456)

The spleen, situated in the left hypochondrium, is the largest lymphoid organ in the body. Its main functions are phagocytosis of old red blood cells, immunological defence, and to act as a 'pool' of blood from which cells may be rapidly mobilized. Pluripotential stem cells are present in the spleen and proliferate in severe haematological stress (*extramedullary haemopoiesis*), e.g. haemolytic anaemia.

Hypersplenism

Hypersplenism can result from splenomegaly of any cause (Table 5.12). It results in pancytopenia, increased plasma volume and haemolysis caused by increased destruction of red cells. The normal spleen length on ultrasound examination is < 13 cm.

Table 5.12 Causes of splenomegaly	
Sometimes massive (extending into the right iliac fossa)	**Moderate**
Haematological	Haematological
Chronic myeloid leukaemia	Lymphomas
Myelofibrosis	Leukaemias
	Myeloproliferative disorders
	Haemolytic anaemia
Infections	Infections
Chronic malaria	Acute, e.g. endocarditis, typhoid
Schistosomiasis	Chronic, e.g. tuberculosis, brucellosis
Kala-azar	Parasitic, e.g. malaria
Others	Inflammation
Tropical splenomegaly	Rheumatoid arthritis
Gaucher's disease (rarely)	Sarcoidosis
	Systemic lupus erythematosus
	Others
	Portal hypertension, e.g. cirrhosis
	Amyloidosis
	Gaucher's disease

Splenectomy

This is performed mainly for:

- Trauma
- Idiopathic thrombocytopenic purpura
- Haemolytic anaemias
- Hypersplenism.

The main complications are an increased platelet count (thrombophilia) in the short term and overwhelming infection in the longer term. The main infecting organisms are *Streptococcus pneumoniae*, *Haemophilus influenzae* and the meningococci. Vaccination against *S. pneumoniae* and *H. influenzae* should be given to patients about to undergo splenectomy. Immunization with meningococcal group C vaccine is given to all hyposplenic patients; group A vaccine is given to travellers going to areas where there is an increased risk of group A infection. In addition, lifelong antibiotic prophylaxis (e.g. penicillin V 500 mg twice daily) is recommended.

BLOOD PRODUCTS AND TRANSFUSION

217

The components of whole blood are prepared by differential centrifugation of blood collected from volunteer donors.

- Blood components, such as red cell and platelet concentrates, fresh frozen plasma (FFP) and cryoprecipitate, are prepared from single donors.
- Plasma derivatives, such as coagulation factor concentrates, albumin and immunoglobulin are prepared using plasma from many donors as the starting material.

Whole blood itself is rarely used even for acute blood loss. Use of the required component is a more effective use of a scarce resource.

Packed red cells and red cell concentrates are used for acute bleeds (in combination with crystalloid or colloid) and correction of anaemia. Transfusion of red cells in addition to colloid is usually only necessary when >30% (>1500 mL in an adult) of circulating volume has been lost (p. 550). This degree of blood loss is manifest by reduced systolic and diastolic blood pressure, pulse rate >120/minute, slow capillary refill and respiratory rate >20/minute. The patient will be pale and may be anxious

Blood products and tr...

and aggressive. Transfusion may be required for lesser degrees of blood loss that are superimposed on a pre-existing anaemia or reduced cardiorespiratory reserve capacity. Transfusion of red cells is rarely necessary for correction of chronic anaemia (where the underlying cause should be treated) unless the anaemia is severe and life-threatening.

Platelet concentrates are used to treat or prevent bleeding in patients with severe thrombocytopenia. They are not used in stable chronic thrombocytopenia without bleeding. For platelet transfusion, the ABO and RhD group of the patient must be known and the same bedside checks and monitoring procedures as for red cell transfusion must be used. Usually 1 unit (250 mL of plasma containing $> 40 \times 10^9$/L platelets) is given, and the platelet count should rise by $> 20 \times 10^9$/L.

Fresh frozen plasma (FFP) is separated from blood cells and frozen for storage. It contains all the coagulation factors and is used in acquired coagulation factor deficiencies.

Cryoprecipitate is the supernatant obtained after thawing of FFP at 4°C. It contains fibrinogen, antihaemophilic factor (factor VIII), fibrin stabilizing factor (factor XIII), and von Willebrand factor (vWf). It is used for the replacement of fibrinogen when plasma fibrinogen is < 1.0 g/L.

Albumin is sometimes given to patients with acute severe hypoalbuminaemia.

Immunoglobulins are used in patients with hypo-gammaglobulinaemia to prevent infection and in patients with idiopathic thrombocytopenic purpura. Specific immunoglobulin, e.g. anti-hepatitis B, is used after exposure of a non-immune patient to infections.

Blood groups (*K&C* 6e p. 458)

The blood groups are determined by antigens on the surface of red cells; more than 400 blood groups have been found. The ABO (Table 5.13) and rhesus (Rh) systems are the two most important blood groups, but incompatibilities involving many other blood groups (such as Kell and Duffy) may cause haemolytic transfusion reactions and/or haemolytic disease of the newborn. Compatibility testing is performed by the transfusion service in order to select donor blood of the same ABO and Rh group as the recipient and to screen the patient's serum or plasma for antibodies against other red cell antigens that may cause a reduction in

218

Table 5.13 Antigens and antibodies in the ABO system

Blood group	Serum antibody	UK frequency (%)	Comment
O	Anti-A and Anti-B	44	'Universal donors' are O Rh negative
A	Anti-B	45	
B	Anti-A	8	
AB	None	3	Universal recipients

the survival of the transfused red cells. After a massive bleed when immediate transfusion is necessary, O RhD negative blood can be given without any transfusion investigations being undertaken. It should only need to be used on rare occasions.

Many hospitals have guidelines for the ordering of blood for elective surgery. Operations in which blood is required only occasionally can be classified as 'group and save' in order to conserve blood usage. In this case ABO and Rh testing is performed along with the antibody screen. Should blood unexpectedly be required during the course of the procedure, compatible units can be released within a matter of minutes after an immediate spin crossmatch whereby the patient's serum or plasma is incubated with the donor red cells to confirm ABO compatibility.

Blood transfusion is a potentially hazardous procedure which should only be undertaken when the benefits outweigh the risks. Stringent procedures need to be followed to ensure that the correct blood is given to the correct patient and that any adverse reactions are dealt with promptly and efficiently. The temperature, pulse rate and blood pressure should be recorded before the start of each unit, 15 minutes after the start and at hourly intervals during the transfusion. A temperature rise of 1°C or greater above baseline may indicate an acute haemolytic transfusion reaction due to ABO incompatibility and is an indication to stop the transfusion. The care of patients receiving blood and blood products is illustrated in Table 5.14.

Complications of transfusing red blood cells (*K&C* 6e p. 460)

■ ABO incompatibility is the most serious complication and often results from simple clerical errors, leading to

Table 5.14   Care of the patient receiving a blood transfusion or blood products

1 Taking the blood sample for crossmatching
Identify patient positively by asking their surname, forename, date of birth
Confirm that identification details on hospital wrist band match those on transfusion request form
Label sample tube after blood has been added
Label sample tube with patient identification (full name, date of birth, hospital number), patient location, date of sample and signature of person taking blood

2 Procedure for patient identification before transfusion
Blood must be checked by two qualified nurses, one of whom is a registered nurse, before transfusion
Check the blood bag is not leaking or wet and has a compatibility label attached
Check patient identify by cross-checking the patient's full name, sex, date of birth, hospital number on:
Patient's name band which the patient must be wearing
Blood transfusion request form
Compatibility label attached to the blood pack
Medical case notes
Intravenous fluid prescription chart
Check the expiry date of the unit of blood on:
Compatibility label
Blood bag
Check the blood group (ABO and RhD) and blood pack donation number on:
Blood transfusion request form
Blood pack and compatibility label
Record the blood pack donation number on:
Intravenous fluid prescription chart
Date and time and signature of both nurses on:
Blood transfusion request form
Compatibility label
Intravenous fluid prescription chart

the incorrect labelling and identification of blood and patient's blood sample for crossmatching. There is an immediate reaction, starting within minutes of the transfusion, leading to intravascular haemolysis, rigors, lumbar pain, dyspnoea and hypotension. The transfusion must be stopped and the donor units returned to the blood transfusion laboratory for testing with a new blood sample from the patient. Emergency treatment may be needed to maintain the blood pressure (p. 556). Auto-immune haemolysis may develop about a week after transfusion in patients alloimmunized by previous trans-fusions in whom the antibody level is too low to be detected during compatibility testing.

- Febrile reactions are usually the result of antileucocyte antibodies in the recipient acting against transfused leucocytes, leading to the release of pyrogens. The introduction of leucocyte-depleted blood in the UK in 1999, to minimize the risk of transmission of variant Creutzfeldt–Jakob disease by blood transfusion, has reduced the incidence of febrile reactions.
- Anaphylactic reactions are seen in patients lacking IgA but who produce anti-IgA that reacts with IgA in the transfused blood. This is a medical emergency (p. 555). Urticarial reactions are treated by slowing of the infusion and giving intravenous antihistamines, e.g. chlor-phenamine (chlorpheniramine) 10 mg i.v.
- Transmission of infection has decreased now that donated blood is tested for hepatitis B surface antigen and antibodies to hepatitis C, HIV-1 and HTLV-1 (human T-cell lymphotropic virus). CMV-seronegative blood is given to immunosuppressed patients who are suscep-tible to acquiring CMV (cytomegalovirus).
- Heart failure may occur, particularly in elderly people and those having large transfusions.
- Complications of massive transfusion (> 10 units within 24 hours) include hypocalcaemia, hyperkalaemia and hypothermia. Bleeding may occur as a result of depletion of platelets and clotting factors in stored blood.
- In post-transfusion purpura, severe thrombocytopenia develops 7–10 days after the transfusion. Antibodies develop against the human platelet antigen 1a, leading to immune destruction of the patient's own platelets.

Concerns about the safety of blood transfusion have led to increased interest in strategies for avoiding or reducing the use of donor blood. These include artificial haemoglobin solutions and autologous blood transfusion. The latter is more popular in developing countries and involves col-lection of blood from the donor/patient either preoperatively or by intraoperative blood salvage.

BLEEDING DISORDERS

A bleeding disorder is suggested when the patient has unexplained (i.e. no history of trauma) bruising or bleeding, or prolonged bleeding in response to injury or surgery, e.g. after tooth extraction.

Reactions involved in haemostasis (K&C 6e p. 466)

Haemostasis is the process of blood clot formation at the site of vessel injury. When a blood vessel wall breaks, the haemostatic response must be quick, localized to the site of injury, and carefully regulated. Abnormal bleeding or a propensity to non-physiological thrombosis (i.e. thrombosis not required for haemostatic regulation) may occur when specific elements of these processes are missing or dysfunctional.

Haemostasis is a complex process and depends on interactions between the vessel wall, platelets and coagulation and fibrinolytic mechanisms.

- *Blood vessel damage* leads to immediate vasoconstriction, reducing blood flow to the injured area and allowing contact activation of platelets and coagulation factors.
- *Formation of the platelet plug.* The intact vascular endothelium prevents the adherence of platelets. Intimal injury and exposure of subendothelial elements such as collagen lead to the adherence of platelets on the subendothelial matrix. Platelet *adhesion* to collagen is dependent on platelet membrane receptors, glycoprotein Ia (GPIa), which binds directly to collagen, and glycoprotein Ib (GPIb), which binds to von Willebrand factor (vWF) in the plasma; vWF in turn adheres to collagen. Deficiency of GPIb or vWF leads to congenital bleeding disorders: Bernard–Soulier disease and von Willebrand's disease, respectively. Following adhesion, platelets spread along the subendothelium and *release* the contents of their cytoplasmic granules containing adenosine diphosphate (ADP), serotonin, thromboxane A_2, fibrinogen and other factors. Release of ADP results in both exposure of, and a conformational change in the GP IIb/IIIa receptor on the platelet surface, leading to binding of the divalent molecule, fibrinogen, that bridges the activated platelets (*aggregation*). The importance of GP IIb/IIIa is illustrated by the clinical utility of GP IIb/IIIa antagonists in the treatment of coronary disease

222

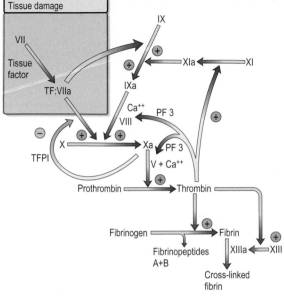

Fig. 5.5 Coagulation mechanism. The in vivo pathway begins with activation of factor IX by factor VIIa. Factor XI is activated by thrombin. TFPI, tissue factor pathway inhibitor; PF 3, platelet factor 3.

(p. 439). During aggregation, platelet membrane receptors are exposed, providing a surface for the interaction of coagulation factors and ultimately the formation of a stable haemostatic plug.

■ *Clotting cascade and propagation of the clot.* Coagulation involves a series of enzymatic reactions leading to the conversion of soluble plasma fibrinogen to fibrin clot (Fig. 5.5). The local generation of fibrin enmeshes and reinforces the platelet plug. All of these proteins are synthesized in the liver except vWf, which is synthesized in megakaryocytes and endothelial cells. The vitamin K-dependent enzymes are prothrombin, factors VII, IX and X. Traditionally, the clotting cascade is depicted as consisting of an intrinsic and an extrinsic pathway. Both pathways converge on the activation of factor X, which then activates prothrombin to thrombin, the final enzyme of the clotting cascade. It is now established that the generation or exposure of tissue factor (TF) at the wound site is the primary physiological event in initiating clotting. Deficiencies in the major proteins involved in the initiation of the intrinsic pathway, such as factor XII, are not associated with excessive bleeding.

Limitation of coagulation

Coagulation would lead to dangerous occlusion of blood vessels if it were not limited to the site of injury by protective mechanisms.

Rapid blood flow   Rapid blood flow at the periphery of the damaged area dilutes and removes coagulation factors.

Circulating inhibitors of the coagulation factors
- Antithrombin binds to and forms stable complexes with coagulation factors. Activity is increased by heparin.
- Active protein C inactivates factors V and VIII.
- Protein S is a cofactor for protein C.

Inherited deficiency or abnormality of these natural anti-coagulant proteins is termed *thrombophilia* and places the patient at increased risk of both arterial and venous thrombosis.

The fibrinolytic system   The plasma protein plasminogen is converted to plasmin by activators present in the tissue and endothelial cells. Plasmin induces lysis of cross-linked (X-linked) fibrin, resulting in the formation of various X-linked fibrin degradation products (FDPs), which include D-dimers which can easily be measured using monoclonal antibodies.

Bleeding disorders are therefore the result of a defect in vessels, platelets or the coagulation pathway (Table 5.15).

Investigation of bleeding disorders

The nature of the defect and therefore the most appropriate initial investigations may be suggested by the history and examination, e.g. family history, intercurrent disease, alcohol consumption, drugs. Vascular/platelet bleeding is characterized by bruising of the skin and bleeding from mucosal membranes. Bleeding into the skin is manifest as petechiae (small capillary haemorrhages of a few mm diameter) and superficial ecchymoses (larger areas of

Table 5.15 Classification of bleeding disorders

Blood vessel defect
Hereditary
  Hereditary haemorrhagic telangiectasia (rare)
  Connective tissue disorders: Marfan's and Ehlers–Danlos
    syndromes
Acquired
  Severe infections: meningococcal, typhoid
  Drugs: steroids
  Allergic: Henoch–Schönlein purpura (mainly children)
  Others: scurvy, senile purpura
  Easy bruising syndrome

Platelet defect
Decreased platelet number or decreased function

Coagulation defect
Hereditary
  Haemophilia A or B, von Willebrand's disease
Acquired
  Anticoagulant treatment, liver disease, disseminated
    intravascular coagulation

bleeding). Haemophilia A and B are typically associated with spontaneous haemarthroses (bleeding into joints) and muscle haematomas. The most common cause of abnormal bleeding is thrombocytopenia.

- Platelet count and blood film will show the number and morphology of platelets and any blood disorder such as leukaemia.
- Coagulation tests are abnormal with deficiencies or inhibitors of the clotting factors. If the abnormal result is corrected by the addition of normal plasma to the patient's plasma in the assay, then the result is abnormal as a result of deficiency and not of inhibitors.
  - The prothrombin time (PT) is prolonged with abnormalities of factors VII, X, V, II or I, liver disease, or if the patient is on warfarin. The international normalized ratio (INR) is the ratio of the patient's PT to a normal control when using the international reference preparation. The advantage of the INR over the PT, is that it uses international standards and thus anticoagulant control can be compared in different hospitals across the world.

- The activated partial thromboplastin time (APTT) is prolonged with deficiencies or inhibitors of one or more of the following factors: XII, XI, IX, VIII, X, V or I (but not factor VII).
- Thrombin time (TT) is prolonged with fibrinogen deficiency, dysfibrinogenaemia (normal levels but abnormal function), heparin treatment or disseminated intravascular coagulation.

The normal ranges of these tests vary from laboratory to laboratory, and patient results must be compared with the testing laboratory's reference range.

- The bleeding time is a measure of the interaction of platelets with the blood vessel wall and is abnormal with von Willebrand's disease, with blood vessel defects, and when there is a decrease in the number or function of platelets.

These tests will localize the site of the problem. Further specialized investigations, e.g. platelet aggregation studies and measurement of fibrinogen, FDPs and individual clotting factors, will be necessary to identify the exact haemostatic defect correctly.

Platelet disorders

Platelet disorders are the result of thrombocytopenia (platelet count $< 150 \times 10^9$/L; Table 5.16) or disorders of platelet function, e.g. those occurring with aspirin treatment and uraemia. Congenital abnormalities of platelet number (e.g. Fanconi's anaemia, Wiskott–Aldrich syndrome) or function (e.g. Bernard–Soulier syndrome) are all extremely rare.

Mild thrombocytopenia can be artefactual and due to platelet clumping or a blood clot in the sample. This is excluded by asking the haematologist to confirm an unexpectedly low count by manual differentiation. Spontaneous bleeding from skin and mucous membranes is unlikely to occur with platelet counts above 20×10^9/L. Increased destruction or decreased production can be differentiated by bone marrow examination, which will show respectively increased or decreased numbers of megakaryocytes (platelet precursors). Platelet transfusion is usually indicated when the platelet count is very low ($< 10 \times 10^9$/L) or to maintain a platelet count of $> 50 \times 10^9$/L in the presence of active bleeding or prior to an invasive procedure.

Table 5.16 Causes of thrombocytopenia	
Impaired production	**Excessive destruction**
Bone marrow failure	**Immune**
Megaloblastic anaemia	Autoimmune thrombocytopenia
Leukaemia	Secondary immune (SLE, CLL,
Myeloma	viruses, drugs, e.g. heparin)
Myelofibrosis	Post-transfusion purpura
Myelodysplasia	
Solid tumour infiltration	**Sequestration**
Aplastic anaemia (Table 5.6)	Hypersplenism
	Dilutional
	Massive transfusion
	Other
	Disseminated intravascular
	coagulation
	Thrombotic thrombocytopenic
	purpura
	Haemolytic uraemic syndrome

SLE, systemic lupus erythematosus; CLL, chronic lymphocytic
leukaemia
Thrombocytopenia due to impaired production is usually also
associated with failure of red and white cell production

Idiopathic thrombocytopenic purpura (K&C 6e p. 470)

Thrombocytopenia results from immune destruction of
platelets. Acute autoimmune thrombocytopenic purpura
(AITP) is seen in children, often following a viral infection.
There is rapid onset of purpura, which is usually self-
limiting and becomes chronic in only about 5% of cases.
Chronic AITP is more commonly seen in adults, and
platelet autoantibodies are detected in 60–70% of patients.

Aetiology

Chronic AITP is usually idiopathic, but may occur with
autoimmune disorders, e.g. systemic lupus erythematosus,
thyroid disease, chronic lymphatic leukaemia and some
viral infections, e.g. HIV. The same drugs that cause
autoimmune haemolytic anaemia (p. 209) may also cause
thrombocytopenia (and neutropenia).

Clinical features

The condition is characteristically seen in young women. There is a fluctuating course, with easy bruising, epistaxis and menorrhagia. Major haemorrhage is rare.

Investigation

There is thrombocytopenia with normal or increased megakaryocytes on bone marrow examination. The detection of antiplatelet autoantibodies is unnecessary in a straightforward case.

Management

Patients with platelet counts greater than 30×10^9/L require no treatment unless they are about to undergo a surgical procedure.

First-line therapy consists of oral corticosteroids but intravenous immunoglobulin (i.v. IgG) is useful where a rapid rise in platelet count is desired, especially before surgery.

Second-line therapy is splenectomy, to which the majority of patients respond. A wide range of treatments are available for chronic AITP. These include high-dose corticosteroids, high-dose i.v. IgG, intravenous anti-D, vinca alkaloids, danazol, immunosuppressive agents such as azathioprine, ciclosporin and dapsone. There is also interest in the use of specific monoclonal antibodies such as rituximab, as well as recombinant thrombopoietin.

Platelet transfusions are reserved for intracranial or other extreme haemorrhage, where emergency splenectomy may be justified.

Thrombotic thrombocytopenic purpura (TTP) (*K&C* 6e pp. 471 & 636)

TTP is a rare, serious condition, in which platelet destruction leads to profound thrombocytopenia. There is a characteristic symptom complex of florid purpura, fever, fluctuating cerebral dysfunction and haemolytic anaemia with red cell fragmentation, often accompanied by renal failure. The coagulation screen is usually normal but lactic dehydrogenase (LDH) levels are markedly raised as a result of haemolysis. The aetiology is poorly understood and treatment is usually with a combination of plasma exchange, oral prednisolone, and aspirin.

Inherited coagulation disorders

Inherited disorders usually involve a deficiency of only one coagulation factor, whereas acquired disorders involve a deficiency of several factors.

Haemophilia A (*K&C* 8e p. 472)

This is the result of a deficiency of factor VIII:C, which is one part of the factor VIII molecule. It is inherited as an X-linked recessive, affecting 1 in 5000 males.

Clinical features

Clinical features depend on the plasma levels of factor VIII:C.

- Levels of less than 1% are associated with frequent spontaneous bleeding into muscles and joints that can lead to a crippling arthropathy.
- Levels of 1–5% are associated with severe bleeding following injury and occasional apparently spontaneous episodes.
- Levels above 5% produce mild disease with bleeding only with trauma or surgery.

The most frequent cause of death in patients with severe haemophilia was cerebral haemorrhage. However, transmission of HIV and hepatic disease (hepatitis C and hepatocellular carcinoma) as a result of plasma-derived therapy are now the most common.

Investigations

The APTT is prolonged and plasma factor VIII:C levels are reduced. The PT and bleeding time are normal.

Management

- Intravenous injection of factor VIII concentrate is the mainstay of treatment. It is given as prophylaxis, e.g. before and after surgery, or to treat an acute bleeding episode. Most severely affected patients are now given prophylaxis three times weekly from early childhood to try to prevent permanent joint damage. Many patients also have a supply of factor VIII concentrate at home to inject at the first sign of bleeding. Recombinant factor VIII is the treatment of choice, though cost constraints

229

have resulted in some patients still being offered treatment with plasma derived concentrates.

■ Synthetic vasopressin (desmopressin) – intravenous, subcutaneous or intranasal administration – raises the level of factor VIII and may be used to treat patients with mild haemophilia.

■ Patients should be vaccinated against hepatitis A and B and encouraged to take part in exercise regimens that avoid contact sport.

Complications

Recurrent bleeding into joints leads to deformity and arthritis. In the past, multiple transfusions of plasma-derived clotting factor concentrates were associated with an increased risk of acquiring hepatitis C and HIV. This risk has been virtually eliminated because of the exclusion of high-risk blood donors, screening of donors and heat treatment of factor VIII concentrates. Ten per cent of people with haemophilia develop antibodies to factor VIII, and may need massive doses to overcome this. Recombinant factor VIIa is used to 'bypass' the inhibitor and shows promise in treating these patients.

Haemophilia B (Christmas disease) (*K&C* 6e p. 474)

This is the result of a deficiency of factor IX, and affects 1 in 30 000 males. Inheritance and clinical features are the same as for haemophilia A. Treatment is with factor IX concentrates. Desmopressin is ineffective.

Von Willebrand's disease (vWD) (*K&C* 6e p. 474)

vWD is the most common inherited bleeding disorder and is caused by an inherited deficiency of von Willebrand factor, an essential cofactor for normal platelet adhesion to damaged subendothelium. This factor also serves as a carrier for factor VIII:C to form the whole VIII complex and protecting VIII:C from inactivation and clearance.

Clinical features

Types 1 and 2 are mild forms, with autosomal dominant inheritance and characterized by mucosal bleeding (nose bleeds and gastrointestinal bleeding) and prolonged bleeding after dental treatment or surgery.

Type 3 patients have more severe bleeding, but rarely experience the joint and muscle bleeds seen in haemophilia A.

Investigations

Prolonged bleeding time reflects a defect in platelet adhesion. There is a prolonged APTT, normal PT and decreased plasma levels of VIII:C and VIII:vWF.

Management

This depends on the severity of the bleeding, and includes treatment with desmopressin and factor VIII concentrates.

Acquired coagulation disorders

Disseminated intravascular coagulation (DIC) (*K&C* 6e p. 475)
There is widespread generation of fibrin within blood vessels, caused by initiation of the coagulation pathway. There is consumption of platelets and coagulation factors, and secondary activation of fibrinolysis leading to production of fibrin degradation products (FDPs), which contribute to coagulation by inhibiting fibrin polymerization.

Aetiology

DIC results from massive activation of the clotting cascade. The major initiating factors are the release or expression of tissue factor, extensive damage to vascular endothelium exposing tissue factor or enhanced expression of tissue factor by monocytes in response to cytokines. The most common causes of DIC are sepsis, major trauma and tissue destruction (surgery, burns), advanced cancer and obstetric complications (amniotic fluid embolism, abruptio placentae). DIC occurs in most cases of acute promyelocytic leukaemia due to generation of procoagulant substances in the blood.

Clinical features

The presentation varies from no bleeding at all to complete haemostatic failure, with bleeding from venepuncture sites and the nose and mouth. Thrombotic events may occur as a result of vessel occlusion by platelets and fibrin.

Investigations

The diagnosis is suggested by the history (e.g. severe sepsis, trauma, malignancy), the clinical presentation and the presence of moderate to severe thrombocytopenia. It is confirmed by finding a prolonged PT, APTT and TT, decreased fibrinogen and elevated FDPs. The blood film shows fragmented red cells. In mild cases with compensatory increase of coagulation factors, the only abnormality may be an increase in the FDPs, or in the D-dimer fragment reflecting accelerated fibrinolysis.

Management

- Treat the underlying condition.
- Platelets (to maintain count $> 50 \times 10^9/\text{L}$), fresh frozen plasma, cryoprecipitate and red cell concentrates are indicated in patients who are bleeding.

Vitamin K deficiency (*K&C* 6e pp. 242 & 475)

Vitamin K is needed for the formation of active factors II, VII, IX and X. Deficiency, which occurs in malabsorption of vitamin K and with warfarin treatment (an inhibitor of vitamin K synthesis), leads to an increase in PT and APTT. Treatment, if required, is with parenteral phytomenadione (vitamin K).

Liver disease (*K&C* 6e p. 475)

Liver disease results in a number of defects of haemostasis: vitamin K deficiency in cholestasis, reduced synthesis of clotting factors, thrombocytopenia and functional abnormalities of platelets. DIC may occur in acute liver failure.

THROMBOSIS

A thrombus is defined as a solid mass formed in the circulation from the constituents of the blood during life. Fragments of thrombi (emboli) may break off and block vessels downstream.

Arterial thrombosis (*K&C* 6e p. 476)

Arterial thrombosis is usually the result of atheroma, which forms particularly in areas of turbulent blood flow, such as the bifurcation of arteries. Platelets adhere to the damaged vascular endothelium and aggregate in response to ADP and thromboxane A_2. This may stimulate blood coagulation, leading to complete occlusion of the vessel, or embolization resulting in distal obstruction.

Prevention and treatment of arterial thrombosis

Prevention of thrombosis is with antiplatelet drugs

- Aspirin inhibits cyclo-oxygenase (COX) reducing production of thromboxane A_2 (p. 222). It is the most commonly used antiplatelet drug.
- Dipyridamole inhibits phosphodiesterase-mediated breakdown of cyclic AMP, which prevents platelet activation.
- Clopidogrel and ticlopidine block platelet aggregation and prolong platelet survival by inhibiting the binding of ADP to its platelet receptor. Ticlopidine has been associated with granulocytopenia and thrombotic thrombocytopenic purpura.
- Antibodies (e.g. abciximab), peptides (e.g. eptifibatide), and non-peptide antagonists (e.g. tirofiban) block the receptor of glycoprotein IIb/IIIa, inhibiting the final common pathway of platelet aggregation. Excessive bleeding has been a problem and research continues to identify their clinical role.
- *Epoprostenol* is a prostacyclin which is used to inhibit platelet aggregation during renal dialysis (with or without heparin) and is also used in primary pulmonary hypertension.

233

Treatment of thrombosis (thrombolytic therapy)

- Streptokinase is a purified fraction of the filtrate obtained from cultures of haemolytic streptococci. It forms a complex with plasminogen which activates other plasminogen molecules to form plasmin. The dose in myocardial infarction is 1.5 million units given by infusion over 1 hour. The main disadvantage of streptokinase is the indiscriminate activation of plasminogen both in clots and in the circulation, leading to an increased risk of haemorrhage. Nevertheless, this is currently the thrombolytic agent of choice in acute myocardial infarction.
- Tissue-type plasminogen activators such as alteplase (t-PA), tenecteplase (TNK-PA) and reteplase(r-PA) are produced using recombinant gene technology. Unlike streptokinase, they are not antigenic and do not give allergic reactions, though they have a slightly higher risk of intracerebral haemorrhage.

The use of thrombolytic therapy in myocardial infarction, pulmonary embolism and ischaemic stroke is discussed on pages 446, 469, and 730. The main risk of thrombolysis is bleeding. Contraindications are prolonged or traumatic cardiopulmonary resuscitation, trauma, a recent major bleed, stroke within the previous 6 months (other than acutely in ischaemic stroke), uncontrolled hypertension, surgery or other invasive procedures within the previous 2 weeks, and bleeding disorders.

Venous thrombosis (K&C 6e p. 477)

Unlike arterial thrombosis, venous thrombosis usually occurs in normal vessels, often in the deep veins of the leg. It originates around the valves as red thrombi consisting of red cells and fibrin. Propagation occurs, inducing a risk of embolization to the pulmonary vessels. Chronic venous obstruction in the leg results in a permanently swollen leg which is prone to ulceration (post-phlebitic syndrome). Factors predisposing to venous thromboembolism are listed in Table 5.17. The clinical features and investigation of deep venous thrombosis (DVT) and pulmonary embolism are discussed on pages 484 and 466.

234

Prevention and treatment of venous thromboembolism (K&C 6e p. 479)

Heparin and warfarin are the two drugs used most frequently in the prevention and treatment of thrombo-embolism (Table 5.18). In general, prophylaxis of venous thromboembolism relies on measures that prevent stasis, such as early mobilization, elevation of the legs and compression stockings, with heparin reserved for higher-risk patients. Low-molecular-weight (LMW) heparins (e.g. enoxaparin 20–40 mg s.c. daily depending on risk), produced by the enzymatic or chemical breakdown of the heparin molecule, are now preferred to conventional heparin for venous prophylaxis in most cases. These can be administered on a once-daily basis, have greater efficacy than conventional heparin in high-risk patients, and do not require monitoring of clotting times. For patients at high risk of bleeding, unfractionated heparin is more suitable because its effect can be terminated rapidly by stopping the infusion.

Table 5.17 **Risk factors for venous thromboembolism**

Major risk factors (relative risk 5–20)	Minor risk factors (relative risk 2–4)
Major abdominal/pelvic surgery	Cardiac failure
Recent hip/knee replacement	Recent myocardial infarction
Postoperative intensive care	Hypertension
Late pregnancy	Superficial venous thrombosis
Caesarean section	Indwelling central vein catheter
Puerperium	Oral contraceptive
Lower limb fracture	Hormone replacement therapy
Varicose veins	COPD
Abdominal/pelvic malignancy	Occult malignancy
Advanced malignancy	Long-distance sedentary travel
Immobility (hospitalization/institutional care)	Thrombophilia
Previous venous thromboembolism	Antithrombin deficiency
	Protein C or S deficiency
	Resistance to activated protein C (factor V Leiden mutation)
	Prothrombin gene variant
	Homocysteinaemia
	Antiphospholipid antibody
	Serious infection
	Inflammatory bowel disease
	Nephrotic syndrome
	Polycythaemia
	Thrombocythaemia
	Paroxysmal nocturnal haemoglobinuria
	Sickle cell anaemia
	Obesity

235

Treatment of established thromboembolism:

- Obtain objective evidence of thrombosis as soon as possible; heparin treatment is often started on the basis of clinical suspicion.
- Perform a coagulation screen and platelet count before starting treatment to exclude a pre-existing thrombotic tendency.
- Heparin treatment:
  - Low-molecular-weight heparin, (e.g. tinzaparin 175 units/kg s.c. daily). Where feasible, selected patients with DVT can be safely treated with LMW heparin as outpatients.

Table 5.18	Anticoagulant treatment	
	Heparin	**Warfarin**
Route of administration	s.c./i.v.	Oral
Half-life	2 hours, longer for LMWH	2 days
Mode of action	Potentiates antithrombotic effects of antithrombin	Inhibits vitamin K-dependent gamma carboxylation of factors II, VII, IX and X
Monitoring	APPT Not necessary for LMW heparin	PT/INR
Reversal of anticoagulation (usually only if patient is bleeding)	Stop heparin Intravenous protamine sulphate 20–50 mg over 10 min (less useful with LMWH) FFP if life-threatening bleed	Stop warfarin Vitamin K, 1 mg by slow intravenous injection FFP 15 mL/kg

OR

- Give 5000 units of standard (unfractionated) heparin intravenously (10 000 units in severe pulmonary embolism) as a loading dose and continue with an intravenous infusion of 1000–2000 units per hour, or subcutaneous injections of 15 000 units every 12 hours. Check the APPT daily 4–6 hours after dose of heparin. Adjust the heparin dose to maintain an APPT of 1.5 to 2.5 times control.

- Warfarin 5–10 mg orally is started at the same time as the heparin.

- The dose of warfarin is adjusted to maintain the INR usually at two to three times the control value.

- Heparin is overlapped with warfarin for a *minimum* of 5 days and continued until the INR is in the therapeutic range (Table 5.19).

Table 5.19	Indications for oral anticoagulation and target INR
Target INR	
2.5	Pulmonary embolism, deep vein thrombosis, symptomatic inherited thrombophilia, atrial fibrillation, cardioversion, mural thrombus, cardiomyopathy
3.5	Recurrence of venous thromboembolism while on warfarin therapy, antiphospholipid syndrome, mechanical prosthetic heart valve, coronary artery graft thrombosis

- Major side-effects of heparin therapy are bleeding and thrombocytopenia. The platelet count should be measured in all patients receiving heparin for more than 5 days.

Anticoagulation for 6 weeks is sufficient for patients after their first thrombosis with a precipitating cause, provided there are no persisting risk factors. Long-term anticoagulation is required for those with repeated episodes or continuing risk factors.

Ximelagatran This oral direct thrombin inhibitor is a potential alternative to warfarin and has already been evaluated in patients with venous thromboembolism, atrial fibrillation and myocardial infarction. It has a rapid onset of action and can be administered in a fixed dose without the need for monitoring. Drug interactions are also less than for warfarin but elimination is primarily renal, and abnormalities of liver function have been described during its use.

THE HAEMATOLOGICAL MALIGNANCIES

The leukaemias (*K&C* 6e p. 501)

The leukaemias are malignant neoplasms of the haemopoietic stem cells, characterized by diffuse replacement of the bone marrow by neoplastic cells. In most cases, the leukaemic cells spill over into the blood, where they may be seen in large numbers. The cells may also infiltrate the liver, spleen, lymph nodes and other tissues throughout the body. They are relatively rare diseases with an overall incidence of 10 per 100 000 per year.

General classification The characteristics of leukaemic cells can be assessed by light microscopy, expression of cytosolic enzymes and expression of surface antigens. These will reflect the lineage and degree of maturity of the leukaemic clone. Thus, leukaemia can be divided on the basis of the speed of evolution of the disease into acute or chronic. Each of these is then further subdivided into myeloid or lymphoid, according to the cell type involved:

- Acute myelogenous leukaemia (AML)
- Acute lymphoblastic leukaemia (ALL)
- Chronic myeloid leukaemia (CML)
- Chronic lymphocytic leukaemia (CLL).

Aetiology

In most cases the aetiology is unknown though several factors are associated.

Genetic factors Genetic factors are suggested by the increased incidence in patients with chromosomal disorders (e.g. Down's syndrome) and in identical twins of affected patients. Chromosomal abnormalities have been described in patients with leukaemia. The earliest described was the Philadelphia (Ph) chromosome, found in 95% of cases with CML and some patients with ALL. In the Ph chromosome the long arm of chromosome 22 is shortened by reciprocal translocation to the long arm of chromosome 9 (t(9;22)). The resulting chimeric protein, BCR-ABL, has tyrosine kinase activity, and enhanced phosphorylating activity compared with the normal protein, resulting in altered cell growth, stromal attachment and apoptosis.

The leukaemic cells of most patients with acute promyelocytic leukaemia have the translocation t(15;17) involving the retinoic acid receptor alpha (*RARa*) on chromosome 17 and the promyelocytic leukaemia gene (*PML*) on chromosome 15. The resulting PML-RARa fusion protein shows reduced sensitivity to retinoic acid and prevents differentiation of myeloid cells.

Environmental factors
- Chemicals, e.g. benzene compounds used in industry.
- Drugs, e.g. chemotherapy using chlorambucil, procarbazine, melphalan.
- Radiation exposure, e.g. nuclear generators and treatment for Hodgkin's disease.

Treatment of haematological malignancies

The treatment of the haematological malignances is based on the use of chemotherapy and radiotherapy. Surgery and other treatments (e.g. steroids and interferon) are used less often.

Chemotherapeutic agents (*K&C* 6e p. 492)

There are many chemotherapy drugs in common use. They directly damage DNA and RNA and kill cells by promoting apoptosis and sometimes cell necrosis. They therefore affect not only tumour cells, but also the rapidly dividing normal cells of the bone marrow, gastrointestinal tract and germinal epithelium. The principal side-effects are:

■ Bone marrow suppression, leading to anaemia, thrombo-cytopenia and infection
■ Mucositis, causing mouth ulceration
■ Loss of hair (alopecia)
■ Sterility, which can be irreversible.

To minimize these side-effects, chemotherapy is given at intervals to allow some recovery of normal cell function between cycles. Nausea and vomiting may be severe with some drugs, such as cisplatin, and are related to the direct actions of cytotoxic agents on the brainstem chemoreceptor trigger zone. Antiemetics such as metoclopramide and domperidone are used initially, but the serotonin $5\text{-}HT_3$ antagonists (ondansetron and granisetron) combined with dexamethasone are used for severe vomiting. Chemo-therapy drugs may themselves cause cancer, particularly acute leukaemia presenting years after treatment. Finally there are additional side-effects that are specific to one class of drug, e.g. cardiotoxicity with the anthracyclines such as doxorubicin.

Radiotherapy (*K&C* 6e p. 499)

Radiation induces strand breaks in DNA and induces apoptosis. The complications of radiotherapy depend on the radiosensitivity of normal tissue in the path of the radiation field. General side-effects are lethargy and loss of energy. There may be damage to the skin (erythema and desquamation), gut (nausea, mucosal ulceration and diarrhoea), testes (sterility) and bone marrow (anaemia, leucopenia).

239

Biological therapy (*K&C* 6e p. 497)

The group includes a range of protein molecules, from small peptide chemokines and larger cytokines to complex antibody molecules, made available by genetic engineering. For example interferons such as alpha-interferon (IFN-α) have many actions in treatment of malignant disease, with both antiproliferative activity and stimulation of humoral and cell-mediated immune responses to the tumour that can result in an antitumour effect if the host effector mechanisms are present and fully competent. Haemopoietic growth factors such as erythropoietin and granulocyte colony-stimulating factor (G-CSF) are used to treat anaemia or to reduce the duration of neutropenia following chemotherapy. Humanized monoclonal antibodies such as rituximab and bevacizumab, directed against tumour cell surface antigens, are being increasingly employed as primary treatment for haematological malignancies and solid tumours.

Acute leukaemia (*K&C* 6e p. 502)

The acute leukaemias are characterized by a clonal pro-liferation of myeloid or lymphoid precursors with reduced capacity to differentiate into more mature cellular elements. There is accumulation of leukaemic cells in the bone marrow, peripheral blood and other tissues with a reduction in red cells, platelets and neutrophils.

Epidemiology

Both types of acute leukaemia can occur in all age groups, but ALL is predominantly a disease of childhood, whereas AML is seen most frequently in older adults (middle-aged and elderly).

Clinical features

These are the result of marrow failure: anaemia, bleeding and infection, e.g. sore throat and pneumonia. Sometimes there is peripheral lymphadenopathy and hepatospleno-megaly.

Investigations

A definitive diagnosis is made on the peripheral blood film and a bone marrow aspirate. The various subtypes

Table 5.20 The World Health Organization classification of acute leukaemia

a. AML (acute myeloid leukaemia)
1. AML with recurrent cytogenetic abnormalities (including acute promyelocytic leukaemia with t(15;17) or variants
2. AML with multilineage dysplasia (usually secondary to a pre-existing myelodysplastic syndrome)
3. Therapy-related AML, i.e. occurring after chemotherapy or radiotherapy
4. AML – other (including minimally differentiated AML)
5. Acute biphenotypic leukaemia (acute leukaemia expressing both lymphoid and myeloid phenotype)

b. ALL (acute lymphoblastic leukaemia)
1. Precursor B acute lymphoblastic leukaemia
2. Burkitt cell leukaemia
3. Precursor T acute lymphoblastic leukaemia

(Table 5.20) are classified on the basis of morphology and immunophenotyping, and cytogenetic studies of blast cells. However, the presence of Auer rods (a rod-like conglomeration of granules in the cytoplasm) within blast cells is pathognomonic of AML. If the patient has a fever, blood cultures and chest radiograph are essential.

- The full blood count shows anaemia and thrombocytopenia. The white cell count is usually raised, but may be normal or low.
- The peripheral blood film shows characteristic leukaemic blast cells.
- Bone marrow aspirate usually shows increased cellularity, with a high percentage of abnormal lymphoid or myeloid blast cells.

Management

The initial requirement of therapy is to return the peripheral blood and bone marrow to normal (complete remission; CR) with 'induction chemotherapy' tailored to the particular leukaemia and the individual patient's risk factors. The risk of failure of treatment is based on the cytogenetic pattern (K&C 6e p 503). Successful remission induction is always followed by further treatment (consolidation), the details being determined by the type of leukaemia and the patient's

241

risk factors (and the patient's tolerance of treatment). Recurrence is almost invariable if 'consolidation' therapy is not given.

General Before starting treatment the following need to be considered:

- Correction of anaemia and thrombocytopenia by administration of blood and platelets
- Treatment of infection with intravenous antibiotics
- Prevention of the acute tumour lysis syndrome (ATLS) with adequate hydration and allopurinol. ATLS results from a massive release of cellular breakdown products consequent upon tumour cell death following effective therapy. The biochemical disturbances include hyperkalaemia, hyperuricaemia, hyperphosphataemia and hypocalcaemia (due to precipitation of calcium phosphate).

Treatment of AML (K&C 6e p. 504)

Treatment with curative intent is undertaken in the majority of adults below the age of 60 years, provided there is no significant co-morbidity.

- Patients at low risk are treated with an aggressive combination of intravenous chemotherapy, e.g. cytosine arabinoside (cytarabine) and daunorubicin given at intervals to allow marrow recovery in between. This is followed by consolidation therapy with a minimum of four cycles of treatment given at 3- to 4-week intervals.
- Patients at intermediate risk should be given consolidating chemotherapy to induce remission followed by sibling matched allogeneic transplantation, despite its attendant risks.
- Patients at high risk of treatment failure may only be treated with curative intent if an HLA-identified sibling is available for stem cell transplantation.

Prognosis

Complete remission will be achieved in about three-quarters of patients under the age of 60, failure being due to either resistant leukaemia or death due to infection or (rarely) bleeding. It may be expected that approximately 50% of those entering complete remission will be cured. (i.e. approximately 30% overall). The management of recurrence is undertaken on an individual basis, since the overall prognosis is very poor despite the fact that second remissions may be achieved. Long survival following recurrence is rarely achieved without allogeneic transplantation.

Treatment of acute promyelocytic leukaemia (APML) (*K&C* 6e p. 504)

Acute promyelocytic leukaemia is specifically associated with disseminated intravascular coagulation (DIC), which may worsen when treatment is started. Management of DIC is discussed on page 232. The empirical discovery that all-*trans*-retinoic acid (ATRA) causes differentiation of promyelocytes and rapid reversal of the bleeding tendency was a major breakthrough. It is now conventional to treat APML with ATRA combined with chemotherapy and to follow successful remission induction with maintenance ATRA. Remission induction therapy as in other forms of AML is also necessary for long-term survival.

Treatment of acute lymphoblastic leukaemia (ALL) (*K&C* 6e p. 505)

The principles of treatment differ from those for AML in several important areas. Remission induction is undertaken with combination chemotherapy including vincristine, prednisolone asparaginase and daunorubicin. Details of consolidation will be determined by the anticipated risk of failure. In addition, ALL has a propensity to involve the CNS, so treatment also includes prophylactic intrathecal drugs, methotrexate or cytosine arabinoside (cytarabine). Cranial irradiation is used in those at very high risk or those with symptoms.

The prognosis in children with ALL is excellent with almost all achieving complete remission and with 80% being alive and disease free at 5 years. The results in adults are not so good, the prognosis getting worse with advancing years. Overall about 70–80% achieve complete remission with only about 30% being cured.

Chronic myeloid leukaemia (*K&C* 6e p. 505)

Clinical features

Chronic myeloid leukaemia (CML) occurs most commonly in middle age. There is an insidious onset, with fever, weight loss, sweating and symptoms of anaemia. Massive splenomegaly is characteristic.

Untreated, this chronic phase lasts 3–4 years. This is usually followed by blast transformation, with the development of acute leukaemia (usually acute myeloid) and, commonly, rapid death. Less frequently, CML transforms into myelofibrosis, death ensuing from bone marrow failure.

Investigations

- Blood count usually shows anaemia and a raised white cell count (often $> 100 \times 10^9$/L). The platelet count may be low, normal or raised.
- Bone marrow aspirate shows a hypercellular marrow with an increase in myeloid progenitors. On cytogenetic analysis the Ph chromosome (p. 238) is present in all patients. The *BCR-ABL* oncogene can be detected by reverse transcriptase polymerase chain reaction (RT-PCR) in all patients.

Management

244

Imatinib, a tyrosine kinase inhibitor that specifically blocks the enzymatic action of the BCR-ABL fusion protein is first-line treatment for the chronic phase. It has replaced alpha-interferon. Imatinib produces a complete haematological response in over 95% of patients, and 70–80% of these have no detectable *BCR-ABL* transcripts in the blood. Event-free, and overall, survival appear to be better than for other treatments. Imatinib can be continued indefinitely.

In the acute phase (blast transformation) most patients have only a short-lived response to imatinib, and other treatments such as allogeneic haemopoietic stem cell transplantation are required (see p. 250).

Chronic lymphocytic leukaemia (*K&C* 6e p. 506)

CLL is an incurable disease of older people, characterized by an uncontrolled proliferation and accumulation of mature B lymphocytes (although T cell CLL does occur).

Clinical features

CLL usually follows an indolent course. Early CLL is generally asymptomatic and isolated peripheral blood lymphocytosis is frequent. Symptoms are a consequence of bone marrow failure: anaemia, infections and bleeding. An autoimmune haemolysis contributes to the anaemia. Some patients may be asymptomatic, the diagnosis being a chance finding on the basis of a blood count done for a different reason. There may be lymphadenopathy and, in advanced disease, hepatosplenomegaly.

Investigations

- Blood count shows a raised white cell count $> 15 \times 10^9/\text{L}$, of which at least 40% are lymphocytes. There may be anaemia and thrombocytopenia.
- Blood film shows small lymphocytes of mature appearance with 'smear cells', an artefactual finding due to cell rupture while the film is being made.
- Bone marrow reflects peripheral blood usually heavily infiltrated with lymphocytes.
- Immunophenotyping is essential to exclude reactive lymphocytosis and other lymphoid neoplasms.
- Cytogenetics to characterize the specific mutation can be helpful in assessing prognosis.

Management

The decision to treat depends on the stage of the disease and more recently on cytogenetic markers (*K&C* 6e p. 506). Early-stage disease is treated expectantly whereas advanced-stage disease is always treated immediately. Other indications for treatment include anaemia, recurrent infections, splenic discomfort and progressive disease.

Oral chlorambucil, with or without prednisolone, reduces the blood count and decreases lymphadenopathy and splenomegaly, and successfully palliates the disease. The bone marrow rarely returns to normal.

The purine analogue fludarabine alone or in combination with cyclophosphamide or mitoxantrone (mitozantrone) has a much greater impact on the bone marrow and can induce complete remission. Recent studies suggest that the addition of the monoclonal antibody rituximab can further enhance response rates.

Prognosis

The median survival from diagnosis is very variable and correlates closely with disease stage at diagnosis and cytogenetic findings. This can vary from normal life expectancy in some groups to rapid progression in others.

THE LYMPHOMAS

The lymphomas are neoplastic transformations of normal B or T cells which reside predominantly in lymphoid tissues. They are commoner than the leukaemias and are increasing in incidence for reasons which are unclear. The disease is classified on the basis of histological appearance into Hodgkin's disease and non-Hodgkin's lymphoma (NHL).

Hodgkin's disease (*K&C* 6e p. 508)

Aetiology

The cause is unknown though there is evidence to link previous infection with Epstein Barr Virus (EBV).

Clinical features

Hodgkin's disease is primarily a disease of young adults. The most common presentation is painless lymph node enlargement (most often cervical nodes). Systemic symptoms, known as 'B' symptoms, are fever, night sweats and weight loss. Other constitutional symptoms may occur, such as pruritus, fatigue, anorexia and alcohol-induced pain at the site of the enlarged lymph nodes.

On examination enlarged nodes are typically non-tender, discrete and with a rubbery consistency. There may be hepatosplenomegaly.

Investigations

- Blood count may be normal or show a normochromic, normocytic anaemia.
- The ESR is usually raised and is an indicator of disease activity.
- Liver biochemistry may be abnormal, with or without liver involvement.
- Serum lactic dehydrogenase (LDH) if raised is an adverse prognostic marker.
- Chest X-ray and CT are necessary for staging and may show mediastinal, intrathoracic or abdominal lymphadenopathy.
- Lymph node biopsy and histological examination are required for a definitive diagnosis. Classically, Sternberg–

Table 5.21 Differential diagnosis of lymphadenopathy

Localized	Generalized
Local infection	Infection
Pyogenic infection, e.g.	Epstein–Barr virus
tonsillitis	Cytomegalovirus
Tuberculosis	*Toxoplasma* sp.
	Tuberculosis
	HIV infection
Lymphoma	Lymphoma
Secondary carcinoma	Leukaemia
	Systemic disease
	Systemic lupus
	erythematosus
	Sarcoidosis
	Rheumatoid arthritis
	Drug reaction, e.g. phenytoin

Reed cells (binucleate or multinucleate malignant B lymphocytes) are present, with a characteristic admixture of lymphocytes and histiocytes.

■ Bone marrow aspirate and trephine biopsy may show involvement in patients with advanced disease.

Differential diagnosis

This includes any other cause of lymphadenopathy (Table 5.21). The management of persistently enlarged lymph nodes includes surgical excision for histological and microbiological examination for diagnostic purposes.

Management

Treatment is always given with a curative intent and consists of radiotherapy, cyclical combination chemotherapy or both. The choice of treatment depends on:

■ Stage (Table 5.22)
■ Involved sites
■ 'Bulk' of lymph nodes involved
■ Presence or absence of 'B' symptoms.

Stage IA and stage IIA disease are treated with brief chemotherapy followed by involved field irradiation. All other stages are usually treated with cyclical combination chemo-

Table 5.22 Staging classification of Hodgkin's disease*

Stage	Definition
I	Involvement of a single lymph node region or a single extralymphatic organ or site
II	Involvement of two or more lymph node regions on the same side of the diaphragm, or localized involvement of an extralymphatic organ or site and of one or more lymph node regions on the same side of the diaphragm
III	Involvement of lymph node regions on both sides of the diaphragm, which may also be accompanied by involvement of the spleen or by localized involvement of an extralymphatic organ or site or both
IV	Diffuse or disseminated involvement of one or more extralymphatic organs or tissues, with or without associated lymph node involvement

*Each stage is subdivided into A (no systemic symptoms) and B (unexplained fever, night sweats and weight loss > 10% of bodyweight)

therapy with or without irradiation to sites of 'bulk' disease. The prognosis is related to the stage of the disease, with a 5-year survival rate of approximately 90% in stage I. The presence of B symptoms indicates more severe disease with a worse prognosis.

Non-Hodgkin's lymphoma (K&C 6e p. 512)

This is a heterogeneous group of disorders which encompasses many different histological subtypes. Subdivisions of the lymphomas into 'low grade' and 'high grade' reflects the rate at which the cells are dividing and thus the clinical progression of the disease. Paradoxically, high-grade lymphomas (rapidly dividing cells) are potentially curable, whereas low-grade lymphomas are generally considered to be incurable with conventional chemotherapy (Table 5.23). The classification of non-Hodgkin's lymphoma is currently based on histological, cytogenetic and immunochemical information.

Clinical features

Non-Hodgkin's lymphoma (NHL) is rare before the age of 40. The presentation can be very varied and almost any

follicular lymphoma — low grade
but bulky.

Table 5.23 Non-Hodgkin's lymphoma: low grade and high grade	
Low grade	**High grade**
Middle-aged/older people	Any age group
Bone marrow infiltration common	Bone marrow infiltration unusual
Incurable with conventional chemotherapy	Potentially curable

organ in the body can be involved. Peripheral lymph node enlargement is the most common clinical presentation. Systemic symptoms as in Hodgkin's disease may occur. Bone marrow infiltration, leading to anaemia, recurrent infections and bleeding, is often seen in low-grade lymphoma.

Investigations

- Blood count may show anaemia. An elevated white cell count or thrombocytopenia suggests bone marrow involvement. The ESR may be raised.
- Liver biochemistry may be abnormal if the liver is involved.
- Serum lactate dehydrogenase and β_2-microglobulin are prognostic indicators.
- Chest X-ray, CT, PET and gallium scans are of help in staging.
- Bone marrow aspiration and trephine biopsy will confirm marrow involvement.
- Lymph node biopsy is required for definitive diagnosis and subtype classification.

Management

Treatment depends on the grade and histological subtype.

- Low-grade disease in general is not curable. However, patients may survive for many years and usually experience several remissions with relatively simple treatment such as chlorambucil, or radiotherapy in localized disease.
- High-grade disease requires combination chemotherapy. Modern regimens, e.g. doxorubicin, cyclophosphamide,

vincristine, prednisolone and rituximab (CHOP+R), achieve a 60–70% response rate, and cure in about 40%. Some patients with localized disease can be cured with local radiotherapy.

Primary gastric lymphoma

In a high proportion of cases this lymphoma is associated with *Helicobacter pylori* infection. Treatment to eradicate the infection is usually all that is required provided there is no evidence of disease outside the stomach. This is followed by close endoscopic surveillance.

Mycosis fungoides and Sézary syndrome (*K&C* 6e p. 1352)

These are rare cutaneous T cell lymphomas that may spread in the later stages to involve lymph nodes and other organs.

Burkitt's lymphoma (*K&C* 6e p. 515)

This is a form of NHL occurring mainly in African children, and is associated with Epstein–Barr virus infection. Jaw tumours are common, usually with gastrointestinal involvement. Treatment is with radiotherapy and chemotherapy.

MYELOABLATIVE THERAPY WITH BONE MARROW TRANSPLANTATION

Myeloablative therapy is a term used for treatment that employs high-dose chemotherapy or chemotherapy plus radiation, with the aim of clearing the bone marrow completely of both benign and malignant cells. Without bone marrow replacement or 'transplantation', the patient would die of bone marrow failure. Approaches to restore bone marrow function include the following:

- *Allogeneic* bone marrow transplantation (BMT) bone marrow or peripheral blood stem cells *from another individual*, usually an HLA-identical sibling, are infused intravenously following myeloablative therapy. Immunosuppression is required to prevent host rejection and graft-versus-host disease (GVHD). The latter is a syndrome in which donor T lymphocytes infiltrate the skin, gut and liver, causing a maculopapular rash, diarrhoea and liver necrosis. This occurs in 30–50% of transplant recipients and is potentially fatal in some cases. Following allogeneic BMT the blood count usually recovers within 3–4 weeks. The mortality rate is 20–40%, depending on the person's age, and is often a result of infection or GVHD.

- *Autologous* (the patient acts as his or her own source of stem cells) peripheral blood progenitor cells (PBPCs) have virtually replaced autologous BMT as support for myeloablative therapy. With this technique it is possible, by using chemotherapy followed by the growth factor granulocyte colony-stimulating factor (G-CSF), to stimulate haemopoietic progenitor cells in the marrow to proliferate so that they can be collected from the peripheral blood. They are stored and re-infused after myeloablative therapy. The main advantage is the short time for blood count recovery because PBPCs are more differentiated. This technique has been particularly effective in relapsed leukaemias, lymphomas and in myeloma.
- *Syngeneic*: donor cells are from an identical twin.
- *From umbilical cord blood*. This is increasingly being used for adult and childhood leukaemia.

THE PARAPROTEINAEMIAS

Multiple myeloma (*K&C* 6e p. 517)

Multiple myeloma is a malignant disease of the plasma cells of bone marrow, accounting for 1% of all malignant disease. There is clonal proliferation of bone marrow plasma cells usually capable of producing monoclonal immunoglobulins (M proteins or paraproteins), which in most cases are IgG or IgA. The paraprotein may be associated with excretion of light chains in the urine, which are either κ or λ; the excess light chains are known as Bence Jones protein.

Clinical features

The peak age of presentation is 60 years. The neoplastic clone of cells induces excess osteoclastic activity, which results in osteoporosis, osteolytic lesions, pathological fractures and hypercalcaemia. Bone pain is the most common presenting symptom. Progressive marrow infiltration results in anaemia, infections and bleeding. Renal failure has multiple causes: deposition of light chains in the tubules, hypercalcaemia, hyperuricaemia and amyloid deposition in the kidneys. Paraproteins may form aggregates in the blood, which greatly increase the viscosity, leading to blurred vision, gangrene and bleeding.

Investigations

Two out of three diagnostic features should be present:

- Plasma cell infiltration on bone marrow aspirate or trephine biopsy
- Osteolytic bone lesions (often in the skull) on skeletal survey
- Monoclonal ('M') bands on serum protein electrophoresis, or Bence Jones protein in the urine. There is also a reduction in the normal polyclonal immunoglobulins (immune paresis).

Other essential investigations are as follows:

- Blood count, which may show anaemia, thrombocytopenia and leucopenia. The ESR is almost always high.
- Serum biochemistry may show evidence of renal failure and hypercalcaemia. The alkaline phosphatase is usually normal.
- DEXA scanning (p. 257) is valuable for follow-up of treatment.
- 24-hour urine immunofixation is used for assessment of light-chain excretion.

Management

With good supportive care and chemotherapy with autologous or allogeneic stem cell transplantation, median survival is now 5 years with some patients surviving to 10 years. Young patients receiving more intensive therapy may live longer.

Supportive therapy includes correction of anaemia with blood transfusion or erythropoietin, prompt treatment of infections, and treatment of bone pain with radiotherapy or NSAIDs. Renal failure (p. 369) and hypercalcaemia (p. 636) may be corrected by adequate hydration alone. In addition, bony complications may be reduced in patients in 'plateau phase' by long-term administration of bisphosphonates. Hyperviscosity is treated by plasmapheresis together with systemic therapy.

Specific treatment involves combination chemotherapy with alkylating agents (melphalan or cyclophosphamide) given in conjunction with prednisolone. Selected patients are treated with high dose melphalan supported by autologous BMT or PBPC. Newer approaches that show promise include thalidomide and the proteosome inhibitor bortezomib.

Waldenström's macroglobulinaemia

As in myeloma the neoplastic B cells secrete a monoclonal immunoglobulin. However, unlike myeloma, but similar to lymphoma, the tumour infiltrates the lymphoid tissues, including bone marrow, spleen and lymph nodes.

Clinical features

The most common features are malaise, weight loss, lymph node enlargement and symptoms of hyperviscosity.

Investigations

- Blood count may show a normal or low Hb and WCC, although the ESR is almost always high.
- Protein electrophoresis shows an IgM paraprotein.
- Bone marrow aspirate shows infiltration with lympho-plasmacytoid cells.

Management

Treatment is with alkylating agents or doxorubicin-containing regimens. Hyperviscosity is treated with plasmapheresis.

Monoclonal gammopathy of undetermined significance (K&C 6e p. 518)

This is usually seen in older patients, where a raised level of paraprotein (usually IgA) is found in the blood, but without other features of myeloma. Patients are often asymptomatic and no treatment is required. Regular follow-up is usually indicated in case they later develop lymphoma or myeloma.

Rheumatology 6

Musculoskeletal problems are common and account for about one in six GP consultations. Most of these are non-articular problems. Osteoarthritis and rheumatoid arthritis are more commonly seen in hospital clinics. Pain, stiffness and swelling are the most common presenting symptoms of joint disease and may be localized to a single joint or affect many joints.

Arthralgia describes joint pains when the joint appears normal on examination. *Arthritis* is the term used when there is objective evidence of joint inflammation (swelling, deformity or an effusion). In a patient presenting with joint pains, the history and examination must assess the distribution of joints affected (symmetrical?, axial or peripheral?), the presence of morning stiffness (common in inflammatory arthropathies), aggravating and relieving factors, past medical history and family history. Table 6.1 lists the likely causes of joint pains based on the age and sex of the patient.

Pain in or around a single joint may arise from the joint itself (articular problem) or from structures surrounding the joint (periarticular problem). Enthesitis (inflammation at the site of attachment of ligaments, tendons and joint capsules), bursitis and tendinitis are all causes of periarticular pain. Pain arising from the joint may be the result of a mechanical problem (e.g. torn meniscus) or an inflammatory problem.

The causes of a large joint monoarthritis include osteo-arthritis, gout, pseudogout, trauma and septic arthritis (p. 277). Disseminated gonococcal infection is a common cause of acute non-traumatic monoarthritis or oligoarthritis in young adults. Less common causes are rheumatoid arthritis, the spondyloarthropathies, tuberculous infection and haemarthrosis (e.g. in haemophilia, or on warfarin). Acute monoarthritis requires urgent investigation and treatment (p. 278). The key investigation is synovial fluid aspiration with Gram stain and culture and analysis for crystals in gout and pseudogout.

Table 6.1 Differential diagnosis of polyarticular disease presenting in adults in the UK

Age	Predominantly males		Predominantly females
Young	Reiter's syndrome Reactive arthritis Ankylosing spondylitis		SLE Rheumatoid arthritis Sjögren's syndrome
		Psoriatic arthropathy Enteropathic arthropathy	
Middle age	Gout	Generalized osteo- arthritis	Rheumatoid arthritis
Elderly		Generalized osteo- arthritis Polymyalgia rheumatica Pseudogout	

Uncommon arthropathies: Malignancy (hypertrophic pulmonary osteoarthropathy), Lyme disease, rheumatic fever, Henoch–Schönlein purpura, Behçet's syndrome

COMMON INVESTIGATIONS OF MUSCULOSKELETAL DISEASE

Blood tests

Simple blood tests   will usually show evidence of a non-specific acute-phase response with inflammatory arthritides and connective tissue diseases. Normochromic, normocytic anaemia is common, though hypochromic, microcytic anaemia may be present indicating iron deficiency, often due to non-steroidal anti-inflammatory drug (NSAID) induced gastrointestinal bleeding. ESR (p. 955) and CRP (p. 952) are the most widely used indicators of the acute-phase response and are frequently used to monitor disease activity. A raised alkaline phosphatase may indicate bony disease (p. 127).

Autoantibodies (*K&C* 6e p. 533)   Autoantibodies (see rheumatoid factor and Table 6.6) may be non-specific and found in normal individuals. At high titre (> 1 : 160) their disease specificity increases and they help to establish a diagnosis in patients with clinical features suggestive of an autoimmune disease. They can sometimes be used to monitor disease activity and provide prognostic data, e.g. a patient with rheumatoid arthritis and positive rheumatoid factor may have more erosive joint disease and extra-articular manifestations.

Imaging (K&C 6e p. 535)

Plain X-rays   may show fractures, deformity, soft tissue swelling, decreased bone density, osteolytic and osteosclerotic areas suggestive of metastases, joint erosions, joint space narrowing and new bone formation. X-rays may be normal in early inflammatory arthritis but are used as a baseline for later comparison.

Technetium bone scan   uses a tracer (^{99}Tc-bisphosphonate) which following intravenous injection localizes to sites of increased bone turnover. 'Hot spots' are non-specific and occur in osteomyelitis, septic arthritis, following surgery or trauma, cancer and Paget's disease.

Ultrasound   is useful for assessment of soft tissue and periarticular changes such as hip joint effusion, Baker's cyst and inflamed/damaged tendons. Quantitative ultrasound of the heel may prove a convenient and portable means of assessing bone density.

MRI (p. 959)   is particularly useful in the investigation of articular disease and spinal disorders. It is not indicated in patients with uncomplicated mechanical low back pain.

DEXA   (dual energy X-ray absorptiometry) is the current method of choice to measure bone mineral density (BMD) in the diagnosis and treatment response of osteoporosis. Osteoporosis is diagnosed when the BMD T-score falls below − 2.5. The T-score measures by how many standard deviations the patient's BMD differs from the population average for young healthy individuals.

Arthroscopy   is a direct means of visualizing the inside of a joint, particularly the knee or shoulder. Biopsies can be taken, surgery performed in certain conditions (e.g. repair or trimming of meniscal tears), and loose bodies removed.

Synovial fluid analysis (*K&C* 6e p. 534)

A needle is inserted into a joint for three main reasons: aspiration of synovial fluid for diagnosis, aspiration of fluid to relieve pressure, and injection of corticosteroid or local anaesthetic. The most common indications for joint aspiration are evaluation for sepsis in a single inflamed joint (p. 278) and confirmation of gout and pseudogout by polarized light. Synovial fluid should be analysed for colour, viscosity, cell count, culture, glucose and protein.

Investigation of suspected muscle disease

See page 706.

OSTEOARTHRITIS (*K&C* 6e p. 550)

Osteoarthritis (OA) is the most common form of arthritis. It is a disease of synovial joints characterized by articular cartilage loss with an accompanying periarticular bone response. Radiological changes of OA are seen in about 10% of the population, and in 50% of those aged over 60, although only a proportion of these have symptoms.

258

Epidemiology

OA occurs world-wide, although it is uncommon in the black population. It is twice as common in women as in men, and there is a marked familial tendency. The prevalence increases with age, and primary OA is uncommon before the age of 50 years.

Pathology and pathogenesis

OA is the result of active, sometimes inflammatory but potentially reparative processes, rather than the inevitable result of trauma and ageing. It is characterized by a progressive destruction and loss of articular cartilage. The exposed subchondral bone becomes sclerotic, with increased vascularity and cyst formation. Attempts at repair produce cartilaginous growths at the margins of the joint which later become calcified (osteophytes).

Several mechanisms have been suggested for the pathogenesis:

- Metalloproteinases, such as stromelysin and collagenase, degrade the cartilage components, collagen and proteoglycans

- Inflammatory mediators such as interleukin-1 and tumour necrosis factor-α stimulate metalloproteinase production and inhibit collagen production
- Deficiency of growth factors such as insulin-like growth factor and transforming growth factor impairs matrix repair
- Genetic susceptibility (35–65% influence) from multiple genes, currently unidentified, rather than a single gene defect.

Most OA is primary with no obvious predisposing factor. Secondary OA occurs in joints that have been damaged in some way (e.g. intra-articular fractures, avascular necrosis) or are congenitally abnormal (e.g. slipped femoral epiphysis).

Clinical features

Pain is the main symptom, made worse by movement and relieved by rest. Stiffness occurs after rest ('gelling') and in contrast to inflammatory arthritis there is only transient (< 30 minutes) morning stiffness. The joints most commonly involved are the distal interphalangeal joints (DIPJ) and first carpometacarpal joint of the hands, first metatarsophalangeal joint of the foot and the weight-bearing joints – vertebrae, hips and knees. Elbows, wrists and ankles are rarely affected. On examination there is deformity and bony enlargement of the joints, limited joint movement and muscle wasting of surrounding muscle groups. Crepitus (grating) is a common finding and is probably due to the disruption of the normally smooth articulating surfaces of the joints. There may be a joint effusion. Heberden's nodes are bony swellings at the DIPJ. Bouchard's nodes are similar but occur at the proximal IPJ. In the knee, cartilage loss due to OA can result in deformity with varus ('bow-legged') or valgus ('knock-kneed') angulation. A fluctuant swelling along the posterior aspect of the knee, popliteal or Baker's cyst, occurs in some patients with a knee effusion.

Differential diagnosis

OA is differentiated from rheumatoid arthritis by the pattern of joint involvement (Fig. 6.1) and the absence of the systemic features and marked early morning stiffness that occur in rheumatoid arthritis. Pyrophosphate arthropathy (p. 276) affects an age group similar to that of OA but the

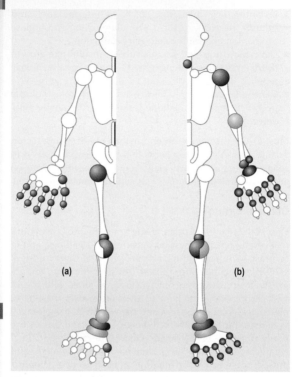

Fig. 6.1 **The pattern of joint involvement in (a) osteoarthritis compared with (b) rheumatoid arthritis.** Joint involvement in RA is usually symmetrical, whereas asymmetry is frequent in OA, especially of the large joints.

wrists are usually involved. Chronic tophaceous gout (p. 274) and psoriatic arthritis affecting the DIPJ (p. 271) may mimic OA.

Investigations

■ FBC and ESR are normal. Rheumatoid factor is negative, but positive low-titre tests may occur incidentally in elderly people.
■ X-rays are only abnormal in advanced disease and show narrowing of the joint space (resulting from loss of

cartilage), osteophytes, subchondral sclerosis and cyst formation.

■ MRI demonstrates early cartilage changes. It is not necessary for most patients with suggestive symptoms and typical plain X-ray features.

■ Arthroscopy reveals early fissuring and surface erosion of the cartilage, but is unnecessary for diagnosis.

Management

Treatment should focus on the symptoms and disability, not the radiological appearances. There are three main types of treatment: patient education and non-pharmacological measures, drugs and surgery. Obese patients should be encouraged to lose weight, particularly if weight-bearing joints are affected.

■ Patient education and non-pharmacological measures are the keystone of OA treatment. Local strengthening and aerobic exercises (little and often with graded increases) maintain muscle power and improve the mobility of weight-bearing joints. Heat applied to an affected joint may provide pain relief. Hydrotherapy may be helpful. A walking stick used correctly reduces hip loading by up to 20%.

■ Drugs. Paracetamol is the initial drug of choice for pain relief. Non-steroidal anti-inflammatory drugs (NSAIDs), e.g. ibuprofen, are indicated in those patients who do not respond to simple analgesia and should ideally be used on an intermittent rather than a continuous basis. NSAIDs inhibit cyclo-oxygenase (COX, prostaglandin synthase) with reduced production of prostaglandins, thromboxane and prostacyclin. NSAIDs inhibit all three isoforms of the enzyme: COX-1 (expressed in most tissues), COX-2 (expressed in the kidney and at sites of inflammation) and COX-3 (expressed in the brain and responsible for central mediation of pain and pyrexia). Inhibition of COX-1 in the gastroduodenal mucosa leads to reduced production of protective prostaglandins and an increased rate of mucosal damage with peptic ulceration. The selective COX 2 inhibitors, e.g. celecoxib, valdecoxib, have a reduced rate of peptic ulceration compared to non-selective NSAIDs. Other side-effects of NSAIDs include fluid retention and chronic tubulo-interstitial nephritis.

Inflammatory arthritis

- Intra-articular steroids can be used for inflammatory exacerbations, but systemic corticosteroids are not used.
- Surgery should be considered in patients with severe symptomatic OA who have failed to respond to drugs and physical therapy. Surgical intervention may involve the realignment, fusion or replacement of joints with prosthetic implants.

INFLAMMATORY ARTHRITIS (K&C 6e p. 554)

Inflammatory arthritis includes a large number of arthritic conditions in which the predominant feature is synovial inflammation. There is joint pain and stiffness after rest and in the morning. Morning stiffness may last several hours. Blood tests often show a normochromic normocytic anaemia and raised inflammatory markers (ESR and CRP).

Rheumatoid arthritis (K&C 6e p. 555)

Rheumatoid arthritis (RA) is a chronic symmetrical poly-arthritis of unknown cause. It is a systemic autoimmune disorder associated with extra-articular involvement, e.g. the lungs and many other organs.

Epidemiology

RA affects 0.5–3% of the population world-wide, with a peak prevalence between the ages of 30 and 50 years. Women are affected three times more often than men before the menopause, with an equal sex incidence thereafter. There is an increased incidence in those with a family history of RA. HLA-DR4 occurs in 50–75% of patients (20–25% of the normal population) and is associated with development of more severe erosive disease.

Aetiology

The cause is unknown. The initiating event in RA is thought to be activation of synovial T cells by an unknown antigen in the immunogenetically susceptible host. Chronic synovitis is maintained by rheumatoid factors (see below) and by the continuous stimulation of macrophages with production of cytokines (IL-1, IL-8, TNF-α, granulocyte–macrophage colony-stimulating factor) and chemokines (macrophage inflammatory protein (MIP)). Synovial fibroblasts produce IL-6.

Pathology

RA is characterized by synovitis (inflammation of the synovial lining of joints, tendon sheaths or bursae). There is synovial infiltration by chronic inflammatory cells: lymphocytes, plasma cells and macrophages with secretion of pro-inflammatory cytokines and autoantibody production with formation of immune complexes. Generation of new synovial blood vessels is induced by angiogenic cytokines, and activated endothelial cells produce adhesion molecules such as vascular cell adhesion molecule-1 (VCAM-1) which expedite extravasation of leucocytes into the synovium. The synovium proliferates and grows out over the surface of cartilage, producing a tumour-like mass called 'pannus'. Pannus destroys the articular cartilage and subchondral bone, producing bony erosions. Rheumatoid factors (RhF) are antibodies directed against the Fc portion of immuno-globulin. Production of RhF by plasma cells in the synovium and self-aggregation with formation of immune complexes plays a part in the maintenance of synovitis.

Subcutaneous nodules (rheumatoid nodules) have a characteristic microscopic appearance with a central area of necrosis surrounded by macrophages and fibrous tissue. Similar lesions occur in the pleura, pericardium and lung.

Clinical features

The typical presentation is with an insidious onset of pain, early-morning stiffness (lasting more than 30 minutes) and swelling in the small joints of the hands and feet. There is spindling of the fingers caused by swelling of the proximal but not distal interphalangeal joints. The metacarpo-phalangeal and wrist joints are also swollen. As the disease progresses there is weakening of joint capsules, causing joint instability, subluxation (partial dislocation) and deformity. The characteristic deformities of the rheumatoid hand are shown in Figure 6.2. Most patients eventually have many joints involved, including the wrists, elbows, shoulders, cervical spine, knees, ankles and feet. The dorsal and lumbar spine are not involved. Joint effusions and wasting of muscles around the affected joints are early features. Less common presentations are 'explosive' (sudden onset of widespread arthritis), palindromic (relapsing and remitting monoarthritis of different large joints), or with a systemic illness with few joint symptoms initially.

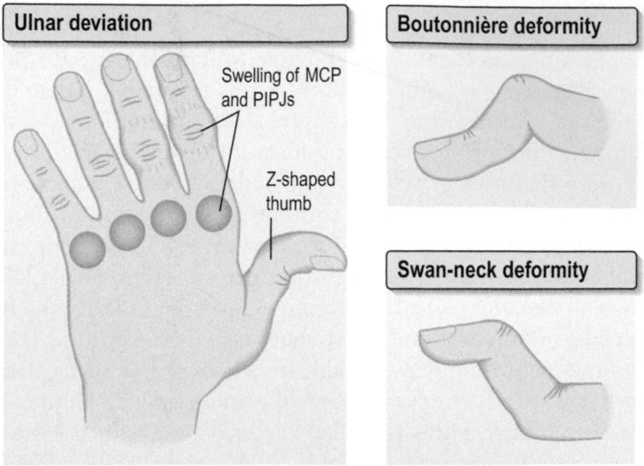

Fig. 6.2 **Characteristic hand deformities in rheumatoid arthritis.** MCP, metacarpophalanges; PIPJs, proximal interphalangeal joints.

264

In patients presenting with disproportionate involvement of a single joint, septic arthritis (p. 277) must be excluded before the symptoms are attributed to a disease flare-up.

Extra-articular manifestations

Periarticular features of RA include bursitis, tenosynovitis, muscle wasting and subcutaneous nodule formation. Rheumatoid nodules are found in about 20% of cases, usually over pressure points, typically the extensor surface of the ulnar, the finger joints and Achilles tendon. Patients with nodules are usually seropositive, i.e. they have circulating RhF.

Other extra-articular disease manifestations are summarized in Table 6.2. The most common manifestations are highlighted; these may be present but cause few symptoms, e.g. atlantoaxial subluxation is commonly seen on a cervical spine X-ray, but much less commonly causes problems.

Patients with RA also have a greater risk of infection, osteoporosis and cardiovascular disease. The systemic inflammation that characterizes RA may play a role in the excess atherosclerosis.

Table 6.2 **Extra-articular manifestations of rheumatoid arthritis**

Systemic	**Fever**
	Fatigue
	Weight loss
Eyes	**Sjögren's syndrome**
	Scleritis
	Scleromalacia perforans (perforation of the eye)
Neurological	**Carpal tunnel syndrome**
	Atlanto-axial subluxation
	Cord compression
	Polyneuropathy, predominantly sensory
	Mononeuritis multiplex
Reticuloendothelial	**Lymphadenopathy**
	Felty's syndrome (RA, splenomegaly, neutropenia)
Blood	**Anaemia caused by:**
	Chronic disease
	NSAID-induced gastrointestinal blood loss
	Haemolysis
	Hypersplenism
	Thrombocytosis
Pulmonary	Pleural effusion
	Fibrosing alveolitis
	Rheumatoid nodules
	Rheumatoid pneumoconiosis (Caplan's syndrome)
	Obliterative bronchiolitis
Heart and peripheral vessels	**Pericarditis (rarely clinically apparent)**
	Pericardial effusion
	Raynaud's syndrome
Kidneys	Amyloidosis
	Analgesic nephropathy
Vasculitis	Leg ulcers
	Nail fold infarcts
	Gangrene of fingers and toes

The most common manifestations are in bold

Investigations

The diagnosis of RA cannot be established by a single laboratory test and is usually made clinically. Appropriate investigations include:

- Blood count. There is a normochromic, normocytic anaemia and thrombocytosis which correlates with disease activity. Other forms of anaemia may also occur (Table 6.2). The ESR and CRP are raised in proportion to the activity of the inflammatory process.
- Serum autoantibodies. RhF (p. 963) is positive in 70% of cases and antinuclear factor in 30% (p. 280). RhF is not specific for RA and may occur in connective tissue diseases and some infections. Anti-citrulline-containing peptide (CCP) antibodies have high specificity (90%) and sensitivity (60%) for RA and are useful to distinguish RA from acute transient synovitis.
- Radiology. X-ray of the affected joints shows soft tissue swelling in early disease and later joint narrowing, erosions at the joint margins and porosis of periarticular bone and cysts. Representative films of the hands and feet are usually sufficient.
- Synovial fluid is sterile with a high neutrophil count in uncomplicated disease.

Differential diagnosis

In the patient with symmetrical peripheral polyarthritis, prolonged morning stiffness (> 1 hour), rheumatoid nodules and positive RhF, the diagnosis is straightforward. RA must be distinguished from the symmetrical seronegative arthropathy occurring in psoriasis. Severe RA can also mimic a form of psoriatic arthritis known as 'arthritis mutilans' (p. 272). In a young woman presenting with joint pains SLE must be considered, but characteristically the joints look normal on examination in this condition.

Management

No treatment cures RA; therefore the therapeutic goals are remission of symptoms, a return of full function and the maintenance of remission with disease-modifying agents. Effective management of RA requires a multidisciplinary approach, with input from rheumatologists, orthopaedic surgeons (joint replacement, arthroplasty), occupational therapists (aids to reduce disability) and physiotherapists (improvement of muscle power and maintenance of mobility to prevent flexion deformities). Patients should be advised to stop smoking to reduce the risk of cardiovascular disease. **NSAIDs** (p. 261) are effective in relieving the joint pain and stiffness of RA, but they do not slow disease progression. Individual response to NSAIDs varies considerably and it is reasonable to try several drugs in a particular patient to find the most suitable. Slow-release preparations (e.g. slow-release diclofenac) taken at night may produce dramatic relief of symptoms on the following day.

Disease-modifying drugs (DMARDs) should be used early (within 3 months of diagnosis) in disease onset to prevent the irreversible effects of long-term inflammation on the joints. These drugs act mainly through inhibition of inflammatory cytokines, and reduce inflammation and slow the development of joint erosions. They may take up to 6 months to achieve maximum effect. Hydroxychloroquine and sulfasalazine are used in patients with mild to moderate disease respectively. Hydroxychloroquine may produce corneal deposits (which disappear when treatment is stopped) and rarely retinopathy, which may be permanent. Visual acuity must be checked and ophthalmoscopy performed 6 monthly. Methotrexate is the drug of choice for patients with more active disease. Leflunomide blocks T cell proliferation. It has a similar initial response rate to sulfasalazine but improvement continues and it is better sustained at 2 years. It is used alone or in combination with methotrexate. All drugs can have serious side-effects (Table 6.3) so careful monitoring with blood tests is necessary. Azathioprine, gold (intramuscular or oral) and penicillamine are used less frequently.

Anti-cytokine agents ('biologics') that inhibit the action of tumour necrosis factor-α (e.g. etanercept, a soluble TNF-α receptor fusion protein that binds TNF-α; infliximab, a chimeric (human/mouse) antibody to TNF-α, and adalimumab, a fully human anti-TNF monoclonal antibody to TNF) have had a major impact in the treatment of RA and slow or halt erosion formation in up to 70% of patients. TNF-blocking agents are used in patients who have active disease despite adequate treatment with at least two DMARDs, including methotreaxate. One recombinant human interleukin-1 receptor antagonist, anakinra, is also licensed for use. The cost of these agents and the lack of long-term data remain barriers to their more widespread use.

Corticosteroids suppress disease activity but the dose required is often large, with the considerable risk of long-term toxicity (p. 625). They are seldom used except in the elderly patient with explosive RA or in patients with severe

Table 6.3 Side-effects of drugs commonly used in long-term suppressive therapy for rheumatoid arthritis

All may cause **myelosuppression** (with neutropenia, thrombocytopenia and anaemia) and regular check of the full blood count is indicated together with other specific monitoring. Rash and nausea are additional side-effects of most of the drugs listed

Drug	Side-effects
Sulfasalazine	Mouth ulcers
	Hepatitis
	Male infertility (reversible)
Methotrexate	Mouth ulcers and diarrhoea
	Liver fibrosis
	Pulmonary fibrosis
	Renal impairment
Leflunamide	Diarrhoea
	Hypertension
	Hepatitis
	Alopecia
TNF blockers	Infusion reactions (infliximab)
	Infections particularly reactivation of latent TB. Often extrapulmonary
	Demyelinating disease
	Exacerbation of heart failure
	Lupus-like syndrome
	Drug antibodies
	Lymphoproliferative disease

extra-articular manifestations. Local injection of a troublesome joint (see below) with a long-acting corticosteroid improves pain, synovitis and effusion. Repeated injections into an individual joint are possible, but usually limited to four a year because too-frequent injections may accelerate joint damage.

Surgery is often beneficial to prevent joint destruction and deformity (e.g. synovectomy) or to restore function with joint replacement.

Prognosis

The prognosis is variable. After 10 years 10% of patients will be severely disabled and 25% will have minimal if any symptoms. Other patients lie between these two extremes.

Table 6.4 **Seronegative spondyloarthropathies**

Ankylosing spondylitis (AS)
Psoriatic arthritis
Reactive arthritis
    Sexually acquired (Reiter's disease)
    Post-dysenteric reactive arthritis
Enteropathic arthritis (ulcerative colitis/Crohn's disease)

THE SERONEGATIVE SPONDYLOARTHROPATHIES (*K&C* 6e p. 564)

This title describes a group of conditions (Table 6.4) that share certain clinical features:

- A predilection for axial (spinal and sacroiliac) inflammation
- Asymmetrical peripheral arthritis
- Absence of rheumatoid factor, hence 'seronegative'
- Inflammation of the enthesis (junction of ligament or tendon and bone)
- A strong association with HLA-B27. The explanation for the association with HLA-B27 is unknown and testing for HLA-B27 is not usually performed as part of the investigation of these diseases.

Ankylosing spondylitis (*K&C* 6e p. 564)

Ankylosing spondylitis (AS) is an inflammatory disorder of the back, affecting mainly young adults. Men are affected more severely than women and so more likely to present with symptoms of the disease.

Clinical features

The typical patient with AS is a young man (late teens, early 20s) who presents with increasing pain and morning stiffness (usually lasting more than 30 minutes) in the lower back. Pain and stiffness improve with exercise but not with rest. There is a progressive loss of spinal movement. Inspection of the spine reveals two characteristic abnormalities:

- Loss of lumbar lordosis and increased kyphosis (Fig. 6.3).
- Limitation of lumbar spine mobility in both sagittal and frontal planes. Reduced spinal flexion is demonstrated

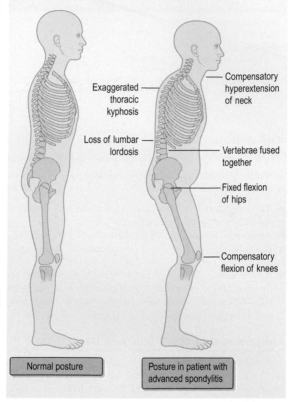

Normal posture

Posture in patient with
advanced spondylitis

Compensatory
hyperextension
of neck

Exaggerated
thoracic
kyphosis

Vertebrae fused
together

Loss of lumbar
lordosis

Fixed flexion
of hips

Compensatory
flexion of knees

Fig. 6.3 **Ankylosing spondylitis – the typical posture in advanced cases compared to normal posture.**

by the Schober test. A mark is made at the 5th lumbar spinous process and 10 cm above, with the patient in the erect position. On bending forward, the distance should increase to > 15 cm in normal individuals.

■ Reduction in chest expansion (< 2.5 cm on deep inspiration measured at the 4th intercostal space).

Other features include Achilles tendinitis and plantar fasciitis (enthesitis) and tenderness around the pelvis and chest wall.

Non-articular features include iritis (in 25%) and, rarely, aortic incompetence, cardiac conduction defects and apical lung fibrosis.

Investigations

- The ESR and CRP are often raised.
- X-rays may be normal or show erosion and sclerosis of the margins of the sacroiliac joints, proceeding to ankylosis (immobility and consolidation of the joint). In the spinal column, squaring of the vertebrae (caused by erosion of the corners) and progressive calcification of the interspinous ligaments produce the 'bamboo spine'.
- MR imaging shows early changes with increased signal from bone and bone marrow suggestive of osteitis and oedema.

Management

- Twice-daily exercises are essential to maintain posture and mobility.
- Slow-release NSAIDs taken at night are particularly effective in relieving night pain and morning stiffness. Sulfasalazine or methotrexate may help the peripheral arthritis but there is little evidence that they control the spinal disease. TNF-α-blocking drugs (see RA) are highly effective in active inflammatory disease and improve both spinal and peripheral joint inflammation. In the UK, NICE recommend TNF-blocking drugs in AS for patients who have clinical evidence of active inflammatory disease and who have failed conventional treatment with two or more NSAIDs at maximum tolerated/recommended dose for 4 weeks.

271

Prognosis

Most patients are able to lead a normal active life and remain at work. In severe cases the spine becomes completely fused and brittle, with a risk of fracture (on minimal trauma) and cord compression. The fixed kyphosis of the cervical and thoracic spine may impair ventilation.

Psoriatic arthritis *(K&C 6e p. 566)*

Arthritis occurs in 5–8% of patients with psoriasis, particularly in those with nail disease (p. 787) and may precede the skin disease.

Clinical features

There are several types:

- *Asymmetrical involvement* of the small joints of the hand, including the distal interphalangeal joints
- *Symmetrical seronegative polyarthritis* resembling rheumatoid arthritis
- *Arthritis mutilans*, a severe form with destruction of the small bones in the hands and feet
- *Ankylosing spondylitis* occurs with increased frequency in patients with psoriasis.

Investigations

- Routine blood tests are unhelpful in the diagnosis. The ESR is often normal.
- X-rays may show erosions and periarticular osteoporosis in the terminal interphalangeal joints.

Treatment

This is with analgesia and NSAIDs. Local synovitis responds to intra-articular corticosteroid injections. In severe cases methotrexate, ciclosporin or anti-TNF agents are used, as they control both the arthritis and the skin lesions.

Reactive arthritis (*K&C* 6e p. 566)

Reactive arthritis is a sterile synovitis, which occurs following an infection, either:

- Gastrointestinal infection with *Shigella*, *Salmonella*, *Yersinia* or *Campylobacter*
- Sexually acquired infection – non-specific urethritis in the male or cervicitis in the female due to infection with *Chlamydia trachomatis* or *Ureaplasma urealyticum*.

Persistent bacterial antigen in the inflamed synovium of affected joints is thought to drive the inflammatory process.

Clinical features

The typical case is a young man who presents with an acute arthritis shortly (within 4 weeks) after an enteric or venereal infection, which may have been mild or asymptomatic. The joints of the lower limbs are particularly affected in an asymmetrical pattern; the knees, ankles and feet are the most common sites.

The skin lesions resemble psoriasis. Circinate balanitis causes superficial ulcers around the penile meatus which harden to a crust in the circumcised male. Red plaques and pustules that resemble pustular psoriasis (keratoderma blenorrhagica) are found on the palms and soles of the feet. Nail dystrophy may also occur.

Additional features are acute anterior uveitis, enthesitis (plantar fasciitis, Achilles tendonitis) and the classical triad of Reiter's syndrome (urethritis, reactive arthritis and conjunctivitis).

Investigations

The diagnosis is clinical. The ESR is raised in the acute stage. Aspirated synovial fluid is sterile, with a high neutrophil count.

Management

Three types of therapy are used in the management of Reiter's syndrome: the acute inflammation is treated with NSAIDs together with local joint aspiration and injection of corticosteroid; the infection with antibiotics; and chronic disease with sulfasalazine or azathioprine.

Prognosis

The acute arthritis resolves within a few months. However, 50% of patients develop recurrent arthritis, iritis or ankylosing spondylitis.

Enteropathic arthritis (K&C 6e p. 568)

Enteropathic arthritis is a large joint mono- or asymmetrical oligoarthritis occurring in 10–15% of patients with ulcerative colitis and Crohn's disease. It usually parallels the activity of the inflammatory bowel disease and consequently improves as bowel symptoms improve. Ankylosing spondylitis occurs in 5% of patients with inflammatory bowel disease but is not related to disease activity.

CRYSTAL DEPOSITION DISEASES (K&C 6e p. 568)

Two main types of crystal account for the majority of crystal-induced arthritis: sodium urate and calcium pyrophosphate. Neutrophils ingest the crystals and initiate a pro-inflammatory reaction. Crystals may be found in asymptomatic joints.

Gout (K&C 6e p. 568)

Gout is an abnormality of uric acid metabolism resulting in the deposition of sodium urate crystals in:

- Joints, causing acute arthritis or chronic polyarticular gout; the latter is uncommon in treated patients
- Soft tissue, causing tophi and tenosynovitis
- Urinary tract, causing urate stones and renal failure.

Epidemiology

Gout is common. The disease is 10 times more common in men, occurs rarely before young adulthood (when it suggests a specific enzyme defect), and seldom in premenopausal females. It is more prevalent in the upper social classes. One-third have a positive family history.

Pathogenesis

The biochemical abnormality is hyperuricaemia resulting from overproduction or renal underexcretion of uric acid. Urate is derived from the breakdown of purines (adenine and guanine in DNA and RNA), which are synthesized in the body or ingested (a minor component). The causes of hyperuricaemia are shown in Table 6.5, but not all patients with hyperuricaemia have gout. Idiopathic (primary) gout is the most common form and most have impaired renal excretion of uric acid.

Clinical features

The typical patient is an obese middle-aged man who presents with acute gout, characterized by the sudden onset of severe pain and swelling, most frequently in the meta-tarsophalangeal joint of the big toe. The joint becomes red, hot, swollen and exquisitely tender. The signs of inflammation may extend beyond the joint giving the impression of cellulitis. The attack may be precipitated by a surgical operation, dietary or alcoholic excess, starvation or drugs, particularly thiazide diuretics. In 25% a joint other than in the big toe is affected. Acute attacks must be differentiated

---

Table 6.5 Causes of hyperuricaemia

Impaired excretion of uric acid
Idiopathic (primary) gout
Chronic renal disease (clinical gout unusual)
Drug therapy, e.g. thiazide diuretics, low-dose aspirin
Hypertension
Lead toxicity
Primary hyperparathyroidism
Hypothyroidism
Increased lactic acid production from alcohol, exercise, starvation
Glucose-6-phosphatase deficiency (interferes with renal excretion)

Increased production of uric acid
Increased turnover of purines
   Myeloproliferative disorders, e.g. polycythaemia vera
   Lymphoproliferative disorders, e.g. leukaemia
   Others, e.g. carcinoma, severe psoriasis
Increased de novo purine synthesis (very rare)
   HGPRT deficiency (Lesch–Nyhan syndrome)
   PPS overactivity

HGPRT, hypoxanthine-guanine phosphoribosyltransferase; PPS, phosphoribosyl-pyrophosphate synthetase

275

from other causes of monoarthritis, particularly septic arthritis. Tophaceous urate deposits may develop in skin and around joints and appear as white nodules particularly on the ear, the fingers and on the Achilles tendon.

Investigations

The clinical picture is often diagnostic, as is the rapid response to NSAIDs.

- Serum uric acid is usually raised, but may be normal in acute gout. However, the diagnosis is excluded if the serum uric acid is in the lower half of the normal range. Conversely, asymptomatic hyperuricaemia is common.
- Serum urea and creatinine for signs of renal impairment.
- Joint fluid microscopy is the most specific and diagnostic test, revealing long needle-shaped crystals which are negatively birefringent under polarized light. This is not usually necessary in clinical practice.

Management

Acute attacks are treated with anti-inflammatory drugs:

- NSAIDs, e.g. naproxen, are the treatment of choice.
- Colchicine, given orally, may be useful if NSAIDs are contraindicated, e.g. active peptic ulceration.
- Corticosteroids: intramuscular or intra-articular depot methylprednisolone is used in difficult cases.

To reduce uric acid levels obese patients should lose weight, alcohol consumption should be reduced, and drugs such as thiazides and salicylates should be withdrawn. A diet which reduces total calorie and cholesterol intake and avoids purine-rich foods (offal, some fish and shellfish and spinach) is advised.

Long-term therapy to reduce serum uric acid is used for patients with frequent attacks (> 2 per year) despite dietary changes or with gouty tophi or renal impairment. Allopurinol inhibits xanthine oxidase (an enzyme in the purine break-down pathway) and reduces serum urate levels rapidly. Paradoxically it may provoke an acute attack. Treatment is not started within 1 month after an acute attack and NSAIDs or colchicine are given for 4 weeks before and after starting allopurinol. The angiotensin II receptor antagonist, losartan, is uricosuric and may be an option for hyper-tensive patients.

Pyrophosphate arthropathy (pseudogout) (*K&C* 6e p. 571)

This condition is associated with the deposition of calcium pyrophosphate dihydrate in articular cartilage and peri-articular tissue. The acute attacks of synovitis that occur in 25% of patients are known as pseudogout. The aetiology is unknown and it occurs most commonly in elderly women. It may occur secondary to other diseases, including primary hyperparathyroidism, haemochromatosis, hypothyroidism and gout.

Clinical features

The clinical picture is similar to primary osteoarthritis, with acute attacks most commonly involving the knee and wrist. There may be polyarticular involvement.

Investigations

- Blood count may show a raised white cell count
- Synovial fluid examination reveals small brick-shaped pyrophosphate crystals which are positively birefringent under polarized light (compare uric acid).
- X-ray of the knee may show linear calcification parallel to the articular surfaces (chondrocalcinosis).
- Serum calcium is normal.

Management

Rest with joint aspiration and NSAIDs forms the mainstay of treatment. Injection of local corticosteroids may also be useful.

INFECTIVE ARTHRITIS

Joint infection is uncommon but can lead to considerable joint destruction. Infection of the joints is usually caused by bacteria and rarely by spirochaetes and fungi. Some viruses (rubella, mumps and hepatitis B virus infections) are associated with a mild self-limiting arthritis but this is not due to direct joint involvement.

Septic arthritis (*K&C* 6e p. 571)

Septic arthritis is a medical emergency with a mortality of 10%. It results from infection of the joint with pyogenic organisms, most commonly *Staphylococcus aureus*. Most cases arise from haematogenous spread to the joint from a distant site of infection. Bacteraemia is more likely to localize in a joint with pre-existing arthritis. Less commonly, infection is from local spread of adjacent osteomyelitis, or through direct injury or trauma.

Clinical features

Classically there is a hot painful red joint, often the knee, which has developed acutely. There may be fever and evidence of infection elsewhere. Fever and systemic reactions may be absent in those with rheumatoid arthritis or in patients taking corticosteroids. The infection may involve more than one joint.

> **Emergency Box 6.1**
> **Acute monoarthritis**
>
> **Investigations**
> - **Joint aspiration** (US guidance if necessary) and synovial fluid analysis: white cell count and differential (normal < 180/mm³), Gram stain and culture, polarized light microscopy for crystals (in gout and pseudogout). Purulent fluid (white cell count > 50 000/mm³, mostly neutrophils) and/or positive Gram stain indicates bacterial infection.
> - **Bloods**: FBC, ESR, C-reactive protein, blood cultures.
> - **X-rays of the affected joint** play little part in the diagnosis because these only become abnormal when joint destruction has occurred. However, a baseline X-ray may be useful for later comparison.
> - **Swab** of urethra, cervix and anorectum if gonococcal infection a possibility.
>
> **Treatment of acute non-gonococcal bacterial arthritis**
> - Antibiotics for 6 weeks, initial 2 weeks i.v. Treatment depends on the organism concerned, but a suitable 'blind' regimen would be flucloxacillin 1–2 g 6-hourly i.v. (erythromycin if penicillin allergic), together with oral fusidic acid 500 mg 8-hourly. Modify treatment depending on culture and sensitivity.
> - Adequate joint drainage: by needle aspiration, arthroscopy or open drainage. Consider orthopaedic referral.
> - Immobilize joint in acute stages, mobilize early to avoid contractures.
> - NSAIDs for pain relief.

Management

This is summarized in Emergency Box 6.1.

Bone and joint tuberculous infection (K&C 6e p. 572)

Approximately 1% of patients with TB have bone and joint involvement, which is usually caused by haematogenous spread from pulmonary or renal disease.

Clinical features

Spinal involvement is the most common (50%). Tuberculous arthritis tends to occur in the weight-bearing joints. There is an insidious onset of pain, swelling and dysfunction. Constitutional symptoms such as fever and weight loss are often not present.

Diagnosis

Culture of the synovial fluid may give the diagnosis. Occasionally, synovial biopsy is required.

Treatment

Treatment is as for tuberculosis elsewhere (see p. 527), in addition to joint rest and immobilization.

Meningococcal arthritis (*K&C* 6e p. 572)

Meningococcal arthritis usually occurs as part of a meningococcal septicaemia and results from the deposition of circulating immune complexes containing meningococcal antigens. It is a migratory polyarthritis, not associated with joint destruction. Treatment is with penicillin.

Gonococcal arthritis (*K&C* 6e p. 572)

Gonococcal arthritis occurs secondary to genital or oral infection (often asymptomatic) and presents with a mild inflammatory polyarthritis. Concomitant skin involvement is common (maculopapular pustules). It affects particularly young women and homosexual men. The organism can usually be cultured from the bloodstream, and from the joints. Treatment is with penicillin.

Salmonella arthritis

Salmonella arthritis presents as a mild polyarthritis and occurs with types of salmonellae that invade the bloodstream rather than staying within the gastrointestinal tract. Gastrointestinal symptoms are not always present. Treatment is with amoxicillin.

AUTOIMMUNE DISEASES (CONNECTIVE TISSUE DISEASE) (*K&C* 6e p. 573)

Autoimmune disease is a pathological condition caused by an immune response directed against an antigen within the host, i.e. a self-antigen. The autoimmune response may, however, be triggered by an exogenous, i.e. foreign, antigen. Organ-specific autoimmune diseases include Graves' disease, Hashimoto's thyroiditis, pernicious anaemia and insulin-dependent diabetes mellitus. In the autoimmune rheumatic diseases the autoantibodies are not organ-

Table 6.6   Association of autoantibodies with the connective tissue diseases

Antibody	Disease
Antinuclear antibodies	Non-specific – connective tissue diseases, organ specific autoimmune disease, infections, normal individuals
Anti-double-stranded DNA (dsDNA)	SLE
Anti-extractable nuclear antigens	
Anti-Smith (Sm)	SLE
Anti-ribonucleoprotein (RNP)	SLE, mixed connective tissue disease
Anti-Ro/SSA	Primary Sjögren's syndrome, SLE
Anti-La/SSB	Occur in association with Anti-Ro/SSA antibodies
Anti-topoisomerase I (Scl-70)	Diffuse cutaneous scleroderma
Anti-RNA polymerase antibodies I, and III	Diffuse cutaneous scleroderma
Anticentromere antibodies	Limited cutaneous scleroderma
Anti-Jo-1	Polymyositis and dermatomyositis
Antiphospholipid	Antiphospholipid syndrome, SLE

specific. Rheumatoid arthritis (p. 262) is the most common autoimmune rheumatic disease.

The diseases discussed in this section are also referred to as connective tissue diseases and have a number of features in common, including arthritis, immune complex deposition and vasculitis. There are four connective tissue diseases:

■ Systemic lupus erythematosus (SLE)
■ Systemic sclerosis (scleroderma)
■ Polymyositis and dermatomyositis
■ 'Overlap' syndrome.

Antinuclear antibodies (ANA) are serological hallmarks of patients with connective tissue disease. However, they are found at low titre in normal individuals (particularly elderly women) and patients with chronic infections and organ-specific autoimmune disease. The different types of autoantibodies are defined by their target antigen and some are relatively specific for a particular disease (Table 6.6).

Systemic lupus erythematosus (K&C 6e p. 574)

SLE is the most common of the connective tissue disorders and is characterized by the presence of serum antibodies against nuclear components. It is a multisystem disease and has a varied clinical presentation.

Epidemiology

It is a disease mostly of young women, with a peak age of onset between 20 and 40 years. It affects about 0.1% of the population but is more common in African American women with a prevalence of 1 in 250.

Aetiology

The cause of the disease is unknown but is probably multifactorial. Factors that are thought to play a role include the following:

- *Genetic factors.* There is a 25% concordance for SLE between identical twins, and an increased incidence of HLA-B8 and -DR3 in Caucasian and DR2 in Japanese patients.
- *Immunological factors.* Antinuclear antibodies are present which are thought to result from polyclonal activation of B cells by an antigenic stimulus, possible viral antigens. This may be associated with impaired T cell regulation and deficiencies in complement. Most of the visceral lesions are mediated by vascular immune complex (DNA–anti-DNA) deposition.
- *Drugs.* Hydralazine, isoniazid, procainamide and anti-TNF therapy with etanercept and infliximab cause a mild lupus-like syndrome, which often resolves after the drug is withdrawn.
- *Infection.* Viral infections may be responsible.
- *Sex hormone status.* The higher incidence in premenopausal women and males with Klinefelter's (XXY) suggests an oestrogen hormonal effect.

Pathogenesis

Patients with lupus appear to have a defect in apoptosis resulting in abnormal programmed cell death. Apoptotic cells and cell fragments are poorly cleared and certain antigens, especially nuclear, are processed by antigen-presenting cells with stimulation of the immune response to autoantigens. UV light, a trigger for lupus flares, probably acts via increased apoptosis. Most of the clinical manifestations of SLE are mediated directly or indirectly by antibody formation and the development and deposition of immune complexes and complement activation.

Clinical features

Clinical manifestations are varied (Table 6.7). A symmetrical small joint arthralgia is one of the most common presenting features. Synovitis and joint effusions are uncommon and joint destruction is very rare. Non-specific features such as fever, malaise and depression can dominate the clinical picture.

Discoid lupus is a benign variant of the disease, in which skin involvement may be the only feature. There is a characteristic facial rash with erythematous plaques which progress to scarring and pigmentation. Sunlight is an exacerbating factor in most patients.

Investigations

- Blood count usually shows a normochromic, normocytic anaemia, often with neutropenia/lymphopenia and thrombocytopenia. The ESR is raised but the CRP is usually normal.
- Serum autoantibodies: antinuclear antibodies are positive in almost all cases. Double-stranded DNA (dsDNA) binding is specific for SLE but is positive in only 50% of cases. Rheumatoid factor is positive in 25% of cases.
- Serum complement levels are reduced in active disease. Isolated C4 deficiency may be a genetic variant.
- Anticardiolipin antibodies (p. 284) are present in 35–45%.
- Histological examination, for example of a renal biopsy, shows a vasculitis.

Management

Treatment depends on the symptoms and severity of disease. Patients should be advised to avoid excessive sunlight and reduce cardiovascular factors, e.g. cessation of smoking.

- NSAIDs are useful for patients with mild disease and with arthralgia.

Table 6.7 Clinical features of SLE

Musculoskeletal
Small joint arthralgia*
Myalgia*
Aseptic necrosis of hip or knee

General*
Tiredness
Fever
Depression

Skin*
'Butterfly' rash – erythematous rash on cheeks and bridge of nose
Vasculitis
Urticaria
Photosensitivity
Alopecia
Raynaud's phenomenon

Blood*
Anaemia
Leucopenia/lymphopenia
Thrombocytopenia

Lungs
Pleurisy*
Pleural effusions (exudates)*
Restrictive defect (rare)

Heart and cardiovascular system
Pericarditis and pericardial effusions
Myocarditis
Aortic valve lesions
Thrombosis – arterial and venous
Accelerated atherosclerosis

Kidneys
Glomerulonephritis (all types)

Nervous system
Epilepsy
Migraine
Cerebellar ataxia
Aseptic meningitis
Cranial nerve lesions
Polyneuropathy

*Indicates common manifestations occurring in > 50% of patients

- Chloroquine and hydroxychloroquine are used for mild disease when symptoms cannot be controlled with NSAIDs, or for cutaneous disease.
- Corticosteroids form the mainstay of treatment, particularly in moderate to severe disease. The aim is to control disease activity (e.g. prednisolone 30 mg/day for 4 weeks) before gradually reducing the dose.
- Immunosuppressives (e.g. azathioprine, cyclophosphamide), usually in combination with corticosteroids, are used for patients with severe manifestations, e.g. renal or cerebral disease.
- Topical steroids are used for discoid lupus.

Prognosis

The disease is characterized by relapses and remissions even in severe disease. The 10-year survival is about 90%, although much lower if there is major organ involvement.

Antiphospholipid syndrome (APS) (K&C 6e p. 577)

This syndrome is characterized by autoantibodies directed against either phospholipids or plasma proteins bound to anionic phospholipids. Three types of antibodies have been described: lupus anticoagulant, anticardiolipin and β_2-glycoprotein I antibodies. The antibodies are thought to play a role in thrombosis by reacting with plasma proteins and phospholipids with an effect on platelet membranes, endothelial cells and clotting compounds such as prothrombin, protein C and protein S (p. 224). Although first described in patients with SLE, it is more common than SLE, and most patients (often young women) with the syndrome do not have SLE.

Clinical features

The major clinical features are the result of thrombosis:

- In arteries: stroke, transient ischaemic attacks, myocardial infarction
- In veins: deep vein thrombosis, Budd–Chiari syndrome (p. 164)
- In the placenta: recurrent abortions.

Other features include valvular heart disease, migraine, epilepsy and thrombocytopenia.

Investigations

The diagnosis is made on finding one or more of the specific serum antibodies (see above) in a patient with thrombosis or recurrent abortion.

Management

Warfarin is given for patients with APS who have had a thrombosis. Aspirin may be given as prophylaxis to patients with APS who have no history of thrombosis.

Systemic sclerosis (K&C 6e pp. 577 & 1343)

Systemic sclerosis (scleroderma) is a chronic multisystem disease which predominantly affects the skin and is usually accompanied by Raynaud's phenomenon (p. 483). It is three to five times more common in women than in men, and usually presents between the ages of 30 and 50 years

Aetiology

The pathogenesis of systemic sclerosis is complex and not completely understood. Altered vascular tone (mediated by endothelin, nitric oxide and superoxide anions) and cytotoxic damage to vascular endothelial cells are early changes. Activation of endothelial cells results in upregulation of adhesion molecules (E-selectin, VCAM, ICAM-1), cell adhesion (T and B cells, monocytes, neutrophils) and migration through the leaky endothelium and into the extracellular matrix. These cell–cell and cell–matrix interactions stimulate the production of cytokines and growth factors which mediate the proliferation and activation of vascular and connective tissue cells, particularly fibroblasts. The end result is uncontrolled and irreversible proliferation of connective tissue, and thickening of vascular walls with narrowing of the lumen.

285

Clinical features

Limited cutaneous scleroderma (60% of cases) This starts initially with Raynaud's phenomenon (p. 483), often prior to the development of cutaneous manifestations. The skin changes that dominate this disease are limited to the hands, face, feet and forearms. The skin is thickened, bound down to underlying structures, and the fingers taper (sclerodactyly). There is often a characteristic facial appearance, with beaking of the nose, a fixed expression, radial furrowing of the lips and limitation of mouth movements. There may be telangiectasia and palpable subcutaneous nodules of calcium deposition in the fingers (calcinosis). The CREST syndrome (Calcinosis, Raynaud's phenomenon, oEsophageal involvement, Sclerodactyly, Telangiectasia) was the term previously used to describe this syndrome.

Diffuse cutaneous scleroderma (40% of cases) The skin changes develop more rapidly after the development of Raynaud's phenomenon and are more widespread than in limited cutaneous scleroderma. There is early involvement of other organs. Heartburn and dysphagia occur in most patients and involvement of the small intestine leads to dilatation and atony with bacterial overgrowth. Pulmonary fibrosis and pulmonary vascular disease resulting in pulmonary hypertension are common and second only in frequency to oesophageal involvement. Abrupt onset of hypertension and acute renal failure develop in 10–15% of patients. Chronic renal failure may also occur. Cardiac disease occurs secondary to systemic or pulmonary hypertension, and direct cardiac manifestations include pericarditis, pericardial effusion, myocarditis and arrhythmias.

286

Investigations

The diagnosis of scleroderma is primarily based upon the presence of characteristic skin changes.

- Blood count shows a normochromic, normocytic anaemia and the ESR may be raised.
- Serum autoantibodies. Antinuclear antibodies are often positive. Anti-topoisomerase 1 (Scl 70) and anti-RNA polymerase I and III antibodies are highly specific for patients with diffuse cutaneous scleroderma. Anti-centromere antibodies occur in limited cutaneous scleroderma. Autoantibodies do not occur in all patients.
- Radiology. An X-ray of the hands may show deposits of calcium around the fingers, and there may be erosion and resorption of the tufts of the distal phalanges. High-resolution CT demonstrates fibrotic lung involvement. Barium swallow shows impaired oesophageal motility.
- Oesophageal manometry demonstrates failure of peristalsis in the distal oesophagus, with reduced oesophageal sphincter pressure.

Management

Management is symptomatic. There is no specific treatment. ACE inhibitors are the drug of first choice to treat hypertension and to prevent further kidney damage.

Prognosis

The 10-year survival is 70% and 55% in limited cutaneous and diffuse cutaneous disease respectively. Pulmonary fibrosis and pulmonary hypertension are the major cause of death.

Polymyositis and dermatomyositis *(K&C 6e p. 579)*

Polymyositis is a rare muscle disorder of unknown aetiology in which there is inflammation and necrosis of skeletal muscle fibres. When accompanied by a rash it is called dermatomyositis.

Clinical features

Peak ages of onset are in childhood and in the fifth and sixth decades. There is symmetrical progressive muscle weakness and wasting affecting the proximal muscles of the shoulder and pelvic girdle. Patients have difficulty squatting, going upstairs, rising from a chair and raising their hands above the head. Pain and tenderness are uncommon. Involvement of pharyngeal, laryngeal and respiratory muscles can lead to dysphagia, dysphonia and respiratory failure. The skin changes of dermatomyositis are characteristic: a heliotrope (purple) periorbital skin rash and scaly erythematous plaques over the dorsal aspects of the fingers and knuckles (collodion patches). Other features include arthralgia or arthritis, dysphagia resulting from oesophageal muscle involvement, and Raynaud's phenomenon. Dermatomyositis is associated with an increased incidence of underlying malignancy, particularly in the older age groups.

287

Investigations

- Muscle biopsy is the definitive test in establishing the diagnosis and in excluding other causes of myopathy. There is inflammatory cell infiltration and necrosis of muscle cells.
- Serum muscle enzymes (creatine kinase, aminotransferases, aldolase) are elevated.

- Anti-Jo-1 antibodies (anti-histidyl-tRNA synthetase) are positive.
- ESR is elevated in 5% of cases.
- Electromyography (EMG) shows characteristic changes.
- MRI can demonstrate areas of muscle inflammation.

Management

Oral prednisolone is the treatment of choice. Sometimes, immunosuppressive therapy with azathioprine or methotrexate is required.

Prognosis

Fifty per cent of affected children die within 2 years. In adults the prognosis is better, except in association with malignancy.

Sjögren's syndrome (K&C 6e p. 581)

Sjögren's syndrome is a chronic autoimmune disorder predominantly affecting middle-aged women. It is characterized by immunologically mediated destruction of epithelial exocrine glands, especially the lacrimal and salivary glands.

Clinical features

The main features are dry eyes (keratoconjunctivitis sicca) and dry mouth (xerostomia). Clinical clues are difficulty eating a dry biscuit and absence of pooling of the saliva when the tongue is lifted. It occurs as an isolated disorder (primary Sjögren's syndrome), also known as the sicca syndrome, or in association with another systemic disease (secondary Sjögren's syndrome), commonly rheumatoid arthritis, SLE, and primary biliary cirrhosis. Other features of primary Sjögren's syndrome are arthritis, Raynaud's phenomenon and interstitial nephritis. Six per cent develop lymphomas.

Investigations

- Antinuclear antibodies are found in 60–70% of patients. Anti-Ro and anti-La antibodies are present in 70% of patients with primary Sjögren's syndrome.
- Labial gland biopsy shows characteristic changes of lymphocyte infiltration and destruction of acinar tissue.

- A positive Schirmer test (a standard strip of filter paper is placed on the inside of the lower eyelid; wetting of less than 10 mm in 5 min is positive) confirms defective tear production.

Management

Treatment is symptomatic with artificial tears for dry eyes.

Overlap syndrome (K&C 6e p. 581)

This rare disorder combines features of more than one of the connective tissue diseases. Cerebral and renal disease is unusual and the prognosis is good. High titres of antibodies to extractable nuclear antigens (p. 280) such as ribonucleo-protein (RNP) are commonly found.

VASCULITIS (K&C 6e p. 581)

Vasculitis is inflammation of the blood vessel walls and may be associated with SLE, rheumatoid arthritis, poly-myositis and some allergic drug reactions. The term 'systemic vasculitides' describes a group of multisystem disorders in which vasculitis is the principal feature. These disorders are all rare except for giant cell (temporal) arteritis. Classification of the systemic vasculitides is based on the size of the vessels affected (Table 6.8).

Polymyalgia and giant cell arteritis (temporal arteritis) (K&C 6e p. 582)

Polymyalgia and giant cell arteritis are clinical syndromes affecting elderly people. Both are associated with the finding of a giant cell arteritis on temporal artery biopsy. Patients may have symptoms and signs limited to polymyalgia or to giant cell arteritis throughout the course of their illness while others have manifestations of both.

Clinical features

Polymyalgia is characterized by an abrupt onset of stiffness and intense pain in the proximal muscles of the shoulder and pelvic girdle. Significant objective weakness is un-common. There may be constitutional symptoms, with malaise, fever, weight loss and anorexia. Arteritic involve-ment by inflammation is most frequently noticed in the

Table 6.8 Classification of vasculitis

Large-vessel vasculitis (aorta and its major branches)
Giant-cell arteritis
Takayasu's arteritis (affects young women, causing coronary and CNS ischaemia)

Medium-sized-vessel vasculitis (main visceral vessels, e.g. renal, coronary)
Classic polyarteritis nodosa
Kawasaki's disease (affects young children)

Small-vessel vasculitis (small arteries, arterioles, venules and capillaries)
ANCA positive
Microscopic polyangiitis
Wegener's granulomatosis (p. 533)
Churg–Strauss syndrome

ANCA negative
Henoch–Schönlein purpura
Cutaneous leucocytoclastic angiitis
Essential cryoglobulinaemia

ANCA, antineutrophil cytoplasmic antibodies (p. 948)

superficial temporal arteries and causes localized headache, temporal artery tenderness and loss of pulsation (p. 762). Giant cell arteritis affecting the vertebrobasilar, and sometimes the carotid, circulation may result in stroke.

Investigations

The diagnosis is usually based on clinical findings.

■ Blood count usually shows a very high ESR (around 100 mm/h) and a normochromic, normocytic anaemia.
■ Temporal artery biopsy is performed if arteritis is suspected and should be performed before or within a week of starting corticosteroids.

Management

Treatment of polymyalgia rheumatica and giant cell arteritis is with corticosteroids. The usual starting dose is 15 mg/day for polymyalgia and 60 mg/day for temporal arteritis. The dose is gradually reduced by weekly decrements of 5 mg. Once 10 mg is reached a reduction of 1 mg every 2–4 weeks is usually sufficient. The dose is titrated against symptoms and the ESR. Prophylaxis against steroid-induced osteoporosis should be given (p. 301). The disease may relapse when steroid treatment is stopped.

Polyarteritis nodosa (classic polyarteritis nodosa) (*K&C* 6e p. 583)

Polyarteritis nodosa (PAN) predominantly affects middle-aged men. Hepatitis B surface antigen is detected in some patients and may be involved in the pathogenesis. There is a necrotizing arteritis associated with microaneurysm formation, thrombosis and infarction. Clinical features include fever, malaise, weight loss, mononeuritis multiplex, abdominal pain (resulting from visceral infarcts), renal impairment and hypertension. The diagnosis is made by biopsy of a clinically affected organ, often the kidney, which shows pathognomonic inflammation of the medium-sized arteries. Mesenteric or renal arteriography shows micro-aneurysms.

Microscopic polyangiitis (*K&C* 6e p. 938)

A focal necrotizing glomerulonephritis causes haematuria, proteinuria and sometimes progressive renal failure. Other features include arthralgia and purpuric rashes. Diagnosis is by renal biopsy and measurement of serum perinuclear antineutrophil cytoplasmic antibodies (pANCA, present in 60%; see p. 948). Treatment is similar to Churg–Strauss syndrome (see below).

Churg–Strauss syndrome (*K&C* 6e p. 938)

This is rare and characterized by a triad of asthma, eosinophilia and a systemic vasculitis. The treatments for Churg–Strauss syndrome, PAN and microscopic polyangiitis are similar, using prednisolone, azathioprine and cyclo-phosphamide.

Henoch–Schönlein purpura (*K&C* 6e pp. 587 & 629)

This condition is most commonly seen in children and presents as a purpuric rash, mainly on the legs and buttocks. The rash is caused by a vasculitis with intradermal bleeding. Abdominal pain, arthritis, haematuria and nephritis also occur. It is characterized by vascular deposition of IgA-dominant immune complexes, and the onset is often preceded by an acute upper respiratory tract infection. Recovery is usually spontaneous.

Behçet's disease (K&C 6e p. 584)

This is a rare multisystem chronic disease of unknown cause, characterized by recurrent oral ulceration. Diagnosis is clinical and requires the presence of oral ulceration and any two of the following:

- Genital ulcers
- Eye lesions (uveitis, retinal vascular lesions)
- Skin lesions (erythema nodosum, papulopustular lesions)
- Positive skin pathergy test (skin injury, e.g. needle prick, leads to pustule formation in 48 h).

Other features include arthritis, gastrointestinal ulceration with pain and diarrhoea, pulmonary and renal lesions, meningoencephalitis, and organic confusional states.

Treatment is with immunosuppressive therapy (steroids, azathioprine, ciclosporin). Thalidomide may be useful in some cases although side-effects of drowsiness and peripheral neuropathy are common. It should not be used in pregnant women because of phocomelia (limb abnormalities).

Arthritis in children

There are three main types: juvenile chronic arthritis, juvenile rheumatoid arthritis and juvenile ankylosing spondylitis discussed in detail in *Clinical Medicine* (K&C 6e p. 586).

BACK PAIN

Lumbar back pain (K&C 6e p. 540)

Lumbar back pain is an extremely common symptom experienced by most people at some time in their lives. Only a few patients have a serious underlying disorder. Mechanical back pain is a common cause in young people. It starts suddenly, is often unilateral, and may be helped by rest. It may arise from the facet joints, spinal ligaments or muscle. The history, physical examination and simple

Table 6.9	Causes of lumbar back pain	
		History and examination
Mechanical	Prolapsed intervertebral disc Osteoarthritis Fractures Spondylolisthesis Spinal stenosis	Often sudden onset Pain worse in the evening Morning stiffness is absent Exercise aggravates pain
Inflammatory	Ankylosing spondylitis Infection (see below)	Gradual onset Pain worse in the morning Morning stiffness is present Exercise relieves pain
Serious causes	Metastatic carcinoma Myeloma Tuberculosis osteomyelitis Bacterial osteomyelitis Cord or cauda equina compression	Age < 20 or > 50 years Constant pain without relief History of TB, HIV, carcinoma, steroid use Systemically unwell: fever, weight loss Localized bone tenderness Bilateral signs in the legs Neurological deficit involving more than one root level Bladder, bowel or sexual function deficits
Others	Osteomalacia, Paget's disease, referred pain from pelvic/abdominal disease	

Text in red indicates the 'red flags' in a patient with lumbar back pain. Onset of thoracic pain is also a 'red flag'

293

investigations will also often identify the minority of patients with other causes of back pain (Table 6.9).

The age of the patient helps in deciding the aetiology of back pain because certain causes are more common in particular age groups. These are illustrated in Table 6.10.

Investigations

A detailed history and physical examination (see Table 6.9) will lead to the diagnosis in many cases. The key points are

Table 6.10 Low back pain – disorders most commonly found in specific age groups

15–30 years	30–50 years	50 years and over
Mechanical	Mechanical	Degenerative joint disease
Prolapsed intervertebral disc	Prolapsed intervertebral disc	Osteoporosis
Ankylosing spondylitis	Degenerative joint disease	Paget's disease
Spondylolisthesis	Malignancy	Malignancy
		Myeloma
Fractures (all ages)		
Infective lesions (all ages)		

age, speed of onset, the presence of motor or sensory symptoms, involvement of the bladder or bowel, and the presence of stiffness and the effect of exercise. Young adults with a history suggestive of mechanical back pain and with no physical signs do not need further investigation.

- Blood count is usually normal. The ESR may be raised with inflammatory back pain and tumours.
- Serum biochemistry. A raised calcium and alkaline phosphatase suggest metastases. Typically with myeloma the calcium is raised, with a normal alkaline phosphatase. A raised alkaline phosphatase with a normal calcium occurs with metabolic bone disease. Prostate-specific antigen should be measured if secondary prostatic disease is suspected.
- Radiology. X-rays may be useful for excluding serious disease, although they may be misleading, e.g. degenerative disease is virtually always present in older people.
- Technetium bone scan (p. 257) will show increased uptake with infection or malignancy.
- MRI is useful when neurological symptoms and signs are present. It is useful for the detection of disc and cord lesions.

Management

The treatment depends on the cause. Mechanical back pain is managed with analgesia, brief rest and physiotherapy. Exercise programmes reduce long-term problems.

INTERVERTEBRAL DISC DISEASE

Acute disc disease *(K&C 6e p 542)*

Acute disc disease is a syndrome in which there is prolapse of the intervertebral disc resulting in acute back pain (lumbago), with or without radiation of the pain to areas supplied by the sciatic nerve (sciatica). It is a disease of younger people (20–40 years) because the disc degenerates with age and in elderly people is no longer capable of prolapse. In older patients sciatica is more likely to be the result of compression of the nerve root by osteophytes in the lateral recess of the spinal canal.

Clinical features

There is a sudden onset of severe back pain, often following a strenuous activity. The pain is often clearly related to position and is aggravated by movement. Muscle spasm leads to a sideways tilt when standing. The radiation of the pain and the clinical findings depend on the disc affected (Table 6.11), the lowest three discs being those most commonly affected.

Investigations

Investigations are of very limited value in acute disc disease and X-rays are often normal. MRI is usually reserved for patients in whom surgery is being considered (see later).

Management

Treatment is aimed at the relief of symptoms and has little effect on the duration of the disease. In the acute stage, treatment consists of bed rest on a firm mattress, analgesia, and occasionally epidural corticosteroid injection in severe disease. Surgery is only considered for severe or increasing neurological impairment, e.g. foot drop or bladder symptoms. Physiotherapy is used in the recovery phase, helping to correct posture and restore movement.

Chronic disc disease

This common syndrome is characterized by the presence of chronic lower back pain associated with 'degenerative' changes in the lower lumbar discs and apophyseal joints. Pain is usually of the mechanical type (see above). Sciatic radiation may occur with pain in the buttocks radiating into

Intervertebral disc disease

Table 6.11	Symptoms and signs of common root compression syndromes produced by lumbar disc prolapse				
Root lesion	Pain	Sensory loss	Motor weakness	Reflex lost	Other signs
S1	From buttock down back of thigh and leg to ankle and foot	Sole of foot and posterior calf	Plantar flexion of ankle and toes	Ankle jerk	Diminished straight leg raising
L5	From buttock to lateral aspect of leg and dorsum of foot	Dorsum of foot and anterolateral aspect of lower leg	Dorsiflexion of foot and toes	None	As above
L4	Lateral aspect of thigh to medial side of calf	Medial aspect of calf and shin	Dorsiflexion and inversion of ankle; extension of knee	Knee jerk	Positive femoral stretch test

296

the posterior thigh. Usually the pain is long-standing and the prospects for cure are limited. However, measures that have been found useful include NSAIDs, physiotherapy and weight reduction. Surgery can be considered when pain arises from a single identifiable level and has failed to respond to conservative measures. Fusion at this level, with decompression of the affected nerve roots, can be successful.

Mechanical problems

Spondylolisthesis (*K&C* 6e p. 543)

Spondylolisthesis is characterized by a slipping forward of one vertebra on another, most commonly at L4/L5. It arises because of a defect in the pars interarticularis of the vertebra, and may be either congenital or acquired (e.g. trauma). The condition is associated with mechanical pain which worsens throughout the day. The pain may radiate to one or other leg and there may be signs of nerve root irritation. Small spondylolistheses, often associated with degenerative disease of the lumbar spine, may be treated conservatively with simple analgesics. A large spondylolisthesis causing severe symptoms should be treated with spinal fusion.

Spinal stenosis (*K&C* 6e p. 542)

Narrowing of the lower spinal canal compresses the cauda equina, resulting in back and buttock pain, typically coming on after a period of walking and easing with rest. Accordingly it is sometimes called spinal claudication. Causes include disc prolapse, degenerative osteophyte formation, tumour and congenital narrowing of the spinal canal. CT and MRI will demonstrate cord compression, and treatment is by surgical decompression.

Neck pain (*K&C* 6e p. 536)

Pain in the neck may be caused by rheumatoid arthritis, ankylosing spondylitis or fibrositis (chronic muscle pain in young women with no underlying cause; large psychological overlay in some patients). In addition, disc disease, both acute and chronic, the latter in association with osteoarthritis, may occur in the neck as well as in the lumbar spine. The three lowest cervical discs are most often affected, and there is pain and stiffness of the neck with or without root pain radiating to the arm. Chronic cervical disc disease is known as cervical spondylosis.

BONE DISEASE

Bone normally consists of 70% mineral and 30% organic matrix (mostly type 1 collagen fibres). The mineral component consists mostly of a complex crystalline salt of calcium and phosphate called hydroxyapatite. Although major skeletal growth occurs in childhood, adult bone is continuously being remodelled, with bone formation and resorption. Two major cell types are involved in bone remodelling:

- Osteoblasts produce type 1 collagen and growth factors, and also regulate osteoclast activity.
- Osteoclasts produce lysosomal enzymes which degrade collagen matrix (K&C 6e p. 591).

Control of calcium and bone metabolism (K&C 6e p. 591)

Vitamin D and parathyroid hormone (PTH) are the major factors that control plasma calcium concentration and bone turnover. Bone metabolism is also controlled by calcitonin, glucocorticoids, sex hormones, growth hormone and thyroid hormone.

298

Vitamin D

The metabolism and actions of vitamin D are shown in Figure 6.4.

Parathyroid hormone (PTH)

PTH is secreted from chief cells of the parathyroid gland. Plasma levels rise in response to a fall in serum ionized calcium. The effects are several, all serving to increase plasma calcium and decrease plasma phosphate:

- Increased osteoclastic resorption of bone
- Increased intestinal absorption of calcium
- Increased synthesis of $1,25\text{-}(OH)_2D_3$
- Increased renal tubular reabsorption of calcium.

Osteoporosis (K&C 6e p. 594)

Osteoporosis means thin bone and the term implies a reduction in bone mass, including all components of bone, not just calcium. The bone is fragile, with an increased risk of fracture. Osteoporosis is defined as a bone density more than 2.5 standard deviations (SDs) below the young adult mean value (T-score < −2.5). Values between 1 and 2.5 SDs below the young adult mean are termed 'osteopenia'.

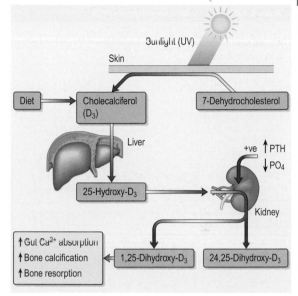

Fig. 6.4 **The metabolism and actions of vitamin D.**
Cholecalciferol is predominantly formed from photoactivation of
7-dehydrocholesterol in the skin. In the liver, cholecalciferol is
converted to 25-hydroxycholecalciferol, which is then converted
to the much more active form, 1,25-dihydroxycholecalciferol, in
the kidney. This latter step can also occur in lymphomatous and
sarcoid tissue, resulting in the hypercalcaemia that may
complicate these diseases.

Aetiology

Bone resorption is part of the normal ageing process,
occurring more in women than in men, largely as a result of
postmenopausal oestrogen deficiency. The risk factors for
osteoporosis are those that cause a reduction in peak bone
mass attained in adult life or those that cause increased
bone loss (Table 6.12).

Clinical features

Symptoms of osteoporosis are the result of fractures, which
typically occur at three sites: the thoracic and lumbar
vertebrae, neck of the femur and the distal radius (Colles'

Bone disease

Table 6.12 **Risk factors for osteoporosis**

Increasing age
Female sex
Early menopause
Oophorectomy
Slender habitus
Smoking
Excess alcohol
Low dietary calcium
Vitamin D deficiency
Lack of exercise
Family history
White race
Drugs (corticosteroids, heparin, ciclosporin, anticonvulsants)
Endocrine disease (Cushing's syndrome, hyperparathyroidism,
    acromegaly)
Other chronic disease (IBD, coeliac disease, chronic liver and
    renal disease)

fracture). Vertebral fractures may lead to kyphosis and loss
of height.

Investigations

- Bone densitometry. Dual-energy X-ray absorptiometry
  (DXA) measures real bone density, usually of the lumbar
  spine and proximal femur. It is the gold standard in
  osteoporosis diagnosis and reflects fracture risk which
  may influence treatment decisions. Quantitative ultrasound
  of the heel may prove a convenient and portable means
  of assessing bone density.
- Radiology. X-rays are relatively insensitive for detecting
  osteopenia but will demonstrate fractures if present.
- Serum biochemistry. Calcium, phosphate and alkaline
  phosphatase are normal.
- Secondary causes of osteoporosis such as thyrotoxicosis,
  myeloma, primary hyperparathyroidism and hypogonadism should be excluded in men and premenopausal women.

Management

Prevention is better than treatment of established disease.
Predisposing factors should be addressed and those at risk
(Table 6.12) identified for DXA.

Those with mild osteopenia (T-score – 1.0–2.5) should be given lifestyle advice such as stopping smoking, reducing alcohol intake, adequate intake of calcium (1500 mg/day) and vitamin D (400–800 IU/day) and regular weight-bearing exercises, and reassessed after 2 years. In the elderly, physiotherapy and assessment of home safety are done to reduce the risk of falls. Hip protectors may reduce the risk of hip fracture in residential care.

Management of established osteoporosis involves lifestyle advice as above and drug treatment.

- Bisphosphonates (e.g. alendronate, risedronate) are the treatment of choice in both women and men with osteoporosis. They inhibit bone resorption through inhibition of osteoclast activity, increase bone mass at the hip and spine and most have been shown to reduce fracture incidence. Optimal duration of therapy is unknown.
- Raloxifene, a selective oestrogen-receptor modulator (SERM), activates oestrogen receptors on bone while having no stimulatory effect on endometrium. It has been shown to reduce bone mineral density loss at spine and hip, though fracture rates are reduced only in the spine. It is used in patients who cannot tolerate or do not respond to bisphosphonates.

- Recombinant human parathyroid peptide 1-34 (teriparatide) stimulates bone formation. It is mainly indicated for very severe cases of osteoporosis or in women who are intolerant of, or fail to respond to other therapies.
- Oestrogen therapy as hormone-replacement therapy (HRT) is now regarded as second-line therapy because of adverse effects on breast cancer and cardiovascular disease risk with long-term use (see p. 599). It is used for women who are intolerant of other therapies or perimenopausal women who have menopausal symptoms.
- Testosterone is given to men with biochemical evidence of hypogonadism.

Prevention of osteoporosis in patients receiving corticosteroids

Oral corticosteroids are associated with a significant fracture risk at the hip and spine. General measures to reduce the fracture risk include reduction of the dose of corticosteroids to a minimum, an alternative route of administration (e.g.

rectal steroids in distal ulcerative colitis) and prescription of alternative immunosuppressive agents. All patients should be given calcium and vitamin D supplements and lifestyle advice as above. In addition all patients over the age of 65 years or with a previous fragility fracture are given drug treatment as above; only bisphosphonates are licensed in the UK for this purpose. Drug treatment is given to younger patients based on the results of a DXA scan.

Paget's disease (K&C 6e p. 599)

Paget's disease is characterized by excessive osteoclastic bone resorption followed by disordered osteoblastic activity, leading to abundant new bone formation which is structurally abnormal and weak.

Aetiology

A gene predisposing to Paget's disease has been identified on chromosome 18q. Osteoclasts contain viral inclusion bodies, suggesting a possible 'slow viral' aetiology.

Epidemiology

The incidence increases with age; it is rare in the under-40s and affects up to 10% of adults by the age of 90.

Clinical features

The most common sites are the pelvis, lumbosacral spine, femur, skull and tibia, although any bone can be involved. Most cases are asymptomatic, but features include the following:

- Bone pain
- Apparent joint pain when the involved bone is close to a joint
- Deformities: enlargement of the skull, bowing of the tibia
- Complications: nerve compression (deafness, paraparesis), fractures, rarely cardiac failure and osteogenic sarcoma.

Investigations

The diagnosis is often clinical and supported by:

- Serum biochemistry, shows a raised alkaline phosphatase concentration (reflects level of bone formation), often > 1000 U/L, with a normal calcium and phosphate.

- X-rays showing characteristic changes, most often in the pelvis, skull or spine. There is localized bony enlargement and distortion, sclerotic changes (increased density) and osteolytic areas (loss of bone and reduced density).
- Radionuclide bone scans showing increased uptake of bone-seeking radionuclides, which is due to increased bone formation. The appearances on bone scans and plain X-rays may be difficult to distinguish from metastatic carcinoma, especially sclerotic secondaries seen with breast and prostate cancer.

Treatment

Bisphosphonates inhibit bone resorption by decreasing osteoclastic activity, and form the mainstay of treatment. They are indicated for symptomatic patients and asymptomatic patients at risk of complications (e.g. fracture, nerve entrapment). Disease activity is monitored by symptoms and measurement of serum alkaline phosphatase.

Neoplastic disease of bone (K&C 6e p. 588)

Primary bone tumours are uncommon malignancies and most present with localized pain and swelling. Metastases are the most common bone tumour, particularly in the elderly. Tumours of the breast, prostate, thyroid, lung, kidney and pancreas account for most patients presenting with metastatic bone disease. In addition, most patients with multiple myeloma will have skeletal abnormalities on imaging (osteopenia, punched-out lytic lesions, fractures) at diagnosis. Metastatic bone disease presents with pain, fractures (which may occur in the absence of trauma) and neurological symptoms due to nerve root or spinal cord compression.

The diagnosis is suspected on the basis of the history and plain X-rays showing osteolytic areas with bony destruction. Osteosclerotic metastases are characteristic of prostate carcinoma. Serum alkaline phosphatase is raised and there may be hypercalcaemia. An isotope bone scan will show bony metastases as 'hot areas' and is more sensitive than plain X-rays. Treatment of bony metastases involves pain control (analgesia, nerve blockade, local radiotherapy), surgery (for fractures, spinal cord compression) and management of the primary lesion. Recent studies have also shown that intravenous bisphosphonates reduce the risk of skeletal complications (fractures, hypercalcaemia, cord compression) in women with breast cancer and skeletal metastases.

Osteomalacia (K&C 6e p. 600)

Inadequate mineralization of the osteoid framework, leading to soft bones, produces rickets during bone growth in children and osteomalacia following epiphyseal closure in adults.

Aetiology

- Deficiency of vitamin D as a result of a combination of poor diet and inadequate sunlight. This is seen in immobile elderly people and in female Asian immigrants in the UK.
- Malabsorption, e.g. coeliac disease and small bowel resection.
- Renal disease leading to inadequate conversion of $25\text{-}(OH)D_3$ to $1,25\text{-}(OH)_2D_3$ (Fig. 6.4).
- Other causes include liver failure, renal phosphate loss and anticonvulsant therapy (caused by increased vitamin D inactivation).

Clinical features

In the adult osteomalacia produces muscle and bone pain and fractures. In addition, a proximal myopathy leads to a 'waddling' gait and difficulty in rising from a chair. The principal differential diagnosis in a patient presenting with bone pain, bone fractures and osteopenia on the X-ray is osteoporosis versus osteomalacia. The distinction can usually be made from the history, physical examination and a combination of laboratory and radiological studies.

Investigations

- Serum biochemistry shows a low phosphate, low or low–normal calcium and increased alkaline phosphatase.
- Serum 25-hydroxyvitamin D_3 is usually low.
- Radiology. X-ray appearance is characteristic, showing defective mineralization and Looser's zones (low-density bands extending from the cortex inwards in the shafts of the long bones).

Table 6.13 Treatment of osteomalacia	
Vitamin D deficiency	Vitamin D_2 10 µg (400 U) daily
Malabsorption	Vitamin D_2 1 2.5 mg (40 000–100 000 U) daily
Renal failure	1α-Hydroxycholecalciferol (alfacalcidol or 1α-$(OH)D_3$) or 1,25-dihydroxycholecalciferol (calcitriol or 1,25-$(OH_2)D_3$)

- Bone biopsy is the definitive investigation and shows increased non-mineralized bone. However, this procedure is uncomfortable and rarely necessary.

Management

The treatment is with oral vitamin D; the dose and formulation depend on the cause (Table 6.13). Treatment is monitored by measurement of serum alkaline phosphatase and calcium.

Water and electrolytes 7

WATER AND ELECTROLYTE REQUIREMENTS

In health, the volume and biochemical composition of both extracellular and intracellular fluid compartments in the body remains remarkably constant. Maintenance of the total amount depends on the balance between intake and loss. Water and electrolytes are taken in as food and water, and lost in urine, sweat and faeces (Table 7.1). In addition, about 500 mL of water are lost daily in expired air.

In certain disease states the intake and loss of water and electrolytes is altered and this factor must be taken into account when providing fluid replacements. For instance, a patient who is losing gastric secretions via a nasogastric tube will be losing additional sodium (25–80 mmol/L), potassium (5–20 mmol/L), chloride (100–150 mmol/L) and hydrogen (40–60 mmol/L) ions each day which will need to be replaced together with normal daily requirements.

BODY FLUID COMPARTMENTS (K&C 6e p. 689)

In healthy adult males about 60% of bodyweight is water; females have proportionately more body fat than males and

Table 7.1 The normal daily water and sodium balance in a 75-kg man

Input		Output	
Water (mL)		**Water (mL)**	
Drink	1500	Urine	1500
Food	800	Insensible loss (skin, lungs)	800
Metabolism	200	Faeces	200
Total	2500		2500
Sodium (mmol)		**Sodium (mmol)**	
Food and drink	140	Urine	140
		Sweat	Negligible
		Faeces	Negligible

Table 7.2 **Normal adult electrolyte concentrations of intracellular and extracellular fluids**

	Plasma (mmol/L)	Interstitial fluid (mmol/L)	Intracellular fluid (mmol/L)
Na^+	142	144	10
K^+	4	4	160
Ca^{2+}	2.5	2.5	1.5
Mg^{2+}	1.0	0.5	13
Cl^-	102	114	2
HCO_3^-	26	30	8
PO_4^{2-}	1.0	1.0	57
SO_4^{2-}	0.5	0.5	10
Organic acid	3	4	3
Protein	16	0	55

total body water is about 55% of bodyweight. In a healthy 70-kg man, total body water is approximately 42 L. The total body water is distributed into two main compartments:

■ Intracellular fluid – 65% of total body water
■ Extracellular fluid – 35% of total body water. The extracellular component is divided into the interstitial space that bathes the cells (25% of total body water) and the intravascular water or plasma (10% of total body water).

The cell membrane separates the intracellular and extracellular fluid compartments and maintains, by active and passive transport mechanisms, the different electrolyte compositions within each compartment (Table 7.2).

Osmotic pressure is the primary determinant of the distribution of water among the three major compartments. Osmolality is determined by the concentration of osmotically active particles. Thus 1 mole of sodium chloride dissolved in 1 kg of water has an osmolality of 2 mmol/kg, as sodium chloride freely dissociates into two particles, the sodium ion Na^+ and the chloride ion Cl^-. One mole of urea (which does not dissociate) in 1 kg of water has an osmolality of 1 mmol/kg. Sodium and chloride are the major extracellular ions and therefore the main determinants of interstitial fluid and plasma osmolality, whilst that of the intracellular fluid is determined by the concentrations of potassium, magnesium, phosphate and sulphate (Table 7.2). A change in osmolality in one compartment will trigger water

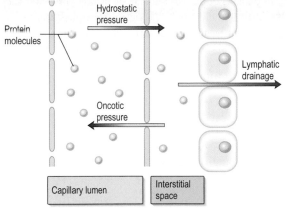

Fig. 7.1 **Distribution of water between the vascular and extravascular (interstitial) spaces** This is determined by the equilibrium between hydrostatic pressure, which tends to force fluid out of the capillaries, and oncotic pressure, which acts to retain fluid within the vessel. The net flow of fluid outwards is balanced by 'suction' of fluid into the lymphatics, which returns it to the bloodstream. Similar principles govern the volume of the peritoneal and pleural spaces.

movement across the cell membrane to re-establish osmotic equilibrium.

Distribution of extracellular fluid

The capillary bed separating the intravascular and interstitial spaces is freely permeable to Na^+, K^+ and glucose, and these solutes do not therefore contribute to fluid distribution between these spaces. However, plasma proteins, e.g. albumin, have a limited ability to traverse the capillary bed, and act to hold water in the vascular space. The distribution of extracellular water between vascular and extravascular (interstitial) space is determined by the equilibrium between hydrostatic pressure (i.e. intracapillary blood pressure), which tends to force fluid out of the capillaries, and oncotic pressure (i.e. osmotic pressure exerted by plasma proteins), which acts to retain fluid within the vessel. The net flow of fluid outwards is balanced by 'suction' of fluid into the lymphatics which returns it to the bloodstream (Fig. 7.1).

Oedema is defined as an increase in interstitial fluid and results from:

- Increased hydrostatic pressure, e.g. sodium and water retention in cardiac failure
- Reduced oncotic pressure, e.g. as a result of nephrotic syndrome with hypoalbuminaemia
- Obstruction to lymphatic flow
- Increased permeability of the blood vessel wall, e.g. at a site of inflammation, cytokines lead to an increase in vascular permeability.

Inspection and palpation are usually sufficient to identify oedema. Compression of the skin of the affected area with a finger tip for 10 seconds results in 'pitting'. Localized oedema is most likely to result from a local cause, e.g. venous obstruction. The location of generalized oedema, e.g. with cardiac failure, is often most prominent in the legs and feet in ambulatory patients and in the sacral region in those who are confined to bed.

REGULATION OF BODY FLUID HOMEOSTASIS (*K&C* 6e p. 690)

Maintenance of the effective circulating volume is essential for adequate tissue perfusion and is mainly related to the regulation of sodium balance. In contrast, maintenance of osmolality prevents changes in cell volume and is largely related to the regulation of water balance.

Regulation of extracellular volume

The regulation of extracellular volume is determined by a tight control of the balance of sodium, which is excreted by normal kidneys. The effective circulating volume (ECV) refers to the effective arterial blood volume (EABV) that perfuses tissues. The fullness of the arterial compartment depends upon a normal ratio between cardiac output and peripheral arterial resistance. Thus, diminished EABV is initiated by a fall in cardiac output or a fall in peripheral arterial resistance (an increase in the holding capacity of the arterial vascular tree). When the EABV is expanded this in turn leads to an increase in urinary sodium excretion and vice versa.

Two types of volume receptors sense changes in the EABV:

- Extrarenal: in the large vessels near the heart
- Intrarenal: in the afferent renal arteriole, which controls the renin–angiotensin system via the juxtaglomerular apparatus.

A decreased effective circulating volume leads to activation of these volume receptors, which leads to an increase in sodium (and hence water) reabsorption by the kidney and expansion of the extracellular volume via stimulation of the sympathetic nervous system and activation of the renin–angiotensin system (p. 639). In contrast, atrial natriuretic peptide (ANP), produced by the atria of the heart in response to an increase in blood volume, increases sodium excretion.

Abnormalities of extracellular volume

Increased extracellular volume (*K&C 6e* p. 695)

Extracellular volume expansion is the result of increased sodium (and hence water) reabsorption or impaired excretion by the kidney.

Aetiology

- *Cardiac failure* due to a reduction in cardiac output and impaired perfusion (therefore effective hypovolaemia) of the volume receptors.
- *Nephrotic syndrome.* Two major factors are thought to contribute to oedema formation in the nephrotic syndrome: arterial underfilling as the low plasma oncotic pressure leads to plasma volume depletion; and primary renal sodium retention due to increased sodium reabsorption in the collecting ducts directly induced by the renal disease. Furthermore, in nephrotic syndrome and other hypoalbuminaemic conditions capillary permeability is increased, thus favouring oedema formation.
- *Cirrhosis.* This is through a complex mechanism, but there is vasodilatation and hence underperfusion of the volume receptors. Hypoalbuminaemia may also contribute.
- *Sodium retention.* This may be as a result of renal impairment, where there is a reduction in renal capacity to excrete sodium, or due to drugs such as mineralocorticoids, non-steroidal anti-inflammatory drugs (NSAIDs) and selective cyclo-oxygenase-2 (COX-2)

Regulation of body fluid homeostasis

inhibitors. NSAIDs and COX-2 inhibitors inhibit synthesis of vasodilatory prostaglandins in the kidney with an increase in renal vascular resistance and increase in water and sodium reabsorption.

Clinical features

These depend on the distribution of extracellular water, e.g. with hypoalbuminaemia caused by loss of plasma oncotic pressure there is predominantly interstitial volume overload. Cardiac failure leads to expansion of both compartments:

- *Interstitial volume overload* – ankle oedema, pulmonary oedema, pleural effusion and ascites
- *Intravascular volume overload* – raised jugular venous pressure, cardiomegaly, and a raised arterial pressure in some cases.

This must be differentiated from local causes of oedema (e.g. ankle oedema as a result of venous damage following thrombosis) which do not reflect a disturbance in the control of extracellular volume.

Management

The underlying cause must be treated. The cornerstone of treatment is diuretics, which increase sodium and water excretion in the kidney. There are a number of different classes of diuretic, of which the most potent are the loop diuretics, e.g. furosemide (frusemide) (Table 7.3).

Decreased extracellular volume (*K&C* 6e p. 699)
This may be the result of loss of sodium and water, plasma or blood.

Aetiology

Volume depletion occurs in haemorrhage, plasma loss in extensive burns, or loss of salt and water from the kidneys, gastrointestinal tract or skin (Table 7.4). Signs of volume depletion occur despite a normal or increased body content of sodium and water in sepsis (due to vasodilatation and increased capillary permeability) and diuretic treatment of oedematous states where mobilization of oedema lags behind a rapid reduction in plasma volume due to diuresis.

Table 7.3 The main classes of diuretics in clinical use

Class	Example	Mechanism of action	Relative potency	Side-effects
Loop diuretics	Furosemide (frusemide) Bumetanide	Reduce Na^+ and Cl^- reabsorption in ascending limb of loop of Henle	++++	Urate retention and gout Hypokalaemia and hypomagnesaemia Decreased glucose tolerance Allergic tubulointerstitial nephritis Myalgia Ototoxicity
Thiazides	Bendroflumethiazide (bendrofluazide) Hydrochlorothiazide	Reduce sodium reabsorption in distal convoluted tubule	++	↓ serum K^+ ↓ Ca^{2+} excretion, increased plasma calcium
Potassium-sparing	Spironolactone Amiloride	Aldosterone antagonist Prevents potassium exchange for sodium in distal tubule	+	Gynaecomastia Hyperkalaemia

Table 7.4 Causes of extracellular volume depletion
Haemorrhage External Concealed, e.g. leaking aortic aneurysm
Burns
Gastrointestinal losses Vomiting Diarrhoea Ileostomy losses
Renal losses Diuretic use Impaired tubular sodium conservation, e.g. reflux nephropathy, papillary necrosis

Clinical features

Symptoms include thirst, nausea and postural dizziness. Interstitial fluid loss leads to loss of skin elasticity ('turgor'). Loss of circulating volume causes peripheral vasoconstriction and tachycardia, a low jugular venous pressure and postural hypotension. Severe depletion of circulating volume causes hypotension, which may impair cerebral perfusion, resulting in confusion and eventual coma.

Investigations

The diagnosis is usually made clinically. A central venous line allows the measurement of central venous pressure (p. 803), which helps in assessing the response to treatment. Plasma urea may be raised because of increased urea reabsorption and, later, prerenal failure (when the creatinine rises as well). This is, however, very non-specific. Urinary sodium is low (< 20 mmol/L) if the kidneys are working normally. The urinary sodium can be misleading, however, if the cause of the volume depletion involves the kidneys, e.g. with diuretics or intrinsic renal disease.

Management

The overriding aims of treatment are to replace what has been lost:

Table 7.5 Intravenous fluids in general use*				
	Na$^+$ (mmol/L)	K$^+$ (mmol/L)	HCO$_3^-$ (mmol/L)	Cl$^-$ (mmol/L)
Normal plasma constituents	142	4.5	26	103
Sodium chloride 0.9% (isotonic physiological saline)	150	–	–	150
Glucose 5%	–	–	–	–
Sodium chloride (0.18%) + glucose 4% (1/5 physiological saline)	30	–	–	30

*Accounting for 95% of the fluids used in clinical practice

- Haemorrhage involves the loss of whole blood. The rational treatment of acute haemorrhage is therefore whole blood, or a combination of red cells and a plasma substitute.
- Loss of plasma, as in burns or severe peritonitis, should be treated with human plasma or a plasma substitute (see p. 558).
- Loss of sodium and water, as in vomiting, diarrhoea or excessive renal losses, should be treated with replacement of water and electrolytes. This is best done orally if possible, with an increased intake of water and salt. Glucose–electrolyte solutions are often used to restore fluid balance in patients with diarrhoeal diseases. This is based on the fact that the presence of glucose stimulates intestinal absorption of salt and water (p. 40).
- In the acute situation if there have been large losses of sodium and water, patients are usually treated with intravenous physiological saline (Tables 7.5 and 7.6), and replacement is assessed clinically and by measurement of serum electrolytes.
- Loss of water alone, e.g. diabetes insipidus, only causes extracellular volume depletion in severe cases because the loss is spread evenly over all the compartments of body water. The correct treatment is to give water. If

> **Table 7.6   Guidelines for intravenous fluid administration in maintenance and replacement of losses**
>
> **For maintenance fluid balance**
> Each day 2500 mL fluid containing about 140 mmol sodium and 60 mmol potassium are required to maintain balance in a 75-kg man. A good regimen is 1.5–2 L 5% dextrose and 1 L physiological saline every 24 h
>
> **For hypovolaemic patients**
> An estimate of the losses is made (e.g. in hospital patients from a review of the input/output charts) and these must be given in addition to the normal daily requirements

intravenous treatment is required, water is given as 5% dextrose (pure water is not given because it would cause osmotic lysis of blood cells).

PLASMA OSMOLALITY AND DISORDERS OF SODIUM REGULATION

Water moves freely between compartments and the distribution is determined by the osmotic equilibrium between them. The plasma osmolality can be calculated from the plasma concentrations of sodium, urea and glucose, as follows:

$$\text{Calculated plasma osmolality (mmol)} = (2 \times \text{plasma Na}^+) + [\text{urea}] + [\text{glucose}] \quad \boxed{\text{目}} \; QC\ 7.1$$

The factor of 2 applied to sodium concentration allows for associated anions (chloride and bicarbonate). The other extracellular solutes, e.g. calcium, potassium and magnesium, and their associated anions exist in very low concentrations and contribute so little to osmolality that they can be ignored when calculating the osmolality. The normal plasma osmolality is 285–300 mmol/kg.

The *calculated* osmolality is the same as the osmolality *measured* by the laboratory, unless there is an unmeasured, osmotically active substance present. For instance, plasma alcohol or ethylene glycol concentration (substances sometimes taken in cases of poisoning) can be estimated by subtracting the calculated from the measured osmolality.

Regulation of body water content

Body water is controlled mainly by changes in the plasma osmolality. An increased plasma osmolality, sensed by osmoreceptors in the hypothalamus, causes thirst and the release of antidiuretic hormone (ADH, vasopressin) from the posterior pituitary, which increases water reabsorption from the renal collecting ducts. In addition, nonosmotic stimuli may cause the release of ADH even if serum osmolality is normal or low. These include hypovolaemia, stress (surgery and trauma) and nausea.

As discussed previously, sodium content is regulated by volume receptors, with water content adjusted to maintain a normal osmolality and a normal plasma sodium concentration. Disturbances of sodium concentration are usually caused by disturbances of water balance, rather than an increase or decrease in total body sodium.

Hyponatraemia (K&C 6e p. 701)

Hyponatraemia reflects too much water in relation to sodium; affected patients may or may not have a concurrent abnormality in sodium balance.

Hyponatraemia (serum sodium < 135 mmol/L) may be the result of the following:

317

- Relative water excess (dilutional hyponatraemia); this is the most common cause.
- Salt loss in excess of water, e.g. diarrhoea and renal diseases as described above.
- Pseudohyponatraemia, in which hyperlipidaemia or hyperproteinaemia results in a spuriously low measured sodium concentration. The sodium is confined to the aqueous phase but its concentration is expressed in terms of the total volume of plasma (i.e. water plus lipid). In this situation plasma osmolality is normal and therefore treatment of 'hyponatraemia' is unnecessary.
- True hyponatraemia must be differentiated from artefactual 'hyponatraemia' caused by taking blood from the drip arm into which a fluid of low sodium is being infused.

Once preliminary evaluation reveals that the hyponatraemia reflects hypo-osmolality (i.e. it is not pseudohyponatraemia or artefactual), assessment of the extracellular volume (pp. 312, 314) allows patients to be classified as hypovolaemic, normovolaemic or hypervolaemic (Fig. 7.2).

Plasma osmolality and disorders of sodium regulation

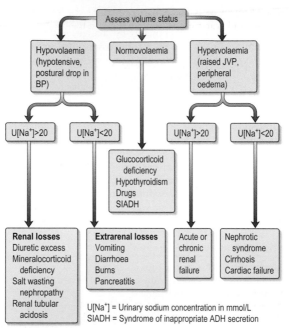

Fig. 7.2   Diagnosis of hyponatraemia.

318

Hyponatraemia resulting from salt loss (hypovolaemic hyponatraemia)

These patients have a deficit of both total body sodium and water, with the sodium deficit exceeding the water deficit. Measurement of urinary sodium will help to differentiate between renal and extrarenal sources of fluid loss (Fig. 7.2). For example, vomiting and diarrhoea are associated with avid sodium retention as the kidney responds to volume contraction by conserving NaCl.

Diuretics are the most common cause of hypovolaemic hyponatraemia with a high urinary sodium concentration ([Na$^+$]).

Clinical features

These are usually a result of the hypovolaemia and extra-cellular volume depletion (p. 314). Symptoms directly related to the hyponatraemia are rare, as the loss of both sodium and water limits osmotic shifts in the brain.

Management

Restoration of extracellular volume with crystalloids or colloids interrupts nonosmotic release of ADH and normalizes serum sodium.

Hyponatraemia resulting from water excess (dilutional hyponatraemia)

An excess of body water relative to sodium is differentiated from hyponatraemia caused by sodium loss, because there are none of the clinical features of extracellular volume depletion. This is the most common mechanism of hyponatraemia seen in hospital patients. The most common iatrogenic cause is overgenerous infusion of 5% glucose into postoperative patients; in this situation it is exacerbated by an increased ADH secretion in response to stress.

Aetiology

Hyponatraemia is often seen in patients with severe cardiac failure, cirrhosis or the nephrotic syndrome, in which there is an inability of the kidney to excrete 'free water'. This is compounded by the use of diuretics. There is evidence of volume overload and the patient is usually oedematous. Where there is no evidence of extracellular volume overload, causes include the syndrome of inappropriate ADH secretion (SIADH) (p. 629), Addison's disease and hypothyroidism.

319

Clinical features

Symptoms rarely occur until the serum sodium is less than 120 mmol/L and are more conspicuous when hyponatraemia has developed rapidly, i.e. over hours. They result from the movement of water into the brain cells (cerebral oedema) in response to the fall in extracellular osmolality, and include headache, confusion, convulsions and coma.

Investigation

Hyponatraemia in association with cardiac failure, cirrhosis or nephrotic syndrome is usually clinically obvious and no further investigation is necessary. If there is no evidence of volume overload the most probable cause is SIADH or

> ! *Emergency Box 7.1*
> **Management of hyponatraemia resulting from water excess**
>
> **Treat the underlying cause.**
>
> **Restrict water intake to 500–1000 mL/day and review diuretic therapy.**
>
> **Correct magnesium and potassium deficiency.**
>
> **With acute symptomatic hyponatraemia and severe neurological signs (fits or coma):**
> - Infuse hypertonic saline 3% (513 mmol/L) at a rate of 1–2 mL/kg/h.
> - Aim to raise serum sodium by 8–10 mmol/L in the first 4 hours and 15–20 mmol/L in the first 48 hours.
> - Give furosemide (frusemide) 40–80 mg i.v. to enhance free water excretion.
> - Serum sodium should not be corrected to greater than 125–130 mmol/L.
> - Hypertonic saline is contraindicated in patients who are fluid overloaded; give 100 mL of 20% mannitol.

diuretic therapy. Serum magnesium and potassium must be checked, as low levels potentiate ADH release and cause diuretic-associated hyponatraemia.

Management

The underlying cause must be corrected where possible. Most cases (those without severe symptoms) are simply managed by water restriction (to 1000 mL or even 500 mL/day) with a review of diuretic treatment. Management of SIADH is described on page 630. Patients with hyponatraemia developing acutely, in less than 48 hours (often a hospital patient on intravenous dextrose), are at the greatest risk of developing cerebral oedema and should be treated more urgently (see Emergency Box 7.1).

Central pontine myelinolysis

Over-rapid correction of the sodium concentration by whatever means must be avoided, as this can result in a severe, neurological syndrome due to local areas of demyelination, called central pontine myelinolysis or the osmotic demyelination syndrome. Features of this include quadriparesis, respiratory arrest, pseudobulbar palsy, mutism, and, rarely, fits. The distribution of the areas of demyelination include most often the pons, but also, in some cases, the basal ganglia, internal capsule, lateral geniculate body, and even the cerebral cortex.

Hypernatraemia (*K&C* 6e p. 703)

Hypernatraemia (serum sodium > 145 mmol/L) is almost always the result of reduced water intake or water loss in excess of sodium. More rarely it is caused by excessive administration of sodium.

Aetiology

Insufficient fluid intake is most often found in elderly people, neonates or unconscious patients when access to water is denied or confusion or coma eliminates the normal response to thirst. The situation is exacerbated by increased losses of fluid, e.g. sweating, diarrhoea.

Water loss relative to sodium occurs in pituitary diabetes insipidus, nephrogenic diabetes insipidus, osmotic diuresis and water loss from the lungs or skin.

Clinical features

Symptoms are non-specific and include nausea, vomiting, fever and confusion.

Investigations

Simultaneous urine and plasma osmolality and sodium should be measured.

The passage of urine with an osmolality lower than that of plasma in this situation is clearly abnormal and indicates diabetes insipidus (p. 630). If urine osmolality is high, this suggests an osmotic diuresis or excessive extrarenal water loss (e.g. heat stroke).

Management

Treatment is that of the underlying cause and replacement of water, either orally if possible or intravenously with 5% dextrose. The aim is to correct sodium concentration over 48 hours, as over-rapid correction may lead to cerebral oedema. In severe hypernatraemia (> 170 mmol/L), 0.9% saline (150 mmol/L) should be used to avoid too rapid a drop in serum sodium. In addition, if there is clinical evidence of volume depletion, this implies that there is a sodium deficit as well as a water deficit, and intravenous 0.9% saline should be used.

DISORDERS OF POTASSIUM REGULATION (*K&C* 6e p. 704)

Dietary intake of potassium varies between 80 and 150 mmol daily, most of which is then excreted in the urine. Potassium is predominantly an intracellular ion, only 2% of total body potassium being extracellular (Table 7.2). Serum levels are controlled by:

- Uptake of K^+ into cells – by altering activity of the Na^+/K^+-ATPase pump in the cell membrane
- Renal excretion – mainly controlled by aldosterone
- Extrarenal losses, e.g. gastrointestinal.

Hypokalaemia (*K&C* 6e p. 704)

This is a serum potassium concentration of < 3.5 mmol/L.

Aetiology

The most common causes of hypokalaemia (Table 7.7) are diuretic treatment and hyperaldosteronism. Blood taken from a drip arm may produce a spurious result.

Clinical features

Hypokalaemia is usually asymptomatic, although muscle weakness may occur if severe. It results in an increased risk of cardiac arrhythmias, particularly in patients with cardiac disease. Hypokalaemia also predisposes to digoxin toxicity.

Management

The underlying cause should be identified and treated where possible. Usually withdrawal of purgatives, assessment of diuretic treatment, and replacement with oral potassium chloride supplements (20–80 mmol/day in divided doses with monitoring of serum K^+ every 1–2 days) is all that is required. Serum magnesium concentrations should be normalized, as hypomagnesaemia makes hypokalaemia difficult or impossible to correct. Indications for the intravenous infusion of potassium chloride include hypokalaemic diabetic ketoacidosis and severe hypokalaemia

Table 7.7 Causes of hypokalaemia

Increased renal excretion (spot urinary K+ > 20 mmol/L)	Diuretics, e.g. thiazides, loop diuretics
	Solute diuresis, e.g. glycosuria
	Hypomagnesaemia
	Increased aldosterone secretion
	Liver failure
	Heart failure
	Nephrotic syndrome
	Cushing's syndrome
	Conn's syndrome
	Exogenous mineralocorticoid
	Corticosteroids
	Carbenoxolone
	Liquorice
	Renal disease
	Renal tubular acidosis: types 1 and 2
	Renal tubular damage
Gastrointestinal losses	Prolonged vomiting*, profuse diarrhoea, villous adenoma, fistulae, ileostomies
Redistribution into cells	Increased activity of Na+/K+ -ATPase
	Alkalosis
	β-Agonists
	Insulin
	Hypokalaemic periodic paralysis (rare, episodic K+ movement into cells leads to profound muscle weakness)
Reduced intake	Severe dietary deficiency
	Inadequate replacement in i.v. fluids

*Hypokalaemia primarily due to increased urinary loss. Loss of gastric acid and associated metabolic acidosis raises plasma bicarbonate and sodium bicarbonate delivery to distal nephron where exchange with potassium takes place

associated with cardiac arrhythmias or muscle weakness. This should be performed slowly, and replacement at rates of greater than 20 mmol/h should only be done with ECG monitoring and hourly measurement of serum potassium. Concentrations over 60 mmol/L should not be given via a

Table 7.8 Causes of hyperkalaemia

Decreased excretion
Acute renal failure
Drugs (potassium-sparing diuretics, ACE inhibitors, NSAIDs, ciclosporin, heparin)
Addison's disease
Hyporeninaemic hypoaldosteronism (type 4 renal tubular acidosis)

Release from cells
Diabetic ketoacidosis
Acidosis
Crush injury
Tumour lysis
Suxamethonium

Increased extraneous load
Potassium chloride
Salt substitutes
Transfusion of stored blood

ACE, angiotensin-converting enzyme inhibitors; NSAIDs, non-steroidal anti-inflammatory drugs

peripheral vein because of local irritation. Ampoules of potassium should be thoroughly mixed in 0.9% saline; glucose solutions should be avoided as this may make hypokalaemia worse.

Hyperkalaemia (*K&C* 6e p.707)

This is defined as a serum potassium concentration of > 5.0 mmol/L. True hyperkalaemia must be differentiated from artefactual hyperkalaemia, which results from lysis of red cells during vigorous phlebotomy or in vitro release from abnormal red cells in some blood disorders, e.g. leukaemia.

Aetiology

The most common causes (Table 7.8) are renal impairment and drug interference with potassium excretion.

Clinical features

Hyperkalaemia usually produces few symptoms or signs until it is high enough to cause cardiac arrest. Symptoms

> **Emergency Box 7.2**
> **Management of hyperkalaemia**

1. **Protect myocardium from hyperkalaemia** (if
   K$^+$ > 7.0 mmol/L or ECG changes present):
   10 mL of 10% calcium gluconate bolus i.v. over 2–3 min
   with ECG monitoring
   Repeat after 5 min if ECG changes persist.
   NB: This treatment does not alter serum K$^+$.
2. **Drive K$^+$ into cells:**
   Soluble insulin 10 units + 50 mL 50% dextrose intravenously
   over 15–30 min and/or correction of severe acidosis
   (pH < 6.9) with 1.26% sodium bicarbonate
   Effect of insulin lasts 1–2 h; repeated doses may be
   necessary.
3. **Deplete body K$^+$** (after emergency treatment):
   Calcium or sodium resonium orally (15 g three times daily
   with laxatives) or rectally (30 g) binds potassium
   Treat the cause
   Stop any extra source of potassium intake or potentiating
   drugs, e.g. NSAIDs and ACE inhibitors
   Haemodialysis or peritoneal dialysis if conservative
   measures fail.
4. **Monitor:**
   Blood glucose (finger-prick Stix testing) hourly during and
   for 6 hours after insulin/dextrose infusion
   Serum K$^+$ every 2–4 hours acutely and daily thereafter.

325

produced by hyperkalaemia are related to impaired neuro-muscular transmission and include muscle weakness and paralysis. It may be associated with metabolic acidosis causing Kussmaul's respiration (low deep sighing inspiration and expiration).

Management

A serum potassium of more than 7 mmol/L is a medical emergency (Emergency Box 7.2) and may be associated with typical ECG changes (Fig. 7.3).

DISORDERS OF MAGNESIUM REGULATION (K&C 6e p. 709)

Disturbance of magnesium balance is uncommon and usually associated with more obvious fluid and electrolyte disturbance. Like potassium, magnesium is mainly an

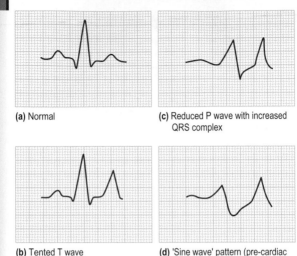

(a) Normal

(c) Reduced P wave with increased QRS complex

(b) Tented T wave

(d) 'Sine wave' pattern (pre-cardiac arrest)

Fig. 7.3 **Progressive ECG changes with increasing hyperkalaemia.**

intracellular cation (Table 7.2) and balance is maintained mainly via the kidney. The average daily magnesium intake is 15 mmol, about one-third of which is absorbed in the small bowel; excretion is via the kidney.

Hypomagnesaemia (*K&C* 6e p. 710)

Aetiology

A low serum magnesium is most often caused by loss of magnesium from the gut or kidney. Gastrointestinal causes include severe diarrhoea, malabsorption, extensive bowel resection and intestinal fistulae. Excessive renal loss of magnesium occurs with diuretics, alcohol abuse, and with an osmotic diuresis such as glycosuria in diabetes mellitus.

Clinical features

Hypomagnesaemia increases renal excretion of potassium, inhibits secretion of parathyroid hormone and leads to parathyroid hormone resistance. Many of the symptoms of hypomagnesaemia are therefore due to hypokalaemia (p. 322) and hypocalcaemia (p. 636).

Management

The underlying cause must be corrected where possible and oral supplements given (magnesium chloride 5–20 mmol daily or magnesium oxide tablets 600 mg four times daily). Symptomatic severe magnesium deficiency should be treated by intravenous infusion (50 mmol of MgCl in 1 L of 5% dextrose over 12–24 h), plus a loading dose (4 mmol over 10 min) if there are seizures or ventricular arrhythmias.

Hypermagnesaemia (*K&C* 6e p. 710)

Hypermagnesaemia is rare and is usually iatrogenic, occurring in patients with renal failure who have been given magnesium-containing laxatives or antacids. Symptoms include neurological and cardiovascular depression, with narcosis, respiratory depression and cardiac conduction defects. The only treatment usually necessary is to stop magnesium treatment. In severe cases, intravenous calcium gluconate may be necessary to reverse the cellular toxic effects of magnesium and dextrose/insulin (as for hyperkalaemia) to lower the plasma magnesium level.

DISORDERS OF ACID–BASE BALANCE (*K&C* 6e p. 712)

The pH (the negative logarithm of $[H^+]$) is maintained at 7.4 (normal range 7.35–7.45). The metabolism of food and endogenous body tissues produces about 70–100 mmol of H^+ each day, which is excreted by the kidneys. Bicarbonate (HCO_3^-) is the main plasma and extracellular fluid buffer. It mops up free H^+ ions and prevents increases in the H^+ concentration (Fig. 7.4). Bicarbonate is filtered at the glomerulus but is then reabsorbed in the proximal and distal renal tubule. The lungs also constantly regulate acid–base balance through the excretion of CO_2. Between production and excretion of H^+ ions there is an extremely

carbonic anhydrase

$$H^+ + HCO_3^- \rightleftharpoons H_2CO_3 \rightleftharpoons H_2O + CO_2$$

Fig. 7.4 **The carbonic anhydrase reaction.**

Disorders of acid-base balance

Table 7.9 Changes in arterial blood gases			
	pH	$P_a\text{CO}_2$	HCO_3^-
Acidosis			
Metabolic	Normal or reduced	Normal or reduced	Reduced ++
Respiratory	Normal or reduced	Increased ++	Normal or increased
Alkalosis			
Metabolic	Normal or increased	Increased	Increased ++
Respiratory	Normal or increased	Reduced ++	Reduced

The pH may be at the limits of the normal range if the acidosis or alkalosis is compensated, e.g. respiratory compensation (hyperventilation) of a metabolic acidosis. The clue to the abnormality from the blood gases will be the abnormal $P_a\text{CO}_2$ and HCO_3^-

effective buffering system maintaining a constant H$^+$ ion concentration inside and outside the cell. Buffers include haemoglobin proteins, bicarbonate and phosphate.

Acid–base disturbances may be caused by:

- Abnormal carbon dioxide removal in the lungs ('respiratory' acidosis and alkalosis)
- Abnormalities in the regulation of bicarbonate and other buffers in the blood ('metabolic' acidosis and alkalosis).

In general, the body compensates to some extent for changes in pH by regulating renal bicarbonate excretion and altering the respiratory rate. For instance, metabolic acidosis causes hyperventilation (via medullary chemoreceptors), leading to increased removal of CO_2 in the lungs and partial compensation for the acidosis. Conversely, respiratory acidosis is accompanied by renal bicarbonate retention, which could be mistaken for primary metabolic alkalosis.

Measurement of pH, $P_a\text{CO}_2$ and [HCO_3^-] will reveal which type of disturbance is present (Table 7.9). These measurements are made on an arterial blood sample (p. 799) using an automated blood gas analyser. Clinical history and examination usually point to the correct diagnosis.

Respiratory acidosis

This is usually associated with ventilatory failure, with retention of carbon dioxide (p. 563). Treatment is of the underlying cause.

Respiratory alkalosis

Hyperventilation results in increased removal of carbon dioxide, resulting in a fall in $P_a co_2$ and $[H^+]$.

Metabolic acidosis (*K&C* 6e p. 716)

This is the result of the accumulation of any acid other than carbonic acid. The most common cause is lactic acidosis following shock or cardiac arrest.

Clinical features

These include hyperventilation, hypotension caused by arteriolar vasodilatation and the negative inotropic effect of acidosis, and cerebral dysfunction associated with confusion and fits.

Differential diagnosis (the anion gap)

The first step is to identify whether the acidosis is the result of retention of HCl or of another acid. This is achieved by measurement of the anion gap. The main electrolytes measured in plasma are sodium, potassium, chloride and bicarbonate. The sum of the cations, sodium and potassium, normally exceeds that of chloride and bicarbonate by 6–12 mmol/L ▦ QC 7.2). This anion gap is usually made up of negatively charged proteins, phosphate and organic acids. If the anion gap is normal in the presence of acidosis, it can be concluded that HCl is being retained or $NaHCO_3$ is being lost. The causes of a normal anion gap acidosis are given in Table 7.10.

If the anion gap is increased (i.e. > 12 mmol/L), the acidosis is the result of an exogenous acid, e.g. salicylates or one of the acids normally present in small unmeasured quantities, such as lactate. Causes of a high anion gap acidosis are given in Table 7.11.

Lactic acidosis (*K&C* 6e p. 719)

Increased production of lactic acid occurs when cellular respiration is abnormal, resulting from either lack of

Table 7.10 Causes of metabolic acidosis with a normal anion gap

Increased gastrointestinal HCO_3^- loss
Diarrhoea
Ileostomy
Ureterosigmoidostomy

Increased HCO_3^- renal loss
Acetazolamide ingestion
Proximal (type 2) renal tubular acidosis
Hyperparathyroidism
Tubular damage, e.g. drugs, heavy metals

Decreased renal H^+ excretion
Distal (type 1) renal tubular acidosis
Type 4 renal tubular acidosis

Increased HCl production
Ammonium chloride ingestion
Increased catabolism of lysine, arginin

Table 7.11 Causes of metabolic acidosis with a high anion gap

Renal failure (sulphate, phosphate)

Ketoacidosis
Diabetes mellitus
Starvation
Alcohol poisoning

Lactic acidosis
Type A
Shock
Severe hypoxia
Methanol
Ethylene glycol
Strenuous exercise

Type B
Acute liver failure
Poisoning: ethanol, paracetamol
Metformin accumulation
Leukaemia, lymphoma

Drug poisoning
Salicylates

oxygen (type A) or a metabolic abnormality (type B). The most common form in clinical practice is type A lactic acidosis, occurring in septicaemic or cardiogenic shock.

Diabetic ketoacidosis (p. 658)

This is a high anion gap acidosis caused by the accumulation of organic acids, acetoacetic acid and hydroxybutyric acid.

Renal tubular acidosis (*K&C* 6e p. 716)

Renal tubular acidosis may occur in the absence of renal failure and is a normal anion gap acidosis. There is failure of the kidney to acidify the urine adequately. This group of disorders is uncommon and only rarely a cause of significant clinical disease.

Type 4 renal tubular acidosis   This is the most common of these disorders and is also known as hyporeninaemic hypoaldosteronism. Typical features are acidosis and hyperkalaemia occurring in the setting of mild chronic renal failure, usually caused by tubulointerstitial disease or diabetes. Plasma aldosterone and renin are low and do not respond to stimulation. Treatment is with fludrocortisone, diuretics, sodium bicarbonate and ion exchange resins for the reduction of serum potassium.

Proximal (type 2) renal tubular acidosis   This is failure to absorb bicarbonate in the proximal tubule. Typical features are hypokalaemia, an inability to produce an acid urine in spite of systemic acidosis, and the appearance of bicarbonate in the urine. This disorder normally occurs as part of a generalized tubular defect, together with other features such as glycosuria and aminoaciduria. Treatment is with oral sodium bicarbonate.

Distal (type 1) renal tubular acidosis   There is failure of H^+ excretion in the distal tubule. Typical features include hypokalaemia and an inability to produce an acid urine in spite of systemic acidosis. Causes include autoimmune diseases, SLE and nephrocalcinosis. Presentation is often with renal stones as a result of hypercalciuria, low urinary citrate (citrate inhibits calcium phosphate precipitation) and alkaline urine (favours precipitation of calcium phosphate). Treatment is with sodium bicarbonate.

Uraemic acidosis (*K&C* 6e p. 719)

Reduction of the capacity to secrete H^+ and NH_4^+, in addition to bicarbonate wasting, contributes to the acidosis of chronic renal failure. Acidosis occurs particularly when there is tubular damage, such as reflux and chronic obstructive nephropathy. It is associated with hypercalciuria and renal osteodystrophy because H^+ ions are buffered by bone in exchange for calcium. Treatment is with calcium or sodium bicarbonate, although acidosis in end-stage renal failure is only usually fully corrected by adequate dialysis.

Metabolic alkalosis (K&C 6e p. 720)

This is much less common than acidosis and is often associated with potassium or volume depletion. The main causes are persistent vomiting, diuretic therapy or hyper-aldosteronism. Vomiting causes alkalosis both by causing volume depletion and through loss of gastric acid.

Clinical features

Cerebral dysfunction is an early feature of alkalosis. Respiration may be depressed.

Management

This includes fluid replacement, if necessary, with replacement of sodium, potassium and chloride. The bicarbonate excess will correct itself.

Renal disease

The kidneys are 11–14 cm in length and lie retroperitoneally on either side of the vertebral column from T12–L3. The functional unit of the kidney is the *nephron*, which is composed of glomerulus, proximal tubule, loop of Henle, distal tubule and collecting duct. The arterial supply of the kidney is via the renal artery, a branch of the abdominal aorta, and venous drainage is via the renal veins to the inferior vena cava. The kidney's principal role is the elimination of waste material and the regulation of the volume and composition of body fluid. Urine is produced by glomerular filtration, which depends on the maintenance of a relatively high perfusion pressure within the glomerular capillary and an adequate renal blood flow (the kidney normally receives 25% of cardiac output). In health, glomerular blood flow is autoregulated by the preglomerular arteriole and remains relatively constant within a range of mean arterial pressures. The proximal renal tubules reabsorb most of the filtered solute required to maintain fluid and electrolyte balance, but elimination of potassium, water and non-volatile hydrogen ions is regulated in the distal tubules. As renal perfusion and glomerular filtration fall, reabsorption of water and sodium by the proximal tubules increases so that minimal fluid reaches the distal tubule. Hence hypotensive or hypovolaemic patients cannot excrete potassium and hydrogen ions. Patients with distal tubular damage, e.g. caused by drugs, also cannot excrete potassium and hydrogen ions. The kidney also acts as an endocrine organ and produces erythropoietin, renin and vitamin D in its active form (*K&C* 6e p. 610).

PRESENTING FEATURES OF RENAL DISEASE

The most common diseases of the kidney and urinary tract are benign prostatic hypertrophy in men and urinary tract infection (UTI) in women. The symptoms suggesting renal tract disease are frequency of micturition, dysuria, haematuria, urinary retention and alteration of urine volume (either polyuria or oliguria). In addition there may be pain situated anywhere along the renal tract, from loin to groin. Non-specific symptoms, e.g. lethargy, anorexia and pruritus, may be the presenting features of chronic renal failure. Renal disease may be asymptomatic and discovered by the incidental finding of hypertension, a raised serum urea, or proteinuria and haematuria on Stix testing.

Dysuria   ⟶ investigated + found HPT

Dysuria (pain on micturition) is caused by:

- Inflammation involving the urethra (urethritis) or bladder (cystitis). Dysuria is common in adult women and is usually due to lower urinary tract bacterial infection (p. 354) with inflammation of the urethra and bladder. Other causes of urethritis include infection with *Chlamydia trachomatis* or *Neisseria gonorrhoeae* (p. 45).
- Inflammation involving the vagina in women or glans penis in men. Causes include infection with *Candida albicans* and *Gardnerella vaginalis*.

Polyuria and nocturia

Polyuria can be arbitrarily defined as a urine output exceeding 3 L in 24 hours. It must be differentiated from the more common complaints of urinary frequency and nocturia, which are not necessarily associated with an increase in the total urine output. The causes of polyuria include polydipsia, solute diuresis (e.g. hyperglycaemia with glycosuria), diabetes insipidus and chronic renal failure. Nocturia is most often due to drinking before bed or, in men over 50 years, prostatic enlargement (p. 389).

Oliguria

Oliguria (low urine output) is defined as a urine output of less than 300 mL in 24 hours. It may be 'physiological', as in patients with hypotension and hypovolaemia, where urine is maximally concentrated in an attempt to conserve water. It may also be due to intrinsic renal disease or urinary tract obstruction. Anuria (no urine) suggests bilateral ureteric or bladder outflow obstruction. Management of the oliguric patient is in three steps:

1. *Exclude obstruction.* The patient with outflow obstruction (acute retention of urine) is typically in great discomfort with an intense desire to micturate. The bladder is palpable as a tender mass that is dull to percussion, arising out of the pelvis. The diagnosis is confirmed by passing a urethral catheter and releasing a large volume of urine. If the patient is already catheterized, the catheter should be flushed with sterile saline to relieve any blockage. Obstruction proximal to the bladder (e.g. ureteric obstruction) is often painless, and ultrasound examination is indicated to exclude pelvicalyceal dilatation.

2. *Assess for hypovolaemia.* Once obstruction has been excluded, the patient must be assessed for evidence of hypovolaemia by measurement of blood pressure, pulse, jugular venous pressure (JVP), and urinary electrolytes (p. 314). If the patient is hypovolaemic, the urine output in response to a fluid challenge (500 mL saline intravenously over 30 minutes) should be assessed.

3. *Management of established acute renal failure* (p. 369) once obstruction and hypovolaemia have been excluded.

INVESTIGATION OF RENAL DISEASE

Once renal disease is suspected, the purpose of investigations is to determine the presence or degree of renal dysfunction and the cause of the renal disease. Estimation of the glomerular filtration rate (GFR, see below) is used clinically to determine the degree of renal dysfunction. The clinical history and examination together with Stix testing and microscopy of urine are the starting points for determining the cause.

Blood tests

The serum urea or creatinine concentration represents the dynamic equilibrium between production and elimination but levels do not rise above the normal range until there is a reduction of 50–60% in the GFR. The serum urea concentration is increased by a high-protein diet, increased tissue catabolism (surgery, trauma, infection) and gastrointestinal bleeding, whereas the level of creatinine is much less dependent on diet but is more related to age, sex and muscle mass. Once it is elevated, serum creatinine is a

Renal disease

better guide to GFR than urea, though a normal level is not synonymous with a normal GFR.

Glomerular filtration rate (GFR) (*K&C* 6e p. 608)

Measurement of the GFR is necessary to define the exact level of renal function, Creatinine clearance is a reasonably accurate measure of GFR and is measured from a 24-hour urine collection for volume and creatinine concentration and measurement of a single serum creatinine value during the 24-hour period. Measurement of the creatinine clearance is cumbersome and is inaccurate if urine collection is incomplete. Several formulae have been developed that allow a prediction of creatinine clearance and GFR from serum creatinine and demographics.

Calculation of creatinine clearance using the Cockroft–Gault equation (▦ QC 8.1)
Men

$$\text{Creatinine clearance} = \frac{1.23 \times (140 - \text{Age}) \times (\text{Weight in kg})}{\text{Serum creatinine } (\mu\text{mol/L})}$$

Women Use the same equation but multiply by 1.04 instead of 1.23.

The modification of diet in renal disease (MDRD) is a new prediction equation (▦ QC 8.2 and http://www.nephron.com) that, unlike the Cockroft–Gault equation, takes into account racial background and makes it more reliable in an ethnically diverse population.

Urine Stix testing (*K&C* 6e p. 613)

Commercial reagent Stix detect the presence of protein, glucose, ketones, bilirubin, urobilinogen and blood in the urine. They also measure urine pH, which is useful in the investigation and management of renal tubular acidosis (p. 331). Each test is based on a colour change in a strip of absorbent cellulose impregnated with the appropriate reagent. The Stix is dipped briefly into a fresh specimen of urine collected in a clean container and the colour changes compared with the manufacturer's colour charts on the reagent strip container. The degree of colour change is a semi-quantitative assessment of the amount of substance present. Haematuria or proteinuria suggests renal tract disease. Dipsticks are also available for testing for urinary nitrites, which if present indicate bacteriuria (p. 355).

Proteinuria

The glomerular ultrafiltrate normally contains a small amount of protein, most of which is absorbed in the proximal renal tubule and only small amounts (up to 200mg/24h) appear in the urine. Most reagent Stix can detect a protein concentration of 200mg/L or more in the urine (300mg per 24 hours if urine volume is normal). Pyrexia, exercise and adoption of the upright posture may all produce a mild increase in urinary protein output. 'Postural proteinuria' is the term used when proteinuria occurs in the upright posture but not when supine. It may be diagnosed by testing for protein in several early morning urine samples passed after overnight recumbency, and then testing several samples after being up and about. The condition is usually benign and the amount of protein excreted small.

Persistent proteinuria (Fig. 8.1) detected on Stix testing requires full investigation. The first step is to quantify protein excretion by a 24-hour urine collection, or more simple and almost as accurate is to calculate a spot urine protein : creatinine ratio from a single (preferably early-morning) urine specimen. The 24-hour urinary protein excretion (mg/24 h) can be approximated as (mg/L protein) ÷ (mmol/L creatinine) × 10. More than 150 mg protein excretion in 24 hours is abnormal. Proteinuria greater than 2 g/24 h is usually the result of glomerular disease (p. 343), and greater than 3.5 g/24 h may result in the nephrotic syndrome (p. 351). Proteinuria caused by failure of proximal tubular reabsorption is uncommon and is seldom an isolated defect: there are usually multiple proximal tubular defects causing glycosuria, aminoaciduria, phosphaturia and renal tubular acidosis (Fanconi's syndrome). Bence Jones proteins (immunoglobulin light chains in patients with myeloma) are not detected by Stix and are identified by immunoelectrophoresis of urine.

Microalbuminuria is defined as an increase above the normal range in urinary albumin excretion (normal less than 30 mg in 24 hours) but undetectable by conventional dipsticks. It is now known to be an early indicator of diabetic glomerular disease and is widely used as a

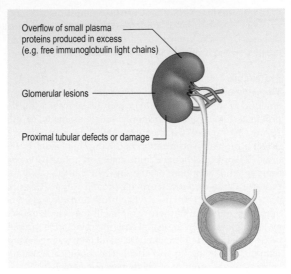

Fig. 8.1 **Sources of urinary protein.** (Adapted from Mallick N P. Presenting features of renal disease. *Medicine* 1995 23:3: 91–96 by kind permission of The Medicine Publishing Company.)

In the figure, the labels read:
- Overflow of small plasma proteins produced in excess (e.g. free immunoglobulin light chains)
- Glomerular lesions
- Proximal tubular defects or damage

predictor of the development of nephropathy in diabetics. Microalbuminuria is detected by measurement of the albumin in a 24-hour urine collection or by comparison of albumin concentration to creatinine concentration in a random urine sample. generally an albumin : creatinine ratio of 2.5 : 20 corresponds to albuminuria of 30–300 mg per 24 hours.

Haematuria

Haematuria arises from any site in the kidney or urinary tract (Fig. 8.2) and may be macroscopic, with bloody urine, or microscopic and found only on Stix testing. Vaginal bleeding is a common source of a positive test and does not need further renal investigations. A positive Stix test must always be followed by careful microscopy of fresh urine to confirm the presence of red cells, to look for red cell casts and to exclude haemoglobinuria or myoglobinuria, which are uncommon but also result in a positive result on Stix testing. Signs of glomerular bleeding are red cell casts, proteinuria and renal impairment, and these patients

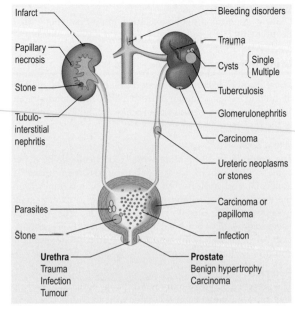

Infarct

Papillary
necrosis

Stone

Tubulo-
interstitial
nephritis

Parasites

Stone

Urethra
Trauma
Infection
Tumour

Bleeding disorders

Trauma

Cysts { Single
Multiple

Tuberculosis

Glomerulonephritis

Carcinoma

Ureteric neoplasms
or stones

Carcinoma or
papilloma

Infection

Prostate
Benign hypertrophy
Carcinoma

Fig. 8.2 **Sites and causes of bleeding from the urinary
tract.**

should be investigated for glomerulonephritis (see later). In
the absence of indicators of glomerular bleeding further
investigations, such as urine cytology, renal ultrasound,
excretion urography and cystoscopy, are required to define
the site of bleeding. Patients with isolated haematuria and
negative radiological and cystoscopic evaluation are likely
to have glomerular disease (often IgA nephropathy), and
referral should be made to a renal physician for consideration of renal biopsy (not usually performed) and long-term
follow-up.

With macroscopic haematuria, the source of bleeding
may be suggested by a careful history. Haematuria that is
only apparent at the start of micturition is usually
associated with urethral disease. Haematuria that occurs at
the end of micturition suggests bleeding from the prostate
or bladder base, whereas blood seen as an even discoloration throughout the urine suggests bleeding from a
source in the bladder or above.

Glycosuria

Diabetes mellitus must be excluded in any patients with a positive Stix test for glucose.

Urine microscopy (*K&C* 6e p. 614)

Microscopy of urine is performed on all patients suspected of having renal disease. A fresh clean-catch mid-stream specimen of urine is essential to make a valid interpretation of the results.

White cells

The presence of 10 or more white blood cells (WBCs) per cubic millimetre in fresh unspun mid-stream urine is abnormal and indicates an inflammatory reaction within the urinary tract. Usually it is the result of a urinary tract infection (UTI). Sterile pyuria (i.e. pus cells without bacterial infection) occurs in a partially treated UTI, urinary tract tuberculosis, calculi, bladder tumour, papillary necrosis and tubulointerstitial nephritis.

Red cells

The presence of one or more red cells per cubic millimetre is abnormal and must be investigated (see above).

Casts

Mucoprotein precipitated in the renal tubules results in the formation of hyaline casts, which on their own are a normal finding. The incorporation of red cells results in red cell casts, a finding pathognomonic of glomerulonephritis. White cell casts may be seen in acute pyelonephritis. Granular casts result from the disintegration of cellular debris and indicate renal disease.

Bacteria

A reliable indicator of a UTI is a bacterial count over 10^5 or 10^3 pathogenic organisms per mL of urine in a fresh mid-stream specimen in a symptomatic woman or man respectively. In a woman the diagnosis is also made with 10^2 organisms per mL in the presence of pyuria (> 10 white cells/mm^3).

Imaging techniques (*K&C* 6e p. 615)

Plain X-ray is useful to identify renal calcification or radiodense calculi in the kidney, renal pelvis, line of the ureters or bladder.

Intravenous urography (IVU) also known as intravenous pyelography (IVP), still plays a role in renal diagnosis, especially in patients with haematuria and stone disease, but has in part been replaced by ultrasonography and CT scanning. Following intravenous injection of an organic iodine-containing contrast medium, the series is inspected for renal size and position, calyceal dilatation (e.g. due to obstruction), filling defects in renal pelves (e.g. stones, tumour), and ureteric obstruction and displacement. The bladder is examined both pre- and postmicturition for abnormalities of contour and residual volume. Contrast medium may cause an 'allergic' reaction (bronchospasm, urticaria, rarely hypotension), and renal damage (contrast nephropathy, *K&C* 6e p. 664) in patients with impaired renal function.

Ultrasonography of the kidneys is the method of choice for assessing renal size, checking for pelvicalyceal dilatation as an indication of renal obstruction, characterizing renal masses, diagnosing polycystic kidney disease, and detecting intrarenal and/or perinephric fluid (e.g. pus, blood). It has the advantage over X-ray techniques of avoiding ionizing radiation and intravascular contrast medium. Doppler ultrasonography is used to demonstrate renal artery perfusion and detect renal vein thrombosis.

Computed tomography is used increasingly as a first-line investigation in cases of suspected ureteric colic. It is also used to characterize renal masses which are indeterminate at ultrasonography, to stage renal, bladder and prostate tumours, and to detect 'lucent' calculi; low-density calculi which are lucent on plain films (e.g. uric acid stones) are well seen on CT.

Magnetic resonance imaging (MRI) is used to characterize renal masses as an alternative to CT, to stage renal, prostate and bladder cancer and also to image the renal arteries by magnetic resonance angiography with gadolinium as contrast medium. In experienced hands its sensitivity and specificity approaches renal angiography.

Renal arteriography remains the 'gold standard' for the diagnosis of renal artery disease. The technique requires cannulation of the femoral artery, and the contrast injected may cause kidney damage.

Antegrade pyelography involves percutaneous puncture of a pelvicalyceal system with a needle and the injection of contrast medium to outline the pelvicalyceal system and ureter to the level of obstruction. It is used when ultra-sonography has shown a dilated pelvicalyceal system in a patient with suspected obstruction. Antegrade pyelography is the preliminary to percutaneous placing of a drainage catheter or ureteric stent in the obstructed pelvicalyceal system (percutaneous nephrostomy).

Retrograde pyelography Following cystoscopy, prefer-ably under screening control, a catheter is either impacted in the ureteral orifice or passed a short distance up the ureter, and contrast medium is injected. Retrograde pyelography is mainly used to investigate lesions of the ureter and to define the lower level of ureteral obstruction shown on excretion urography or ultrasound plus ante-grade studies. It is invasive, commonly requires a general anaesthetic, and may result in the introduction of infection.

Renal scintigraphy (*K&C* 6e p. 617)
Dynamic renal scintigraphy provides functional inform-ation about each renal tract. The isotopes most commonly used are: diethylenetriaminepentaacetic acid (DPTA) labelled with technetium-99m, mercaptoacetylglycine (MAG3) labelled with technetium-99m, hippuran labelled with iodine-131. Dynamic scanning is used to assess renal blood flow in suspected renal artery stenosis, renal function in obstruction, and in detection of vesicoureteric reflux.

Static renal scintigraphy provides morphological inform-ation on each kidney. It is most commonly performed using technetium-99m labelled dimercaptosuccinic acid (DMSA), which becomes fixed in the proximal renal tubular cells. DMSA imaging enables assessment of size and position of kidneys, differential function of each kidney and parenchymal defects (scars, ischaemic areas, tumours).

Percutaneous renal biopsy (*K&C* 6e p. 618) is carried out under ultrasound control and requires interpretation by an experienced pathologist. It is indicated in the investigation of the nephritic and nephrotic syndromes, acute and chronic renal failure, haematuria after urological investigations and renal graft dysfunction. Complications include haematuria, which may be profuse, flank pain, and perirenal haematoma formation.

GLOMERULAR DISEASES (K&C 6e p. 619)

Normal glomerular structure

There are about 1 million renal glomeruli in each kidney and each consists of a capillary plexus invaginating the blind end of the proximal renal tubule (Fig. 8.3). The glomerular capillaries are lined by a fenestrated endothelium, which rests on the glomerular basement membrane (GBM). External to the GBM are the visceral epithelial cells (podocytes). These cells only make contact with the GBM by finger-like projections, called foot processes, which are separated from one another by 'slit pores'. This unique structure of the glomerular membrane accounts for its tremendous permeability, allowing 125–200 mL of glomerular filtrate to be formed every minute (this is the glomerular filtration rate or GFR). The composition of the glomerular filtrate is similar to plasma but contains only small amounts of protein (all of low molecular weight), most of which is reabsorbed in the proximal tubule. Tubular reabsorption and secretion normally substantially alter the water and electrolyte composition of the glomerular filtrate until it reaches the renal pelvis as urine. The presence of some form of glomerular disease is usually suspected from the history and from one or more of the following urinary findings: haematuria, red cell casts, and proteinuria which may be in the nephrotic range (> 3 g/day).

Glomerulonephritis (GN) is a general term for a group of disorders in which there is bilateral, symmetrical immunologically mediated injury to the glomerulus.

Pathogenesis

Pathogenetic mechanisms include:

- Deposition or in situ formation of immune complexes. Circulating antigen–antibody complexes are deposited in the kidney, or complexes are formed locally when antigen becomes trapped in the glomerulus. The antigen may be exogenous, e.g. β-haemolytic streptococci, or endogenous, e.g. DNA in systemic lupus erythematosus.
- Deposition of antiglomerular basement membrane antibody (anti-GBM, < 5% of glomerulonephritides). The principal target for the anti-GBM antibodies is the α-3 chain of type IV collagen. The antibody may also react with alveolar capillary basement membrane and can

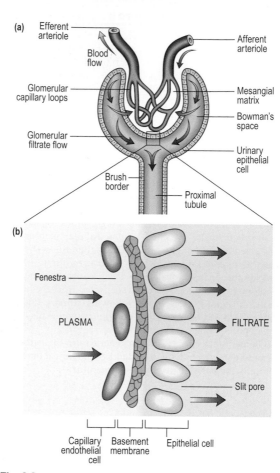

Fig. 8.3 (a) Diagrammatic representation of the normal glomerulus. (b) Components of the glomerular membrane. (Adapted from Read et al 1993 *Essential Medicine*. Churchill Livingstone, Edinburgh; Guyton (1987) *Human Physiology and Mechanisms of Disease*, 4th edn. WB Saunders, London.)

cause both lung haemorrhage and glomerulonephritis (Goodpasture's syndrome).

■ Deposition of an immunoglobulin of atypical configuration in glomerular mesangium. IgA nephropathy is the commonest type of glomerulonephritis world-wide. Presentation is with microscopic or macroscopic haematuria with or without proteinuria. The prognosis is usually good but some patients will progress to end-stage renal failure.

In some glomerulonephritides, e.g. associated with Wegener's granulomatosis and microscopic polyangiitis, there is no evidence of immune complex deposition. Injury is mediated by a vasculitis causing a focal segmental necrotizing glomerulonephritis with haematuria, proteinuria and deteriorating renal function.

Deposition of immune complexes in the glomerulus leads to an inflammatory response, which triggers secondary mechanisms of glomerular injury. These include complement activation, fibrin deposition, platelet aggregation and activation of kinin systems. The histological response to immune complex deposition is very variable.

Renal tissue, obtained at transcutaneous renal biopsy, is examined by light microscopy, electron microscopy and immunofluorescence to determine the extent and type of disease and to assess the type of immunological injury. The main forms of histopathologically identified glomerulonephritis and the clinical features most often associated with each are listed in Table 8.1. The terms 'focal' and 'diffuse' refer to the kidney as a whole, and 'segmental' and 'global' refer to the glomeruli. Thus in focal segmental glomerulonephritis only some glomeruli are affected and only a part of the glomerulus.

Aetiology

In most patients with immune complex-mediated glomerulonephritis the cause is unknown, i.e. the nature of the antigen is not determined. In a minority of cases antigens derived from viruses, bacteria, parasites, drugs and from the host may be involved (Table 8.2).

Table 8.1 Classification of glomerulopathies related to clinical syndromes presenting in adult life

Glomerular syndrome	Glomerular disease	Light microscopic appearance
Nephrotic syndrome		
Without red cell casts	*Primary glomerular disease*	
	Minimal change glomerular lesion	Normal (fusion of epithelial cell foot processes on EM)
	Focal segmental glomerulo-sclerosis	Segmental glomerulo-sclerosis
	Membranous nephropathy	Thickening of capillary basement membrane
	Secondary glomerular disease	
	Amyloidosis	Amyloid deposits (p. 680) in mesangium, capillaries
	Diabetic nephropathy	Thickening of the GBM and mesangial expansion. Later glomerulo-sclerosis with nodules (Kimmelstein–Wilson lesion) and hyaline deposits in glomerular arterioles
With red cell casts	*Primary glomerular disease*	
	Mesangiocapillary glomerulo-nephritis	Mesangial cell proliferation
	Mesangial proliferative glomerulo-nephritis	Only minor changes on light microscopy

Table 8.1 Classification of glomerulopathies related to clinical syndromes presenting in adult life—cont'd

Glomerular syndrome	Glomerular disease	Light microscopic appearance
	Secondary glomerular disease	
	Systemic lupus erythematosus	Variable from normal to advanced sclerosis
	Cryoglobulinaemia disease	Resembles mesangio-capillary glomerulo-nephritis
	Henoch–Schönlein syndrome	Focal segmental proliferative glomerulo-nephritis
	Immunotactoid glomerulopathy	Variable and seen with other glomerulo-pathies
Acute glomerulo-nephritis (acute nephritic syndrome)	Post-streptococcal glomerulo-nephritis	Cellular proliferation (mesangial and endothelial) and inflammatory cell infiltration (neutrophils and macrophages)
	Non-streptococcal post-infectious glomerulo-nephritis	
	Infective endocarditis	
	Systemic lupus erythematosus	
	Cryoglobulinaemia disease	
	Henoch–Schönlein syndrome	
Rapidly progressive glomerulo-nephritis	Goodpasture's syndrome	Focal glomerular necrosis with or without glomerular crescent formation
	Idiopathic	
	Associated with other primary glomerulopathy	

Continued

Glomerular diseases

Table 8.1 **Classification of glomerulopathies related to clinical syndromes presenting in adult life—cont'd**

Glomerular syndrome	Glomerular disease	Light microscopic appearance
	Any of the causes of acute GN ANCA-associated systemic vasculitis	(aggregates of macrophages and epithelial cells in Bowman's space)
Asymptomatic haematuria, proteinuria or both	Early presentation of any of the glomerulo-pathies	

Table 8.2 **Some causes of immune complex-mediated glomerulonephritis**

Infections
Lancefield group A β-haemolytic streptococci
Streptococcus viridans (infective endocarditis)
Mumps virus
Legionella
Hepatitis B and C virus
Tropical infections: schistosomiasis, *Plasmodium malariae*, filariasis

Systemic disease
Systemic lupus erythematosus (SLE)

Malignant tumours

Drugs
Penicillamine, gold, NSAIDs, captopril

NSAIDs, non-steroidal anti-inflammatory drugs

Clinical features

Glomerulonephritis presents in one of four ways:

- Acute nephritic syndrome
- Nephrotic syndrome
- Renal failure, acute and chronic (p. 369)
- Asymptomatic proteinuria and/or microscopic haematuria (p. 337).

Acute nephritic syndrome (*K&C* 6e p. 629)

Diffuse proliferative glomerulonephritis underlies many of the cases of acute nephritic syndrome in adults and children. The prototype exogenous pattern is post-streptococcal glomerulonephritis, whereas that produced by an endogenous antigen is lupus nephritis, seen in systemic lupus erythematosus (SLE). Acute nephritic syndrome may also follow other infections (Table 8.2). The typical case of post-streptococcal glomerulonephritis develops in a child 1–3 weeks after a streptococcal infection (pharyngitis or cellulitis) with a Lancefield group A β-haemolytic streptococcus. The bacterial antigen becomes trapped in the glomerulus, leading to an acute diffuse proliferative glomerulonephritis.

Clinical features

The syndrome comprises:

- Haematuria (macroscopic or microscopic)
- Proteinuria (usually < 2 g in 24 hours)
- Hypertension caused by salt and water retention
- Oedema (periorbital, leg or sacral)
- Oliguria
- Uraemia.

Investigations

A thorough history and examination are essential to assess the severity of the illness and to determine any associated underlying conditions. The investigations to consider in the nephritic syndrome are listed in Table 8.3. If the clinical diagnosis of a nephritic illness is clear-cut, e.g. in post-streptococcal glomerulonephritis, renal ultrasonography and renal biopsy are usually unnecessary.

Management

Post-streptococcal glomerulonephritis usually has a good prognosis, and supportive measures are often all that is required until spontaneous recovery takes place. Hypertension is treated with salt restriction, loop diuretics and vasodilators. Fluid balance is monitored by daily weighing and daily recording of fluid input and output. In oliguric patients with evidence of fluid overload (e.g. oedema,

Table 8.3 Investigations indicated in glomerular disease

Investigations	Significance
Baseline measurements	
Creatinine clearance as a measure of GFR	To determine current status, monitor progress and response to treatment
24-hour urinary protein excretion	
Serum urea and electrolytes	
Serum albumin	
Diagnostically useful tests	
Urine microscopy	Red cell casts indicate glomerulonephritis
Culture (swab from throat or infected skin)	Diagnosis of recent streptococcal infection
Serum antistreptolysin-O titre	
Blood glucose	Diagnosis of diabetes mellitus
Serum tests:	
Antinuclear and anti-DNA antibodies	Present in significant titre in SLE
Antineutrophil cytoplasmic antibodies (ANCA)	Wegener's granulomatosis and other types of vasculitis
Antiglomerular basement membrane antibody	Present in Goodpasture's syndrome
Hepatitis B surface antigen	Hepatitis B infection
Hepatitis C antibody	Hepatitis C infection
HIV antibody	HIV infection
Cryoglobulins	Increased in cryoglobulinaemia
Chest X-ray	Cavities in Wegener's granulomatosis, malignancy
Renal biopsy	Indicated in some adults with nephrotic or nephritic syndrome

SLE, systemic lupus erythematosus

pulmonary congestion and severe hypertension) fluid restriction is necessary. The management of life-threatening complications such as hypertensive encephalopathy (see p. 482), pulmonary oedema (p. 432) and severe uraemia (p. 375) is discussed in the appropriate chapters. In glomerulonephritis complicating SLE or the systemic vasculitides (see below), immunosuppression with prednisolone, cyclophosphamide or azathioprine improves renal function.

NEPHROTIC SYNDROME (*K&C* 6e p. 620)

Nephrotic syndrome consists of heavy proteinuria (> 3.5 g / 24 h), hypoalbuminaemia and oedema. Hyper lipidaemia and thrombotic disease are also frequently observed. Structural damage to the glomerular basement membrane leads to loss of electrostatic and physical barriers, which normally prevent the passage of large-molecular-weight proteins into the glomerular filtrate. Increased protein loss, in addition to increased catabolism of protein in the kidney, leads to hypoalbuminaemia. The pathogenesis of oedema in the nephrotic syndrome is poorly understood. The classic explanation is that intra-vascular hypovolaemia (hypoalbuminaemia reduces plasma oncotic pressure, salt and water move into the extravascular compartment) results in activation of the renin–angiotensin–aldosterone system, which promotes sodium and water reabsorption in the distal nephron. However, it seems probable that there is also a primary intrarenal defect in sodium excretion.

Aetiology

Nephrotic syndrome with 'bland' urine sediments

In Europe and the USA, membranous glomerular disease is the most common cause in adults and minimal-change nephropathy in children. Membranous glomerulonephritis is usually idiopathic but may occur in association with drugs, neoplasms, infections (Table 8.2), sarcoidosis and sickle cell disease. Focal segmental glomerulosclerosis also presents with nephrotic syndrome and may be idiopathic or secondary to HIV infection.

Minimal change nephropathy occurs most commonly in boys under 5 years of age. It accounts for 90% of cases of nephrotic syndrome in children and 20–25% in adults; however, it is rare in black African populations. The patho-genesis of this condition is not known; immune complexes are absent on immunofluorescence but the increase in glomerular permeability is thought to be immunologically mediated in some way.

Amyloid (p. 680) involving the kidneys and diabetes mellitus (p. 665) are also causes of the nephrotic syndrome but, unlike minimal change and membranous glomerulo-nephritis, the mechanism is not immune mediated. Other renal diseases, e.g. polycystic kidneys, reflux nephropathy, may cause proteinuria, but are rarely severe enough to cause the nephrotic syndrome.

Nephrotic syndrome with 'active' urine sediments (mixed nephritic/nephritic)

Mesangiocapillary (membranoproliferative glomerulonephritis) may be idiopathic or may occur with chronic infection (abscesses, infective endocarditis, infected ventriculoperitoneal shunt) or cryoglobulinaemia secondary to hepatitis C infection. A different type may occur with partial lipodystrophy (loss of subcutaneous fat on face and upper trunk). Most patients develop renal failure over several years. Mesangial proliferative GN presents with heavy proteinuria with minimal changes on light microscopy. There are deposits in the glomerular mesangium of IgM and complement (IgM nephropathy) or C1q (C1q nephropathy). Some patients respond to steroids and some will progress to renal failure.

Clinical features

Oedema of the ankles, genitals and abdomen is the principal finding. The face (periorbital oedema) and arms may also be involved in severe cases.

Differential diagnoses

Nephrotic syndrome must be differentiated from other causes of oedema and hypoalbuminaemia. In congestive cardiac failure (p. 425) there is oedema and a raised jugular venous pressure (JVP). In nephrotic syndrome the JVP is normal or low unless there is concomitant renal failure and oliguria. Hypoalbuminaemia and oedema occur in cirrhosis, but there are usually signs of chronic liver disease on examination (p. 141).

Investigations

The diagnosis is established by demonstrating:

- Heavy proteinuria (> 3.5 g/24 h in adults)
- Hypoalbuminaemia (serum albumin < 30 g/L).

Hyperlipidaemia is common in the nephrotic syndrome and is the result of increased hepatic synthesis of cholesterol and triglycerides, which accompanies hepatic albumin synthesis. Further investigations are listed in Table 8.3.

In the UK most cases of childhood nephrotic syndrome are caused by minimal change nephropathy, and therefore treatment is usually started with corticosteroids without recourse to a renal biopsy. In adults a renal biopsy is performed unless the diagnosis is clear-cut, e.g. nephrotic syndrome in a patient with long-standing diabetes mellitus must be advanced diabetic glomerulopathy. If a drug is implicated, e.g. penicillamine, the correct management is to stop the drug.

Management

General Oedema is treated with bed rest, dietary salt restriction and a thiazide diuretic (p. 313) followed by furosemide (frusemide) and amiloride for unresponsive patients. Intravenous diuretics and occasionally intravenous salt-poor albumin are required to initiate a diuresis which, once established, can usually be maintained with oral diuretics alone. If diuresis is too vigorous it may precipitate circulatory collapse and acute renal failure. Patients should be offered influenza vaccination (p. 495).

Specific treatment Minimal change nephropathy is almost always steroid responsive in children, although less commonly in adults. High-dose prednisolone therapy (40–60 mg daily) should be given over a period of 8 weeks and then reduced slowly. Of patients who enter remission 30–50% will have a relapse within 3 years, and this is treated with a further course of steroids. In patients with frequent relapses and in steroid-unresponsive patients, immunosuppressive therapy with cyclophosphamide or ciclosporin is used.

The benefits of immunosuppressive therapy in membranous glomerulonephritis remain contentious. In other types of glomerulonephritis remission may occur if the underlying disease can be treated, e.g. in patients with SLE, treatment with steroids or cyclophosphamide may induce long-term remission.

Complications

- *Venous thrombosis.* Hypovolaemia and a hypercoagulable state predispose to thrombus formation in both renal (seen on ultrasonography) and peripheral veins. Prolonged bed rest should be avoided but, if necessary,

353

patients should receive prophylactic anticoagulation with subcutaneous heparin (p. 234). Renal vein thrombosis presents with renal pain, haematuria and a deterioration in renal function.

- *Sepsis.* Loss of immunoglobulin in the urine increases the susceptibility to infection which is a cause of death in these patients.
- *Acute renal failure* is rarely the result of progression of the underlying renal disease. However, acute renal failure occurs as a result of hypovolaemia (particularly after diuretic therapy) or with renal vein thrombosis.

URINARY TRACT INFECTION (*K&C* 6e p. 637)

Urinary tract infection (UTI) is common in women, with about 35% having symptoms of a UTI at some time in their lives. It is uncommon in children and in men, when it usually indicates an underlying renal tract abnormality.

Pathogenesis

Infection of the urinary tract is most often via the ascending transurethral route, and this is facilitated by sexual intercourse and urethral catheterization. Women are more susceptible to infection because the short urethra and its proximity to the anus facilitates the transfer of bowel organisms to the bladder. Infection is most often caused by bacteria from the patient's own bowel flora (Table 8.4), but in 20–30% of young women it is caused by skin organisms: *Staphylococcus saprophyticus* or *Staph. epidermidis*.

Table 8.4 Organisms causing urinary tract infection in domiciliary practice

Organism	Approximate frequency (%)
Escherichia coli and other coliforms	68+
Proteus mirabilis	12
*Klebsiella aerogenes**	4
*Enterococcus faecalis**	6
Staphylococcus saprophyticus or *Staph. epidermidis*†	10

*More common in hospital practice
†More common in women

Abnormalities that encourage bladder infection (*cystitis*) include:

- Urinary obstruction or stasis
- Previous damage to the bladder epithelium
- Bladder stones
- Poor bladder emptying.

Ascending infection of the ureters results in renal parenchymal infection (*acute pyelonephritis*). This is facilitated by vesicoureteric reflux and dilated hypotonic ureters. Reflux nephropathy (previously called chronic pyelonephritis or atrophic pyelonephritis) arises from childhood UTIs in combination with vesicoureteric reflux, leading to progressive renal scarring. It presents as hypertension or chronic renal failure in childhood and adult life.

Clinical features

The most common symptoms of lower urinary tract infection are frequency of micturition, dysuria, suprapubic pain and tenderness, haematuria and smelly urine. In acute pyelonephritis there may also be loin pain and tenderness, with fever and systemic upset. However, localization of infection on the basis of symptoms alone is unreliable. In elderly people the symptoms may be atypical, with incontinence, nocturia or just a vague change in well-being.

355

Investigations

- Dipstick tests can be used to detect the presence of urinary nitrites (produced by reduction of urinary nitrates by bacteria) and elastase (produced by neutrophils). Dipstick tests positive for both nitrite and elastase are highly predictive of acute infection.
- Urine microscopy and culture and antimicrobial susceptibility testing of pathogens. The criteria for diagnosis of a UTI are listed on page 340. Mixed growths are of uncertain significance and the test should be repeated. Rarely and if in doubt, urine must be obtained by suprapubic bladder aspiration, where any growth of a uropathogenic organism is evidence of infection.
- Intravenous urography and ultrasound (pp. 340, 341) are performed to look for physiological and anatomical abnormalities of the urinary tract that predispose to UTI.

Radiological investigation is indicated in the following circumstances:

- Women with a *relapse* of infection defined as a recurrent UTI with the same organism within 7 days of completion of antibacterial treatment
- Women with *repeated* infections (more than two in 6 months) defined as a recurrent UTI arising more than 2 weeks after treatment
- After a single infection in children and men.

Management

A 3- to 5-day course of oral amoxicillin, nitrofurantoin or trimethoprim is usually effective. The treatment regimen may be modified in light of the result of urine culture and sensitivity testing and the clinical response. A high fluid intake (2 L daily) should be encouraged during treatment and for some weeks afterwards. In women with relapsing infection, low-dose prophylactic antibiotics are required for a period of 6–12 months. Patients with acute pyelonephritis are often acutely ill and usually require initial treatment with parenteral antibiotics, such as intravenous cefuroxime, ciprofloxacin or an aminoglycoside (e.g. gentamicin) and total treatment duration of 14 days. In patients with an indwelling catheter, antibiotic treatment is indicated only in the presence of symptoms, and should be accompanied by replacement of the catheter.

In patients with a *relapse* of infection the underlying cause should be treated if possible, e.g. removal of stones, and intensive (1 week intravenous) or prolonged (6 weeks oral) antibiotics are required. *Recurrent* infections where there is usually no underlying renal tract abnormality are managed initially with lifestyle advice: voiding before bedtime and after intercourse, avoidance of spermicidal jellies and constipation, 2 L daily fluid intake.

Complications

Acute cystitis in the otherwise healthy non-pregnant adult woman is generally considered to be uncomplicated and will rarely result in serious kidney damage. Patients with abnormal urinary tracts (e.g. stones) or systemic disease involving the kidney (e.g. diabetes mellitus), are considered to have *complicated* infection and are more likely to fail treatment and develop complications which include renal papillary necrosis (p. 358) and the development of a renal or perinephric abscess with the risk of Gram-negative septicaemia. Abscesses can be seen on ultrasonography and usually require surgical drainage as well as antibiotic therapy.

Urinary tract infection in pregnancy (*K&C* 6e p. 642)

Approximately 6% of pregnant women have significant bacteriuria in pregnancy; if untreated, 20% of these will develop acute pyelonephritis with significant risk to both mother and fetus (e.g. septic shock, low birthweight and prematurity). Early detection of asymptomatic bacteriuria and treatment is necessary.

Abacteriuric frequency or dysuria ('urethral syndrome') (*K&C* 6e p. 640)

The urethral syndrome occurs in women and presents with dysuria and frequency but in the absence of bacteriuria. It may be associated with vaginitis in postmenopausal women, irritant chemicals (e.g. soaps) and sexual intercourse.

Tuberculosis of the urinary tract (*K&C* 6e p. 642)

Tuberculosis (TB) of the urinary tract may present with all the symptoms of a UTI, i.e. dysuria, frequency or haematuria, and should be considered particularly in the Asian immigrant population of the UK and in countries with a high prevalence of TB. Classically, there is sterile pyuria (p. 340). Diagnosis depends on culture of mycobacteria from early-morning urine samples. Treatment is as for pulmonary tuberculosis (p. 527).

TUBULOINTERSTITIAL NEPHRITIS (*K&C* 6e p. 643)

Interstitial inflammation with tubular damage is a regular feature of bacterial pyelonephritis but it rarely, if ever, leads to chronic renal damage in the absence of reflux, obstruction or other complicating factors. The importance of other factors, particularly drugs, in the causation of this disorder has now been realized.

Acute tubulointerstitial nephritis

Acute tubulointerstitial nephritis is the result of a hypersensitivity reaction to drugs in approximately 70% of cases

Table 8.5	Common causes of drug-induced acute tubulointerstitial nephritis

Penicillins
NSAIDs
Sulfonamides
Allopurinol
Cephalosporins
Rifampicin
Diuretics – furosemide (frusemide), thiazides
Cimetidine
Phenytoin

(Table 8.5), most commonly drugs of the penicillin family and non-steroidal anti-inflammatory drugs (NSAIDs). Patients present with fever, eosinophilia and eosinophiluria, normal or only mildly increased urine protein excretion (< 1 g/day) and acute renal failure. Renal biopsy shows an intense interstitial cellular infiltrate, predominantly eosinophils, and variable tubular necrosis. Management involves withdrawal of the offending drug and treatment of acute renal failure (p. 375). High-dose prednisolone therapy is often used, although its value has not been proven. The prognosis is generally good; patients should avoid further exposure to the offending drug.

Occasionally, acute tubulointerstitial nephritis can complicate systemic infections with viruses (hantavirus, Epstein–Barr virus, HIV, measles, adenovirus), bacteria (*Legionella*, *Leptospira*, streptococci, *Mycoplasma*, *Brucella*, *Chlamydia*) and others (*Leishmania*, *Toxoplasma*). Treatment involves eradication of infection by appropriate antibiotics or antiviral agents.

Chronic tubulointerstitial nephritis

The most common cause of chronic tubulointerstitial nephritis is prolonged consumption of large amounts of analgesic drugs, particularly NSAIDs ('analgesic nephropathy'). Some causes are shown in Table 8.6. Presentation is usually with polyuria, proteinuria (usually < 1 g/day) or uraemia. Polyuria and nocturia are the result of tubular damage in the medullary area of the kidney, leading to defects in the renal concentrating ability. Necrosis of the

---

Table 8.6 Causes of chronic tubulointerstitial nephritis

Reflux nephropathy
NSAIDs
Diabetes mellitus
Sickle cell disease
Sjögren's syndrome
Hyperuricaemic nephropathy

---

papillae, which may subsequently slough off and be passed in the urine, sometimes causes ureteric colic or acute ureteral obstruction. Management is largely supportive. In cases of analgesic nephropathy the drug should be stopped and replaced if necessary with paracetamol or dihydrocodeine.

HYPERTENSION AND THE KIDNEY *(K&C 6e p.645)*

Hypertension can be the cause or the result of renal disease, and it is often difficult to differentiate between the two on clinical grounds. Investigations, as described on page 478, should be performed on all patients, although renal imaging is usually unnecessary.

Essential hypertension

Hypertension leads to characteristic histological changes in the renal vessels and intrarenal vasculature over time. These include intimal thickening with reduplication of the elastic lamina, reduction in kidney size, and an increase in the proportion of sclerotic glomeruli. The changes are usually accompanied by some deterioration in renal function.

Accelerated or malignant-phase hypertension is marked by the development of fibrinoid necrosis in afferent glomerular arterioles and fibrin deposition in arteriolar walls. A rapid rise in blood pressure may trigger these arteriolar lesions, and a vicious circle is then established whereby fibrin deposition leads to renal damage, increased renin release and a further increase in blood pressure.

Treatment of hypertension is described on page 478. The outlook is good if treatment is started before renal impairment has occurred.

Renal hypertension (K&C 6e p. 646)

Bilateral renal disease

Hypertension commonly complicates bilateral renal disease, such as in chronic glomerulonephritis, reflux nephropathy or analgesic nephropathy. Two main mechanisms are responsible:

- Activation of the renin–angiotensin–aldosterone system
- Retention of salt and water, leading to an increase in blood volume and hence blood pressure.

Good control of blood pressure will prevent further deterioration in renal function, with angiotensin-converting enzyme (ACE) inhibitors or angiotensin II blockers being the drugs of choice. These drugs confer an additional renoprotective effect for a given degree of blood pressure control when compared with other hypotensive drugs.

Unilateral renal disease

Hypertension may arise as a result of unilateral renal artery stenosis (caused by fibromuscular hyperplasia in young women, or atheroma in people with evidence of atherosclerosis elsewhere) or unilateral reflux nephropathy. The mechanism of hypertension with renal artery stenosis is illustrated in Figure 8.4.

Imaging for renal artery stenosis is necessary in the following circumstances:

- Patients with hypertension or progressive chronic renal failure who also have evidence of atheromatous vascular disease elsewhere
- A rise in the serum creatinine by more than 30% after introduction of an ACE inhibitor or angiotensin II receptor antagonist (an increase of 30% is acceptable and reflects reduction of glomerular perfusion)
- Abdominal bruits
- Recurrent flash pulmonary oedema without cardio-pulmonary disease
- Renal asymmetry of > 1.5 cm on imaging.

Screening for unilateral renal disease

- *MR angiography* is a non-invasive technique for visualizing the renal arteries, with close correlation with conventional angiography.
- *Helical (spiral) CT scanning* with intravenous contrast injection (CT angiography) also permits non-invasive

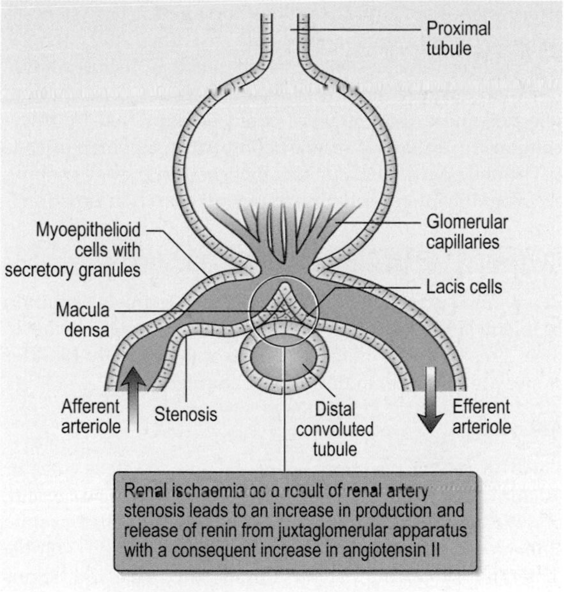

Fig. 8.4 The mechanism of hypertension in unilateral renal artery stenosis. (Adapted from Davidson (1991) *Principles and Practice of Medicine*. Churchill Livingstone, Edinburgh.)

imaging of the renal arteries, though it exposes the patient to ionizing radiation and to a large volume of contrast which may be harmful to patients with poor renal function.

- *Renal arteriography* remains the 'gold standard' for the diagnosis of renal artery disease, though the technique is invasive and requires cannulation of the femoral artery.
- *Radionuclide studies* using ^{99m}[TC]DTPA (p. 342). With significant renal artery stenosis, a fall in uptake of isotope on the affected side follows administration of an angiotensin-converting enzyme (ACE) inhibitor, such as captopril. A completely normal result renders the diagnosis unlikely.

Management

Most patients do well with hypotensive therapy without the need for surgery. ACE inhibitors are avoided because they can lead to acute renal failure in the presence of renal artery stenosis. Surgical options for renal artery stenosis include transluminal angioplasty to dilate the stenotic region, insertion of a stent across the stenosis, reconstructive vascular surgery and nephrectomy. With good patient selection more than 50% are cured or improved by intervention. In unilateral reflux nephropathy, nephrectomy is advocated, particularly if the abnormal kidney is making an insignificant contribution to overall excretion function.

RENAL STONE DISEASE (K&C 6e p. 648)

Renal and ureteral stones (urolithiasis) are a common problem affecting 2% of the population at some time in their life. There is a male:female ratio of 2:1. Bladder stones are common in developing countries.

Aetiology

Most stones are composed of calcium oxalate and/or calcium phosphate. The other main types include uric acid, struvite (magnesium ammonium phosphate), and cystine stones. Stone formation occurs when normally soluble material (e.g. calcium) supersaturates the urine and begins the process of crystal formation. In normal urine, inhibitors of crystal formation also prevent stone formation.

Hypercalciuria

More than half of all patients with calcium oxalate stones have idiopathic hypercalciuria in which there is increased absorption of calcium from the gut and a defect in renal calcium absorption. Serum calcium levels are normal. Less common causes of hypercalciuria are:

■ Hypercalcaemia (p. 633). Most patients with hypercalcaemia who form stones have primary hyperparathyroidism.
■ Excessive dietary intake of calcium.
■ Excessive resorption of calcium from the skeleton, as occurs with prolonged immobilization or weightlessness.

Hyperoxaluria

Increased oxalate excretion favours the formation of calcium oxalate, even if calcium excretion is normal. The causes are:

■ Dietary hyperoxaluria from excessive ingestion of high-oxalate-containing foods (e.g. spinach, rhubarb and tea), or from dietary calcium restriction with compensatory increased absorption of oxalate.

■ Enteric hyperoxaluria: small bowel disease, e.g. Crohn's disease or resection, is associated with increased absorption of oxalate from the colon. Dehydration secondary to fluid loss from the gut also plays a part in stone formation.

■ Primary hyperoxaluria is a rare autosomal recessive enzyme deficiency leading to increased oxalate production and corresponding oxalate excretion. There is widespread calcium oxalate crystal deposition in the kidneys, and later in other tissues (myocardium, tissues and bone). Renal failure typically develops in the late teens or early 20s.

Primary renal disease may lead to calcium stone formation. Medullary sponge kidney is associated with hypercalciuria and a tendency to develop stones (p. 387). The alkaline urine seen in the renal tubular acidoses favours the precipitation of calcium phosphate.

Uric acid stones

These are sometimes associated with hyperuricaemia (p. 275) with or without clinical gout. Patients with ileostomies are also at risk of developing urate stones, as loss of bicarbonate from gastrointestinal secretions results in the production of an acid urine (uric acid is more soluble in an alkaline than in an acid medium).

Infection-induced stones

Urinary tract infection with organisms that produce urease (*Proteus*, *Klebsiella* and *Pseudomonas* spp.) is associated with stones containing ammonium, magnesium and calcium. Urease hydrolyses urea to ammonia and thus raises the urine pH. An alkaline urine and high ammonia concentration favour stone formation. These stones are often large and fill the pelvi-calyceal system, producing the typical radio-opaque staghorn calculus.

Cystine stones

These may occur with cystinuria, an autosomal recessive condition affecting cystine and dibasic amino acid transport (lysine, ornithine and arginine) in the epithelial cells of renal tubules and the gastrointestinal tract. The excessive urinary excretion of cystine, which is the least soluble of the naturally occurring amino acids, leads to the formation of crystals and calculi.

Table 8.7	Clinical features of urinary tract calculi
Asymptomatic	
Pain	
Haematuria	
Urinary tract infection	
Urinary tract obstruction	

Clinical features (Table 8.7)

Most people with urinary tract calculi are asymptomatic; pain is the most common symptom. Large staghorn renal calculi may cause loin pain. *Ureteric stones* cause renal colic, a severe intermittent pain lasting for hours. The pain is felt anywhere between the loin and the groin, and may radiate into the scrotum or labium or into the tip of the penis. Nausea and vomiting are common. Microscopic haematuria is almost always present. The patient will be pyrexial only if there is a UTI associated with the stone. *Bladder stones* present with urinary frequency and haematuria. *Urethral stones* may cause bladder outflow obstruction, resulting in anuria and painful bladder distension.

Differential diagnosis

Bleeding within the kidney, e.g. after renal biopsy, can produce clots that lodge temporarily in the ureter and produce ureteric colic. Pain may also occur from sloughed necrotic renal papillae (p. 358). Pain from an ectopic pregnancy or leaking aortic aneurysm may be mistaken for renal colic.

Investigations

These should include a mid-stream specimen of urine for culture and measurement of serum urea, electrolyte, creatinine and calcium levels. The urine should be sieved to trap any stones for chemical analysis. A plain abdominal X-ray (KUB: kidney, ureters and bladder) and excretion urography are still used widely for diagnosis, although unenhanced helical (spiral) CT is the best diagnostic test available. Ureteric stones can be missed by ultrasound.

Ninety per cent of renal stones are radio-opaque, and calcification may be seen in the line of the renal tract.

Table 8.8 Investigations in a patient with urinary calculi

First line	Second line in recurrent stone formers
Urine	
Chemical analysis of any stone passed	24-h urine collection for calcium, oxalate, and uric acid
MSU for culture and sensitivity	Screening test for cystinuria (purple colour of urine after addition of sodium nitroprusside)
Blood	
Serum urea and electrolytes	
Serum calcium	
Serum urate	
Serum bicarbonate (low in renal tubular acidosis)	
Radiography	
Plain film	
Intravenous (excretion) urography	
Helical CT scanning	

Excretion urography shows a delayed nephrogram (opacification of the renal parenchyma) on the side of the stone and may identify the site and degree of obstruction. A normal examination during an episode of pain excludes stones as the cause of symptoms.

A detailed history may reveal possible aetiological factors for stone formation, e.g. vitamin D consumption, gouty arthritis, recurrent UTIs, intestinal resection. The subsequent work-up for a renal calculus is indicated in Table 8.8.

Management

Initial treatment A strong analgesic, e.g. diclofenac 75 mg i.v. should be given to relieve the pain of renal colic. Patients can be managed at home if there is no evidence of sepsis and they are able to take oral medications and fluids. Most ureteric stones that are 5 mm or less in diameter will pass spontaneously. Indications for intervention include persistent pain, infection above the site of obstruction, and failure of the stone to pass down the ureter. The options for stone removal include the following:

- Extracorporeal shock wave lithotripsy (ESWL) is the treatment of choice in 85% of patients and is particularly good for stones in the renal pelvis and upper ureter. Shock wave lithotripsy fragments the stones and allows them to pass spontaneously down the urethra.
- Endoscopy (ureteroscopy) and some form of in situ stone fragmentation are used for ureteric calculi. Bladder stones are removed at cystoscopy.
- Percutaneous nephrolithotomy for stones in the renal pelvis and calyces. Stones are removed by creating a percutaneous track followed by endoscopic removal of stones along this track.
- Open surgery for very large stones.

Prevention of recurrence   Further therapy depends on the type of stone and any underlying condition identified during screening investigations. For prevention of all stones whatever the cause, a high intake of fluid (to produce a urine volume of 2–2.5 L/day) must be maintained, particularly during the summer months. When no metabolic or renal abnormality has been identified ('idiopathic stone formers') adequate hydration is the mainstay of treatment.

- *Idiopathic hypercalciuria.* Reduction of dietary intake of calcium by avoiding milk, cheese and white bread. A water softener may be helpful for patients who live in hard water areas. If hypercalciuria persists, a thiazide diuretic, e.g. bendroflumethiazide (bendrofluazide), will reduce urinary calcium excretion.
- *Mixed infective stones.* Recurrent stones should be prevented by maintenance of a high fluid intake and measures to stop bacteriuria. This will require long-term follow-up and may demand the use of long-term, low-dose, prophylactic antibiotics.
- *Uric acid stones* are prevented by the long-term use of the xanthine oxidase inhibitor, allopurinol, which allows the excretion of the soluble precursor compound, hypoxanthine, in preference to uric acid. Oral sodium bicarbonate supplements to maintain an alkaline urine, and hence increased solubility of uric acid, are an alternative approach in those patients unable to tolerate allopurinol.
- *Cystine stones.* Patients may be unable to tolerate the very high fluid intake (5 litres of water in 24 hours) needed to maintain solubility of cystine in the urine. An alternative

Table 8.9 Common causes of nephrocalcinosis
Mainly medullary
Hypercalcaemia
Renal tubular acidosis
Primary hyperoxaluria
Medullary sponge kidney
Tuberculosis
Mainly cortical (rare)
Renal cortical necrosis

is D-penicillamine, which chelates cystine, forming a more soluble complex.

Nephrocalcinosis (Table 8.9) (*K&C* 6e p. 653)

The term 'nephrocalcinosis' means diffuse renal parenchymal calcification that is detectable radiologically. The condition is typically painless. Hypertension and renal impairment commonly occur. The treatment is of the underlying cause.

URINARY TRACT OBSTRUCTION (*K&C* 6e p. 654)

The urinary tract may be obstructed at any point along its length between the kidney and the urethral meatus. This results in dilatation of the tract above the obstruction. Dilatation of the renal pelvis is known as *hydronephrosis*.

Aetiology

The causes of obstruction may be classified into three groups (Table 8.10). In adults the most common causes are prostatic hypertrophy or tumour, gynaecological cancer and calculi.

Clinical features

- *Upper urinary tract obstruction* results in a dull ache in the flank or loin, which may be provoked by an increase in urine volume, e.g. high fluid intake or diuretics. Complete anuria is strongly suggestive of complete bilateral obstruction or complete obstruction of a single functioning kidney. Partial obstruction causes polyuria as a result of tubular damage and impairment of concentrating mechanisms.

Table 8.10 Causes of urinary tract obstruction

Within the lumen
Calculi
Tumour
Blood clots
Sloughed renal papillae (diabetes, NSAIDs, sickle cell disease or trait)

Within the wall
Stricture: ureteric or urethral
Neuropathic bladder
Pelviureteric junction obstruction (functional disturbance in peristalsis of collecting system)
Obstructive megaureter (defective peristalsis at lower end of ureter)

Outside the wall
Prostatic hypertrophy/tumour
Pelvic tumours
Phimosis
Retroperitoneal fibrosis (chronic periaortitis)
Accidental surgical ligation of the ureter

- *Bladder outlet obstruction* results in hesitancy, poor stream, terminal dribbling and a sense of incomplete emptying. Retention with overflow is characterized by the frequent passage of small quantities of urine. Infection commonly occurs and may precipitate acute retention of urine.

Depending on the site of obstruction an enlarged bladder or hydronephrotic kidney may be felt on examination. Pelvic (for malignancy) and rectal examination (for prostate enlargement) is essential in determining the cause of obstruction.

Investigations

Imaging studies are performed to identify the site and nature of the obstruction and, together with serum biochemistry, to assess function of the affected kidney.

- Ultrasonography and intravenous urography are the initial investigations. Ultrasonography confirms the diagnosis of obstruction and may show hydronephrosis. Excretion urography identifies the site of obstruction and shows a characteristic appearance (a delayed nephrogram, which eventually becomes denser than the non-obstructed side).

- Radionuclide studies (p. 342) are of no value in the investigation of acute obstruction but may help, in long-standing obstruction, to differentiate true obstructive uropathy from retention of tracer in a baggy low-pressure unobstructed pelvicalyceal system.
- Subsequent investigations may include helical (spiral) CT scanning, retrograde and antegrade pyelography (p. 341), cystoscopy and pressure–flow studies during bladder filling and voiding.

Management

Surgery is the usual treatment for persistent urinary tract obstruction. Elimination of the obstruction may be associated with a massive postoperative diuresis, resulting partly from a solute diuresis from salt and urea retained during obstruction and partly from the renal concentrating defect. In some cases definitive relief of obstruction is not possible and urinary diversion may be required. This may be simply an indwelling urethral catheter, a stent placed across the obstructing lesion, or the formation of an ileal conduit.

RENAL FAILURE

The term 'renal failure' means failure of renal excretory function as a result of the depression of the glomerular filtration rate (GFR). This is accompanied to a variable extent by failure of erythropoietin production, vitamin D hydroxylation, regulation of acid–base balance, regulation of salt and water balance and blood pressure control.

- *Acute renal failure* (ARF) is a sudden and rapid decline in renal function which lasts days to weeks. It is usually but not invariably reversible or self-limiting.
- *Chronic renal failure* (CRF) develops over months or years. It is usually not reversible but treatment may slow progression.

Acute renal failure (K&C 6e p. 659)

Acute renal failure (ARF) can be defined as an abrupt sustained rise in serum urea and creatinine due to a rapid decline in glomerular filtration rate leading to loss of normal water and solute homeostasis. There is no universally accepted biochemical definition of ARF, but commonly used definitions include an increase in the serum creatinine of more than 44 μmol/L or more than 50% over the baseline value.

Aetiology

ARF may be:

- Prerenal
- Renal
- Postrenal.

It may also result from a combination of these factors, e.g. in post-surgical ARF, fluid depletion (prerenal), systemic infection and nephrotoxic drugs (renal) may all play a role. ARF may also complicate chronic renal failure ('*acute-on-chronic*').

Prerenal failure

There is failure of perfusion of the kidneys with blood in prerenal failure. The kidney is able to maintain glomerular filtration close to normal in spite of wide variations in the renal perfusion pressure and volume status – so-called 'autoregulation'. Maintenance of a normal GFR in the face of decreased systemic pressure depends on the intrarenal production of prostaglandins and angiotensin II. With severe or prolonged hypovolaemia there is eventually a drop in glomerular filtration, termed 'prerenal failure'. Drugs that impair renal autoregulation, such as angiotensin-converting enzyme (ACE) inhibitors, and non-steroidal anti-inflammatory drugs, increase the risk of prerenal failure in hypovolaemia. ACE inhibitors may also cause renal failure (ischaemic nephropathy) in patients with atherosclerotic renal artery stenosis (p. 360).

Prerenal failure is most commonly the result of hypovolaemia (Table 8.11), and is characterized in the early stages by lack of structural damage and rapid reversibility once normal renal perfusion has been restored. Hypovolaemia is identified from the clinical history and, on physical examination, by the presence of hypotension, a postural drop in blood pressure, a low jugular venous pressure (JVP) and reduced tissue turgor.

A number of criteria have been proposed to differentiate between prerenal and intrinsic renal causes of uraemia (Table 8.12).

- *Urine specific gravity and urine osmolality* are easily obtained measures of concentrating ability but are un-

Table 8.11 Prerenal causes of acute renal failure

Hypovolaemia
Haemorrhage
Diarrhoea
Diuretics
Pancreatitis
Diabetic ketoacidosis
Sepsis
Burns

Decreased cardiac output
Myocardial infarction
Massive pulmonary embolism
Congestive cardiac failure

Severe liver failure (hepatorenal syndrome)

Renal artery obstruction
Stenosis
Thrombosis
Embolization

Table 8.12 Criteria for distinction between prerenal and intrinsic causes of renal dysfunction

	Prerenal	Intrinsic
Urine specific gravity	> 1.020	< 1.010
Urine osmolality (mOsm/kg)	> 500	< 350
Urine sodium (mmol/L)	< 20	> 40
Fractional excretion of sodium (Na^+)	< 1%	> 1%

Fractional excretion of $Na^+ = \dfrac{[\text{urine } Na^+ \times \text{plasma Cr}]}{[\text{plasma } Na^+ \times \text{urine Cr}]} \times 100\%$

where Cr is creatinine concentration

reliable in the presence of glycosuria or other osmotically
active substances in the urine.
- *Urine sodium* is low if there is avid tubular reabsorption,
  but may be increased by diuretics or dopamine.
- *Fractional excretion of sodium (FE_{Na})*, the ratio of sodium
  clearance to creatinine clearance, increases the reliability
  of this index but may remain low in some 'intrinsic'
  renal diseases, including contrast nephropathy and
  myoglobinuria.

The urinary indices do not, however, completely segregate the two conditions and they are no substitute for a proper clinical assessment.

Management of prenatal failure If, on the basis of the history and clinical examination, prerenal (hypovolaemia) failure is diagnosed or strongly suspected, the effect of volume repletion on renal function must be tested. Volume repletion should be with an appropriate fluid: blood in the case of post-haemorrhagic shock and physiological saline if fluid depletion is caused by vomiting, diarrhoea or polyuria. In some cases, e.g. with a very sick patient, volume replacement is guided by measurement of the central venous pressure (CVP) (p. 803). With pure prerenal failure, urine output should increase with volume replacement. If hypovolaemia is corrected (i.e. the JVP or CVP is normal) and urine output does not increase, the kidneys may respond to a strong diuretic stimulus (e.g. furosemide (frusemide) 120 mg i.v. over 10 minutes, which may be repeated once if there is no response). If urine output does not increase with these measures, then the patient has progressed to acute tubular necrosis (ATN) and the management is that of established intrinsic renal failure (see later).

Postrenal failure

Postrenal ARF occurs when both urinary outflow tracts are obstructed or when one tract is obstructed in a patient with a single functional kidney (p. 368). It is usually quickly reversed if the obstruction is relieved. All patients with ARF must be examined for evidence of obstruction (enlarged palpable kidneys or bladder, large prostate on rectal examination, pelvic masses on vaginal examination in women) and undergo renal ultrasonography to look for hydronephrosis and dilated ureters. Bladder outflow obstruction is ruled out by flushing of an existing catheter or insertion of a urethral catheter, which should then be removed unless a large volume of urine is obtained. Treatment of obstruction is usually by a temporary measure, e.g. urethral/suprapubic catheterization or percutaneous nephrostomy, until definitive treatment of the obstructing lesion can be undertaken (p. 369).

Intrinsic renal failure

Intrinsic renal diseases that result in ARF are categorized according to the primary site of injury: tubules, interstitium,

---

Table 8.13 Causes of intrinsic renal failure

Acute tubular necrosis*
Ischaemia
Exogenous nephrotoxins: gentamicin, cefaloridine, intravenous
  contrast agents
Endogenous nephrotoxins: Bence Jones protein, uric acid,
  myoglobin (secondary to rhabdomyolysis)

Acute tubulointerstitial nephritis
Drug hypersensitivity
Infections

Large renal vessels
Renal artery thrombosis
Renal vein thrombosis

Small renal vessels
Vasculitis
Malignant hypertension
Haemolytic uraemic syndrome/thrombotic thrombocytopenic
  purpura

Acute glomerulonephritis

---

*Accounts for about 90% of intrinsic ARF

renal vessels or glomerulus (Table 8.13). Injury to the tubules is most often ischaemic or toxic in origin. Prerenal ARF and ischaemic tubular necrosis represent a continuum, with the former leading to the latter when blood flow is sufficiently compromised to result in the death of tubular cells. In established renal failure the kidney loses its ability to concentrate the urine and conserve sodium. This may, in addition to clinical examination, be useful in differentiating renal from prerenal failure where the kidney is able to concentrate the urine and conserve sodium (see Table 8.12).

Clinical features of established ARF

The early stages of renal failure are often completely asymptomatic. Symptoms are common when the plasma urea concentration is over 40 mmol/L, but many patients develop uraemic symptoms at lower levels of plasma urea. It is not the accumulation of urea itself that causes symptoms, but a combination of many different metabolic abnormalities.

373

- *Alteration of urine volume.* Oliguria (urinary output < 300 mL/day) usually occurs with acute renal failure, but there may be polyuria with the passage of large quantities of dilute urine.
- *Neurological.* Weakness, fatigue and lassitude occur. Mental confusion, seizures and coma may also occur with severe uraemia, but this is less commonly seen since the introduction of effective renal replacement therapy.
- *Skin.* Symptoms include pallor, pruritus, pigmentation and bruising.
- *Cardiopulmonary.* Breathlessness occurs from a combination of anaemia and pulmonary oedema secondary to volume overload. There may be deep sighing respiration (Kussmaul's respiration) resulting from systemic metabolic acidosis. Pericarditis occurs with severe untreated uraemia and may be complicated by a pericardial effusion and tamponade.
- *Gastrointestinal.* Nausea, anorexia and vomiting are common.
- *Haematological.* Anaemia is most commonly seen in chronic renal failure but occurs in ARF. Impaired platelet function causes bruising and exacerbates gastrointestinal bleeding.

Investigation of the uraemic emergency

The purpose of investigation, together with clinical examination, is threefold:

1. To differentiate acute from chronic renal failure (see p. 380).
2. To document the degree of renal impairment and obtain baseline values so that the response to treatment can be monitored. This is accomplished by measurement of serum urea and electrolytes and creatinine clearance (p. 336).
3. To establish whether ARF is prerenal, renal or postrenal, and to determine the underlying cause so that specific treatment (e.g. intensive immunosuppression in Wegener's granulomatosis) may be instituted as early as possible and thus prevent progression to irreversible renal failure.

Investigations include:

- Blood count: anaemia, a very high ESR, or eosinophilia may suggest myeloma or a vasculitis
- Urine and blood cultures to exclude infection.
- Urine Stix testing and microscopy: glomerulonephritis is suggested by haematuria and proteinuria on urine Stix testing and by the presence of red cell casts on urine microscopy (p. 340).
- Urinary electrolytes: measurement of urinary electrolytes (see Table 8.12) may help to exclude a significant prerenal element to ARF.
- Serum calcium, phosphate and uric acid.
- Renal ultrasound can exclude obstruction and give an assessment of renal size; CT is useful for the diagnosis of retroperitoneal fibrosis and some other causes of urinary obstruction, and may also indicate cortical scarring.
- Histological investigations: renal biopsy should be performed in every patient with unexplained renal failure and normal-sized kidneys.
- Optional investigations (depending on the case):
  - Serum protein electrophoresis for myeloma
  - Serum autoantibodies, ANCAs (p. 948) and complement
  - Antibodies to hepatitis B and C point to polyarteritis or cryoglobulinaemia
  - Antibodies to HIV point to HIV-related renal disease.

Management

The principles of management of established ARF are summarized in Emergency Box 8.1. In all patients with intrinsic renal failure, hypovolaemia and obstruction must be excluded as contributing factors.

Indications for dialysis include:

- Hyperkalaemia not controlled by conservative measures
- Severe metabolic acidosis
- Pulmonary oedema
- Progressive uraemia with encephalopathy or pericarditis.

Whether haemodialysis, haemofiltration or peritoneal dialysis (p. 383) is used depends on the facilities available and the clinical circumstances, e.g. haemodialysis requires anticoagulation and thus would be inappropriate in a patient with recent haemorrhage from peptic ulceration.

> !
>
> *Emergency Box 8.1*
> **Principles of management of a patient with acute
> renal failure**
>
> **Emergency resuscitation**
> To prevent death from hyperkalaemia (p. 325) or pulmonary
> oedema (p. 433).
>
> **Establish the aetiology and treat the underlying cause**
> - History, including family history, systemic disease, use of
>   nephrotoxic drugs.
> - Examination includes assessment of haemodynamic status,
>   pelvic and rectal examination.
> - Investigations, including bladder catheterization or flush of
>   existing catheter.
>
> **Prevention of further renal damage**
> Early detection of infection and prompt treatment with
> antibiotics. Avoid hypovolaemia, nephrotoxic drugs, NSAIDs
> and ACE inhibitors.
>
> **Management of established renal failure**
> - Seek advice from a nephrologist.
> - Once fluid balance has been corrected, the daily fluid intake
>   should equal fluid lost on the previous day plus insensible
>   losses (approximately 500 mL).
> - Adequate nutrition – enteral route preferred over parenteral.
> - Nursing care, e.g. prevention of pressure sores.
> - Adjust doses of drugs that are excreted by the kidney, and
>   monitor serum drug levels where appropriate (refer to
>   *National Formulary* for guidance).
> - Monitor daily: urine volume, serum biochemistry,
>   bodyweight.
> - Frequent review regarding the need for dialysis.
>
> **Careful fluid and electrolyte balance during recovery phase**
> The patient may pass large volumes of dilute urine until the
> kidney recovers its concentrating ability.

NSAIDs, non-steroidal anti-inflammatory drugs; ACE, angiotensin-converting
enzyme

Prognosis

The prognosis depends on the underlying cause. The most
common cause of death is sepsis as a result of impaired
immune defence (from uraemia and malnutrition) and
instrumentation (dialysis and urinary catheters and
vascular lines). In those who survive, renal function usually
begins to recover within 2–3 weeks. ARF is irreversible in a

Table 8.14 Causes of end-stage renal failure

Congenital and hereditary disease
Polycystic kidneys

Glomerular disease
Primary glomerular disease
Secondary glomerular disease, e.g. diabetes mellitus,
    amyloidosis, systemic lupus

Tubulointerstitial disease
Reflux nephropathy
Tuberculosis
Nephrocalcinosis
Interstitial nephritis, e.g. drugs, idiopathic

Vascular disease
Atherosclerotic renal artery stenosis
Hypertensive nephropathy
Vasculitis

Urinary tract obstruction

Other
HIV-associated nephropathy

---

few patients, probably because of cortical necrosis which,
unlike tubules, which regenerate, heals with the formation
of scar tissue.

Chronic renal failure (K&C 6e p. 665)

Aetiology

The causes of chronic renal failure (CRF) are listed in Table
8.14. In European countries diabetes mellitus is the single
most common cause of end-stage renal failure. Hypertensive nephropathy and glomerulonephritis are other
common causes. Regardless of the underlying cause, fibrosis
of the remaining tubules, glomeruli and small blood vessels
results in progressive renal scarring and eventually end-
stage renal failure.

Clinical features and investigations

Clinical features are summarized in Table 8.15. Investigations
are similar to those in ARF (p. 374).

Table 8.15 Symptoms and signs of chronic renal failure

Anaemia
Pallor, lethargy, breathlessness on exercise

Platelet abnormality
Epistaxis, bruising

Skin
Pigmentation
Pruritus

Gastrointestinal tract
Anorexia, nausea, vomiting, diarrhoea

Endocrine/gonads
Amenorrhoea, erectile dysfunction, infertility

Central nervous system
Confusion, coma, fits (in severe uraemia)

Cardiovascular system
Uraemic pericarditis, hypertension, peripheral vascular disease,
  heart failure

Renal
Nocturia, polyuria, salt and water retention causing oedema

Renal osteodystrophy
Osteomalacia, muscle weakness, bone pain, hyperparathyroidism,
  osteosclerosis

In addition there may be symptoms and signs resulting from the long-term complications of CRF.

Anaemia   This is present in the great majority of patients with CRF. The pathogenesis is multifactorial:

- Decreased erythropoietin production by the diseased kidney
- Depressed bone marrow activity
- Shortened red cell survival
- Increased blood loss (from the gut, during haemodialysis and as a result of repeated sampling)
- Dietary deficiency of haematinics (iron and folate).

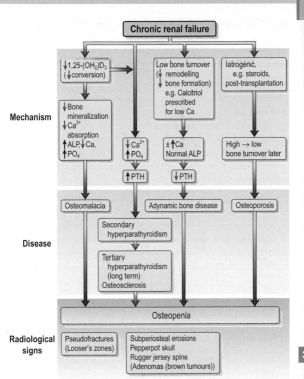

Fig. 8.5 Pathogenesis and radiological features of renal osteodystrophy.

Bone disease The term 'renal osteodystrophy' embraces the various forms of bone disease that develop in CRF, i.e. osteomalacia, osteoporosis, secondary and tertiary hyperparathyroidism, and osteosclerosis. Renal phosphate retention and impaired production of 1,25-dihydroxyvitamin D (the active hormonal form of vitamin D) lead to a fall in serum calcium concentration and hence to a compensatory increase in parathyroid hormone (PTH) secretion. A sustained excess of PTH results in skeletal decalcification with the classic radiological features described in Figure 8.5. Osteosclerosis (hardening of bone) may be a result of hyperparathyroidism. Alternate bands of sclerotic and porotic bone in the vertebra produce the characteristic 'rugger jersey spine' radiographic appearance.

Neurological A motor and sensory neuropathy may occur in uraemia. Most commonly the sensory neuropathy may manifest as peripheral paraesthesiae. Median nerve compression in the carpal tunnel is common and is usually caused by β_2-microglobulin-related amyloidosis (see later). Autonomic dysfunction may present as postural hypotension and disturbed gastrointestinal motility. Dialysis produces an improvement in neuropathy.

Cardiovascular disease The highest mortality in CRF is from cardiovascular disease, which is increased as a result of the presence of hypertension, abnormalities of lipid metabolism and vascular calcification. Renal disease also results in a form of cardiomyopathy with both systolic and diastolic dysfunction.

Other complications include an increased risk of peptic ulceration, acute pancreatitis, hyperuricaemia, erectile dysfunction and, in children, failure to thrive.

Differentiating ARF from CRF

Distinction between ARF and CRF depends on the history, duration of symptoms and previous urinalysis or measurement of renal function. A normochromic anaemia, small kidneys on ultrasonography and the presence of renal osteodystrophy (see below) favour a chronic process.

Management

The underlying cause of renal disease should be treated aggressively wherever possible, e.g. tight metabolic control in diabetes.

Renoprotection

The goal of treatment should be to maintain the blood pressure at less than 120/80 and to maintain a urinary protein concentration of less than 0.3 g/24 hours. Good blood pressure control may slow the decline in renal function.

Patients with chronic renal failure and proteinuria > 1 g/24 hours should receive:

- ACE inhibitor increasing to maximum dose
- Angiotensin receptor antagonist if goals are not achieved (in type 2 diabetes start with angiotensin receptor antagonist)
- Diuretic to prevent hyperkalaemia and help to control BP
- Calcium-channel blocker (verapamil or diltiazem) if goals not achieved.

Additional measures
- Statins to lower cholesterol to < 4.5 mmol/L
- Stop smoking (threefold higher rate of deterioration in CRF)
- Treat diabetes (HbA_{1c} < 7%)
- Reduce protein intake (0.8–1 g/kg bodyweight/day)
- Patients should be offered influenza immunization (p. 495).

Correction of complications

Hyperkalaemia often responds to dietary restriction of potassium intake. Drugs which cause potassium retention should be stopped. Occasionally it is necessary to prescribe ion-exchange resins to remove potassium in the gastro-intestinal tract. Emergency treatment of severe hyper-kalaemia is described on page 325.

Calcium and phosphate Hyperphosphataemia is treated by dietary restriction and administration of oral phosphate-binding agents such as calcium carbonate. Newer phosphate binders such as sevelamar and lanthanum carbonate are currently being evaluated. The serum calcium should be maintained in the normal range through the use of synthetic vitamin D analogues such as 1_α-colecalciferol or the vitamin D metabolite 1,25-dihydroxyvitamin D_3 $(1,25\text{-}(OH)_2D_3)$.

Anaemia Recombinant human erythropoietin is a very effective but expensive treatment for the anaemia of CRF and has largely replaced repeated blood transfusions. It is administered subcutaneously or intravenously three times weekly. Failure to respond may be the result of haematinic deficiency, bleeding, malignancy or infection. The dis-advantages of treatment are that erythropoietin may accelerate hypertension and, rarely, lead to encephalopathy with convulsions.

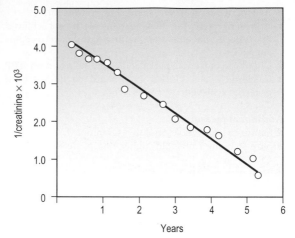

Fig. 8.6 **A reciprocal plot of serum creatinine against time.**
Such a slope is particular to an individual patient. It may be used
to predict the time of onset of end-stage renal failure and thus
prepare the patient for dialysis, e.g. the formation of an
arteriovenous fistula.

Acidosis Systemic acidosis accompanies the decline in
renal function and may contribute to increased serum
potassium levels as well as dyspnoea and lethargy. Treatment is with oral sodium bicarbonate; the increased sodium
load may exacerbate oedema and reduce blood pressure
control.

Preparation for dialysis and transplantation
In most patients with CRF there is a progressive loss of
renal function, which proceeds at a constant rate for that
patient (Fig. 8.6). The graph of the reciprocal creatinine
concentration plotted against time may be used to predict
when the patient is likely to develop end-stage renal failure
and thus require a form of renal replacement therapy. This
may be haemodialysis, chronic ambulatory peritoneal
dialysis or renal transplantation. Patients should be referred
to a nephrologist by the time the serum creatinine reaches
350 mmol/L (250 mmol/L in diabetics), or earlier if the
primary diagnosis is unknown.

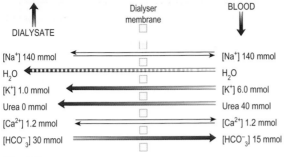

Fig. 8.7 The principle of haemodialysis.

RENAL REPLACEMENT THERAPY (K&C 6e p. 673)

Dialysis

'Uraemic toxins' can be efficiently removed from the blood by the process of diffusion across a semipermeable membrane towards the low concentrations present in dialysis fluid (Fig. 8.7). The gradient is maintained by replacing used dialysis fluid with fresh solution. In haemodialysis, blood in an extracorporeal circulation is exposed to dialysis fluid separated by an artificial semipermeable membrane. In peritoneal dialysis the peritoneum is used as the semipermeable membrane and dialysis fluid is instilled into the peritoneal cavity.

Haemodialysis

Adequate dialysis requires a blood flow of at least 200 mL/min and the most reliable way of achieving this is by surgical construction of an arteriovenous fistula, usually in the forearm. This provides a permanent and easily accessible site for the insertion of needles. An adult of average size usually requires 4–5 hours of haemodialysis three times a week, which may be performed in hospital; in the UK some patients have self-supervised home haemodialysis. All patients are anticoagulated during treatment (usually with heparin) because contact of blood with foreign surfaces activates the clotting cascade. The most common acute complication of haemodialysis is hypotension, caused in part by excessive removal of extracellular fluid.

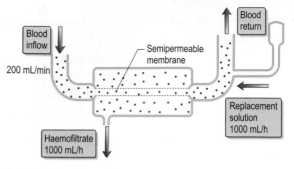

Fig. 8.8 **Principles of haemofiltration.**

Haemofiltration

Haemofiltration involves the removal of plasma water and its dissolved constituents (e.g. Na^+, K^+, urea, phosphate) and replacing it with a solution of the desired biochemical composition. The procedure employs a highly permeable membrane, which allows large amounts of fluid and solute to be removed from the patient (Fig. 8.8). The procedure is costly, and only a tiny minority of patients with end-stage renal failure are managed in this way. However, it is readily performed in intensive care units on very sick patients, as haemofiltration can be managed by ITU nursing staff rather than renal unit nurses.

Peritoneal dialysis

- *Continuous ambulatory peritoneal dialysis* (CAPD) requires the insertion of a permanent catheter (Tenkoff catheter) into the peritoneal cavity via a subcutaneous tunnel. Up to 3 litres of dialysate are introduced and exchanged three to five times a day.
- *Intermittent peritoneal dialysis.* Dialysate is introduced into the peritoneal cavity via a catheter and exchanged every 60–120 minutes, requiring the patient to remain in bed during treatment. It is mainly used in ARF.

Peritonitis is the most common serious complication of peritoneal dialysis. Infection with *Staph. epidermidis* accounts for 50% of cases. Treatment is with appropriate antibiotics, which are often given intraperitoneally.

Long-term complications of dialysis (K&C 6e p. 677)

Cardiovascular disease (as a result of atheroma) and sepsis are the leading causes of death in long-term dialysis patients. Causes of fatal sepsis include peritonitis complicating peritoneal dialysis and *Staph. aureus* infection (including endocarditis) complicating the use of indwelling access devices for haemodialysis. Amyloidosis is the result of the accumulation and polymerization of β_2-microglobulin. This molecule (a component of HLA proteins on most cell membranes) is normally excreted by the kidneys, but is not removed by dialysis membranes. Deposition results in the carpal tunnel syndrome and joint pains, particularly of the shoulders.

Transplantation (K&C 6e p. 678)

Successful renal transplantation offers the potential for complete rehabilitation in end-stage renal failure. It allows freedom from dietary and fluid restriction, anaemia and infertility are corrected and the need for parathyroidectomy reduced. In the best centres graft survival is 80% at 10 years. Kidneys are obtained from cadavers or, less frequently, from healthy close relatives. The donor must be ABO compatible, and good HLA matching increases the chances of successful transplantation. The donor kidney is placed in the iliac fossa and anastomosed to the iliac vessels of the recipient; the donor ureter is placed into the recipient's bladder.

Long-term immunosuppressive treatment is employed in all cases (unless the donor is an identical twin, i.e. genetically identical) to reduce the incidence of graft rejection. This treatment comprises corticosteroids, azathioprine or mycophenolate mofetil and ciclosporin or tacrolimus. Monoclonal and polyclonal antibodies such as antilymphocyte and anti-thymocyte globulin or basiliximab and dacluzimab are potent immunosuppressives and are increasingly being used for the treatment of steroid-resistant rejections and as an induction therapy for high immunological risk patients (previously sensitized with circulating anti-HLA antibodies).

The complications of renal transplantation and immuno-suppression include opportunistic infection (e.g. *Pneumocystis carinii*), hypertension, the development of tumours (skin malignancies and lymphomas) and, occasionally, recurrence of the renal disease (e.g. Goodpasture's syndrome).

CYSTIC RENAL DISEASE

Solitary and multiple renal cysts

Renal cysts are common, particularly with advancing age. They are usually asymptomatic and discovered incidentally on ultrasonography or excretion urography performed for some other reason. Occasionally they may cause pain and/or haematuria.

Adult polycystic disease (K&C 6e p. 681)

Adult polycystic disease (APCD) is a common (1 : 1000) autosomal dominantly inherited condition in which multiple cysts develop throughout both kidneys. Cysts increase in size with advancing age and lead to renal enlargement and the progressive destruction of normal kidney tissue, with gradual loss of renal function. Most cases are due to a mutation in the *PKD1* gene (short arm of chromosome 16), which encodes for a protein, polycystin, an integral membrane protein thought to be involved in cell adhesion. The underlying mechanism by which cysts form remains unclear.

Clinical features

The disease presents at any age after the second decade. Presenting symptoms include the following:

- Acute loin pain and/or haematuria as a result of haemorrhage into a cyst
- Abdominal discomfort caused by renal enlargement
- Development of hypertension or symptoms of uraemia.

About 30% of patients will develop hepatic cysts, which are usually clinically insignificant. More rarely cysts develop in the pancreas, spleen, ovary and other organs. Berry aneurysms of the cerebral vessels are found in 8% of patients; these may result in subarachnoid haemorrhage.

Diagnosis

Clinical examination commonly reveals large irregular kidneys, hypertension and possibly hepatomegaly. A definitive diagnosis is established by ultrasonography.

Management

Treatment involves careful control of blood pressure, and salt replacement if necessary. As the disease is always progressive, many patients will require renal replacement by dialysis and/or transplantation. Children and siblings of patients with the disease should be offered renal ultra-sonographic screening. This is carried out in the second decade because diagnosis before this age is difficult and hypertension is rare in the very young.

Medullary sponge kidney (*K&C* 6e p. 683)

Medullary sponge kidney is an uncommon condition characterized by dilatation of the collecting ducts in the papillae with associated stasis of urine. In severe cases there are numerous cysts and the medullary area has a sponge-like appearance. In 20% of patients there is hypercalciuria or renal tubular acidosis (see p. 331). Most patients have intermittent colic, with the passage of small stones, or haematuria with well-preserved renal function. The diagnosis is made by excretion urography.

TUMOURS OF THE KIDNEY AND GENITOURINARY TRACT

Renal cell carcinoma (*K&C* 6e p. 683)

387

Renal cell carcinomas are the most common renal tumours in adults, presenting most commonly in the fifth decade, with a male : female ratio of 2 : 1. They arise from the proximal tubular epithelium and may be solitary, multiple and occasionally bilateral.

Clinical features

Haematuria, loin pain and a mass in the flank are the most common presenting features. Other features include malaise, weight loss, fever and occasionally polycythaemia (p. 211). Twenty-five per cent have metastases at presentation to bone, liver and the lung, where they are often solitary and large ('cannonball' metastases).

Investigations

■ Excretion urography will reveal a space-occupying lesion in the kidney.

- Ultrasonography will demonstrate a solid lesion and can assess the patency of the renal vein and inferior vena cava.
- MRI and CT are useful for tumour staging.

Management

Surgery forms the mainstay of treatment. Nephrectomy is carried out unless there is bilateral involvement or the contralateral kidney functions poorly. Medroxyprogesterone may be of value in controlling metastatic disease. Treatment with interleukin-2 and alpha-interferon produces a remission in about 20% of cases.

Prognosis

The 5-year survival rate is 60–70% when the tumour is confined to the renal parenchyma, but less than 5% in those with distant metastases.

Urothelial tumours (*K&C* 6e p. 684)

The calyces, renal pelvis, ureter, bladder and urethra are lined by transitional cell epithelium. Bladder tumours are the most common form of transitional cell malignancy. They occur most commonly after the age of 40 years and are four times more common in males. Predisposing factors for bladder cancer include:

- Cigarette smoking
- Industrial chemicals, e.g. β-naphthylamine, benzidine
- Drugs, e.g. phenacetin, cyclophosphamide
- Chronic inflammation, e.g. schistosomiasis.

Clinical features

Painless haematuria is the most common symptom of bladder cancer, although pain sometimes occurs from clot retention. Transitional cell cancers of the kidney and ureters present with haematuria and flank pain.

Investigations

- Cytology of the urine may show malignant cells.
- Excretion urography shows filling defects, but small tumours may not be seen.
- Cystoscopy if no evidence of upper urinary tract pathology has been found.

Management

Pelvic and ureteric tumours are treated with surgical resection. Treatment of bladder tumours depends on the stage, but options include local diathermy or cystoscopic resection, bladder resection, radiotherapy, and local and systemic chemotherapy.

DISEASES OF THE PROSTATE GLAND

Prostate-specific antigen (PSA) is a glycoprotein that is expressed by normal and neoplastic prostate tissue and secreted into the bloodstream. Plasma PSA concentration increases yearly in men over the age of 40 years, and different normal reference ranges may be appropriate based upon a man's age. The main causes of an elevated serum PSA are benign prostatic enlargement, prostate cancer, prostate inflammation, perineal trauma and mechanical manipulation of the prostate (cystoscopy, prostate biopsy or surgery). In the latter three conditions the elevation is transient. Serum PSA levels overlap considerably in men with benign prostatic hypertrophy and those with prostate cancer and levels may be within the reference range in men with prostate cancer. For instance, just less than one in three men with an elevated serum PSA (above $4 \mu g/L$) will have prostate cancer on biopsy.

Benign enlargement of the prostate gland (K&C 6e p. 685)

Benign prostatic enlargement (hypertrophy, BPH) is extremely common, occurring most commonly after the age of 60 years. There is hyperplasia of both glandular and connective tissue elements of the gland, although the aetiology of the condition remains unknown.

Clinical features

Frequency of micturition, nocturia, delay in initiation of micturition and post-void dribbling are common symptoms. Acute urinary retention or retention with overflow incontinence also occurs. An enlarged smooth prostate may be felt on rectal examination.

Investigations

Serum electrolytes and renal ultrasonography are performed to exclude renal damage resulting from obstruction. Prostate-specific antigen (PSA) is raised in patients with BPH and prostate cancer and both may present with similar symptoms.

Management

Patients with mild or moderate symptoms require no treatment or medical treatment only. Selective α_1-adrenoceptor antagonists such as tamsulosin relax smooth muscle in the bladder neck and prostate. 5α-Reductase inhibitors such as finasteride block the conversion of testosterone to dihydro-testosterone – the latter is thought to be responsible for the development of prostatic hypertrophy. α-Blockers provide better symptom relief than finasteride. Patients with acute retention of urine or retention with overflow require urethral catheterization or, if this is not possible, suprapubic catheter drainage. Patients with persistent severe symptoms or with dilatation of the upper urinary tract require surgery, most commonly with transurethral resection of the prostate (TURP).

Prostatic carcinoma (K&C 6e p. 685)

Prostatic adenocarcinoma is common, accounting for 7% of all cancers in men. Malignant change within the prostate is increasingly common with increasing age, being present in 80% of men aged 80 and over. In most cases these malignant foci remain dormant.

Clinical features

In developed countries most patients now present as a result of screening for prostate cancer by measurement of serum PSA. Presentation is also with symptoms of bladder outflow obstruction identical to those of benign prostatic hypertrophy. Occasionally, presenting symptoms are due to metastases, particularly to bone. In some cases malignancy is unsuspected until histological investigation is carried out on the resected specimen after prostatectomy. Rectal examination may reveal a hard irregular gland.

Investigation

Investigation is as for benign prostatic enlargement, with measurement of serum PSA. If metastases are present serum PSA is usually markedly elevated (> 16 µg/L). Supplemental tests include transrectal ultrasonography, which helps in tumour staging, and transrectal prostate biopsy for histological confirmation.

Management

Microscopic tumour is sometimes managed by watchful waiting. Treatment of disease confined to the gland is radical prostatectomy or radiotherapy, both resulting in 80–90% 5-year survival. The treatment of metastatic disease depends on removing androgenic drive to the tumour. This is achieved by bilateral orchidectomy, synthetic luteinizing hormone-releasing hormone analogues, e.g. goserelin, or antiandrogens, e.g. cyproterone acetate.

Screening

The value or otherwise of screening for prostate cancer remains uncertain. Annual measurement of PSA in asymptomatic men results in earlier diagnosis, and large-scale trials are in progress to determine the potential benefits (i.e. increased survival) and drawbacks of screening (expense, side-effects of treatment, emotional impact of a positive result).

TESTICULAR TUMOURS (K&C 6e p. 522)

Testicular cancer is the most common cancer in young men. More than 96% of testicular tumours arise from germ cells. There are two main types: seminomas and teratomas. The aetiology is unknown and the risk of malignant change is greater in undescended testes.

Clinical features

Typically the man or his partner finds a painless lump in the testicle. Presentation may also be with metastases in the lungs causing cough and dyspnoea, or para-aortic lymph nodes causing back pain.

Investigations

- Ultrasound scanning will help to differentiate between masses in the body of the testes and other intrascrotal swellings.
- Serum concentrations of the tumour markers α-fetoprotein (AFP) and/or the beta subunit of human chorionic gonadotrophin (β-HCG) are elevated in most men with teratomas. They are used to help make the diagnosis, to assess response to treatment and in following up patients. β-HCG is elevated in a minority of men with seminomas, and AFP is not elevated in men with pure seminomas.
- Tumour staging is assessed by chest X-ray and CT scanning of the chest, abdomen and pelvis.

Treatment

Orchidectomy is performed to permit histological evaluation of the primary tumour and to provide local tumour control. Seminomas with metastases below the diaphragm only are treated by radiotherapy. More widespread tumours are treated with chemotherapy. Teratomas with metastases are also treated with chemotherapy. Sperm banking should be offered prior to therapy to men who wish to preserve fertility.

392

URINARY INCONTINENCE (K&C 6e p. 686)

Normal bladder physiology

As the bladder fills with urine, two factors act to ensure continence until it is next emptied:

- Intravesical pressure remains low as a result of stretching of the bladder wall and the stability of the bladder muscle (detrusor), which does not contract involuntarily.
- The sphincter mechanisms of the bladder neck and urethral muscles.

At the onset of voiding the sphincters relax (mediated by decreased sympathetic activity) and the detrusor muscle contracts (mediated by increased parasympathetic activity). Overall control and coordination of micturition is by higher brain centres, which include the cerebral cortex and the pons.

Stress incontinence

Stress incontinence occurs as a result of sphincter weakness, which may be iatrogenic in men (post-prostatectomy) or the result of childbirth in women. There is a small leak of urine when intra-abdominal pressure rises, e.g. with coughing, laughing or standing up. In young women pelvic floor exercises may help. In postmenopausal women the contributing factor of urethral atrophy may be helped by oestrogen creams.

Urge incontinence

In urge incontinence there is a strong desire to void and the patient may be unable to hold his or her urine. The usual cause is detrusor instability, which occurs most often in women, and the aetiology is not known. Mild cases may respond to bladder retraining (gradually increasing the time interval between voids). More severe cases are treated with anticholinergic agents, e.g. oxybutynin, which decrease detrusor excitability. Less commonly, urge incontinence is caused by bladder hypersensitivity from local pathology (e.g. UTI, bladder stones, tumours) and treatment is then of the underlying cause.

Overflow incontinence

Overflow incontinence is most often seen in men with prostatic hypertrophy causing outflow obstruction. There is leakage of small amounts of urine, and on abdominal examination the distended bladder is felt rising out of the pelvis. If the obstruction is not relieved with urethral or suprapubic catheterization then renal damage will develop.

Neurological causes (*K&C* 6e p. 1201)

These are usually apparent from the history and examination, which reveal accompanying neurological deficits. Brainstem damage, e.g. trauma, may lead to incoordination of detrusor muscle activity and sphincter relaxation, so that the two contract together during voiding. This results in a high-pressure system with the risk of obstructive uropathy. The aim of treatment is to reduce outflow pressure, either with α-adrenergic blockers or by sphincterotomy. Autonomic neuropathy, e.g. in diabetic individuals, decreases detrusor excitability and results in a distended atonic bladder with a large residual urine which is liable to infection. Permanent catheterization may be necessary.

In elderly people incontinence may be the result of a combination of factors: diuretic treatment, dementia (antisocial incontinence) and difficulty in getting to the toilet because of immobility.

Cardiovascular disease 9

COMMON PRESENTING SYMPTOMS OF HEART DISEASE

The common symptoms of heart disease are chest pain, breathlessness, palpitations, syncope, fatigue and peripheral oedema. Careful history taking is important as there is overlap between symptoms arising from cardiovascular disease and those from other pathology. The severity of anginal pain, dyspnoea, palpitations or fatigue may be classified according to the New York Heart Association grading of 'cardiac status' (Table 9.1).

Chest pain (*K&C* 6e p. 732)

Acute central chest pain or discomfort is a common presenting symptom of cardiovascular disease and must be differentiated from non-cardiac causes. The site of pain, its character, radiation and associated symptoms will often point to the cause (Table 9.2).

Dyspnoea (*K&C* 6e p. 733)

Dyspnoea is an abnormal awareness of breathlessness. The causes are discussed on page 487. Left heart failure is the most common cardiac cause of exertional dyspnoea.

Orthopnoea (*K&C* 6e p. 733) refers to breathlessness on lying flat, as a result of gravitational redistribution of blood leading to increased pulmonary blood volume. *Paroxysmal nocturnal dyspnoea* occurs when there is an accumulation of

Table 9.1	The New York Heart Association grading of 'cardiac status'
Grade 1	Uncompromised
Grade 2	Slightly compromised
Grade 3	Moderately compromised
Grade 4	Severely compromised

Table 9.2 Common causes of chest pain	
Usually retrosternal	
Angina pectoris	Crushing pain on exercise, relieved by rest. May radiate to jaw or arms
Myocardial infarction	Similar in character to angina but more severe, occurs at rest, lasts longer
Pericarditis	Sharp pain aggravated by movement, respiration and changes in posture
Aortic dissection	Severe tearing chest pain which radiates to the back
Reflux oesophagitis	Pain may occur at night and when bending or lying down. Pain may radiate into the neck
Other sites: usually lateral	
Pulmonary infarct ⎫ Pneumonia ⎬ Pneumothorax ⎭	Typically pleuritic in nature, i.e. sharp, well-localized pain aggravated by inspiration, coughing and movement
Costochondritis ⎫ Fractured rib ⎬	Musculoskeletal pain is usually a sharp, well-localized pain with a tender area on palpation

fluid in the lungs at night causing the patient to awake suddenly from sleep.

Palpitations (*K&C* 6e p. 733)

A palpitation is an awareness of the heartbeat. The normal heartbeat is sensed when the patient is anxious, excited, exercising or lying on the left side. In other circumstances it usually indicates a cardiac arrhythmia, commonly ectopic beats or a paroxysmal tachycardia (p. 412).

Syncope and dizziness (*K&C* 6e p. 734)

Syncope means a temporary impairment of consciousness due to inadequate cerebral blood flow. There are many causes, but the most common is a simple faint or vasovagal attack (p. 697). The cardiac causes of syncope are the result of either very fast (e.g. ventricular tachycardia) or very slow heart rates (e.g. complete heart block) which are unable to maintain an adequate cardiac output. Attacks occur suddenly and without warning. They last only 1 or 2 minutes, with complete recovery in seconds (compare with epilepsy, where complete recovery may be delayed for some hours). Obstruction to ventricular outflow also causes syncope (e.g. aortic stenosis, hypertrophic cardiomyopathy), which typically occurs on exercise when the requirements for increased cardiac output cannot be met.

Other symptoms

Tiredness, lethargy and exertional fatigue occur with heart failure and result from poor perfusion of brain and skeletal muscle. Heart failure also causes salt and water retention, leading to oedema, which in ambulant patients is most prominent over the ankles. In severe cases it may involve the genitalia and thighs.

INVESTIGATIONS IN CARDIAC DISEASE

The chest X-ray (K&C 6e p. 741)

This is usually taken in the postero-anterior (PA) direction at maximum inspiration. A PA chest film can aid the identification of cardiomegaly, pericardial effusions, dissection or dilatation of the aorta, and calcification of the pericardium or heart valves. Cardiomegaly is indicated by a cardiothoracic width ratio > 50% (maximum transverse diameter of the heart compared to maximum transverse diameter of the thorax measured from the inside of the ribs). Examination of the lung fields may show signs of left ventricular failure (Fig. 9.1), valvular heart disease (Fig. 9.2) or pulmonary oligaemia (reduction of vascular markings) associated with pulmonary embolic disease.

The electrocardiogram (K&C 6e p. 744)

The electrocardiogram (ECG) is a recording from the body surface of the electrical activity of the heart. Each cardiac cell generates an action potential as it becomes depolarized and then repolarized during a normal cycle. Depolarization of cardiac cells proceeds in an orderly fashion in the normal situation, beginning in the sinus node (lying in the junction between superior vena cava and right atrium) and then spreading sequentially through the atria, AV node (lying beneath the right atrial endocardium within the lower inter-atrial septum), and the His bundle in the interventricular

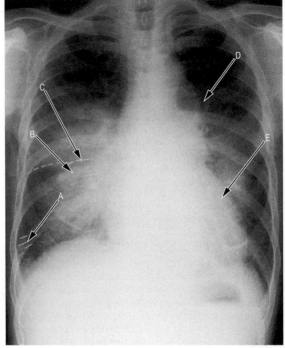

Fig. 9.1 **The chest X-ray in left ventricular failure.** A, Kerley B lines; B, hilar haziness; C, fluid in the right horizontal interlobar fissure; D, upper lobe venous engorgement; E, cardiomegaly.

septum, which divides into right and left bundle branches (Fig. 9.3). The bundle branches spread throughout the subendocardial surface of the right ventricle and left ventricle respectively. The main left bundle divides into an anterior superior division (the anterior hemi-bundle) and a posterior inferior division (the posterior hemi-bundle).

The standard ECG has 12 leads:

- Chest leads, V_1–V_6, look at the heart in a *horizontal plane* (Fig. 9.4).
- Limb leads look at the heart in a *vertical plane* (Fig. 9.5). Limb leads are unipolar (AVR, AVL and AVF) or bipolar (I, II, III).

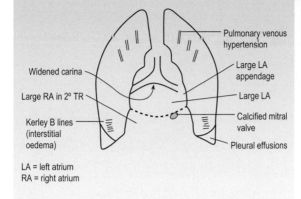

Fig. 9.2 Schematic representation of the chest X-ray in mitral stenosis. LA, left atrium; RA, right atrium; TR, tricuspid regurgitation.

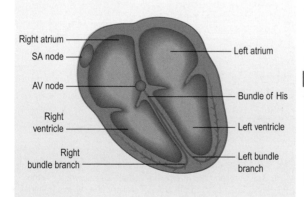

Fig. 9.3 The normal cardiac conduction system. In normal circumstances only the specialized conducting tissues of the heart undergo spontaneous depolarization (automaticity) which initiates an action potential. The sinus (SA) node discharges more rapidly than the other cells and is the normal pacemaker of the heart. The impulse generated by the sinus node spreads first through the atria, producing atrial systole, and then through the atrioventricular (AV) node to the His–Purkinje system, producing ventricular systole.

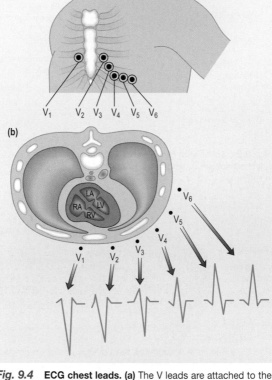

Fig. 9.4 **ECG chest leads. (a)** The V leads are attached to the chest wall overlying the intercostal spaces as shown: V_4 in the mid-clavicular line, V_5 in the anterior axillary line, V_6 in the mid-axillary line. **(b)** Leads V_1 and V_2 look at the right ventricle, V_3 and V_4 at the interventricular septum, and V_5 and V_6 at the left ventricle. The normal QRS complex in each lead is shown. The R wave in the chest (precordial) leads steadily increases in amplitude from lead V_1 to V_6 with a corresponding decrease in S wave depth, culminating in a predominantly positive complex in V_6.

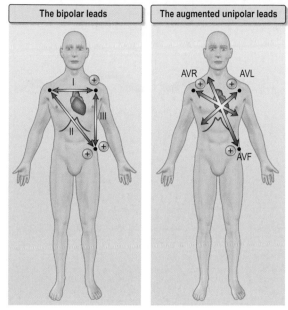

The bipolar leads	The augmented unipolar leads

Fig. 9.5 ECG limb leads. Lead I is derived from electrodes on the right arm (negative pole) and left arm (positive pole), lead II is derived from electrodes on the right arm (negative pole) and left leg (positive pole), and lead III from electrodes on the left arm (negative pole) and the left leg (positive pole).

The ECG machine is arranged so that when a depolarization wave spreads towards a lead the needle moves upwards on the trace (i.e. a positive deflection), and when it spreads away from the lead the needle moves downwards.

ECG waveform and definitions (Fig. 9.6)

The *heart rate*. At normal paper speed (usually 25 mm/s) each 'big square' measures 5 mm wide and is equivalent to 0.2 s. The heart rate (if the rhythm is regular) is calculated by counting the number of big squares between two consecutive R waves and dividing into 300.

The *P wave* is the first deflection and is caused by atrial depolarization. When abnormal it may be:

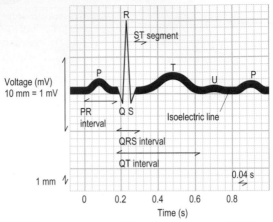

Fig. 9.6 The waves and elaboration of the normal ECG.
(From Goldman MJ (1976) *Principles of Clinical Electrocardiography*, 9th edn. Los Altos: Lange.)

■ Broad and notched (> 0.12 s, i.e. 3 small squares) in left atrial enlargement ('P mitrale', e.g. mitral stenosis)
■ Tall and peaked (> 2.5 mm) in right atrial enlargement ('P pulmonale', e.g. pulmonary hypertension)
■ Replaced by flutter or fibrillation waves (p. 414)
■ Absent in sinoatrial block (p. 409).

The *QRS complex* represents ventricular depolarization:

■ A negative (downward) deflection preceding an R wave is called a Q wave. Normal Q waves are small and narrow; deep (> 2 mm), wide (> 1 mm) Q waves (except in AVR and V_1) indicate myocardial infarction (p. 443).
■ A deflection upwards is called an R wave whether or not it is preceded by a Q wave.
■ A negative deflection following an R wave is termed an S wave.

Ventricular depolarization starts in the septum and spreads from left to right (Fig. 9.3). Subsequently the main free walls of the ventricles are depolarized. Thus, in the right ventricular leads (V_1 and V_2) the first deflection is upwards (R wave) as the septal depolarization wave spreads towards those leads. The second deflection is downwards (S wave) as the bigger left ventricle (in which depolarization is spreading away) outweighs the effect of the right ventricle (see Fig. 9.4). The opposite pattern is seen in the left ventricular leads (V_5 and V_6), with an initial downwards deflection (small Q wave reflecting septal depolarization) followed by a large R wave caused by left ventricular depolarization.

Left ventricular hypertrophy. The increased bulk of the left ventricular myocardium in left ventricular hypertrophy (e.g. with systemic hypertension) increases the voltage-induced depolarization of the free wall of the left ventricle. This gives rise to tall R waves (> 25 mm) in the left ventricular leads (V_5, V_6) and/or deep S waves (> 30 mm) in the right ventricular leads (V_1, V_2). The sum of the R wave in the left ventricular leads and the S wave in the right ventricular leads exceeds 40 mm. In addition to these changes there may also be ST-segment depression and T wave flattening or inversion in the left ventricular leads.

Right ventricular hypertrophy (e.g. in pulmonary hypertension) causes tall R waves in the right ventricular leads.

The QRS duration reflects the time that excitation takes to spread through the ventricle. A wide QRS complex (> 0.10 s, 2.5 small squares) occurs if conduction is delayed, e.g. with right or left bundle branch block, or if conduction is through a pathway other than the right and left bundle branches, e.g. an impulse generated by an abnormal focus of activity in the ventricle (ventricular ectopic).

T waves result from ventricular repolarization. In general the direction of the T wave is the same as that of the QRS complex. Inverted T waves occur in many conditions and, although usually abnormal, they are a non-specific finding.

The *PR interval* is measured from the start of the P wave to the start of the QRS complex whether this is a Q wave or an R wave. It is the time taken for excitation to pass from the sinus node, through the atrium, atrioventricular node and His–Purkinje system to the ventricle. A prolonged PR interval (> 0.22 s) indicates heart block (p. 410).

The *ST segment* is the period between the end of the QRS complex and the start of the T wave. ST elevation (> 1 mm above the isoelectric line) occurs in the early stages of myocardial infarction (p. 443) and with acute pericarditis. ST segment depression (> 0.5 mm below the isoelectric line) indicates myocardial ischaemia.

The *QT interval* extends from the start of the QRS complex to the end of the T wave. It is primarily a measure of the time taken for repolarization of the ventricular myocardium, which is dependent on heart rate (shorter at faster heart rates). The QT interval is therefore corrected for heart rate (QT_c) and normally is ≤ 0.44 s. The long QT syndrome may be congenital or acquired (hypokalaemia or hypomagnesaemia, drugs e.g. quinidine, sotalol, chlorpromazine) and is associated with an increased risk of torsades de pointes ventricular tachycardia (p. 420) and sudden death.

$$QT_c = QT \text{ interval} \div \text{Square root of the RR interval}$$
(in seconds) (▦ QC 9.1)

The *cardiac axis* refers to the overall direction of the wave of ventricular depolarization in the vertical plane measured from a zero reference point (Fig. 9.7). The normal range for the cardiac axis is between $-30°$ and $+90°$. An axis more negative than $-30°$ is termed left axis deviation whereas an axis more positive than $+90°$ is termed right axis deviation. A simple method to calculate the axis is by inspection of the QRS complex in leads I, II and III. The axis is normal if leads I and II are positive; there is right axis deviation if lead I is negative and lead III positive, and left axis deviation if lead I is positive and leads II and III negative. Left axis deviation occurs due to a block of the anterior bundle of the main left bundle conducting system (p. 399), inferior myocardial infarction and the Wolff–Parkinson–White syndrome. Right axis deviation may be normal and occurs in conditions in which there is right ventricular overload, dextrocardia, Wolff–Parkinson–White syndrome and left posterior hemiblock.

Exercise electrocardiography (*K&C* 6e p. 746)

This is a technique used to assess the cardiac response to exercise. The 12-lead ECG is recorded whilst the patient walks or runs on a motorized treadmill, and the test should be performed according to a standardized method (e.g. the Bruce protocol). Myocardial ischaemia provoked by exertion results in ST segment depression (> 1 mm) in leads facing the affected area of ischaemic cardiac muscle. During an exercise test the blood pressure and rhythm responses to exercise are also assessed. Exercise normally causes an increase in heart rate and blood pressure. A sustained fall in

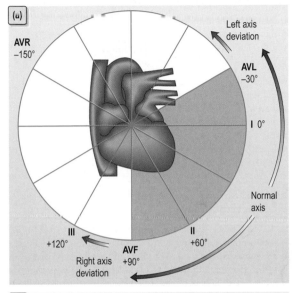

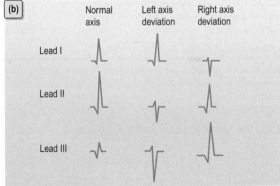

Fig. 9.7 Cardiac vectors. **(a) The hexaxial reference system**, illustrating the six leads in the frontal plane, e.g. lead I is 0°, lead II is +60°, lead III is 120°. **(b)** ECG leads showing the predominant positive and negative deflection with axis deviation.

blood pressure usually indicates severe coronary artery disease. A slow recovery of the heart rate to basal levels has also been reported to be a predictor of mortality. Contra-indications include recent myocardial infarction (within 6 days), unstable angina, severe hypertrophic cardiomyo-pathy, severe aortic stenosis and malignant hypertension. A positive test and indications for stopping the test are:

- Chest pain
- ST segment depression or elevation > 1 mm
- Fall in systolic blood pressure > 20 mmHg
- Fall in heart rate despite an increase in workload
- BP > 240/110
- Significant arrhythmias or increased frequency of ventricular ectopics.

24-Hour ambulatory taped (Holter) electrocardiography

A 12-lead ECG is recorded continuously over a 24-hour period and is used to record transient changes such as a brief paroxysm of tachycardia, an occasional pause in rhythm or intermittent ST segment shifts. *Event recording* is used to record less frequent arrhythmias in which the patient triggers ECG recording at the time of symptoms. They are both outpatient investigations.

Echocardiography (*K&C* 6e p. 749)

This is a non-invasive method of recording the position and motion of the structures of the heart by echo obtained from beams of ultrasonic waves directed at a particular region of the heart.

- *Transthoracic echo* involves the placement of a handheld transducer on the chest wall. Ultrasound pulses are emitted through various body tissues, and reflected waves are detected by the transducer as an echo. The commonest reasons for undertaking an echocardiogram are to assess left ventricular function in patients with symptoms suggestive of left heart failure, or to assess valvular disease. Left ventricular function is assessed by the ejection fraction, which is the percentage of blood ejected from the left ventricle with each heart beat and normally is more than 50%.

- *Transoesophageal echo* uses miniaturized transducers incorporated into special endoscopes. It allows better visualization of some structures and pathology, e.g. aortic dissection, prosthetic valve endocarditis.
- *Doppler echocardiography* uses the Doppler principle (in this case, the frequency of ultrasonic waves reflected from blood cells is related to their velocity and direction of flow) to identify and assess the severity of valve lesions.
- *Stress (exercise or pharmacological) echocardiography* is used to assess myocardial wall motion as a surrogate for coronary artery perfusion. It is used in the detection of coronary artery disease, assessment of risk post-myocardial infarction and perioperatively, and in patients in whom routine exercise testing is non-diagnostic. For those who cannot exercise, pharmacological intervention with dobutamine is used to increase myocardial oxygen demand.

Cardiac nuclear imaging (*K&C* 6e p. 755)

Nuclear imaging is used to detect myocardial infarction or to measure myocardial function, perfusion or viability, depending on the radiopharmaceutical used and the technique of imaging. A variety of radiotracers can be injected intravenously and these diffuse freely into myocardial tissue or attach to red blood cells.

Thallium-201 is taken up by cardiac myocytes. Ischaemic areas (produced by exercising the patient) with reduced tracer uptake are seen as 'cold spots' when imaged with a γ camera.

Technetium-99m is used to label red blood cells and produce images of the left ventricle during systole and diastole.

Cardiac catheterization (*K&C* 6e p. 757)

A small catheter is passed through a peripheral vein (for study of right-sided heart structures) or artery (for study of left-sided heart structures) into the heart, permitting the securing of blood samples, measurement of intracardiac pressures and determination of cardiac anomalies. Specially designed catheters are then used to selectively engage the left and right coronary arteries, and contrast cine-angiograms are taken in order to define the coronary circulation and identify the presence and severity of any coronary artery disease.

Cardiovascular magnetic resonance (CMR) (K&C 6e p. 758)

This is a non-invasive imaging technique that does not involve harmful radiation. It is increasingly utilized in cardiology to provide both anatomical and functional information.

CARDIAC ARRHYTHMIAS (K&C 6e p. 764)

An abnormality of cardiac rhythm is called a cardiac arrhythmia. Arrhythmia may cause sudden death, syncope, dizziness, palpitations or no symptoms at all.

Paroxysmal arrhythmias may not be detected on a single ECG recording. Twenty-four-hour ambulatory ECG monitoring and event recorders (p. 406) are often used to detect arrhythmias causing intermittent symptoms.

There are two main types of arrhythmia:

- *Bradycardia,* where the heart rate is slow (< 60 beats/min). Slower heart rates are more likely to cause symptomatic arrhythmias.

- *Tachycardia,* where the heart rate is fast (> 100 beats/min). Tachycardias are more likely to be symptomatic when the arrhythmia is fast and sustained. They are subdivided into *supraventricular tachycardias* (SVTs), which arise from the atrium or the atrioventricular junction, and *ventricular tachycardias,* which arise from the ventricles.

Arrhythmias and conduction disturbances complicating acute myocardial infarction are discussed on page 448.

General principles of management of arrhythmias

Patients with adverse symptoms and signs (ongoing chest pain, low cardiac output with cold clammy extremities, hypotension, impaired consciousness, and severe pulmonary oedema) require urgent treatment of their arrhythmia. Oxygen is given to all patients, intravenous access established and serum electrolyte abnormalities (potassium, magnesium, calcium) are corrected.

Sinus rhythms (K&C 6e p. 764)

Sinus arrhythmia

Fluctuations of autonomic tone result in phasic changes in the sinus discharge rate. During inspiration parasympathetic tone falls and the heart rate quickens, and on expiration the heart rate falls. This variation is normal, particularly in children and young adults, and typically results in a regularly irregular pulse.

Sinus bradycardia

Sinus bradycardia is normal during sleep and in well-trained athletes. During the acute phase of a myocardial infarction it often reflects ischaemia of the sinus node. Other causes include hypothermia, hypothyroidism, cholestatic jaundice, raised intracranial pressure, and drug therapy with β-blockers, digitalis and other antiarrhythmic drugs. Patients with persistent symptomatic bradycardia are treated with a permanent cardiac pacemaker. Intravenous atropine is used in the acute situation.

Sinus tachycardia

Sinus tachycardia is a physiological response during exercise and excitement. It may also occur with fever, anaemia, heart failure, thyrotoxicosis and drugs (e.g. catecholamines and atropine). Treatment is aimed at correction of the underlying cause. If necessary, β-blockers may be used to slow the sinus rate, e.g. in hyperthyroidism.

Pathological bradycardias (K&C 6e p. 766)

Bradycardias may be due to sinus node dysfunction (failure of impulse formation) or atrioventricular block (failure of impulse conduction from the atria to the ventricles). Bradycardia also occurs during a vasovagal attack (fainting, p. 697).

Sinus node dysfunction

Most cases of chronic sinus node dysfunction are the result of idiopathic fibrosis occurring in elderly people (sick sinus syndrome). Bradycardia is caused by intermittent failure of sinus node depolarization (sinus arrest) or failure of the sinus impulse to propagate through the perinodal tissue to the atria (sinoatrial block). This is seen on the ECG as intermittent long pauses between consecutive P waves (> 2 s). The slow heart rate predisposes to ectopic pacemaker activity and tachyarrhythmias are common (tachy–brady syndrome).

Insertion of a permanent pacemaker is only indicated in symptomatic patients to prevent dizzy spells and black-outs. Antiarrhythmic drugs are used to treat tachycardias. Thromboembolism is common in sinus node dysfunction and patients are anticoagulated unless there is a contra-indication.

Atrioventricular block

The common causes of atrioventricular block are coronary artery disease, cardiomyopathy and, particularly in elderly people, fibrosis of the conducting tissue.

There are three forms:

■ *First-degree atrioventricular (AV) block* is the result of delayed atrioventricular conduction and reflected by a prolonged PR interval (> 0.22 s) on the ECG. No change in heart rate occurs and treatment is unnecessary.

■ *Second-degree (partial) AV block* occurs when some atrial impulses fail to reach the ventricles. There are several forms (Fig. 9.8):

  - Mobitz type 1 block (Wenckebach block phenomenon) is progressive PR interval prolongation until a P wave fails to conduct, i.e. absent QRS after the P wave. The PR interval then returns to normal and the cycle repeats itself.

  - Mobitz type II block occurs when a dropped QRS complex is not preceded by progressive PR prolongation.

  - A 2 : 1 or 3 : 1 block occurs when only every second or third P wave conducts to the ventricles. A 4 : 1 or 5 : 1 block can also occur.

  Progression to complete heart block occurs more frequently following anterior myocardial infarction and in Mobitz type II block, and treatment with pacing is usually indicated. Patients with Wenckebach AV block or those with second-degree block following acute inferior infarction are usually monitored.

■ *Third-degree AV block (complete heart block).* There is no association between atrial and ventricular activity and ventricular contractions are maintained by a spontaneous escape rhythm (usually about 40/min) from an automatic centre below the site of the block. The ECG shows regular P waves and QRS complexes which occur independently of one another. The usual symptoms are dizziness and blackouts (Stokes–Adams attacks). If the ventricular rate is very slow, heart failure may occur. Insertion of a

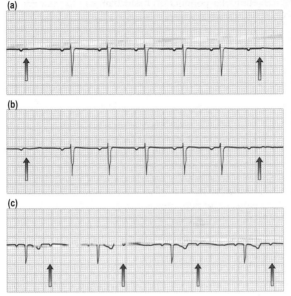

Fig. 9.8 **Three varieties of second-degree atrioventricular
(AV) block. (a)** Wenckebach (Mobitz type I) AV block. The PR
interval gradually prolongs until the P wave does not conduct to
the ventricles (arrows). **(b)** Mobitz type II AV block. The P waves
that do not conduct to the ventricles (arrows) are not preceded
by gradual PR interval prolongation. **(c)** Two P waves to each
QRS complex. The PR interval prior to the dropped P wave is
always the same. It is not possible to define this type of AV block
as type I or type II Mobitz block and it is, therefore, a third variety
of second-degree AV block (arrows show P waves), not
conducted to the ventricles.

permanent pacemaker is always required for sustained
complete heart block. In the acute situation, e.g. myocardial infarction, recovery may be expected and a
temporary transvenous pacing wire is only necessary for
patients with adverse symptoms and signs (p. 408) or
who are at risk of asystole (wide QRS complexes,
ventricular pauses of > 3 s). Interim measures before
placement of the wire include administration of atropine
(500 µg i.v. repeating to a maximum of 3 mg) or
transcutaneous external pacing.

Intraventricular conduction disturbances

Complete block of a bundle branch (p. 397 and Fig. 9.3) is associated with a wide QRS complex (0.12 s or more) with an abnormal pattern. The shape of the QRS depends on whether the right or the left bundle is blocked. In right bundle branch block (RBBB) the right bundle branch no longer conducts an impulse and the two ventricles do not receive an impulse simultaneously. There is sequential spread of an impulse (i.e. first the left ventricle and then the right) resulting in a secondary R wave (RSR') in V1 and a slurred S wave in V5 and V6. The opposite is true in LBBB with an RSR' pattern in the left ventricular leads (I, AVL, V4–V6) and deep slurred S waves in V1 and V2. RBBB occurs in normal healthy individuals, pulmonary embolus, right ventricular hypertrophy and ischaemic heart disease. LBBB indicates underlying cardiac pathology and occurs in ischaemic heart disease, left ventricular hypertrophy, aortic valve disease and following cardiac surgery.

Pathological tachycardias

Tachyarrhythmias can be divided into two broad categories: supraventricular (SVT) and ventricular (VT). VT gives rise to a broad complex (QRS complex > 120 ms) tachycardia. SVT may be narrow complex (QRS < 120 ms) or broad complex if coupled with bundle branch block.

Mechanisms of arrhythmia production

Most tachyarrhythmias are a result of abnormal automaticity or atrioventricular nodal re-entry.

- *Abnormal automaticity* arises if there is enhanced automaticity of the normal conducting tissue or automaticity is acquired by damaged cells of the atria or ventricles; this causes ectopic beats and, if sustained, tachyarrhythmias.
- *Re-entry* may occur if there are two separate pathways for impulse conduction (Fig. 9.9).

Supraventricular tachycardia

Atrial tachyarrhythmias (*K&C* 6e p. 773)

Atrial fibrillation, atrial flutter, atrial tachycardia and atrial ectopic beats all arise from the atrial myocardium. They share common aetiologies, which are listed in Table 9.3.

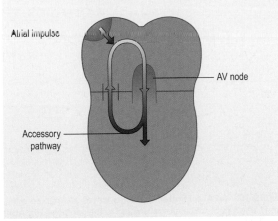

Fig. 9.9 **A re-entry circuit.** The impulse is conducted normally through the AV node and initiates ventricular depolarization. In certain circumstances the accessory pathway is able to transmit the impulse retrogradely back into the atria, thus completing a circuit and initiating a self-sustaining re-entry tachycardia.

Table 9.3 **Causes of atrial arrhythmias**

Ischaemic heart disease
Rheumatic heart disease
Thyrotoxicosis
Cardiomyopathy
Lone atrial fibrillation (i.e. no cause discovered)
Wolff–Parkinson–White syndrome
Pneumonia
Atrial septal defect
Carcinoma of the bronchus
Pericarditis
Pulmonary embolus
Acute and chronic alcohol abuse
Cardiac surgery

Atrial fibrillation (AF) (*K&C* 6e p. 773)

This is a common arrhythmia, occurring in 5–10% of patients over 65 years of age. It also occurs, particularly in a paroxysmal form, in younger patients. Atrial activity is

(a)

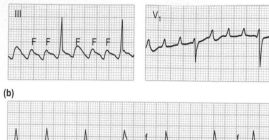

(b)

Fig. 9.10 **(a) Atrial flutter.** The flutter waves are marked with an F, only half of which are transmitted to the ventricles. **(b) Atrial fibrillation.** There are no P waves; the ventricular response is fast and irregular.

chaotic and mechanically ineffective. The AV node conducts a proportion of the atrial impulses to produce an irregular ventricular response. In some patients it is an incidental finding; in others symptoms range from palpitations and fatigue to acute pulmonary oedema. There are no clear P waves on the ECG (Fig. 9.10b), only a fine oscillation of the baseline (so-called fibrillation or f waves).

Management

When AF is caused by an acute precipitating event, such as alcohol toxicity, chest infection or thyrotoxicosis, the underlying cause should be treated initially. Patients with adverse symptoms and signs (see above) require immediate heparinization and attempted cardioversion with a synchronized DC shock (p. 804). If cardioversion fails or AF recurs, amiodarone 300 mg is given over 1 hour before a further attempt at cardioversion. A second dose of amiodarone can be given.

In patients without adverse symptoms and signs and in whom AF arises in an apparently normal heart it is sometimes possible to convert to sinus rhythm, either electrically (by cardioversion, p. 804) or chemically (with class Ic or III drugs – Table 9.4).

Table 9.4 Vaughan Williams' classification of antiarrhythmic drug therapy

Class	Mechanism of action	Individual drugs
I	Membrane-stabilizing action	
Ia		Disopyramide, procainamide, quinidine
Ib		Lidocaine (lignocaine), mexiletine
Ic		Flecainide, propafenone
II	β-Adrenergic blockers	Metoprolol, atenolol, propranolol
III	Prolong action potential	Amiodarone, sotalol
IV	Calcium-channel blocking agents	Verapamil, diltiazem
Other		Adenosine, digoxin

These drugs all have proarrhythmic side-effects (among others) and should be used with caution
All except amiodarone are negatively inotropic and may exacerbate heart failure

Strategies for the long-term management of atrial fibrillation include:

- Maintenance of sinus rhythm with antiarrhythmic drugs after cardioversion

- Rate control and consideration of anticoagulation (e.g. β-blockers/verapamil/digoxin and warfarin).

Atrial fibrillation is associated with an increased risk of thromboembolism, and anticoagulation with warfarin should be given for at least 3 weeks before (with the exception of those who require immediate cardioversion) and 4 weeks after cardioversion. Most patients with chronic AF should also be anticoagulated (INR 2.0–3.0). The exception is young patients (< 65 years) with lone AF, i.e. in the absence of demonstrable cardiac disease, diabetes or hypertension. This group has a low incidence of thromboembolism and is treated with aspirin alone.

Atrial flutter (*K&C* 6e p. 775)
Atrial flutter is often associated with atrial fibrillation and usually associated with organic disease of the heart. The atrial rate is usually 300 beats/min. The AV node usually

conducts every second flutter beat, giving a ventricular rate of 150 beats/min. The ECG (Fig. 9.10a) characteristically shows 'sawtooth' flutter waves (F waves), which are most clearly seen when AV conduction is transiently impaired by carotid sinus massage or drugs. Treatment of an acute paroxysm is electrical synchronized cardioversion (p. 804). Prophylaxis is achieved with class Ic or III drugs (Table 9.4). Rate control of a chronic arrhythmia is with AV nodal blocking drugs, e.g. β-blockers or digoxin. Recurrent atrial flutter is best treated with radiofrequency catheter ablation of focal arrhythmogenic sites.

Atrial ectopic beats (K&C 6e p. 776)

These are caused by premature discharge of an ectopic atrial focus. On the ECG this produces an early and abnormal P wave, usually followed by a normal QRS complex. Treatment is not usually required unless they cause troublesome palpitations or are responsible for provoking more significant arrhythmias when β-blockade may be effective.

Atrioventricular junctional tachycardias

In these tachycardias the AV node is an essential part of the re-entry circuit. They are often seen in young patients with no evidence of structural heart disease.

Atrioventricular nodal reciprocating tachycardia (AVNRT) is the commonest type of SVT. It is due to the presence of two functionally and anatomically distinct conducting pathways in the atrioventricular (AV) node. One of these is fast-conducting, the other slow-conducting. During an episode of SVT one of these acts as the antegrade limb of a re-entry circuit, while the other acts as the retrograde limb. AVNRT is the most common form of SVT. The usual history is of a sudden onset of fast (140–280/min) regular palpitations. On the ECG the P waves may be seen very close to the QRS complex, or are not seen at all. The QRS complex is usually of normal shape because the ventricles are activated in the normal way, down the bundle of His. Occasionally the QRS complex is wide, because of a rate-related bundle branch block, and it may be difficult to distinguish from ventricular tachycardia.

Atrioventricular reciprocating tachycardia (AVRT) is due to the presence of an accessory pathway that connects the atria and ventricles, but that lies outside the AV node.

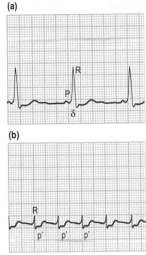

Fig. 9.11 **(a) An ECG showing Wolff–Parkinson–White syndrome.** There is an abnormal connection, termed an accessory pathway, between the atria and ventricles. The accessory pathway has a more rapid rate of conduction from the atria to the ventricles than does the normal AV node and ventricular depolarization occurs sooner than expected. Such pre-excitation is apparent on the ECG during sinus rhythm as a short PR interval and wide QRS complex with a 'slurred' upstroke (δ wave). **(b) A trace demonstrating the paroxysmal tachycardia which may result from this syndrome.** Note the tachycardia p wave visible between QRS and T wave complexes.

Accessory pathways may be capable of antegrade or retrograde conduction, or both. Wolff–Parkinson–White (WPW) syndrome is the best-known type of AVRT in which there is an accessory pathway (bundle of Kent) between atria and ventricles (Fig. 9.11). The resting ECG in WPW shows evidence of the pathway's existence if the path allows some of the atrial depolarization to pass quickly to the ventricle before it gets though the AV node. The early depolarization of part of the ventricle leads to a shortened PR interval and a slurred start to the QRS (delta wave). The QRS is narrow.

Acute management

Emergency cardioversion is required in patients whose arrhythmia is accompanied by adverse symptoms and signs (p. 408).

In the haemodynamically stable patient, manoeuvres that increase vagal stimulation of the sinus node such as the Valsalva manoeuvre (ask the patient to blow into a 20-mL syringe with enough force to push back the plunger), carotid sinus massage (contraindicated in the presence of a carotid bruit), or ocular pressure should be attempted.

Drug treatment is used if physical manoeuvres are ineffective: Adenosine is a very short-acting AV nodal-blocking drug given as a 3-mg bolus dose intravenously. It will terminate most junctional tachycardias. If there is no response after 1–2 minutes, a further bolus of 6 mg is given. Up to three boluses of 12 mg each at 1- to 2-minute intervals may be given if there is still no response. Transient side-effects include complete heart block, hypotension, broncho-spasm, nausea, flushing and chest discomfort. The patient should be warned in advance to expect the latter three. Asthma and second- or third-degree AV block are contraindications to adenosine. An alternative treatment is intravenous verapamil 5–10 mg i.v. over 5–10 minutes (contraindicated if the QRS complex is wide and therefore differentiation from ventricular tachycardia difficult). Other treatments of the tachycardia are with type Ic agents (propafenone or flecainide) or type Ia agents (procainamide or quinidine). Digoxin, verapamil, and diltiazem are contraindicated in the presence of AF and an accessory pathway as they block the AV node but not the accessory pathway and will exacerbate the arrhythmia.

Long-term managements

- Radiofrequency ablation of the accessory pathway via a cardiac catheter is successful in about 95% of cases.
- Flecainide, disopyramide, amiodarone and β-blockers are the drugs most commonly used.

Ventricular arrhythmias (K&C 6e p. 776)

Ventricular ectopic beats (extrasystoles, premature beats) (K&C 6e p. 779)

Ventricular ectopic beats may be asymptomatic or patients may complain of extra beats, missed beats or heavy beats.

418

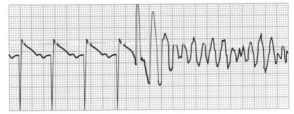

Fig. 9.12 **A rhythm strip demonstrating four beats of sinus rhythm followed by a ventricular ectopic beat that initiates ventricular fibrillation.** The ST segment is elevated owing to acute myocardial infarction.

The ectopic electrical activity is not conducted to the ventricles through the normal conducting tissue and thus the QRS complex on the ECG is widened, with a bizarre configuration (Fig. 9.12). In normal individuals ectopic beats are of no significance, but treatment is sometimes given for symptoms. In patients with heart disease they are associated with an increased risk of sudden death. Prophylaxis with amiodarone may reduce mortality by preventing arrhythmias and sudden death.

Ventricular tachycardia (*K&C* 6e p. 776)
Ventricular tachycardia and ventricular fibrillation are usually associated with underlying heart disease, e.g. ischaemia, cardiomyopathy and hypertensive heart disease. Ventricular tachycardia is defined as three or more consecutive ventricular beats occurring at a rate of 120/min or more. The ECG shows a rapid ventricular rhythm with broad abnormal QRS complexes, which can sometimes be confused with a broad complex junctional tachycardia. Urgent DC cardioversion is necessary if there are adverse symptoms or signs with arrhythmia (p. 408). If there is no haemodynamic compromise, treatment is usually with intravenous lidocaine (lignocaine) (50–100 mg i.v. over 5 min followed by an intravenous infusion of 2–4 mg/min). Prophylaxis is with mexiletine, disopyramide, flecainide or amiodarone. Patients who are refractory to all medical treatment may need an implantable cardioverter–defibrillator (ICD). This is a small device implanted behind the rectus abdominis and connected to the heart; it recognizes ventricular tachycardia or ventricular fibrillation and automatically delivers a defibrillation shock to the heart.

Ventricular fibrillation (*K&C* 6e p. 776)

This is a very rapid and irregular ventricular activation (see Fig. 9.12) with no mechanical effect and hence no cardiac output. The patient is pulseless and becomes rapidly unconscious, and respiration ceases (cardiac arrest). Ventricular fibrillation rarely reverts spontaneously and management is immediate cardioversion (Emergency Box 9.1). Survivors of ventricular fibrillation are, in the absence of an identifiable reversible cause (e.g. acute myocardial infarction, severe metabolic disturbance), at high risk of sudden death. Implantable cardioverter–defibrillators are first-line therapy in the management of these patients.

Torsades de pointes (*K&C* 6e p. 777)

This uncommon arrhythmia is characterized by rapid irregular sharp QRS complexes that continuously change from an upright to an inverted position on the ECG. It arises when ventricular repolarization (QT interval) is greatly prolonged – the so-called long QT syndrome (p. 404). Torsades de pointes causes palpitations and syncope and usually terminates spontaneously. It can, however, degenerate to ventricular fibrillation and cause sudden death.

Cardiac arrest (*K&C* 6e p. 759)

In cardiac arrest there is no effective cardiac output. The patient is unconscious and apnoeic with absent arterial pulses (best felt in the carotid artery in the neck). Irreversible brain damage occurs within 3 minutes if an adequate circulation is not established. Management of a cardiac arrest is described in Emergency Box 9.1.

Prognosis of cardiac arrest In many patients resuscitation is unsuccessful, particularly in those who collapse out of hospital and are brought into hospital in an arrested state. In patients who are successfully resuscitated the prognosis is often poor because they have severe underlying heart disease. The exception is those who are successfully resuscitated from a ventricular fibrillation arrest in the early stages of myocardial infarction, when the prognosis is much the same as for other patients with an infarct.

Emergency Box 9.1
Basic life support (BLS)

- Call for help.
- Thump the chest firmly over the sternum; occasionally reverts VT/VF to sinus rhythm.

AIRWAY
- Place patient on his or her back on a firm surface.
- Remove obstructing material, e.g. blood and vomit.
- Open the airway by flexing the neck and extending the head.

BREATHING
- Give four breaths in quick succession of mouth-to-mouth resuscitation. Watch for the rise and fall of the patient's chest, indicating adequate ventilation.

CIRCULATION
- Circulation is achieved by external chest compression.
- The heel of one hand is placed over the lower half of the victim's sternum and the heel of the second hand is placed over the first with the fingers interlocked. With straight arms, the sternum is depressed by 4–5 cm (1–2 inches).
- Compressions : respiration in a ratio of 30 : 2 with 100 compressions per minute.

Advanced life support (ALS)
- Institute as soon as help arrives; continue cardiac massage throughout except during defibrillation.
- Defibrillate immediately (ventricular fibrillation is the most common arrhythmia in cardiac arrest).
- Give 100% O_2 via Ambu-bag, intubate as soon as possible and initiate positive-pressure ventilation.
- Establish intravenous access and connect ECG leads.
- Drugs administered by the peripheral route should be followed by a flush of 20 mL of 0.9% saline.
- If intravenous access not possible, give drugs via endotracheal tube (3 × intravenous dose) diluted to 10 mL with 0.9% saline.

Universal advanced life-support algorithm*

Continued

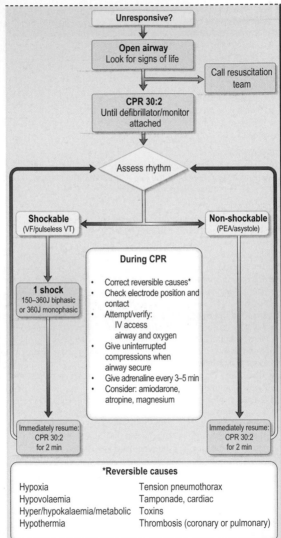

*Reproduced by permission of the European Resuscitation Council and Laerdal Medical Ltd

CPR, cardiopulmonary resuscitation; PEA, pulseless electrical activity (loss of a palpable pulse in the presence of recordable electrical activity); VF/VT, ventricular fibrillation/ventricular tachycardia

HEART FAILURE (*K&C* 6e p. 784)

Heart failure is a complex syndrome that can result from any structural or functional cardiac disorder that impairs the ability of the heart to function as a pump and maintain sufficient cardiac output to meet the demands of the body. It is a common condition, with an estimated annual incidence of 10% in patients over 65 years. The long-term outcome is poor and approximately 50% of patients are dead within 5 years.

Aetiology

The causes of heart failure are given in Table 9.5. Ischaemic heart disease is the commonest cause in western countries. Any factor that increases myocardial work may aggravate existing heart failure or initiate failure. These include arrhythmias, anaemia, thyrotoxicosis, pregnancy and obesity.

Pathophysiology

When the heart fails, compensatory mechanisms attempt to maintain cardiac output and peripheral perfusion. However, as heart failure progresses the mechanisms are over-whelmed and become pathophysiological. These mechanisms involve the following.

Table 9.5 **Causes of heart failure**

Main causes
Ischaemic heart disease
Dilated cardiomyopathy
Systemic hypertension

Other causes
Cardiomyopathy (hypertrophic, restrictive)
Valvular heart disease (mitral, aortic, tricuspid)
Congenital heart disease (atrial septal defect, ventricular septal defect)
Alcohol
Chemotherapeutic drugs
Hyperdynamic circulation (anaemia, thyrotoxicosis, Paget's disease)
Right heart failure (RV infarct, pulmonary hypertension, pulmonary embolism, cor pulmonale, COPD)
Severe bradycardia or tachycardia
Pericardial disease (constrictive pericarditis, pericardial effusion)

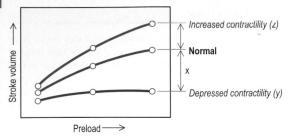

Fig. 9.13 **The Starling curve.** Starling's law states that the
stroke volume is directly proportional to the diastolic filling (i.e.
the preload or ventricular end-diastolic pressure). As the preload
is increased, the stroke volume rises (normal). Increasing
contractility (e.g. increased with sympathetic stimulation) shifts
the curve upwards and to the left (z). If the ventricle is
overstretched the stroke volume will fall (x). In heart failure (y) the
ventricular function curve is relatively flat so that increasing the
preload has only a small effect on cardiac output.

Sympathetic nervous system Activation of the
sympathetic nervous system improves ventricular function
by increasing heart rate and myocardial contractility.
Constriction of venous capacitance vessels redistributes
flow centrally, and the increased venous return to the heart
(preload) further augments ventricular function via the
Starling mechanism (Fig. 9.13). Sympathetic stimulation,
however, also leads to arteriolar constriction, this increasing
the afterload which would eventually reduce cardiac
output.

Renin–angiotensin system The fall in cardiac output
and increased sympathetic tone lead to diminished renal
perfusion, activation of the renin–angiotensin system, and
hence increased fluid retention. Salt and water retention
further increases venous pressure and maintains stroke
volume by the Starling mechanism (Fig. 9.13). As salt and
water retention increases, however, peripheral and
pulmonary congestion cause oedema and contribute to
dyspnoea. Angiotensin II also causes arteriolar constriction,
thus increasing the afterload and the work of the heart.

Natriuretic peptides are released from the atria (atrial
natriuretic peptide, ANP), ventricles (BNP – so called

because it was first discovered in the brain) and vascular endothelium (C-type peptide). They have diuretic, natriuretic and hypotensive properties. The effect of their action may represent a beneficial, albeit inadequate, compensatory response leading to reduced cardiac load (preload and afterload).

Ventricular dilatation Myocardial failure leads to a reduction of the volume of blood ejected with each heart-beat, and thus an increase in the volume of blood remaining after systole. The increased diastolic volume stretches the myocardial fibres and, as Starling's law would suggest, myocardial contraction is restored. Once heart failure is established, however, the compensatory effects of cardiac dilatation become limited by the flattened contour of Starling's curve. Eventually the increased venous pressure contributes to the development of pulmonary and peripheral oedema. In addition, as ventricular diameter increases, greater tension is required in the myocardium to expel a given volume of blood, and oxygen requirements increase.

Clinical features

It is clinically useful to divide heart failure into the syndromes of right, left and biventricular (congestive) heart failure, but it is rare for any one part of the heart to fail in isolation. Biventricular heart failure is the most common manifestation of heart failure.

425

Left heart failure The most common cause of left heart failure is ischaemic heart disease. Other causes are systemic hypertension, mitral and aortic valve disease and cardiomyopathies. Mitral stenosis causes the signs of left heart failure but does not itself cause failure of the left ventricle. The clinical features are largely the result of pulmonary congestion, with symptoms of fatigue, exertional dyspnoea, orthopnoea and paroxysmal nocturnal dyspnoea (p. 395). Physical signs include tachypnoea, tachycardia, a displaced apex beat and basal lung crackles. A third heart sound occurs and is the result of rapid filling of the ventricles. In severe failure, dilatation of the mitral annulus results in functional mitral regurgitation.

Right heart failure The most frequent cause of chronic right heart failure is secondary to left heart failure. Other causes are indicated in Table 9.5. There is jugular venous distension, hepatomegaly and dependent pitting oedema (over the ankles and calves in ambulant patients, over the sacrum in bed-bound patients). Less frequently ascites or pleural effusions occur. Dilatation of the right ventricle may give rise to functional tricuspid incompetence, with giant 'V' waves in the JVP and a tender pulsatile liver. Non-specific features include fatigue, anorexia and nausea.

Biventricular failure (congestive) This term is used variously but is best restricted to cases where right heart failure is a result of pre-existing left heart failure. The physical signs are thus a combination of the above syndromes.

Systolic versus diastolic heart failure Systolic ventricular dysfunction is most commonly due to coronary artery disease. The left ventricle is dilated and fails to contract normally. In diastolic dysfunction there is impaired myocardial relaxation and left ventricular filling is impaired; left ventricular systolic function is normal (defined as a left ventricular ejection fraction > 50%, see p. 406 for definition). About one-third of patients with heart failure have diastolic dysfunction, and it is most common in the elderly. Coronary artery disease, hypertension with left ventricular hypertrophy, hypertrophic cardiomyopathy and restrictive cardiomyopathy are the major causes of diastolic heart failure. Presentation and management are similar to systolic heart failure but there may be an additional place for calcium-channel blockers.

Acute heart failure This is a medical emergency, with left or right heart failure developing over minutes or hours. It most commonly occurs in the setting of myocardial infarction and can also occur following an acute pulmonary embolus or cardiac tamponade.

Investigations

The investigation of patients with suspected heart failure is summarized in Figure 9.14. The underlying cause should be established in all patients.

■ *Chest X-ray* is usually unhelpful in determining the cause of heart failure, but shows cardiac enlargement (cardio-thoracic ratio > 50% on a postero-anterior chest film) and characteristic appearances in left heart failure (Fig. 9.1). The chest X-ray can be normal.

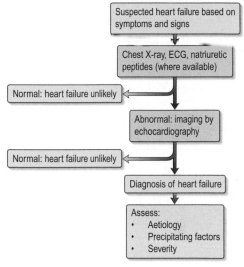

Fig. 9.14 Algorithm for the diagnosis of heart failure.

- *ECG* may show evidence of underlying causes, e.g. arrhythmias, ischaemia, left ventricular hypertrophy in hypertension.
- *Blood tests*. These include full blood count (to look for anaemia which may exacerbate heart failure), liver biochemistry (may be altered due to hepatic congestion), blood glucose (for diabetes), urea and electrolytes (as a baseline before starting diuretics and ACE inhibitors), and sometimes thyroid function tests.
- *Two-dimensional and Doppler echocardiography* is performed in all patients with new onset heart failure. It allows an assessment of ventricular systolic and diastolic function, and may reveal the aetiology of heart failure (valve disease, regional wall motion abnormalities in ischaemic heart disease, cardiomyopathy, pericardial disease). An ejection fraction of < 0.45 is usually accepted as evidence for systolic dysfunction.
- *Natriuretic peptide*. BNP or the N terminal fragment (NTproBNP) released from pro-BNP can be used to distinguish heart failure from other causes of dyspnoea. A normal plasma level excludes heart failure.

427

■ *Other investigations.* Cardiac catheterization, thallium perfusion imaging, PET scanning or dobutamine stress echocardiography (p. 407) may be of benefit in selected patients to identify those with *hibernating myocardium* (a region of impaired myocardial contractility due to persistently impaired coronary blood flow) in whom revascularization will improve left ventricular function and long-term prognosis.

Treatment of chronic heart failure

Treatment is aimed at relieving symptoms, retarding disease progression and improving survival (Table 9.6).

General treatment

During exacerbations of heart failure, bed rest is encouraged as it reduces the demands on the heart and promotes a diuresis. Low level endurance exercise is encouraged in compensated heart failure to reverse deconditioning of peripheral muscle metabolism. Large meals and alcohol should be avoided, smoking should be stopped and salt restriction encouraged. Drugs (NSAIDs, calcium-channel blockers, steroids) that worsen heart failure should be discontinued if possible. Patients should be offered influenza immunization.

Drug treatment

Vasodilator therapy   Vasodilators have a beneficial effect in heart failure by reducing venous constriction (reduction of preload) and/or arteriolar constriction (reduction of afterload).

■ *Angiotensin-converting enzyme inhibitors (ACEI),* e.g. captopril, enalapril, lisinopril and quinapril, inhibit the production of angiotensin II, a potent vasoconstrictor, and increase concentrations of the vasodilator bradykinin. They enhance renal salt and water excretion and increase cardiac output by reducing afterload. They improve symptoms, limit the development of progressive heart failure and prolong survival, and should be given to all patients with heart failure. The major side-effect is first-dose hypotension, which is a particular risk in those with severe heart failure receiving large doses of diuretics. Patients should stop potassium supplements and omit or reduce the dose of diuretics for 24 hours before the first dose of ACE inhibitor at bedtime. They should start with

Treatment of chronic heart failure

Table 9.6 **Summary of the management of chronic heart failure**

General measures*
Reduction of physical activity during exacerbations, thus
  reducing the work of the heart
Low-level exercise (20- to 30-min walks 3–5 times weekly)
  encouraged in patients with compensated heart failure
Dietary modification: weight reduction if necessary, no added
  salt diet
Stop smoking
Avoid alcohol, which has negative inotropic effects
Correct aggravating factors, e.g. arrhythmias, anaemia,
  hypertension, pulmonary infections
Vaccinate against pneumococcal disease and influenza
If possible discontinue aggravating drugs

Pharmacological treatment
ACE inhibitor (or angiotensin II receptor antagonist)*
β-Blocker
Diuretic*
Spironolactone
Digoxin
Vasodilators
Inotropic agents
Antiarrhythmic drugs

Non-pharmacological treatment
Revascularization (coronary artery bypass graft)
Biventricular pacing (selected patients not responding to drug
  treatment)
Replacement of diseased valves
Repair of congenital heart disease
Cardiac transplantation
Left ventricular assist device and artificial heart (bridge to
  transplantation)

---

*In all patients

429

a low dose followed by gradual increments every
1–2 weeks with a check on serum potassium and renal
function; creatinine levels normally rise by about 10–15%
during ACE inhibitor therapy. Other side-effects are
prerenal renal failure (p. 370), hyperkalaemia, rash, angio-
edema and persistent cough due to inhibition of bradykinin metabolism.

■ *Angiotensin II type 1 receptor antagonists (ARA)* (e.g. losartan,
  ibersartan, candesartan and valsartan) specifically block

the binding of angiotensin II to the type 1 receptor (AT1). In contrast, the ACE inhibitors inhibit production of angiotensin II and consequently diminish the activity of both AT1 and AT2 receptors. One important consequence of this difference is that angiotensin II receptor antagonists do not affect kinin metabolism and do not cause cough. Both ACE inhibitors and AII receptor antagonists are contraindicated in patients with bilateral renal artery stenosis.

■ *Other vasodilators.* The combination of isosorbide mononitrate (a vasodilator) and hydralazine (arteriolar vasodilator) improves symptoms and survival, and is used when ACE inhibitors or AII receptor antagonists are not tolerated or their use is contraindicated. Calcium-channel blockers, e.g. nifedipine, diltiazem, also reduce afterload but may have a detrimental effect on left ventricular function. The second-generation calcium antagonist amlodipine is safe in heart failure but not of prognostic benefit. Other vasodilators, used less commonly, include prazosin and nitroprusside.

β-blockers Metoprolol, bisoprolol and carvedilol improve symptoms and exercise tolerance in patients with chronic stable heart failure, in addition to improving mortality. This effect is thought to arise through blockade of the chronically activated sympathetic system. Beta-blocker treatment should be initiated in patients with confirmed heart failure due to left ventricular systolic dysfunction after ACE inhibitor therapy, regardless of whether or not symptoms persist. Following the administration of beta-blockers, the ejection fraction may decline, but usually returns to baseline within a month and then increases after 3 months.

Diuretics (Table 7.3, p. 313) are used in patients with signs of sodium and water retention (p. 312). They act by promoting renal sodium excretion, with enhanced water excretion as a secondary effect. The resulting loss of fluid reduces ventricular filling pressures (preload) and thus decreases pulmonary and systemic congestion.

■ *Loop diuretics*, e.g. furosemide (frusemide) and bumetanide, are potent diuretics used in moderate/severe heart failure. When given intravenously, they also induce arteriolar vasodilatation, a beneficial action independent of their diuretic effect.
■ *Thiazide diuretics*, e.g. bendroflumethiazide (bendro-

fluazide), are mild diuretics that inhibit sodium reabsorption in the distal renal tubule. The exception is metolazone, which causes a profound diuresis and is only used in severe and resistant heart failure.

■ *Potassium-sparing diuretics.* Spironolactone is a relatively weak diuretic with a potassium-sparing action. Low-dose spironolactone (25 mg daily) in combination with conventional treatment reduces all-cause mortality by 30% in patients with moderate to severe heart failure and should be given to all these patients. Amiloride and triamterene have a direct action on ion transport in the distal renal tubule and are useful in combination with loop diuretics. They increase renal sodium loss and reduce potassium loss but have not been shown to have a prognostic effect as yet.

Digoxin is of benefit in patients with congestive heart failure and atrial fibrillation. Digoxin is also used in patients in sinus rhythm who remain in severe heart failure despite standard treatment (vasodilators, β-blockers, diuretics).

Dopamine and dobutamine are intravenous adrenergic agonists and used in cardiogenic shock (p. 559).

Antiarrhythmic drugs Arrhythmias are frequent in heart failure and are implicated in sudden death, though the evidence that medical treatment of complex arrhythmias reduces mortality is conflicting. The insertion of an implantable cardioverter–defibrillator (ICD) may be the optimal treatment for patients who have experienced episodes of life-threatening arrhythmias.

Non-pharmacological treatment of heart failure

Revascularization Coronary artery disease is the most common cause of heart failure. Revascularization with angioplasty and stenting or surgery can result in improvement in regional abnormalities in wall motion in up to a third of patients and may thus have an important role to play in some individuals.

Biventricular pacemaker insertion improves symptoms and exercise tolerance in patients with severe heart failure and should be considered in highly symptomatic patients with systolic heart failure not responding to conventional medical therapy.

Cardiac transplantation (*K&C* 6e p. 796) This is the treatment of choice for younger patients with severe intractable heart failure. The expected 1-year survival following transplantation is over 90%, with 75% alive at 5 years. Death is usually the result of operative mortality, organ rejection and overwhelming infection secondary to immunosuppressive treatment. After this time the greatest threat to health is accelerated coronary atherosclerosis, the cause of which is unknown.

Prognosis

There is usually a gradual deterioration necessitating increased doses of diuretics, and sometimes admission to hospital. The prognosis is poor in those with severe heart failure (i.e. breathless at rest or on minimal exertion), with a 1-year survival rate of 50%.

Pulmonary oedema (*K&C* 6e p. 797)

This is a very frightening life-threatening emergency characterized by the rapid onset of extreme breathlessness. Causes include acute, severe left ventricular failure (e.g. myocardial infarction, acute mitral and aortic regurgitation), mitral stenosis and arrhythmias. An acute elevation of left atrial pressure produces corresponding elevation of the pulmonary capillary pressure and increased transudation of fluid into the pulmonary interstitium and alveoli (cardiogenic pulmonary oedema). *Non-cardiogenic pulmonary oedema* (acute lung injury) is seen in very ill patients and is discussed on page 567.

Clinical features

The patient is acutely breathless, wheezing and anxious. There is often a cough productive of frothy blood-tinged (pink) sputum. Increased sympathoadrenal activity leads to profuse sweating, tachycardia and peripheral circulatory shutdown. On auscultation there is a gallop rhythm, and wheezes and crackles are heard throughout the chest.

Investigations

■ Chest X-ray shows distension of the upper lobe veins (indicating a raised pulmonary venous pressure) and bilateral perihilar shadowing in a 'butterfly' or 'bat's

> ### Emergency Box 9.2
> ### Management of pulmonary oedema
>
> Sit the patient up.
> 60% oxygen by face mask.
> Furosemide (frusemide) 40–80 mg i.v.
> Morphine 2.5–10 mg i.v. + an antiemetic, e.g. metoclopramide
>   10 mg i.v.
>
> Consider:
>   Intravenous GTN infusion (50 mg in 50 mL 0.9% saline at
>   2–10 mL/h)
>   Intravenous aminophylline (250 mg over 10 min) to relieve
>   bronchospasm.
>
> Treat exacerbating and precipitating factors:
>   Hypertension
>   Pulmonary infection
>   Arrhythmias.
>
> Mechanical ventilation if no response to treatment.

wing' distribution caused by alveolar fluid. Interstitial pulmonary oedema produces Kerley B lines (see Fig. 9.1).
- ECG and cardiac enzymes may show evidence of a myocardial infarction as the precipitating event.

- Arterial blood gases show hypoxaemia. Initially the $P_a\mathrm{CO_2}$ falls because of overbreathing, but later increases because of impaired gas exchange.

Management

In many cases the patient is so unwell that treatment (Emergency Box 9.2) must begin before investigations are completed. Intravenous opiates, e.g. morphine, and diuretics, are the first-line agents. Morphine relieves dyspnoea by a combination of vasodilatation and relief of anxiety. Respiratory depression can occur with large doses (> 10 mg). Diuretics produce immediate vasodilatation with a reduction in preload, in addition to the more delayed diuretic response. If the patient does not improve and is not hypotensive, intravenous nitrates such as glyceryl trinitrate may be used to reduce the preload. Occasionally, in severe cases which do not respond to treatment, ventilation is necessary.

Cardiogenic shock (*K&C* 6e p. 797)

Cardiogenic shock (pump failure) is an extreme type of heart failure characterized by hypotension, a low cardiac output and signs of poor tissue perfusion, such as oliguria, cold extremities and poor cerebral function. The most common cause is massive myocardial infarction, and management is discussed on page 558.

ISCHAEMIC HEART DISEASE (*K&C* 6e p. 798)

Myocardial ischaemia results from an imbalance between the supply of oxygen to cardiac muscle and myocardial demand. The most common cause is coronary artery atheroma (coronary artery disease), which results in a fixed obstruction to coronary blood flow. Other causes of ischaemia include coronary artery thrombosis, spasm or, rarely, arteritis (e.g. polyarteritis). Increased demand for oxygen due to an increase in cardiac output may occur in thyrotoxicosis or myocardial hypertrophy (e.g. from aortic stenosis or hypertension).

Coronary artery disease (CAD) is the single largest cause of death in the UK, resulting in approximately 60 deaths per 100 000 population per year.

Atheroma consists of atherosclerotic plaques (seen postmortem as raised yellow-white areas covering the intimal surface of the artery) rich in cholesterol and other lipids, surrounded by smooth muscle cells and fibrous tissue. CAD gives rise to a wide variety of clinical presentations, ranging from stable angina to the acute coronary syndromes of unstable angina and myocardial infarction. A number of risk factors have been identified for CAD, some of which are irreversible and some of which can be modified.

Irreversible risk factors

Age   CAD rate increases with age. It rarely presents in the young, except in familial hyperlipidaemia (p. 675).

Gender   Men are more often affected than premenopausal women, although the incidence in women after the menopause is similar to that in men. The cause for this difference is poorly understood, but probably relates to the loss of the protective effect of oestrogen.

Family history   CAD is often present in several members of the same family. It is unclear, however, whether family history is an independent risk factor as so many other factors are familial. A number of genetic risk factors have been associated with CAD. For example, a specific genotype of the *ACE* gene associated with higher circulating ACE levels may be significantly associated with a predisposition to CAD and myocardial infarction.

Potentially reversible risk factors

Hyperlipidaemia   Elevated cholesterol levels increase the risk of premature atherosclerosis, particularly when associated with low levels of high-density lipoproteins (HDLs). High triglyceride levels are also independently linked with coronary atheroma. Lowering serum cholesterol slows the progression of coronary atherosclerosis and causes regression of the disease.

Smoking   In men the risk of developing CAD is directly related to the number of cigarettes smoked. In women this relationship, although still important, is less clear. Stopping smoking reduces the risk but does not eliminate it.

Hypertension   Both systolic and diastolic hypertension are linked to an increased incidence of CAD.

Hyperhomocysteinaemia   Homocysteine is an intermediary amino acid formed by the conversion of methionine to cysteine. It has atherogenic and prothrombotic properties. Elevated levels of homocysteine occur due to genetic defects involved in homocysteine metabolism, to nutritional deficiencies of vitamin cofactors (folic acid, vitamin B_{12} and vitamin B_6) or to some chronic medical conditions and drugs.

Other factors   Diabetes mellitus, an abnormal glucose tolerance, raised fasting glucose, lack of exercise, and obesity have all been linked to an increased incidence of atheroma.

Newer risk factors   A number of other factors, including high alcohol intake and high levels of fibrinogen, C-reactive protein, and lipoprotein (a) in the blood, have been linked to atherosclerosis, although it is unclear whether they are directly linked to the pathogenesis of the disease.

Angina (K&C 6e p. 803)

Angina pectoris is a descriptive term for chest pain arising from the heart as a result of myocardial ischaemia.

Clinical features

Angina is usually described as central, crushing, retrosternal chest pain, coming on with exertion and relieved by rest within a few minutes. It is often exacerbated by cold weather, anger and excitement, and it frequently radiates to the arms and neck. Variants of classic angina include:

- *Decubitus angina* occurs on lying down.
- *Nocturnal angina* occurs at night and may waken the patient from sleep.
- *Variant (Prinzmetal's) angina* is caused by coronary artery spasm and results in angina that occurs without provocation, usually at rest.
- *Unstable angina.* Angina which increases rapidly in severity, occurs at rest, or is of recent onset (less than 1 month) (see Acute coronary syndromes).
- *Cardiac syndrome X* refers to those patients with symptoms of angina, a positive exercise test and normal coronary arteries on angiogram. It is thought to result from functional abnormalities of the coronary microcirculation. The prognostic and therapeutic implications are not known.

Physical examination in patients with angina is often normal but must include a search for risk factors (e.g. hypertension and xanthelasma occurring in hyperlipidaemia). It is essential to look for signs of aortic stenosis as a possible cause for the angina.

Diagnosis

The primary diagnosis is clinical because investigations may be normal. Occasionally chest wall pain or oesophageal reflux causes diagnostic confusion (p. 396).

Investigations

- Resting ECG typically shows ST segment depression and T-wave flattening or inversion during an attack. The ECG is usually normal between attacks.

- Exercise ECG testing is positive (p. 404) in about 75% of people with severe CAD; a normal test does not exclude the diagnosis. ST segment depression (>1 mm) at a low workload (within 6 minutes of starting the Bruce protocol) or a paradoxical fall in blood pressure with exercise usually indicates severe coronary artery disease, and these patients should be considered for coronary angiography.

- Other testing protocols (pharmacological stress testing with myocardial perfusion imaging or stress echocardiography, p. 407) are used in patients who cannot exercise or have baseline ECG abnormalities that can interfere with interpretation of the exercise ECG test. They may also be helpful in patients with an equivocal exercise test.

- Coronary angiography (p. 407) is occasionally used when the diagnosis of angina is uncertain. More commonly it is used to delineate the exact coronary anatomy before coronary artery angioplasty or surgery is considered (K&C 6e p. 805).

Management

Secondary prevention Patients with CAD have a high risk of subsequent cardiovascular events, including myocardial infarction, sudden death and stroke. Modification of risk factors has a beneficial effect on subsequent morbidity and mortality, and includes smoking cessation, control of hypertension, maintaining ideal bodyweight, regular exercise and glycaemic control in diabetes mellitus. In addition, aspirin, statins and β-blockers reduce subsequent risk.

437

- Aspirin (75 mg daily) inhibits platelet cyclo-oxygenase, an enzyme involved in the formation of the aggregating agent thromboxane A_2, and reduces the risk of coronary events in patients with CAD. Clopidogrel (75 mg daily) is an alternative when aspirin is not tolerated, or is contraindicated.

- Lipid-lowering agents reduce mortality and incidence of myocardial infarction in patients with CAD and should be used in patients to achieve a cholesterol level of less than 5.0 mmol/L. Guidelines on introduction of lipid-lowering therapy are illustrated on page 678. A statin is used unless the triglycerides are above 3.5 mmol/L, in which case a fibrate is indicated.

Symptomatic treatment Acute attacks are treated with sublingual glyceryl trinitrate tablet or spray. Patients should be encouraged to use this before exertion, rather than waiting for the pain to develop. The main side-effect is a severe bursting headache, which is relieved by inactivating the tablet either by swallowing or spitting it out.

Most patients will require regular prophylactic therapy. Nitrates, β-blockers or calcium antagonists are most commonly used, with treatment being tailored to the individual patient. Some patients will require combination therapy.

- *β-Adrenergic blocking drugs*, e.g. atenolol 50–100 mg daily and metoprolol 25–50 mg twice daily, reduce heart rate and the force of ventricular contraction, both of which reduce myocardial oxygen demand.
- *Calcium antagonists*, e.g. diltiazem, amlodipine, block calcium influx into the cell and the utilization of calcium within the cell. They relax the coronary arteries and reduce the force of left ventricular contraction, thereby reducing oxygen demand. The side-effects (postural dizziness, headache, ankle oedema) are the result of systemic vasodilatation. High-dose nifedipine increases mortality and should not be used in this situation.
- *Nitrates* reduce venous and intracardiac diastolic pressure, reduce impedance to the emptying of the left ventricle, and dilate coronary arteries. They are available in a variety of slow-release preparations, including infiltrated skin plasters, buccal pellets and long-acting oral nitrate preparations, e.g. isosorbide mononitrate, isosorbide dinitrate. The major side-effect is headache, which tends to diminish with continued use.
- *Nicorandil* combines nitrate-like activity with potassium-channel blockade. It can be useful when there are contraindications to the above agents or in refractory unstable angina.

When angina persists or worsens in spite of general measures and optimal medical treatment, patients should be considered for coronary artery bypass grafting (CABG) or angioplasty.

Coronary angioplasty Localized atheromatous lesions are dilated at cardiac catheterization using small inflatable balloons. This technique is widely applied for angina resulting from isolated, proximal, non-calcified atheromatous plaques. Complications include death (1%), acute myocardial infarction (2%), the need for urgent coronary artery bypass grafting (2%) and restenosis (30% in the first 6 months).

Intracoronary stents reduce the risk of acute vessel closure and restenosis rates but increase the cost of the procedure. Aspirin and other antiplatelet drugs, e.g. clopidogrel, are routinely given, and the use of monoclonal antibodies to the glycoprotein IIb/IIIa platelet receptor (the final common pathway of platelet aggregation) in selected high-risk cases may reduce peri-procedural complications. Drug-eluting stents which release antiproliferative agents (sirolimus, paclitaxel) reduce restenosis rates still further and are the subject of on-going studies.

Coronary artery bypass grafting The left or right internal mammary artery is used to bypass stenoses in the left anterior descending or right coronary artery respectively. Less commonly, the saphenous vein from the leg is anastomosed between the proximal aorta and coronary artery distal to the obstruction. Surgery successfully relieves angina in about 90% of cases and, when performed for left main stem obstruction or three-vessel disease, an improved lifespan and quality of life can be expected. Operative mortality rate is less than 1%. In most patients the angina eventually recurs because of accelerated atherosclerosis in the graft (particularly vein grafts), which can be treated by stenting.

CAD equivalents

Intensive risk factor modification (as described in Secondary prevention above) is also used in patients without known CAD but with a risk of subsequent cardiovascular events that is comparable to that seen in patients with established CAD. These patients are described as *CAD equivalents* and include patients with carotid artery disease, peripheral vascular disease, type 2 diabetes mellitus and chronic renal failure.

439

Acute coronary syndromes (ACS) (K&C 6e p. 808)

ACS include ST-elevation myocardial infarction (STEMI, see below), non-ST-elevation myocardial infarction (NSTEMI) and unstable angina. The common mechanism to all ACS is rupture or erosion of the fibrous cap of a coronary artery plaque with subsequent formation of a platelet-rich clot and vasoconstriction produced by platelet release of serotonin and thromboxane A_2. Unstable angina differs from NSTEMI in that in the latter the ischaemia is severe enough to cause sufficient myocardial damage to cause an elevation in serum markers of myocardial injury (troponin and creatine kinase, see Myocardial infarction). A negative serum troponin at 6 and 12 hours after the onset of chest pain suggests unstable angina rather than NSTEMI. Both unstable angina and NSTEMI may be complicated by myocardial infarction with ST segment elevation if treatment is inadequate. The initial management of patients presenting with suspected ACS is summarized in Emergency Box 9.3.

Immediate investigations in ACS are the same as for myocardial infarction (p. 441).

Treatment

- *Antiplatelet therapy.* In the absence of contraindications, aspirin (300 mg initially, then 75 mg daily) is indicated in all patients with ACS. It reduces the risk of subsequent vascular events and deaths and is continued indefinitely. Clopidogrel (75 mg daily) is also given, and to patients with contraindications or intolerance to aspirin. Platelet glycoprotein IIb/IIIa receptor inhibitors, e.g. abciximab, are sometimes added for high-risk patients (see below).
- *Heparin* (enoxaparin 1 mg/kg s.c. twice daily) interferes with thrombus formation at the site of plaque rupture and reduces the risk of ischaemic events and death.
- *Anti-ischaemia agents.* Nitrates are given sublingually (0.4 mg every 5 min for three doses) or by intravenous infusion with continuing pain (50 mg in 50 mL 0.9% saline at 2–10 mL/h to maintain systolic blood pressure > 90 mmHg) for 24–48 hours. Long-acting oral nitrates are useful for recurrent ischaemia. β-Blockers are given orally or intravenously, e.g. metoprolol 5 mg i.v. over 2 minutes repeated every 5 minutes to a maximum of 15 mg, then 2–50 mg by mouth twice daily.
- *Plaque stabilization.* Statins, e.g. atorvastatin 80 mg daily, and an ACE inhibitor, e.g. ramipril 2.5–10 mg daily are continued long term and reduce future cardiovascular events.

Risk stratification

Patients with unstable angina/NSTEMI present with a wide spectrum of risk for subsequent ischaemic events,

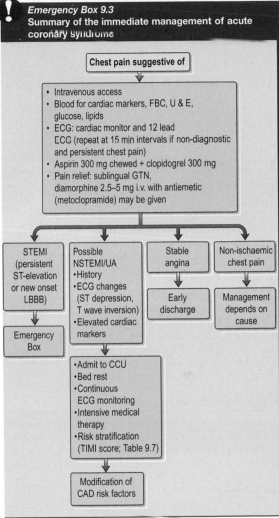

Emergency Box 9.3
Summary of the immediate management of acute coronary syndrome

Chest pain suggestive of

- Intravenous access
- Blood for cardiac markers, FBC, U & E, glucose, lipids
- ECG: cardiac monitor and 12 lead ECG (repeat at 15 min intervals if non-diagnostic and persistent chest pain)
- Aspirin 300 mg chewed + clopidogrel 300 mg
- Pain relief: sublingual GTN, diamorphine 2.5–5 mg i.v. with antiemetic (metoclopramide) may be given

STEMI (persistent ST-elevation or new onset LBBB)

Possible NSTEMI/UA
- History
- ECG changes (ST depression, T wave inversion)
- Elevated cardiac markers

Stable angina

Non-ischaemic chest pain

Emergency Box

Early discharge

Management depends on cause

- Admit to CCU
- Bed rest
- Continuous ECG monitoring
- Intensive medical therapy
- Risk stratification (TIMI score; Table 9.7)

Modification of CAD risk factors

441

GTN, glyceryl trinitrate; STEMI, ST-segment elevation myocardial infarction; NSTEMI, non-STEMI; UA, unstable angina; LBBB, left bundle branch block; CAD, coronary artery disease

Table 9.7 The TIMI risk score in acute coronary syndrome

Risk factor	Score
Age > 65 years	1
More than three coronary artery disease risk factors – hypertension, hyperlipidaemia, family history, diabetes, smoking	1
Prior coronary stenosis of ≥ 50% on angiography	1
Aspirin use in the last 7 days	1
At least two episodes of rest pain in the last 24 hours	1
ST deviation on admission ECG (horizontal ST depression or transient ST elevation > 1 mm)	1
Elevated cardiac markers (CK-MB or troponin)	1

Low risk = score 0–2; Intermediate risk = score 3–4; High risk = score 5–7

myocardial infarction and death. The TIMI risk score is a simple prognostication scheme that categorizes a patient's risk of death and ischaemic events and provides a basis for therapeutic decision-making (Table 9.7). Early coronary angiography with a view to surgery or angioplasty is recommended in patients at high risk and in some at intermediate risk. Coronary stenting may stabilize the disrupted coronary plaque and reduces angiographic restenosis rates compared to angioplasty alone. Low-risk patients should have an exercise ECG test (p. 404) prior to hospital discharge if they remain pain-free with no evidence of ischaemia, heart failure or arrhythmias.

Myocardial infarction (*K&C* 6e p. 812)

Myocardial infarction (MI) is now the most common cause of death in developed countries. It is almost always the result of rupture of an atherosclerotic plaque, with the development of thrombosis and total occlusion of the artery.

Clinical features

Central chest pain similar to that occurring in angina is the most common presenting symptom. Unlike angina it usually occurs at rest, is more severe and lasts for some hours. The pain is often associated with sweating, breathlessness, nausea, vomiting and restlessness. There may be no physical signs unless complications develop (see later), although the patient often appears pale, sweaty and grey. About 20% of patients have no pain, and such 'silent' infarctions either go unnoticed or present with hypotension, arrhythmias or pulmonary oedema. This occurs most commonly in elderly patients or those with diabetes or hypertension.

Investigations

In most cases the diagnosis is made on the basis of the clinical history and early ECG appearances. Serial changes (over 3 days) in the ECG and serum levels of cardiac markers confirm the diagnosis and allow an assessment of infarct size (on the magnitude of the enzyme and protein rise and extent of ECG changes). A normal ECG in the early stages does not exclude the diagnosis.

The ECG usually shows a characteristic pattern. Within hours there is ST segment elevation (> 1 mm in two or more contiguous leads) followed by T-wave flattening or inversion (Fig. 9.15). Pathological Q waves are broad (> 1 mm) and deep (> 2 mm, or > 25% of the amplitude of the following R wave) negative deflections that start the QRS complex. They are seen once full-thickness infarction (as opposed to non-Q-wave or subendocardial infarction) has occurred. They develop because the infarcted muscle is electrically silent so that the recording leads 'look through' the infarcted area. This means that the electrical activity being recorded (on the opposite ventricular wall) is moving away from the electrode and is therefore negative. New left bundle branch block is also an indicator of acute myocardial infarction.

Typically ECG changes are confined to the leads that 'face' the infarct. Leads II, III and AVF are involved in inferior infarcts; I, II and AVL in lateral infarcts; and V_2–V_6 in anterior infarcts. As there are no posterior leads, a posterior wall infarct is diagnosed by the appearance of reciprocal changes in V_1 and V_2 (i.e. the development of tall initial R waves, ST segment depression and tall upright T waves).

Cardiac markers Necrotic cardiac muscle releases several enzymes and proteins into the systemic circulation:

- Troponin T and troponin I are regulatory proteins, highly specific and sensitive for cardiac muscle damage. They

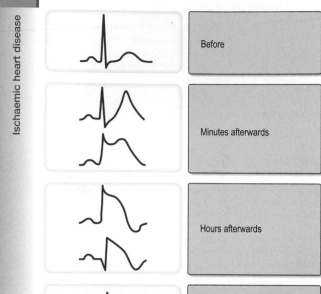

Fig. 9.15 **Electrocardiographic evolution of myocardial infarction.** After the first few minutes the T waves become tall, pointed and upright and there is ST segment elevation. After the first few hours the T waves invert, the R wave voltage is decreased and Q waves develop. After a few days the ST segment returns to normal. After weeks or months the T wave may return to upright but the Q wave remains.

are released early (within 8 hours of event onset) and persist for several days, and are more sensitive and cardiac specific than CK-MB (see below). Measurement of these proteins can be performed at the bedside.

■ Creatine kinase (CK), which is also produced by damaged skeletal muscle and brain, is less sensitive than

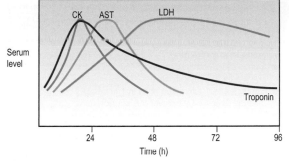

Fig. 9.16 The cardiac enzyme and protein profile in acute myocardial infarction. CK, creatine kinase; AST, aspartate aminotransferase; LDH, lactic dehydrogenase.

troponin for myocardial damage. The myocardial-bound (MB) isoenzyme fraction of CK is specific for heart muscle damage and the size of the enzyme rise is broadly proportional to the infarct size.

■ Aspartate aminotransferase (AST) and lactic dehydrogenase (LDH) are now rarely used for the diagnosis of infarction, but because serum levels remain elevated for up to 10 days after infarction, measurement may be useful in a patient presenting several days after an episode of chest pain.

There is a characteristic time course for the release of the enzymes into the blood, and thus they are usually measured for 3 days following suspected myocardial infarction (Fig. 9.16).

Other investigations These include a chest X-ray, full blood count, serum urea and electrolytes, blood glucose and lipids (lipids taken within the first 12 hours reflect preinfarction levels, but after this time they are altered for up to 6 weeks).

Management

The aims of treatment are relief of pain, limitation of infarct size and treatment of complications. The immediate management and subsequent management are summarized in (Emergency Boxes 9.3 and 9.4).

445

> **Emergency Box 9.4**
> **Summary of the management of myocardial infarction**

Immediate management

- Immediate investigations and treatment as for ischaemic chest pain (Emergency Box 9.3).
- Streptokinase: 1.5 million units in 100 mL 0.9% sodium chloride over 1 h by intravenous infusion pump.
- Metoprolol 5 mg slow i.v. injection if systolic HR > 100 b.p.m. Repeat every 15 min, titrated against heart rate and BP. Do not give if hypotension, heart failure, bradycardia, asthma.
- Insulin infusion if admission blood glucose > 11 mmol/L, aim for blood glucose of 7–10 mmol/L.
- Treat complications (pp. 448–450).
- Treat persistent pain with glyceryl trinitrate infusion 2–10 mg/h titrated against the response; consider angiography and possible angioplasty.

Subsequent management of uncomplicated infarction

- Repeat ECG, serum cardiac markers and electrolytes at 24 and 48 hours after admission.
- Initiate secondary prevention therapy: aspirin, statin, metoprolol, ACE inhibitor and modification of CAD risk factors (as for acute coronary syndrome).
- Transfer from CCU to medical ward after 48 h.
- Mobilize gradually after 24–48 h if pain-free.
- Discharge from hospital after 6 days.
- Submaximal exercise ECG test prior to discharge. Consider angiography if ischaemic ECG changes or chest pain in early stages.
- Refer to rehabilitation nurse. No driving for 1 month; special assessment is required for heavy goods or public service licence holder before driving. Usually return to work in 2 months.

Acute management Thrombolytic therapy (p. 233) is indicated in patients with chest pain consistent with myocardial infarction and ST segment elevation on the ECG. These agents can achieve early reperfusion in 50–70% of patients (compared to a spontaneous reperfusion of less than 30%) and reduce mortality and the extent of myocardial damage. They should be given as soon as possible, although benefit may occur for up to 12 hours after the onset of symptoms. Commonly used thrombolytic agents are streptokinase and recombinant tissue-type plasminogen activator (t-PA). Streptokinase is the cheapest and most commonly used, but may induce the development of antistreptokinase antibodies. This puts the patient at risk of allergic reactions and reduces the effectiveness of subsequent thrombolysis with streptokinase. t-PA is preferred in patients under 50 years of age with anterior MIs, in patients previously treated with streptokinase or when the systolic blood pressure is less than 100 mmHg. t-PA must be followed by low-molecular-weight heparin. The side-effects of and contraindications to thrombolysis are discussed on page 234.

Following initiation of thrombolysis, the patient should be transferred to the coronary care unit where close ECG monitoring and immediate resuscitation are possible. Mortality is increased in diabetic patients with MI, largely owing to the high incidence of heart failure. This is due in part to metabolic changes which occur in the early stages of MI, and is reduced by rigorous control of blood glucose with insulin infusion, and monitoring with 2-hourly BM Stix. This regimen is also indicated in patients not known to be diabetic who have an admission blood glucose of > 11 mmol/L.

β-Blockers reduce infarct size and the incidence of sudden death. Metoprolol (5–10 mg i.v) should be given, particularly if the heart rate is greater than 100 b.p.m. and there is persistent pain.

Recanalization of the infarct-related artery may also be achieved by primary (direct) angioplasty without prior or concomitant thrombolytic therapy; in experienced hands the results are equal or superior to thrombolysis. It is only a therapeutic option when rapid access to a catheterization laboratory is possible, the cardiologist is experienced in interventional cardiology and a full support team is immediately available. Therefore, it is not usually used in preference to thrombolysis but should be considered in patients when thrombolytic therapy is contraindicated (p. 234), or as 'rescue' therapy in patients who have received thrombolysis and who seem on clinical grounds not to have reperfused (ongoing chest pain and < 50% resolution of ST elevation 45–60 minutes after start of thrombolysis).

Subsequent management ACE inhibitors reduce mortality and prevent the development of heart failure and should be started on the first day after MI. Treatment with

447

Ischaemic heart disease

Table 9.8 Complications of myocardial infarction
Heart failure
Rupture of free wall of infarcted ventricle (usually fatal)
Rupture of the interventricular septum
Mitral regurgitation
Arrhythmias
Heart block
Pericarditis
Thromboembolism
Dressler's syndrome*
Ventricular aneurysm*

*May develop weeks or months after MI

ACE inhibitors, aspirin, statin and β-blockers is continued indefinitely. Gradual mobilization takes place on the second day and if the patient is fully ambulant and pain-free, a sub-maximal exercise tolerance test is performed (70% of age-predicted maximal heart rate) before hospital discharge on day 5 or 6 in uncomplicated cases. Patients with test results suggesting ischaemia are referred for coronary angiography.

Complications

The common complications are listed in Table 9.8.

Disturbances of rate, rhythm and conduction (p. 408)

- *Atrial arrhythmias.* Sinus tachycardia is common; treatment is that of the underlying cause, particularly pain, anxiety and heart failure. Sinus bradycardia is especially associated with acute inferior wall myocardial infarction. Treatment is initially with intravenous atropine (0.5 mg repeated up to six times in 4 hours). Temporary trans-cutaneous or transvenous pacemaker insertion may be required if there are adverse signs (heart failure, hypotension, ventricular arrhythmias). Atrial fibrillation occurs in about 10% of cases and is usually a transient rhythm disturbance. Treatment with digoxin or amiodarone is indicated if the fast rate is exacerbating ischaemia or causing heart failure.
- *Ventricular arrhythmias.* Ventricular ectopic beats are very common and may precede the development of ventricular tachycardia or fibrillation. Antiarrhythmic drug treatment has not been shown to affect progression to these more

serious arrhythmias. Ventricular tachycardia (VT) may degenerate into ventricular fibrillation (p. 420) or may itself produce shock or heart failure. Treatment of VT is with intravenous lidocaine (lignocaine) (p. 419) or amiodarone or direct current cardioversion if there is severe hypotension. Ventricular fibrillation (VF) may be primary (occurring in the first 24–48 hours) or secondary (occurring late after infarction and associated with large infarcts and heart failure). Treatment is with immediate DC cardioversion. Recurrences may be prevented with intravenous lidocaine or amiodarone. Late VF is associated with a poor prognosis and a high incidence of sudden death, and prophylactic antiarrhythmic treatment must be continued long term.

■ *Heart block occurring with inferior infarction* is common and usually resolves spontaneously. Some patients respond to intravenous atropine, but a temporary pacemaker may be necessary if the rhythm is very slow or producing symptoms.

■ *Complete heart block occurring with anterior wall infarction* indicates the involvement of both bundle branches by extensive myocardial necrosis, and hence a very poor prognosis. The ventricular rhythm in this case is unreliable and a temporary pacing wire is necessary. Heart block is often permanent and a permanent pacing wire may be necessary.

Heart failure in a mild form occurs in up to 40% of patients following myocardial infarction. Extensive infarction may cause pulmonary oedema (see Emergency Box 9.2), which may also occur following rupture of the ventricular septum or mitral valve papillary muscle. Both conditions present with worsening heart failure, a systolic thrill and a loud pansystolic murmur. Mortality is high, and urgent surgical correction is often needed. Hypotension with a raised JVP is usually a complication of right ventricular infarction, which may occur with inferior wall infarcts. Initial treatment is with volume expansion, and pericardial effusion (which produces similar signs) should be ruled out on an echocardiogram.

Thromboembolism occurs most commonly following prolonged bed rest and with heart failure. Patients at risk of embolism from left ventricular or left atrial clot (those with severe left ventricular dysfunction, persistent AF or mural thrombus on echocardiography) should be anticoagulated with warfarin to achieve a target INR of 2–3.

Pericarditis is characterized by sharp chest pain and a pericardial rub. Treatment is with non-steroidal anti-inflammatory drugs until spontaneous resolution occurs within 1–2 days. Late pericarditis (2–12 weeks after) with fever and a pericardial effusion (Dressler's syndrome) is rare and corticosteroids may be necessary in some patients.

Prognosis

Prognosis is variable depending on factors such as age and size of infarct. Fifty per cent of patients die during the acute event, many before reaching hospital. A further 10% die in hospital, and of the survivors a further 10% die in the next 2 years.

RHEUMATIC FEVER

Rheumatic fever is an inflammatory disease that occurs in children and young adults (the first attack usually occurs between 5–15 years of age) as a result of infection with group A streptococci. It is a complication of less than 1% of streptococcal pharyngitis, developing 2–3 weeks after the onset of sore throat. It is thought to develop because of an autoimmune reaction triggered by the streptococci, and is not the result of direct infection of the heart.

Epidemiology

The incidence in developed countries has decreased dramatically since the 1920s. This is thought to be the result of improved sanitation, a change in the virulence of the organism and the use of antibiotics.

Clinical features

The disease presents suddenly with fever, joint pains and loss of appetite. The major clinical features are as follows:

■ Changing heart murmurs, mitral and aortic regurgitation, heart failure and chest pain, caused by carditis affecting all three layers of the heart
■ Polyarthritis which is classically fleeting and affects the large joints, e.g. knees, ankles and elbows

- Skin manifestations include erythema marginatum (transient pink coalescent rings develop on the trunk) and small non-tender subcutaneous nodules which occur over tendons, joints and bony prominences
- Sydenham's chorea ('St Vitus' dance') refers to involvement of the central nervous system. It develops late after a streptococcal infection. Sufferers are noticeably 'fidgety' and display spasmodic, unintentional movements.

Investigations

Blood count shows a leucocytosis and a raised ESR.

The diagnosis is based on the revised Duckett Jones criteria, which depend on the combination of certain clinical features and evidence of recent streptococcal infection.

Treatment

Treatment is with complete bed rest and high-dose aspirin. Penicillin is given to eradicate residual streptococcal infection, and then long term to all patients with persistent cardiac damage.

Chronic rheumatic heart disease

More than 50% of those who suffer acute rheumatic fever with carditis will later (after 10–20 years) develop chronic rheumatic valvular disease, predominantly affecting the mitral and aortic valves (see below).

451

VALVULAR HEART DISEASE (K&C 6e p. 817)

Cardiac valves may be incompetent (regurgitant), stenotic or both. The most common problems are acquired left-sided valvular lesions: aortic stenosis, mitral stenosis, mitral regurgitation and aortic regurgitation. Abnormal valves produce turbulent blood flow, which is heard as a murmur on auscultation; a few murmurs are also felt as a thrill on palpation. Murmurs may sometimes be heard with normal hearts ('innocent murmurs'), often reflecting a hyperdynamic circulation, e.g. in pregnancy, anaemia and thyrotoxicosis. Benign murmurs are soft, short, systolic, may vary with posture, and are not associated with signs of organic heart disease (K&C 6e p. 740).

Diagnosis of valve dysfunction is made clinically and by echocardiography (K&C 6e p. 749). The severity is assessed by Doppler echocardiography, which measures the direction and velocity of blood flow and allows a calculation to be made of the pressure across a stenotic valve. Transoesophageal echocardiography and invasive cardiac catheterization are usually only necessary to assess complex situations such as coexisting valvular and ischaemic heart disease, or suspected dysfunction of a prosthetic valve. Treatment of valve dysfunction is both medical and surgical; this may be valve replacement, valve repair (some incompetent valves) or valvotomy (the fused cusps of a stenotic valve are separated along the commissures). The timing of surgery is critical and must not be delayed until there is irreversible ventricular dysfunction or pulmonary hypertension.

Prosthetic heart valves

Prosthetic heart valves may be either tissue or mechanical. Tissue valves are fashioned from pig aortic valves (a porcine xenograft), but occasionally a human aortic valve is used (homograft). Tissue valves tend to degenerate within about 10 years but patients do not need long-term anticoagulation. These valves are often used in elderly patients. Mechanical valves last much longer but patients need lifelong anticoagulation. There are several types: a ball-and-cage design (Starr–Edwards valve), a tilting disc (Björk–Shiley valve) or a double tilting disc (St Jude valve). Valves are susceptible to infection and thrombosis and may cause haemolysis or systemic emboli.

The individual valve lesions are considered separately below, but disease may affect more than one valve (particularly in rheumatic heart disease and infective endocarditis), when a combination of clinical features is produced. Damaged and prosthetic valves are at risk of infection during an episode of bacteraemia (e.g. after tooth extraction, endoscopy or surgery), and patients should always receive prophylactic antibiotics to cover these procedures (see p. 464).

Mitral stenosis (*K&C* 6e p. 817)

Aetiology

Most cases of mitral stenosis are a result of rheumatic heart disease, with symptoms appearing many years after the episode of acute rheumatic fever. It primarily affects women. However, a reliable history of rheumatic fever is not always obtained.

Pathophysiology

Thickening and immobility of the valve leaflets leads to obstruction to blood flow from the left atrium to left ventricle. Symptoms are the result of increased left atrial pressure and reduced cardiac output, caused by the mechanical obstruction of filling of the left ventricle. An increase in left atrial pressure leads to left atrial hypertrophy and dilatation. Thrombus may form in the dilated atrium, which is also prone to fibrillate and give rise to systemic emboli (e.g. to the brain, resulting in a stroke). Chronically elevated left atrial pressure leads to an increase in pulmonary capillary pressure and pulmonary oedema. Pulmonary arterial vasoconstriction leads to pulmonary hypertension and eventually right ventricular hypertrophy, dilatation and failure.

Symptoms

Exertional dyspnoea which becomes progressively more severe is usually the first symptom. A cough productive of blood-tinged sputum is common, and frank haemoptysis may occasionally occur. The onset of atrial fibrillation may produce an abrupt deterioration and precipitate pulmonary oedema.

Signs

- Cyanotic or dusky-pink discoloration on the upper cheeks produces the so-called mitral facies or malar flush that occurs with severe stenosis.
- The pulse is often irregular as a result of atrial fibrillation.
- The apex beat is 'tapping' in quality as a result of a combination of a palpable first heart sound and left ventricular backward displacement produced by an enlarging right ventricle.
- Auscultation at the apex reveals a loud first heart sound, an opening snap (when the mitral valve opens) in early diastole, followed by a rumbling mid-diastolic murmur. If the patient is in sinus rhythm the murmur becomes louder when atrial systole occurs (presystolic accentuation), as a result of increased flow across the narrowed valve.

The presence of a loud second heart sound, parasternal heave, elevated JVP, ascites and peripheral oedema indicates that pulmonary hypertension producing right ventricular overload has developed.

Investigations

Investigations are performed to confirm the diagnosis, to estimate the severity of valve stenosis and to look for pulmonary hypertension.

Chest X-ray appearances of mitral stenosis are demonstrated in Figure 9.2.

ECG usually shows atrial fibrillation. In patients in sinus rhythm, left atrial hypertrophy results in a bifid P wave ('P mitrale').

Echocardiography is the most useful investigation to confirm the diagnosis and to assess the severity.

Management

General Treatment is often not required for mild mitral stenosis. Complications are treated medically, e.g. beta-blockers/digoxin for atrial fibrillation, diuretics for heart failure and anticoagulation in patients with atrial fibrillation to prevent clot formation and embolization.

Specific If symptoms are more than mild, or if there is evidence that pulmonary hypertension is beginning to develop, mechanical relief of the mitral stenosis is indicated. In many cases percutaneous balloon valvotomy (access to the mitral valve is obtained via a catheter passed through the femoral vein, right atrium and interatrial septum, and a balloon inflated across the valve to split the commissures) provides relief of symptoms. In other cases commissurotomy (splitting of the valve leaflets) or mitral valve replacement is necessary. The latter is performed if there is associated mitral regurgitation, a badly calcified valve or thrombus in the left atrium despite anticoagulation.

Mitral regurgitation (*K&C* 6e p. 820)

Aetiology

A prolapsing mitral valve and rheumatic heart disease are the most common causes of mitral regurgitation (Table 9.9).

Table 9.9 Causes of mitral regurgitation
Rheumatic heart disease
Mitral valve prolapse
Infective endocarditis*
Ruptured chordae tendineae*
Rupture of the papillary muscle* complicating myocardial infarction
Papillary muscle dysfunction
Dilating left ventricle disease causing 'functional' mitral regurgitation
Hypertrophic cardiomyopathy
Rarely: systemic lupus erythematosus, Marfan's syndrome
Ehlers–Danlos syndrome

*These disorders may produce acute regurgitation

Pathophysiology

The circulatory changes depend on the speed of onset and severity of regurgitation. Long-standing regurgitation produces little increase in the left atrial pressure because flow is accommodated by an enlarged left atrium. With acute mitral regurgitation there is a rise in left atrial pressure, resulting in an increase in pulmonary venous pressure and pulmonary oedema. The left ventricle dilates, but more so with chronic regurgitation.

Symptoms

Acute regurgitation presents as pulmonary oedema. Chronic regurgitation causes progressive exertional dyspnoea, fatigue and lethargy (resulting from reduced cardiac output). Thromboembolism is less common than with mitral stenosis, although infective endocarditis is much more common.

Signs

- The apex beat is displaced laterally, with a diffuse thrusting character.
- The first heart sound is soft.
- There is a pansystolic murmur (palpated as a thrill), loudest at the apex and radiating widely over the precordium and into the axilla.
- A third heart sound is often present, caused by rapid filling of the dilated left ventricle in early diastole.

Investigations

■ Chest X-ray and ECG changes are not sensitive or specific for the diagnosis of mitral regurgitation. On both, evidence of enlargement of the left atrium, the left ventricle or both, is seen late in the course of the disease.
■ Echocardiography confirms the diagnosis and may indicate the cause. The severity of the lesion can usually be assessed from Doppler studies without the need to resort to cardiac catheterization.

Management

Mild mitral regurgitation in the absence of symptoms can be managed conservatively by following the patient with serial echocardiograms every 1–5 years depending on the severity. Patients should be referred for surgery (mitral valve replacement or repair) if more than mild symptoms develop or there is evidence of left ventricular dysfunction (ventricular dilatation or reduced ejection fraction). Emergency valve replacement is necessary with acute severe mitral regurgitation.

Prolapsing mitral valve (*K&C* 6e p. 822)

This is a common condition occurring mainly in young women. One or more of the mitral valve leaflets prolapses back into the left atrium during ventricular systole, producing mitral regurgitation in a few cases.

Aetiology

The cause is unknown but it may be associated with Marfan's syndrome, thyrotoxicosis, and rheumatic or ischaemic heart disease.

Clinical features

Most patients are asymptomatic. Atypical chest pain is the most common symptom. Some patients complain of palpitations caused by atrial and ventricular arrhythmias. The typical finding on examination is a mid-systolic click, which may be followed by a murmur. Occasionally there are features of mitral regurgitation.

Investigation

Echocardiography is diagnostic and shows the prolapsing valve cusps.

Management

Chest pain and palpitations are treated with β-blockers. Anticoagulation to prevent thromboembolism is indicated if there is significant mitral regurgitation and atrial fibrillation. Prophylaxis against endocarditis is advised if there is clinical evidence of mitral regurgitation indicated by a systolic murmur on auscultation.

Aortic stenosis (K&C 6e p. 822)

Aetiology

There are three causes of aortic valve stenosis:

- Degeneration and calcification of a normal valve – presenting in the elderly
- Calcification of a congenital bicuspid valve – presenting in middle age
- Rheumatic heart disease.

Pathophysiology

Obstruction to left ventricular emptying results in left ventricular hypertrophy. In turn this results in increased myocardial oxygen demand, relative ischaemia of the myocardium and consequent angina, arrhythmias and eventually left ventricular failure.

Symptoms

There are usually no symptoms until the stenosis is moderately severe (aortic orifice reduced to a third of its normal size). The classic symptoms are angina, exertional syncope and the symptoms of congestive heart failure. Ventricular arrhythmias may cause sudden death.

Signs

The carotid pulse is slow rising (plateau pulse) and the apex beat thrusting. There is a harsh systolic ejection murmur (palpated as a thrill) at the right upper sternal border and radiating to the neck. The murmur may be preceded by an ejection click, which is the result of sudden opening of a deformed but mobile valve.

Investigations

- Chest X-ray shows a normal heart size, prominence of the ascending aorta (post-stenotic dilatation) and there may be valvular calcification.
- ECG shows evidence of left ventricular hypertrophy and a left ventricular strain pattern when the disease is severe (depressed ST segment and T wave inversion in the leads orientated to the left ventricle, i.e. I, AVL, V_5 and V_6).
- Echocardiography is diagnostic in most cases. Doppler examination of the valve allows an assessment of the pressure gradient across the valve during systole.
- Cardiac catheterization and coronary angiography are used particularly in patients with angina to exclude coronary artery disease, which may coexist in this predominantly elderly population.

Management

The onset of symptoms in a patient with aortic stenosis is an ominous sign: 75% of patients will be dead within 3 years unless the valve is replaced. Thus aortic valve replacement is indicated in symptomatic patients, and some would recommend valve replacement for a critically stenotic valve (valve area ≤ 0.6 cm² or the valve gradient exceeds 50 mmHg on echocardiography) in the absence of symptoms. Balloon aortic valvotomy is sometimes used as a 'bridge' to valve replacement in very sick patients.

Aortic regurgitation (K&C 6e p. 824)

Aetiology

Aortic regurgitation results from either disease of the valve cusps or dilatation of the aortic root and valve ring. The most common causes are rheumatic fever, and infective endocarditis complicating an already damaged valve (Table 9.10).

Pathophysiology

Chronic regurgitation volume loads the left ventricle and results in hypertrophy and dilatation. The stroke volume is

Table 9.10 Causes and associations of aortic regurgitation	
Acute aortic regurgitation	Chronic aortic regurgitation
Infective endocarditis	Chronic rheumatic heart
Acute rheumatic fever	disease
Dissection of the aorta	Syphilis
Ruptured sinus of Valsalva	Arthritides
aneurysm	Reiter's syndrome
Failure of prosthetic heart valve	Ankylosing spondylitis
	Rheumatoid arthritis
	Severe hypertension
	Bicuspid aortic valve
	Aortic endocarditis
	Marfan's syndrome
	Osteogenesis imperfecta

increased, which results in an increased pulse pressure and the myriad of clinical signs described below. Eventually contraction of the ventricle deteriorates, resulting in left ventricular failure. The adaptations to the volume load entering the left ventricle do not occur with acute regurgitation and patients may present with pulmonary oedema and a reduced stroke volume (hence many of the signs of chronic regurgitation are absent).

Symptoms

In chronic regurgitation, patients remain asymptomatic for many years before developing dyspnoea, orthopnoea and fatigue as a result of left ventricular failure.

Signs

- A 'collapsing' (water-hammer) pulse with wide pulse pressure is pathognomonic.
- The apex beat is displaced laterally and is thrusting in quality.
- A blowing early diastolic murmur is heard at the left sternal edge in the fourth intercostal space. It is accentuated when the patient sits forward with the breath held in expiration. Increased stroke volume produces turbulent flow across the aortic valve, heard as a mid-systolic murmur.

■ A mid-diastolic murmur (Austin Flint murmur) may be heard over the cardiac apex and is thought to be produced as a result of the aortic jet impinging on the mitral valve, producing premature closure of the valve and physiological stenosis.

Investigations

■ Chest X-ray shows a large heart and dilatation of the ascending aorta.
■ ECG shows evidence of left ventricular hypertrophy (see aortic stenosis).
■ Echocardiography with Doppler examination of the aortic valve helps estimate the severity of regurgitation.
■ Aortography during cardiac catheterization helps confirm the severity of the disease.

Management

Mild symptoms may respond to the reduction of afterload with vasodilators and diuretics. The timing of surgery and valve replacement is critical and must not be delayed until there is irreversible left ventricular dysfunction.

Tricuspid and pulmonary valve disease (K&C 6e p. 826)

Tricuspid and pulmonary valve disease are both uncommon. Tricuspid stenosis is almost always the result of rheumatic fever and is frequently associated with mitral and aortic valve disease, which tends to dominate the clinical picture.

Tricuspid regurgitation is usually functional and secondary to dilatation of the right ventricle (and hence tricuspid valve ring) in severe right ventricular failure. Much less commonly it is caused by rheumatic heart disease, infective endocarditis or carcinoid syndrome (p. 94). On examination there is a pansystolic murmur heard at the lower left sternal edge, the jugular venous pressure is elevated, with giant 'v' waves (produced by the regurgitant jet through the tricuspid valve in systole), and the liver is enlarged and pulsates in systole. There may be severe peripheral oedema and ascites. In functional tricuspid regurgitation these signs improve with diuretic therapy.

Pulmonary regurgitation results from pulmonary hypertension and dilatation of the valve ring. Occasionally it is the result of endocarditis (usually in intravenous drug abusers). Auscultation reveals an early diastolic murmur heard at the upper left sternal edge (Graham–Steell murmur), similar to that of aortic regurgitation. Usually there are no symptoms and treatment is rarely required. Pulmonary stenosis is usually a congenital lesion but may present in adult life with fatigue, syncope and right ventricular failure.

Infective endocarditis

Infective endocarditis is an infection of the endocardium or vascular endothelium of the heart. It may occur as a fulminating or acute infection, but more commonly runs an insidious course and is known as subacute (bacterial) endocarditis (SBE).

Infection occurs in the following:

- On valves which have a congenital or acquired defect (usually on the left side of the heart). Right-sided endocarditis is more common in intravenous drug addicts.
- On normal valves with virulent organisms such as *Streptococcus pneumoniae* or *Staphylococcus aureus.*
- On prosthetic valves, when infection may be 'early' (acquired at surgery) or 'late' (following bacteraemia). Infected prosthetic valves often need to be replaced.
- In association with a ventricular septal defect or persistent ductus arteriosus.

Aetiology

461

Not all organisms have the same propensity to cause endocarditis. *Strep. viridans*, *Staph. aureus* and enterococci are common causes (Table 9.11). Blood cultures remain negative in 5–10% of patients with infective endocarditis. The usual cause is prior antibiotic therapy and good history taking is vital. Culture-negative endocarditis is particularly likely with the following organisms which are more difficult to isolate in culture: *Coxiella burnetii* (the cause of Q fever), *Chlamydia* spp., *Bartonella* spp. (organisms that cause trench fever and cat scratch disease) and *Legionella*.

Pathology

A mass of fibrin, platelets and infectious organisms forms vegetations along the edges of the valve. Virulent organisms destroy the valve, producing regurgitation and worsening heart failure.

Clinical features

Symptoms and signs result from:

- Systemic features of infection, such as malaise, fever, night sweats, weight loss and anaemia. Slight splenomegaly is common. Clubbing is rare and occurs late.
- Valve destruction, leading to heart failure and new or changing heart murmurs (in 90% of cases).
- Vascular phenomena due to embolization of vegetations and metastatic abscess formation in the brain, spleen and kidney. Embolization from right-sided endocarditis causes pulmonary infarction and pneumonia.
- Immune complex deposition in blood vessels producing a vasculitis and petechial haemorrhages in the skin, under the nails (splinter haemorrhages) and in the retinae (Roth's spots). Osler's nodes (tender subcutaneous nodules in the fingers) and Janeway lesions (painless erythematous macules on the palms) are uncommon. Immune complex deposition in the joints causes arthralgia and, in the kidney, acute glomerulonephritis. Microscopic haematuria occurs in 70% of cases but renal failure is uncommon.

Endocarditis should always be considered in any patient with a heart murmur and fever.

Investigation

- Blood cultures must be taken before antibiotics are started. Three sets (i.e. six bottles) taken over 24 hours will identify the organism in 75% of cases. Special culture techniques and serological tests are occasionally necessary if blood cultures are negative and unusual organisms suspected.
- Echocardiography identifies vegetations and underlying valvular dysfunction. Small vegetations may be missed and a normal echocardiogram does not exclude endocarditis. Transoesophageal echocardiography is more sensitive (but not 100%) particularly in cases of suspected prosthetic valve endocarditis.
- Serological tests may be helpful if unusual organisms are suspected e.g. *Coxiella, Bartonella, Legionella*.
- Chest X-ray may show heart failure or evidence of septic emboli in right-sided endocarditis.

- ECG may show myocardial infarction (emboli to the coronary circulation) or conduction defects (due to extension of the infection to the valve annulus and adjacent septum).
- Blood count shows a normochromic, normocytic anaemia with a raised ESR and often a leucocytosis.
- Urine Stix testing shows haematuria in most cases.
- Serum immunoglobulins are increased and complement levels decreased as a result of immune complex formation.

Diagnostic criteria

The Duke classification for diagnosis of endocarditis relies upon major and minor criteria (Table 9.11). A definite diagnosis of endocarditis requires one of the following:

- Direct evidence of infective endocarditis by histology or culture of organism, e.g. from a vegetation
- Two major criteria
- One major and any three minor criteria
- Five minor criteria.

Possible endocarditis is diagnosed if there is one major and one minor criterion or three minor.

Management

Drug therapy Treatment is with bactericidal antibiotics, given intravenously for the first 2 weeks and by mouth for a further 2–4 weeks. While awaiting the results of blood cultures a combination of intravenous benzylpenicillin and gentamicin is given unless staphylococcal endocarditis is suspected, when vancomycin should be substituted for penicillin. Subsequent treatment depends on the results of blood cultures and the antibiotic sensitivity of the organism. Antibiotic doses are adjusted to ensure adequate bactericidal activity (microbiological assays of minimum bactericidal concentrations). Surgery to replace the valve should be considered when there is severe heart failure, early infection of prosthetic material, worsening renal failure and extensive damage to the valve.

Prophylaxis

Patients at risk of endocarditis should receive antibiotic therapy before undergoing a procedure likely to result in

Table 9.11 Modified Duke criteria for the diagnosis of infective endocarditis

Major criteria
Positive blood cultures for infective endocarditis
Typical microorganism for infective endocarditis from two separate blood cultures in the absence of a primary focus:
  Streptococcus viridans
  Streptococcus bovis
  HACEK group – *Haemophilus* species, *Actinobacillus actinomycetemcomitans*, *Cardiobacterium hominis*, *Eikenella corrodens*, and *Kingella kingae*
  Community-acquired *Staphylococcus aureus* or enterococci
Persistently positive blood cultures, defined as recovery of a microorganism consistent with infective endocarditis from blood cultures drawn more than 12 hours apart *or* all of three or the majority of four or more separate blood cultures, with first and last drawn at least 1 hour apart
Single positive blood culture for *Coxiella burnetii* or antiphase IgG antibody titre > 1 : 800

Evidence for endocardial involvement
TTE (TEE in prosthetic valve) showing oscillating intracardiac mass on a valve or supporting structures, in the path of regurgitant jet or on implanted material, in the absence of an alternative anatomic explanation, *or*
Abscess, *or*
New partial dehiscence of prosthetic valve

Minor criteria
Predisposition, e.g. prosthetic valve, intravenous drug use
Fever – 38.0°C
Vascular phenomena
Immunological phenomena
Microbiological evidence – positive blood culture but not meeting major criteria

TTE, transthoracic echocardiogram; TEE, transoesophageal echocardiogram

bacteraemia. The choice of antibiotic depends on the procedure and the likelihood of endocarditis.

PULMONARY HEART DISEASE

Pulmonary hypertension (*K&C* 6e p. 841)

The lung circulation offers a low resistance to flow and the normal mean pulmonary artery pressure at rest is

10–14 mmHg. An increase in either pulmonary vascular resistance or pulmonary blood flow results in pulmonary hypertension (pulmonary artery pressure > 25 mmHg). The causes are chronic lung disease, increased pulmonary blood flow (which occurs with atrial septal defect, ventricular septal defect and patent ductus arteriosus), left ventricular failure, mitral stenosis, recurrent pulmonary emboli and primary pulmonary hypertension. The latter is a rare condition of unknown aetiology predominantly affecting young women. In primary disease, medial hypertrophy and intimal fibrosis of the small pulmonary vessels leads to vascular obstruction, increased pulmonary vascular resistance and pulmonary hypertension.

Clinical features

Chest pain, fatigue, dyspnoea and syncope are common symptoms. The physical signs include a right parasternal heave (caused by right ventricular hypertrophy) and a loud pulmonary second sound. In advanced disease there is right heart failure. There are also features of the underlying disease.

Investigations

- Chest X-ray shows enlarged proximal pulmonary arteries which taper distally. It may also reveal the underlying cause (e.g. emphysema, calcified mitral valve).
- ECG shows right ventricular hypertrophy and P pulmonale (p. 402).
- Echocardiography shows right ventricular hypertrophy and dilatation, and may reveal the underlying cause of pulmonary hypertension. Pulmonary artery pressure can be measured indirectly with Doppler echocardiography.

Management

The treatment is that of the cause. In primary pulmonary hypertension there is a progressive downhill course which in some patients can be slowed by a combination of warfarin and oral calcium-channel blockers as pulmonary vasodilators. Continuous (a year or more) intravenous infusions of prostacyclin reduce pulmonary resistance and improve symptoms. However, many patients ultimately require heart and lung transplantation.

Pulmonary embolism (*K&C* 6e p. 844)

Pulmonary embolism (PE) is a common condition. Emboli usually arise from thrombi in the iliofemoral veins (deep venous thrombosis, p. 234). The risk factors for thrombo-embolism are listed on page 235. Rarely PE results from clot formation in the right heart.

Pathology

After PE, lung tissue is ventilated but not perfused, resulting in impaired gas exchange. A *massive* embolism obstructs the right ventricular outflow tract and therefore suddenly increases pulmonary vascular resistance, causing acute right heart failure. A *small* embolus impacts in a terminal, peripheral pulmonary vessel and may be clinically silent unless it causes pulmonary infarction.

Clinical features

- Small/medium PEs present with dyspnoea, pleuritic chest pain, and haemoptysis if there is pulmonary infarction. On examination the patient may be tachypnoeic and have a pleural rub and an exudative (occasionally blood-stained) pleural effusion can develop.
- Massive PE presents as a medical emergency: the patient has severe central chest pain and suddenly becomes shocked, pale and sweaty, with marked tachypnoea and tachycardia. Syncope and death may follow rapidly. On examination the patient is shocked, with central cyanosis. There is elevation of the jugular venous pressure, a right ventricular heave, accentuation of the second heart sound and a gallop rhythm (acute right heart failure).
- Multiple recurrent PEs present with symptoms and signs of pulmonary hypertension (see above), developing over weeks to months.

Investigations

An assessment of clinical probability (Table 9.12) of PE is essential in the interpretation of tests used in the diagnosis.

- Chest X-ray, ECG and blood gases may all be normal with small/medium emboli and any abnormalities with massive emboli are non-specific. The chest X-ray and ECG are useful to exclude other conditions that may

Table 9.12 Clinical probability of pulmonary embolism

(1)	One or more clinical features compatible with pulmonary embolism
	Breathlessness
	Pleuritic chest pain
	Haemoptysis
(2)	Absence of another clinical explanation for symptoms
(3)	Presence of a major risk factor for thromboembolism (p. 235)

In the presence of:
(1) only – clinical probability is low
(1) and **(2)** *or* **(3)** – clinical probability is intermediate
(1) and **(2)** and **(3)** – clinical probability is high

present similarly. The chest X-ray may show decreased vascular markings and a raised hemidiaphragm (caused by loss of lung volume). With pulmonary infarction, a late feature is the development of a wedge-shaped opacity adjacent to the pleural edge, sometimes with a pleural effusion. The commonest ECG finding is sinus tachycardia. The features of acute right heart strain may be seen: tall peaked P waves in lead II, right axis deviation and right bundle branch block. Blood gases show hypoxaemia and hypocapnia.

- Plasma D-dimers are a subset of fibrinogen degradation products released into the circulation when a clot begins to dissolve. A negative D-dimer test excludes PE only in those patients who have a low clinical probability (Table 9.12). However, it is not specific and raised levels occur in a variety of conditions.

- Radionuclide lung scan ($\dot{V}/\dot{Q}$ scan) demonstrates areas of ventilated lung with perfusion defects (ventilation–perfusion defects). It is usually the initial diagnostic investigation in patients without coexistent chronic lung disease. Pulmonary embolism is excluded in patients with a normal scan. In patients with coexistent cardiopulmonary disease inconclusive results are frequently obtained and further imaging will be necessary.

- Ultrasound will detect clots in the pelvic or iliofemoral veins.

- Spiral CT with *intravenous* contrast (CT pulmonary angiography, CTPA) images the pulmonary vessels

467

directly and has greater than 90% sensitivity and specificity for medium/large pulmonary emboli. Small emboli may not be detected. However, the likelihood for subsequent thromboembolic events is extremely small following a negative result from a spiral CT scan. CTPA is particularly useful if the $\dot{V}/\dot{Q}$ scan is equivocal or if urgent investigation is necessary.

- MRI gives similar results and is used if CT is contra-indicated.
- Pulmonary angiography is sometimes undertaken if surgery is considered in acute massive embolism. It shows obstructed vessels or obvious filling defects in the artery.
- Echocardiography is diagnostic in massive PE and can be performed at the bedside. It demonstrates proximal thrombus and right ventricular dilatation.

Management

Treatment (Emergency Box 9.5) should be started on the basis of clinical suspicion pending investigation. Anti-coagulation is continued for 6 weeks to 6 months (see p. 237) depending on the likelihood of recurrence of thrombo-embolism, and lifelong treatment is indicated for recurrent emboli. Insertion of a vena caval filter is used to prevent further emboli when emboli recur despite adequate anticoagulation, or in high-risk individuals where anti-coagulation is contraindicated. Surgery is rarely necessary but may be employed in severe cases of acute massive embolism.

Chronic cor pulmonale (K&C 6e p. 843)

Cor pulmonale is right heart failure resulting from chronic pulmonary hypertension.

Aetiology

Chronic obstructive pulmonary disease caused by bronchitis and emphysema is responsible for most cases (Table 9.13). Pulmonary vascular resistance is increased because of destruction of the pulmonary vascular bed and pulmonary vasoconstriction caused by acidosis and hypoxia. Eventually, increased resistance leads to right heart strain and right ventricular failure.

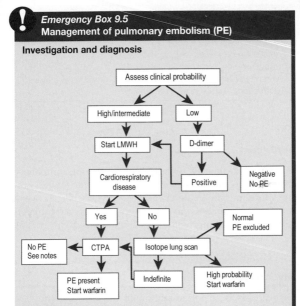

> ! **Emergency Box 9.5**
> **Management of pulmonary embolism (PE)**
>
> **Investigation and diagnosis**

CTPA, CT pulmonary angiogram; LMWH, low-molecular-weight heparin. CTPA is performed as the first-line imaging investigation in preference to isotope lung scan in some centres. NB: In high-probability patients with normal CTPA, further imaging (US legs, pulmonary angiogram) may be necessary.

Treatment
- 60% oxygen if hypoxaemic.
- Dissolution of the thrombus:
  Consider for massive embolism with hypotension and signs of acute right heart strain
  Streptokinase 1.5 million units or alteplase 100 mg by peripheral i.v. infusion over 2 hours.
- Analgesia:
  Morphine (5–10 mg i.v.) to relieve pain and anxiety.
- Prevention of further thrombi:
  LMWH and oral warfarin (p. 235).
- Intravenous fluids (to raise the filling pressure) ± inotropes for patients presenting with moderate/severe embolism.

Table 9.13 Causes of cor pulmonale

Intrinsic lung disease, e.g. COPD, pulmonary fibrosis
Recurrent pulmonary emboli
Skeletal abnormalities, e.g. kyphoscoliosis
Hypoventilation, e.g. morbid obesity
Neuromuscular disease, e.g. poliomyelitis, myasthenia gravis
Obstruction, e.g. sleep apnoea syndrome

Treatment

Treatment is directed towards the underlying pulmonary disease as well as right ventricular failure. Acute chest infections must be treated promptly. Oxygen therapy over a long period may reduce established pulmonary hypertension, with an improvement in overall prognosis (p. 500).

MYOCARDIAL DISEASE

Myocarditis (*K&C* 6e p. 847)

Myocarditis is an inflammation of the myocardium. The most common cause in the UK is viral, particularly Coxsackie virus infection, but it may also occur with diphtheria, rheumatic fever, radiation injury and some drugs.

Clinical features

Patients present with an acute illness characterized by fever and varying degrees of biventricular failure. Cardiac arrhythmias and pericarditis may also occur.

Investigations

■ Chest X-ray may show cardiac enlargement.
■ ECG shows non-specific T-wave and ST changes.
■ The diagnosis is supported by demonstration of an increase in serum viral titres and inflammation on cardiac biopsy. The findings rarely influence management, and biopsy is not usually performed.

Management

Treatment is with bed rest and treatment of heart failure. The prognosis is generally good.

CARDIOMYOPATHY (*K&C* 6e p. 848)

Cardiomyopathies are myocardial disorders that are not secondary to coronary artery disease, hypertension, or congenital, valvular or pericardial abnormalities.

There are four main types:

- Dilated
- Hypertrophic
- Restrictive
- Arrhythmogenic right ventricular.

Dilated cardiomyopathy (*K&C* 6e p. 848)

Dilated cardiomyopathy (DCM) is characterized by a dilated left ventricle which contracts poorly. In about 25% of patients it is a familial disease.

Clinical features

Shortness of breath is usually the first complaint; less often patients present with embolism (from mural thrombus) or arrhythmia. Subsequently there is progressive heart failure with the symptoms and signs of biventricular failure.

Investigations

- Chest X-ray may show cardiac enlargement.
- ECG is often abnormal. The changes are non-specific and include arrhythmias and T-wave flattening.
- Echocardiography shows dilated ventricles with global hypokinesis (compare with ischaemia with regional contractile impairment).

Other tests such as coronary arteriography, viral and auto-immune screen, and endomyocardial biopsy may be needed to exclude other diseases (Table 9.14) that present with the clinical features of DCM.

Management

Heart failure and atrial fibrillation are treated in the conventional way (pp. 428, 414). Disease progression is slowed by ACE-inhibitors, angiotensin II receptor antagonists and spironolactone, which, along with β-blockers, are indicated in most cases. Ventricular tachycardia is not prevented with antiarrhythmic drugs and is best treated with an internal

Table 9.14 Heart muscle disease presenting with features of DCM

Ischaemia
Hypertension
Congenital heart disease
Peripartum cardiomyopathy
Infections, e.g. cytomegalovirus, HIV
Alcohol excess
Muscular dystrophy
Amyloidosis
Haemochromatosis

cardioverter–defibrillator. A history of embolization or AF is an indication for anticoagulation. Severe cardiomyopathy is treated with cardiac transplantation.

Hypertrophic cardiomyopathy (K&C 6e p. 850)

Hypertrophic cardiomyopathy is characterized by marked ventricular hypertrophy of unknown cause, usually with disproportionate involvement of the interventricular septum. The hypertrophic non-compliant ventricles impair diastolic filling, so that stroke volume is reduced. Most cases are familial, autosomal dominant, and caused by mutations in genes coding for proteins that regulate contraction, e.g. troponin T and β-myosin.

Clinical features

Patients may be symptom-free or have dyspnoea, angina or syncope. Atrial and ventricular arrhythmias are common; ventricular tachyarrhythmias are the major cause of sudden death, which is most common in adolescence and young adulthood. The carotid pulse is jerky because of rapid ejection and sudden obstruction to the ventricular outflow during systole. An ejection systolic murmur occurs because of left ventricular outflow obstruction, and the pansystolic murmur of functional mitral regurgitation may also be heard.

Investigations

■ ECG is almost always abnormal. A pattern of left ventricular hypertrophy with no discernible cause is diagnostic.

■ Echocardiography shows ventricular hypertrophy with disproportionate involvement of the septum.

Management

The risk of arrhythmias and sudden death is reduced by amiodarone, but survivors of cardiac arrest need to be fitted with an internal defibrillator. Chest pain and dyspnoea are treated with β-blockers and verapamil. In selected cases outflow tract gradients are reduced by surgical resection or alcohol ablation of the septum, or by dual-chamber pacing.

Family members should be screened for evidence of disease by ECG and echocardiography.

Restrictive cardiomyopathy (*K&C* 6e p. 851)

The rigid myocardium restricts diastolic ventricular filling and the clinical features resemble those of constrictive pericarditis (see later). In the UK the most common cause is amyloidosis. The ECG, chest X-ray and echocardiogram are often abnormal, but the findings are non-specific. Diagnosis is by cardiac catheterization, which shows characteristic pressure changes. An endomyocardial biopsy may be taken during the catheter procedure, thus providing histological diagnosis. There is no specific treatment and the prognosis is poor, with most patients dying less than a year after diagnosis. Cardiac transplantation is performed in selected cases.

Arrhythmogenic right ventricular cardiomyopathy (*K&C* 6e p. 852)

There is progressive fibro-adipose replacement of the wall of the right ventricle. The typical presentation is ventricular tachycardia or sudden death in a young man.

PERICARDIAL DISEASE

The normal pericardium is a fibroelastic sac containing a thin layer of fluid (50 mL) that surrounds the heart and roots of the great vessels.

Acute pericarditis (K&C 6e p. 854)

Aetiology

In the UK, acute inflammation of the pericardium is most commonly due to viral infection (Coxsackie B, echovirus, HIV infection) or follows myocardial infarction. Other causes include uraemia, connective tissue diseases, trauma, infection (bacterial, tuberculosis, fungal), and malignancy (breast, lung, leukaemia and lymphoma).

Clinical features

There is sharp retrosternal chest pain which is characteristically relieved by leaning forward. Pain may be worse on inspiration and radiate to the neck and shoulders. The cardinal clinical sign is a pericardial friction rub, which may be transient.

Diagnosis

The ECG is diagnostic. There is concave upwards (saddle shaped) ST segment elevation and return towards baseline as inflammation subsides. ST segment elevation is convex upwards in infarction.

Management

474

Treatment is of the underlying disorder plus NSAIDs. Systemic corticosteroids are used in resistant cases. NSAIDs should not be used in the few days following myocardial infarction as they are associated with a higher rate of myocardial rupture. Complications of acute pericarditis are pericardial effusion and chronic pericarditis (> 6–12 months).

Pericardial effusion and tamponade (K&C 6e p. 855)

Pericardial effusion is an accumulation of fluid in the pericardial sac which may result from any of the causes of pericarditis. Hypothyroidism also causes a pericardial effusion which rarely compromises ventricular function. Pericardial tamponade is a medical emergency and occurs when a large amount of pericardial fluid (which has often accumulated rapidly) restricts diastolic ventricular filling and causes a marked reduction in cardiac output.

Clinical features

The effusion obscures the apex beat and the heart sounds are soft. The signs of pericardial tamponade are hypotension, tachycardia and an elevated jugular venous pressure, which paradoxically rises with inspiration (Kussmaul's sign). There is invariably pulsus paradoxus (a fall in blood pressure of more than 10 mmHg on inspiration). This is the result of increased venous return to the right side of the heart during inspiration. The increased right ventricular volume thus occupies more space within the rigid pericardium and impairs left ventricular filling.

Investigations

- Chest X-ray shows a large globular heart.
- ECG shows low-voltage complexes.
- Echocardiography is diagnostic, showing an echo-free space around the heart.
- Invasive tests to establish the cause of the effusion may only be necessary with a persistent effusion, if a purulent or tuberculous effusion is suspected, or if the effusion is not known to be secondary to an underlying illness. Pericardiocentesis (aspiration of fluid under echocardiographic guidance) and pericardial biopsy for culture, cytology/histology and PCR (for tuberculosis) gives a greater diagnostic yield with large effusions.

475

Management

The treatment of tamponade is emergency pericardio-centesis. Pericardial fluid is drained percutaneously by introducing a needle into the pericardial sac. If the effusion recurs, in spite of treatment of the underlying cause, excision of a pericardial segment may be necessary. Fluid is then absorbed through the pleural and mediastinal lymphatics.

Constrictive pericarditis (*K&C* 6e p. 856)

In the UK, most cases of constrictive pericarditis are idiopathic in origin or result from intrapericardial haemor-rhage during heart surgery. Tuberculous infection is no longer the most common cause.

Clinical features

The heart becomes encased within a rigid fibrotic pericardial sac which prevents adequate diastolic filling of the
ventricles. The clinical features resemble those of right-
sided heart failure, with jugular venous distension, dependent oedema, hepatomegaly and ascites. Kussmaul's sign
(JVP rises paradoxically with inspiration) is usually present
and there may be pulsus paradoxus, atrial fibrillation and,
on auscultation, a pericardial knock caused by rapid ventricular filling. Clinically, constrictive pericarditis cannot be
distinguished from restrictive cardiomyopathy (p. 473).

Investigations

A chest X-ray shows a normal heart size and pericardial
calcification (best seen on the lateral film). Diagnosis is
made by CT or MRI, which shows pericardial thickening
and calcification.

Management

Treatment is by surgical excision of the pericardium.

SYSTEMIC HYPERTENSION

The level of blood pressure can be said to be abnormal
when it is associated with a clear increase in morbidity and
mortality from heart disease, stroke and renal failure. This
level varies with age, sex, race and country. The definition
of hypertension is over 140/90 mmHg, based on at least
two readings on separate occasions. The validity of a single
blood pressure measurement is unclear (blood pressure
rises acutely in certain situations, e.g. visiting the doctor)
and usually several readings are required to confirm a
diagnosis of hypertension. Occasionally, ambulatory blood
pressure monitoring (blood pressure measured over a
24-hour period using a non-invasive technique) is used if
there is doubt as to the level of blood pressure.

Aetiology

Essential hypertension   More than 90% of cases of
hypertension have no known underlying cause, and the
terms 'primary' or 'essential' hypertension are used.
Several factors may play an aetiological role:

- Genetic factors
- Low birthweight
- Obesity
- High alcohol intake
- High salt intake
- The metabolic syndrome (see p. 162).

Secondary hypertension This should always be considered, particularly in those presenting under the age of 35. Causes of secondary hypertension are the following:

- Renal disease (over 80% of cases of secondary hypertension): diabetic nephropathy, chronic glomerulonephritis, reflux nephropathy, congenital polycystic kidneys and renal artery stenosis are the diseases usually involved
- Endocrine disease (p. 639): Conn's syndrome, Cushing's syndrome, phaeochromocytoma and acromegaly
- Coarctation of the aorta (narrowing of the aorta)
- Pre-eclampsia occurring in the third trimester of pregnancy
- Drugs, including oestrogen-containing oral contraceptives, other steroids, NSAIDs and vasopressin.

Clinical features

Hypertension is generally asymptomatic, although malignant or accelerated hypertension (usually BP > 200/140 mmHg) may present with characteristic symptoms. These include visual impairment, nausea, vomiting, fits, headaches or symptoms of acute heart failure. Secondary causes of hypertension may be suggested by specific features, such as attacks of sweating and tachycardia in phaeochromocytoma.

477

Examination In most patients the only finding is high blood pressure, but in others signs relating to the cause (e.g. abdominal bruit in renal artery stenosis, delayed femoral pulses in coarctation of the aorta) or the end-organ effects of hypertension may be present, e.g. loud second heart sound, left ventricular heave, fourth heart sound in hypertensive heart disease, and retinal abnormalities. The latter are graded according to severity:

- Grade 1 – increased tortuosity and reflectiveness of the retinal arteries (silver wiring)
- Grade 2 – grade 1 plus arteriovenous nipping

■ Grade 3 – grade 2 plus flame-shaped haemorrhages and soft 'cotton wool' exudates
■ Grade 4 – grade 3 plus papilloedema.

Investigations

Investigations are carried out to identify end-organ damage and those patients with secondary causes of hypertension. Routine investigation must include:

■ Serum urea and electrolytes may show evidence of renal impairment, in which case more specific renal investigations are indicated. Hypokalaemia occurs in Conn's syndrome.
■ Urine Stix testing is performed to look for haematuria and proteinuria, which may indicate renal disease (either the cause or the effect of hypertension).
■ Blood glucose.
■ Serum lipids.
■ ECG may show evidence of left ventricular hypertrophy or myocardial ischaemia.

Young patients with hypertension (< 30 years) or those where a secondary cause is suspected (e.g. from clinical examination or abnormal baseline investigations) should undergo further investigation, e.g. urinary/plasma catecholamines for phaeochromocytoma, investigation for renovascular hypertension (p. 360).

Management

Treatment is begun immediately in patients with malignant or very severe hypertension (BP ≥ 220/120 mmHg). In other patients treatment is started if repeated measurements show that sustained hypertension is present. This period of observation varies from 1–12 weeks depending on the original blood pressure reading and presence of additional cardiovascular risk factors.

Non-pharmacological measures in the treatment of hypertension include:

■ Weight reduction (aim for BMI < 25 kg/m^2)
■ Low-fat and low saturated fat diet
■ Low-salt diet (< 6 g sodium chloride per day)
■ Limited alcohol consumption (< 21 units per week for men and < 14 units per week for women)

Table 9.15 Indications for treatment and goal BP (mmHg) based on sustained BP recordings

Category	Systolic BP	Diastolic BP	Intervention	Target BP
Normal	< 130	< 85	Reassess in 5 years	
High normal	130–139	85–89	Lifestyle modification Reassess yearly	
Mild hypertension	≥ 140	≥ 90	Lifestyle modification Reassess yearly	
Mild hypertension with: – end-organ damage or – 10-year cardiovascular risk ≥ 20% or – established cardiovascular disease	≥ 140	≥ 90	Lifestyle modification Drug therapy	< 140/85
Mild hypertension in patients with diabetes mellitus	≥ 140	≥ 90	Lifestyle modification Drug therapy	130/80
Moderate hypertension	≥ 160	≥ 100	Lifestyle modification Drug therapy	< 140/85

479

- Dynamic exercise (at least 30 minutes brisk walk per day)
- Increased fruit and vegetable consumption
- Reduce cardiovascular risk by stopping smoking and increasing oily fish consumption.

The indications for treatment and target goals are listed in Table 9.15. In most hypertensive patients therapy with statins and aspirin is also given to reduce the overall cardiovascular risk burden. Glycaemic control should be

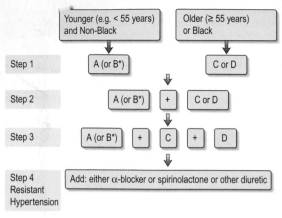

A = ACE inhibitor or angiotensin receptor blocker   B = β-blocker
C = Calcium Channel Blocker   D = Diuretic

- *Combination therapy involving B and D may induce more new onset diabetes compared with other combination therapies
- Fixed drug combinations are recommended to reduce the number of medications, which may improve compliance
- BP measurements are repeated after 4 weeks to assess treatment response unless more urgent control of BP indicated
- Dose titration is needed for most drugs other than thiazide/thiazide-like diuretic

Fig. 9.17 The British Hypertension Society recommendations for combining blood pressure-lowering drugs.

optimized in diabetics (HbA$_{1c}$ < 7%). For each class of anti-hypertensive there will be indications and contraindications in specific patient groups. A single antihypertensive drug is used initially, but combination treatment will be needed in many patients to control blood pressure. In patients without compelling reasons for a particular drug class a treatment algorithm (AB/CD) is used to advise on the sequencing of drugs and logical drug combinations (Fig. 9.17). This algorithm is based on the observation that younger people and Caucasians tend to have higher renin levels compared to older people or the black population.

Thus the A or B drugs which reduce blood pressure at least in part by suppression of the renin–angiotensin system are more effective as initial blood pressure-lowering therapy in younger Caucasian patients.

Diuretics   increase renal sodium and water excretion and directly dilate arterioles (p. 313). Loop diuretics, e.g. furosemide (frusemide), and thiazide diuretics, e.g. bendro-flumethiazide (bendrofluazide), are equally effective in lowering blood pressure, although thiazides are usually preferred, as the duration of action is longer, the diuresis is not so severe and they are cheaper. The major concern with thiazide diuretics is their adverse metabolic effects: increased serum cholesterol, hypokalaemia, hyperuricaemia (may precipitate gout) and impairment of glucose tolerance.

β-Adrenergic blocking agents   The mechanism of action of these agents is unclear. Although they reduce the force of cardiac contraction and renin production, they probably act predominantly via the central nervous system. There are a wide range of β-blocking agents with different properties, such as cardioselectivity, intrinsic sympathomimetic activity and lipid solubility. Complications include bradycardia, bronchospasm, cold extremities, fatigue and weakness.

ACE inhibitors   e.g. captopril, enalapril, lisinopril, and ramipril, block the conversion of angiotensin I to angiotensin II, which is a potent vasoconstrictor, and block degradation of bradykinin, which is a vasodilator. Side-effects include first-dose hypotension and cough, proteinuria, rashes and leucopenia in high doses. ACE inhibitors are contraindicated in renal artery stenosis because inhibition of the renin–angiotensin system in this instance may lead to loss of renal blood flow and infarction of the kidney.

Angiotensin II receptor antagonists   e.g. losartan, valsartan, irbesartan and candesartan, selectively block receptors for angiotensin II. They share some of the actions of ACE inhibitors and are useful in patients who cannot tolerate ACE inhibitors because of cough.

Calcium antagonists   e.g. amlodipine and nifedipine, are increasingly used and act predominantly by dilatation of peripheral arterioles. Side-effects are few and include bradycardia and cardiac conduction defects (verapamil and diltiazem), headaches, flushing and fluid retention.

Other agents α-Blocking agents (e.g. doxazosin), hydralazine, and centrally acting agents (e.g. clonidine, moxonidine) may be indicated in specific circumstances.

Management of severe hypertension

Patients with severe hypertension (diastolic BP > 140 mmHg) or those with severe hypertensive complications such as encephalopathy or heart failure should be admitted to hospital for treatment. The aim should be to reduce the diastolic blood pressure slowly (over 24–48 hours) to about 100–110 mmHg and this is usually achieved with oral antihypertensives, e.g. atenolol or amlodipine. Sublingual and intravenous antihypertensives are not recommended because they may produce a precipitous fall in blood pressure leading to cerebral infarction.

When rapid control of blood pressure is required (e.g. aortic dissection), the agent of choice is intravenous sodium nitroprusside (starting dose 0.3 μg/kg/min, i.e. 100 mg nitroprusside in 250 mL saline at 2–5 mL/h). Alternatively, intravenous labetolol can be used.

ARTERIAL AND VENOUS DISEASE

Aortic aneurysms (K&C 6e p. 868)

An aneurysm refers to an increase in 50% or greater of the normal diameter of the vessel. Aortic aneurysms are usually abdominal and result from atheroma.

Abdominal Abdominal aortic aneurysms may be asymptomatic and found as a pulsating mass on abdominal examination or as calcification on a plain X-ray. An expanding aneurysm may cause epigastric or back pain. A ruptured aortic aneurysm is a surgical emergency presenting with epigastric pain radiating to the back, and hypovolaemic shock. Diagnosis is by ultrasonography or CT scan. Surgical replacement of the aneurysmal segment with a prosthetic graft is indicated for a symptomatic aneurysm or large asymptomatic aneurysms (> 5.5 cm). In patients that are poor surgical risks, endovascular repair with insertion of an aortic stent is being increasingly employed.

Thoracic Cystic medial necrosis and atherosclerosis are the usual causes of thoracic aneurysms. Cardiovascular syphilis is no longer a common cause. Thoracic aneurysms may be asymptomatic, cause pressure on local structures (causing back pain, dysphagia and cough) or result in aortic regurgitation if the aortic root is involved.

Dissecting aortic aneurysm Aortic dissection results from a tear in the intima: blood under high pressure creates a false lumen in the diseased media. Typically there is an abrupt onset of severe, tearing central chest pain, radiating through to the back. Involvement of branch arteries may produce neurological signs, absent pulses and unequal blood pressure in the arms. The chest X-ray shows a widened mediastinum and the diagnosis is confirmed by CT scanning and transoesophageal echocardiography or MRI. Management involves urgent control of blood pressure (p. 482) and surgical repair for proximal aortic dissection.

Raynaud's disease and phenomenon (*K&C* 6e p. 869)

Raynaud's phenomenon consists of intermittent spasm in the arteries supplying the fingers and toes. It is usually precipitated by cold and relieved by heat. There is initial pallor (resulting from vasoconstriction) followed by cyanosis and, finally, redness from hyperaemia. Raynaud's disease (no underlying disorder) occurs most commonly in young women and must be differentiated from secondary causes of Raynaud's phenomenon, e.g. connective tissue diseases and β-blockers. Treatment is by keeping the hands and feet warm, stopping smoking and stopping β-blockers. Medical treatment includes oral nifedipine and occasionally prostacyclin infusions. Lumbar sympathectomy may help lower limb symptoms.

Venous disease (*K&C* 6e p. 870)

Superficial thrombophlebitis This usually occurs in the leg. The vein is painful, tender and hard, with overlying redness. Treatment is with simple analgesia, e.g. NSAIDs. Anticoagulation is not necessary as embolism does not occur.

Deep venous thrombosis Thrombosis can occur in any vein, but those of the pelvis and leg are the most common sites. The risk factors for deep vein thrombosis (DVT) are listed on page 235.

Clinical features

DVT is often asymptomatic but the leg may be warm and swollen, with calf tenderness and superficial venous distension. The differential diagnosis includes ruptured Baker's cyst, oedema from other causes and cellulitis.

Investigations

Diagnosis of iliofemoral thrombosis is made by Doppler ultrasonography. This method is not reliable for calf vein thrombosis, which is diagnosed by venography.

Management

This is discussed on page 237.

The main aim of therapy is to prevent pulmonary embolism, and all patients with thrombi above the knee must be anticoagulated. Anticoagulation for below-knee thrombi is now also recommended for 6 weeks to reduce proximal extension. Anticoagulation is initially with heparin and subsequently with warfarin, continued for 3 months unless there had been a definite risk factor prior to presentation, e.g. bed rest, when treatment is usually for 4 weeks. Thrombolytic therapy is occasionally used for patients with a large iliofemoral thrombosis.

The main complications of DVT are pulmonary embolus, post-thrombotic syndrome (permanent pain, swelling, oedema and sometimes venous eczema may result from destruction of the deep-vein valves) and recurrence of thrombosis. Elastic support stockings are used for the post-thrombotic syndrome.

Respiratory disease 10

BASIC RESPIRATORY SYSTEM STRUCTURE AND FUNCTION (K&C 6e p. 873)

The main function of the lungs is to provide continuous gas exchange between inspired air and the blood in the pulmonary circulation, supplying oxygen and removing carbon dioxide. The lungs are each enclosed within a double membrane (the pleura); visceral pleura covers the surface of the lung and parietal pleura lines the inside of the thoracic cavity. Under normal circumstances the interpleural space between these layers contains only a tiny amount of lubricating fluid. The right lung is the larger and divided into three lobes, while the left is divided into two lobes. The trachea divides at the carina (which lies under the junction of manubrium sterni and second right costal cartilage) into right and left main bronchi. Within the lungs the bronchi branch again, forming secondary and tertiary bronchi, then smaller bronchioles, and finally terminal bronchioles. At the end of the terminal bronchioles are the alveoli.

The larger conducting airways are compliant tubes lined by respiratory mucosa and containing variable amounts of muscle and/or cartilage in their wall. Ciliated columnar cells and mucous (goblet) cells are the two major components of the epithelium. The mucous blanket traps inhaled particulate matter. Cilia move the mucus in a cephalad direction thus clearing the lungs (the mucociliary escalator). Gas exchange occurs in the alveolus where capillary blood flow and inspired air are separated only by a thin wall composed mainly of type 1 pneumocytes and capillary endothelial cells and the capillary and alveolar basement membranes are fused as one.

The lung has a dual blood supply: pulmonary (venous blood) and systemic (arterial blood). The pulmonary circulation delivers deoxygenated blood via the pulmonary artery from the right side of the heart. Oxygen from inhaled air passes through the alveoli into the bloodstream and oxygenated blood is returned to the left heart via the pulmonary veins. The bronchial (systemic) system carries arterial blood from the descending aorta to oxygenate lung tissue primarily along the larger conducting airways. In contrast, carbon dioxide passes from the capillaries which surround the alveoli, into the alveolar spaces, and is breathed out.

In spontaneous respiration, inspiratory flow is achieved by creating a sub-atmospheric pressure in the alveoli by increasing the volume of the thoracic cavity under the action of the inspiratory muscles. The main muscle creating this negative pressure is contraction and descent of the diaphragm (innervated by the phrenic nerve, C3–C5). Additional inspiratory efforts are produced by the external intercostal muscles and the accessory muscles of respiration (sternomastoids and scalenes), although the latter only become important during exercise or respiratory distress. During quiet breathing, expiration is a passive process, relying on the elastic recoil of the lung and chest wall. If ventilation is increased, e.g. during exercise, expiration becomes active, with contraction of the muscles of the abdominal wall and the internal intercostals.

SYMPTOMS OF RESPIRATORY DISEASE (*K&C* 6e p. 882)

The most common symptoms of respiratory disease are cough, sputum production, chest pain (p. 396), breathlessness, haemoptysis and wheeze.

Cough is the most common manifestation of lower respiratory tract disease. It is initiated by stimulation of specialized receptors on the epithelium of the upper and lower respiratory tract. Cough receptors are stimulated by mechanical (e.g. touch and displacement) and chemical (e.g. noxious fumes) stimuli and impulses carried by afferent nerves to a 'cough centre' in the medulla. This generates efferent signals (via phrenic nerve and efferent branches of the vagus) to expiratory musculature to generate a cough. Estimating the duration of cough is useful in making a diagnosis (Table 10.1).

Postnasal drip is the most common cause of persistent cough. Underlying reasons for postnasal drip include rhinitis, acute nasopharyngitis and sinusitis. Symptoms of

Table 10.1	Causes of cough
Acute **< 3 weeks' duration**	**Chronic** **> 3 weeks' duration**

Upper respiratory tract infection
Exacerbation of COPD
Sinusitis
Allergic rhinitis
	Postnasal drip*
	Asthma*
	Gastro-oesophageal reflux
	   disease*
	Lung airway disease: COPD,
	   bronchiectasis, tumour,
	   foreign body
	Lung parenchymal disease:
	   interstitial lung disease,
	   lung abscess
	Drugs: ACE inhibitors

*These causes are responsible for 90% of cases of chronic cough; and responsible for 99% of cases who are non-smokers, not taking ACE inhibitors and with a normal chest X-ray
COPD, chronic obstructive pulmonary disease; ACE, angiotensin-converting enzyme

postnasal drip, other than cough, include nasal discharge, a sensation of liquid dripping back into the throat, and frequent throat clearing. Cough due to asthma is frequently accompanied by intermittent wheezing and breathlessness but it may be the only symptom (cough variant asthma), when it is typically worse at night, on waking and after exercise. Similarly, gastro-oesophageal reflux disease may present with a cough as the only symptom. A chronic cough, sometimes accompanied by sputum production, is common in smokers; however, a worsening cough may be the presenting symptom of bronchial carcinoma and needs investigation.

Dyspnoea This is the subjective sensation of shortness of breath. *Orthopnoea* is breathlessness that occurs when lying flat and is the result both of abdominal contents pushing the diaphragm into the thorax and of redistribution of blood from the lower extremities to the lungs. *Paroxysmal nocturnal dyspnoea* is a manifestation of left heart failure: the patient wakes up gasping for breath and finds some relief by sitting upright. The mechanism is similar to orthopnoea, but because sensory awareness is depressed during sleep, severe interstitial pulmonary oedema can accumulate.

Table 10.2 Differential diagnosis of dyspnoea			
Sudden	**Acute: over hours**	**Over days/months**	**Intermittent**
Upper airway obstruction: Inhaled foreign body Anaphylaxis Pneumothorax Pulmonary embolism Asthma	Asthma Pneumonia Pulmonary oedema Extrinsic allergic alveolitis Cardiac tamponade	Asthma COPD Diffuse parenchymal lung disease Heart failure Pleural effusion Cancer of the bronchus/ trachea Severe anaemia	Asthma Pulmonary oedema

COPD, chronic obstructive pulmonary disease

The speed of onset of breathlessness is useful when formulating a differential diagnosis (Table 10.2). The clinical history and examination will often suggest a probable cause, particularly with sudden and acute breathlessness. In acute breathlessness, appropriate initial investigations include a chest X-ray, pulse oximetry and sometimes arterial blood gases, ECG, full blood count, serum urea and electrolytes, and blood glucose. Pulmonary embolism can be a difficult diagnosis to make and chest X-ray, blood gases and ECG may be normal. Simple lung function tests, pulse oximetry, a full blood count and a chest X-ray are the initial investigations for most patients with chronic breathlessness. Echocardiography is indicated if a cardiac cause for dyspnoea is suspected.

Psychogenic breathlessness is usually described as 'inability to take a deep breath' and rarely disturbs sleep and may be better with exercise. Panic-related hyperventilation must be included in the differential diagnosis of acute breathlessness.

Wheeze Wheezing is the result of airflow limitation of any cause. It may be due to localized obstruction of the airways, e.g. cancer, foreign body, or to generalized obstruction, of which the commonest causes are asthma and chronic obstructive pulmonary disease. Asthma is a common cause of wheezing and considered likely when patients present with episodic wheezing, cough and dyspnoea which responds favourably to inhaled broncho-dilators. Wheeze should be distinguished from stridor which is a harsh inspiratory wheezing sound caused by obstruction of the trachea or major bronchi, e.g. by tumour.

Haemoptysis (coughing blood) requires thorough investigation. The common causes are bronchiectasis, bronchial carcinoma, pulmonary infarction, bronchitis and lung infections including pneumonia, abscess and tuberculosis. Pulmonary oedema is associated with the production of pink frothy sputum. Rust-coloured sputum may occur with pneumococcal pneumonia but haemoptysis should not be attributed to infection without investigation. Less common causes include benign tumours, bleeding disorders and rarely Wegener's granulomatosis (p. 533) and Goodpasture's syndrome (p. 345). A chest X-ray should be performed in all patients, and subsequent investigations (e.g. bronchoscopy, CT of the thorax, ventilation–perfusion scan) decided from the history and examination.

Massive haemoptysis (more than 200 mL in 24 h) is often due to bronchiectasis, TB or cancer. It may be life-threatening due to asphyxiation and is an indication for hospital admission. The initial management includes administration of oxygen, placement of a large-bore intravenous catheter, blood samples (for full blood count, clotting screen, urea and electrolytes), arterial blood gases and chest X-ray. There should be early referral to a respiratory physician and thoracic surgeon.

489

Chest pain (p. 396) The most common chest pain encountered in respiratory disease is a localized sharp pain, typically made worse by deep breathing or coughing. It is commonly referred to as pleuritic pain and is most commonly caused by infection or by pleural irritation from a pulmonary embolism.

INVESTIGATION OF RESPIRATORY DISEASE

Sputum (K&C 6e pp. 882 & 885)

Sputum samples are obtained during the investigation of pneumonia, and suspected tuberculosis and bronchial carcinoma. A 5% saline nebulizer will encourage productive coughing if sputum is difficult to obtain. Inspection of the sputum may indicate infection (yellow/green) or haemoptysis (blood-stained). Sputum is commonly sent for microbiology (Gram stain and culture, Ziehl–Neelsen stain) and cytology (for malignant cells, may be falsely negative).

Respiratory function tests (K&C 6e p. 888)

Respiratory function tests are simple outpatient investigations carried out to assess airflow limitation and lung volumes. The normal values vary for age, sex and height, and between individuals.

Peak expiratory flow rate (PEFR) is measured with a peak flow meter. This records the maximum expiratory flow rate during a forced expiration after full inspiration. It is useful in detecting airflow limitation and in monitoring the response to treatment of acute asthma. It is simple to perform and many patients will monitor their own PEFR at home.

Forced expiratory volume (FEV) and forced vital capacity (FVC) are measured with a spirometer. The patient exhales as fast and as long as possible from a full inspiration; the volume expired in the first second is the FEV_1 and the total volume expired is the FVC. The ratio $FEV_1 : FVC$ is a measure of airflow limitation and is normally about 75%.

■ Airflow limitation: $FEV_1 : FVC < 75\%$
■ Restrictive lung disease: $FEV_1 : FVC > 75\%$.

More sophisticated techniques allow the measurement of total lung capacity (TLC) and residual volume (RV). These are increased in obstructive lung disease, e.g. asthma or COPD, because of air trapping, and reduced in lung fibrosis. Transfer factor (T_{CO}) measures the transfer of a low concentration of added carbon monoxide in the inspired air to haemoglobin. The transfer coefficient (K_{CO}) is the value corrected for differences in lung volume. Gas transfer is reduced early on in emphysema and lung fibrosis.

Assessment of lung function is also made by measuring arterial blood gases (p. 799) and with exercise tests to assess walking distance in a 6-minute period.

Imaging (K&C 6e p. 885)

The 'plain' chest X-ray (K&C 6e p. 885)

Routine films are taken postero-anteriorly (PA), i.e. the film is placed in front of the patient with the X-ray source behind. AP films are taken only in patients who are unable to stand; the cardiac outline appears bigger and the

Table 10.3 Causes of a solitary pulmonary nodule

Benign	Malignant
Infectious granuloma, e.g. TB	Bronchial carcinoma
Other infections, e.g. localized pneumonia, abscess, hydatid cyst	Single metastasis
	Lymphoma
Benign neoplasms	Pulmonary carcinoid
Arteriovenous malformation	
Bronchogenic cyst	
Pulmonary infarct	
Inflammatory, rheumatoid nodule, Wegener's granuloma	

scapulae cannot be moved out of the way. The following should be noted:

■ Patient's name and date of the film
■ Contour of diaphragm and outline of rib cage (? pleural effusion, pneumothorax, raised hemidiaphragm, air under the diaphragm)
■ Bony structure (ribs, clavicles, spine)
■ Size, shape and position of the heart (enlarged heart is > 50% of maximum distance between ribs)
■ Position of trachea (? deviated from midline; a rotated patient will also make the trachea look deviated)
■ Mediastinum (? widened, ? lymphadenopathy)
■ Hilar shadows (? enlarged pulmonary arteries and veins)
■ Lungs (? opacities, consolidation, fluid, nodules). The solitary pulmonary nodule detected on chest X-ray is a common clinical problem (Table 10.3). Risk factors for malignancy in this situation are older age, smoker, occupational exposure to carcinogens, increasing size of lesion (80% > 3 cm), irregular border, eccentric calcification of the lesion and increasing size compared to an old X-ray. CT scan is often necessary for further evaluation.

Computed tomography (CT scan) (*K&C* 6e p. 886)

The initial imaging tool for the lung parenchyma is the chest X-ray. However, a CT scan can detect lung disease in symptomatic patients with a normal chest X-ray. It can be used as a guide to the type and site of lung or pleural biopsy, and is used in the staging of bronchial carcinoma. *High-resolution CT scanning* (sampling lung parenchyma with scans of 1–2 mm thickness at intervals of 10–20 mm) is particularly useful in the detection and evaluation of diffuse parenchymal lung disease and in diagnosis of bronchiectasis. *CT angiography* (helical CT using intravenous contrast) is used in the diagnosis of pulmonary emboli.

Magnetic resonance imaging (MRI) (*K&C* 6e p. 887)

MRI is less useful than CT scanning in the assessment of the lung parenchyma. It is useful to stage lung cancer, for assessing tumour invasion in the mediastinum, lung apex and chest wall. It also provides accurate images of the heart and aorta.

Positron emission tomography (PET) (*K&C* 6e p. 887)

PET scanning (p. 961) is used in the investigation of pulmonary nodules to differentiate benign from malignant, and in the staging of lung cancer.

Scintigraphic imaging (*K&C* 6e p. 887)

Ventilation–perfusion $(\dot{V}/\dot{Q})$ scanning is used in the diagnosis of pulmonary emboli. Xenon-133 gas is inhaled (the ventilation scan) and microaggregates of albumin labelled with technetium-99m are injected intravenously (the perfusion scan). Pulmonary emboli are detected as 'cold areas' on the perfusion scan relative to the ventilation scan. However, many lung diseases affect pulmonary blood flow as well as ventilation and the $\dot{V}/\dot{Q}$ scan is only diagnostic when it is reported as normal (excluding pulmonary embolism (PE)) or high probability (diagnostic of PE).

Pleural aspiration and biopsy (*K&C* 6e p. 891)

See page 806.

Bronchoscopy (*K&C* 6e p. 891)

The trachea and larger bronchi as far as the subsegmental bronchi are inspected using a flexible bronchoscope. The procedure is usually performed with intravenous midazolam sedation, topical lidocaine (lignocaine) anaesthesia and pre-medication with an antimuscarinic agent such as atropine to reduce bronchial secretions. Biopsies and brushings can be taken of macroscopic abnormalities and washings can be taken for appropriate microbiological staining and culture and cytological examination for malignant cells. Diffuse parenchymal lung disease can be investigated using trans-bronchial biopsy. Complications of bronchoscopy ± biopsy include respiratory depression, pneumothorax, respiratory obstruction, cardiac arrhythmias, and haemorrhage.

Arterial blood gases and pulse oximetry (*K&C* 6e pp. 890 & 980)

See page 799.

DISEASES OF THE UPPER RESPIRATORY TRACT

The common cold (acute coryza) (*K&C* 6e p. 895)

The common cold is caused by infection with one of the many strains of rhinovirus. Spread is by droplets and close personal contact. After an incubation period of 12 hours to 5 days the major symptoms are malaise, slight pyrexia, a sore throat and a watery nasal discharge, which becomes mucopurulent after a few days. Treatment is symptomatic. The differential diagnosis is mainly from rhinitis.

Sinusitis (*K&C* 6e p. 1158)

Sinusitis is an infection of one of the paranasal sinuses (maxillary, frontal or ethmoid) and may complicate allergic rhinitis or an upper respiratory tract infection (caused by mucosal oedema and blockage of the ostium). Acute infections are usually caused by *Streptococcus pneumoniae* or *Haemophilus influenzae*. Symptoms are frontal headache, facial pain and tenderness, and nasal discharge. The diagnosis is usually clinical and treatment is with antibiotics, e.g. cefaclor, and nasal treatment with decongestants, e.g. xylometazoline. Rare complications include local and cerebral abscesses. Chronic sinusitis can be a cause of headaches.

Rhinitis (*K&C* 6e p. 895)

The symptoms of rhinitis are sneezing, nasal discharge and blockage. *Perennial rhinitis* occurs throughout the year and may be allergic (the allergens are similar to those for asthma) or non-allergic. Some of these patients develop nasal polyps which may cause nasal obstruction, loss of smell and taste, and mouth breathing. *Seasonal allergic rhinitis* (hay fever) occurs during the summer months and is caused by allergy to grass and tree pollen and a variety of mould spores (e.g. *Aspergillus fumigatus*) which grow on cultivated plants. The diagnosis of rhinitis is clinical. Skin-prick testing or measurement of specific serum IgE antibody against the particular antigen (RAST test) in conjunction with a detailed clinical history will identify causal antigens. The management involves avoidance of allergens if practical, antihistamines, e.g. cetirizine or loratidine tablets, decongestants and topical steroids, e.g. beclometasone spray twice daily. A 2-week course of low-dose oral prednisolone (5–10 mg daily) may be necessary when other treatments fail.

Acute pharyngitis (K&C 6e p. 898)

Viruses, particularly from the adenovirus group, are the most common cause of acute pharyngitis. Symptoms are a sore throat and fever which are self-limiting and only require symptomatic treatment. More persistent and severe pharyngitis may imply bacterial infection, often secondary invaders, of which the most common organisms are haemolytic *Streptococcus*, *Haemophilus influenzae* and *Staphylococcus aureus*. This requires antibiotic treatment such as oral cefaclor.

Acute laryngotracheobronchitis (K&C 6e p. 898)

This is usually the result of infection with one of the parainfluenza viruses or measles virus. Symptoms are most severe in children under 3 years of age. Inflammatory oedema involving the larynx causes a hoarse voice, barking cough (croup) and stridor. Tracheitis produces a burning retrosternal pain. Treatment is with oxygen and inhaled steam; tracheostomy is needed in severe cases.

Influenza (K&C 6e pp. 55 & 898)

The influenza virus belongs to the orthomyxovirus group and exists in two main forms, A and B. The surface of the virion is coated with haemagglutinin (H) and an enzyme, neuraminidase (N), which are necessary for attachment to the host respiratory epithelium. Human immunity develops against the H and N antigens. Influenza A has the capacity to undergo antigenic 'shift', and major changes in the H and N antigens are associated with pandemic infections which may cause millions of deaths world-wide. Minor antigenic 'drifts' are associated with less severe epidemics. In South East Asia an avian strain of influenza has recently been transmitted from poultry to man (avian influenza).

Clinical features

After an incubation period of 1–3 days there is an abrupt onset of fever, generalized aching in the limbs, headache, sore throat and dry cough, which may last several weeks.

Diagnosis

Laboratory diagnosis is not always necessary, but serology shows a fourfold rise in antibody titre over a 2-week period, or the virus can be demonstrated in throat or nasal secretion.

Management

Treatment is usually symptomatic (aspirin, bed rest, maintenance of fluid intake), together with antibiotics for individuals with chronic bronchitis, or heart or renal disease. Neuraminidase inhibitors, e.g. zanamivir and oseltamivir, shorten the duration of symptoms in patients with influenza. They are recommended in the UK for patients over the age of 65 years with suspected influenza and 'at-risk' adults (i.e. with co-morbid disease).

Complications

Pneumonia is the most common complication. This is either viral or the result of secondary infection with bacteria, of which *Staphylococcus aureus* is the most serious, with a mortality rate of up to 20%.

Prophylaxis

Influenza vaccine is prepared from current strains. It is effective in 70% of people and lasts for about a year. It is recommended for the following groups:

■ Individuals over 65 years of age
■ Chronic respiratory disease including asthma needing continuous or repeated use of inhaled or oral steroids
■ Chronic heart disease (congenital heart disease, heart failure, ischaemic heart disease)
■ Chronic liver disease
■ Chronic renal disease (nephrotic syndrome, chronic renal failure, renal transplantation)
■ Diabetes mellitus

- The immunocompromised, including individuals treated, or likely to be treated, with systemic steroids for more than a month at a dose equivalent to 20 mg daily
- Persons who are the main carer for an elderly or disabled person whose welfare may be at risk if the carer falls ill.

Inhalation of foreign bodies (K&C 6e p. 899)

Children inhale foreign bodies – frequently peanuts – more often than do adults. In adults inhalation is usually associated with a depressed conscious level, such as after an alcoholic binge. A large object may totally occlude the airways and rapidly result in death. Smaller objects impact more peripherally (usually in the right main bronchus, because it is more vertical than the left) and cause choking or persistent wheeze, or patients may present at a later stage with persistent suppurative pneumonia or lung abscess. In an emergency the foreign body is dislodged from the airway using the Heimlich manoeuvre: the subject is gripped from behind with the arms around the upper abdomen, a sharp forceful squeeze pushes the diaphragm into the thorax and the rapid airflow generated may be sufficient to force the foreign body out of the trachea or bronchus. In the non-emergency situation bronchoscopy is used to remove the foreign body.

DISEASES OF THE LOWER RESPIRATORY TRACT

Acute bronchitis (K&C 6e p. 899)

Acute bronchitis is usually viral but may be complicated by bacterial infection, particularly in smokers and in patients with chronic airflow limitation. Symptoms are cough, retrosternal discomfort, chest tightness and wheezing, which usually resolve spontaneously over 4–8 days.

Chronic obstructive pulmonary disease (COPD) (K&C 6e p. 900)

COPD is characterized by poorly reversible airflow limitation that is usually progressive and associated with a persistent inflammatory response of the lungs. In developed countries the disease is predominantly caused by smoking. COPD is now the preferred term for patients with airflow obstruction who were previously diagnosed as having chronic bronchitis or emphysema.

Epidemiology

COPD develops over many years and patients are rarely symptomatic before middle age. It is common (18% of male and 14% of female smokers) in the UK, where it is one of the leading causes of lost working days.

Pathology

In chronic bronchitis there is airway narrowing, and hence airflow limitation, as a result of hypertrophy and hyperplasia of mucus-secreting glands of the bronchial tree, bronchial wall inflammation and mucosal oedema. The epithelial cell layer may ulcerate and, when the ulcers heal, squamous epithelium may replace columnar epithelium (squamous metaplasia). Emphysema is defined pathologically as dilatation and destruction of the lung tissue distal to the terminal bronchioles. Emphysematous changes lead to loss of elastic recoil, which normally keeps airways open during expiration; this is associated with expiratory airflow limitation and air trapping. Although it has been suggested that these definitions separate patients into two different clinical groups (the 'pink puffers' with predominant emphysema and the 'blue bloaters' with predominant chronic bronchitis), most have both emphysema and chronic bronchitis, irrespective of the clinical signs.

Aetiology and pathogenesis

- *Smoking* is the dominant causal agent. Cigarette smoke activates macrophages and airway epithelial cells in the respiratory tract, which release neutrophil chemotactic factors, including interleukin-8 and leukotriene B_4. Neutrophils and macrophages then release proteases that break down connective tissue in the lung parenchyma resulting in emphysema, and also stimulate mucus hypersecretion. Proteases are normally counteracted by protease inhibitors, including α_1-antitrypsin, but in COPD the balance is tipped in favour of proteolysis. In contrast to asthma (see p. 509) the bronchiole wall infiltrate is predominantly CD8+ (cytotoxic) T cells. The role of cytotoxic T cells is not yet clear.

- *Atmospheric pollution* plays a minor role compared to smoking.
- α_1-Antitrypsin deficiency (p. 161) is a rare cause of early-onset emphysema.

Clinical features

The characteristic symptoms of COPD are cough with the production of sputum, wheeze and breathlessness following many years of a smoker's cough. Frequent infective exacerbations occur, giving purulent sputum. On examination the patient with severe disease is breathless at rest, with prolonged expiration and using the accessory muscles of respiration (sternomastoids and scalenes); chest expansion is poor and the lungs are hyperinflated. There may be a wheeze or quiet breath sounds. In 'pink puffers' breathlessness is the predominant problem; they are not cyanosed. 'Blue bloaters' hypoventilate; they are cyanosed, may be oedematous and have features of CO_2 retention (warm peripheries with a bounding pulse, flapping tremor of the outstretched hands and confusion in severe cases). Symptoms and signs may help to distinguish COPD from asthma in untreated patients presenting for the first time (Table 10.4).

Table 10.4 **Clinical features differentiating COPD and asthma**

	COPD	Asthma
Smoker or ex-smoker	Most	Possibly
Symptoms under age 35	Rare	Common
Chronic productive cough	Common	Uncommon
Breathlessness	Persistent and progressive	Variable
Waking at night time with breathlessness or wheeze	Uncommon	Common
Significant diurnal or day-to-day variability of symptoms	Uncommon	Common
FEV_1 and FEV_1/FVC ratio return to normal with drug therapy	Never with significant disease	Probably

Chronic obstructive pulmonary disease (COPD)

Investigations

There is no single diagnostic test for COPD. The diagnosis is made on the basis of history (breathlessness and sputum production in a lifetime smoker), physical examination and confirmation of airflow limitation with lung function testing.

- Lung function tests. There is a reduced FEV_1 and reduced FEV_1/FVC ratio usually so that the FEV_1 is < 80% predicted and FEV_1/FVC is less than 0.7. Some patients have partially reversible airflow limitation with an increase in FEV_1 (usually < 15%) following inhalation of a β_2-agonist. Serial peak flow measurements may be necessary to exclude asthma (Table 10.4). Additional testing of lung function is necessary if there is diagnostic uncertainty. Lung volumes are normal or increased, and the loss of alveoli with emphysema results in a decreased gas transfer coefficient of carbon monoxide.
- Chest X-ray. The lungs are hyperinflated, indicated by a low flat diaphragm and a long narrow heart shadow. There are reduced peripheral lung markings and bullae, although the chest X-ray may be normal.
- Haemoglobin and PCV may be high as a result of persistent hypoxaemia and secondary polycythaemia (p. 211).
- Arterial blood gases may be normal or show hypoxia and hypercapnia in advanced cases.
- Serum levels of α_1-antitrypsin if early onset (< 40 years) or family history.
- ECG and echocardiography to assess cardiac status if clinical features of cor pulmonale (p. 468).
- Body mass index (p. 120). Patients are frequently underweight and a low BMI (≤ 21) predicts an accelerated decline in lung function.

Complications

- Respiratory failure (p. 563).
- Cor pulmonale, i.e. right heart failure secondary to lung disease (p. 468).

Management

COPD care should be delivered by a multidisciplinary team to include GP and respiratory physicians, respiratory nurse specialists, physiotherapy, occupational therapy, dietetics and palliative care in end-stage COPD.

Cessation of smoking The most important aspect of management is to persuade the patient to stop smoking, which is the only measure that will slow the rate of deterioration. Smoking withdrawal clinics, nicotine replacement (gum, transdermal patch, or inhaler) or bupropion tablets help.

Bronchodilators Drug therapy is similar to that for asthma (p. 512). Inhaled (with spacer device if necessary) β_2-agonists and the antimuscarinic agent ipratropium bromide may produce symptomatic improvement even with little change in lung function tests. Nebulized therapy may be useful for patients with disabling breathlessness despite inhalers.

Corticosteroids Assessment of reversibility is made with a 2-week course of oral prednisolone (30 mg daily), with measurement of lung function before and after the treatment period. If there is objective evidence of benefit (> 15% improvement in FEV_1), oral steroids are gradually reduced and replaced with inhaled steroids.

Prevention of infection Acute exacerbations of COPD are commonly due to bacterial or viral infection. Patients should receive pneumococcal vaccine and annual influenza vaccination.

Oxygen Long-term domiciliary oxygen therapy is provided by oxygen concentrators. It reduces mortality if given for 19 hours per day (every day) at a flow rate of 1–3 L/min via nasal prongs to increase arterial oxygen saturation to > 90%. It is prescribed to patients who no longer smoke and who have a P_aO_2 < 7.3 kPa when stable on room air or a P_aO_2 < 8.0 kPa when stable with secondary polycythaemia, nocturnal hypoxaemia, peripheral oedema or evidence of pulmonary hypertension. Assessment for home oxygen should include blood gas measurements made 3 weeks apart.

Additional treatments include venesection for polycythaemia, diuretics for oedema, exercise training to improve sense of well-being and breathlessness, and high-calorie dietary supplements in those with low BMI.

Acute exacerbation of COPD

Patients with COPD are prone to acute exacerbations which are diagnosed on the basis of increased breathlessness, wheeze and production of increased volume of purulent sputum. The major complication is respiratory failure. Exacerbations are usually the result of a superimposed viral or bacterial (often *Haemophilus influenzae*) respiratory tract infection and are treated in a similar manner to asthma. Some patients with mild exacerbations may be managed at home by a dedicated multidisciplinary team (including nurses, physiotherapists and occupational therapists). Management of patients admitted to hospital includes the following steps:

■ Oxygen is given to maintain S_aO_2 > 90%. These patients often depend on a degree of hypoxaemia to maintain respiratory drive and therefore, if oxygen is necessary, low concentrations (24%) are given, via a Venturi mask (fixed-performance mask), so as not to reduce respiratory drive and precipitate worsening hypercapnia and respiratory acidosis. The oxygen concentration may be increased in increments (28% and then 35%) if clinical examination and repeated arterial blood gases do not show hypoventilation, carbon dioxide retention and worsening acidosis.

■ Bronchodilators (salbutamol and ipratropium bromide) are given via an air-driven nebulizer together with oral or intravenous corticosteroids.

■ Antibiotics, e.g. cefaclor or co-amoxiclav, are given if there is a history of more purulent sputum production or with chest X-ray changes. Patients should be encouraged to cough up sputum, initially with the help of a physiotherapist. Antibiotic treatment is modified depending on sputum culture results.

■ Patients with life-threatening respiratory failure require ventilatory assistance. Bilevel positive airway pressure (BiPAP, p. 565) will avoid the need for intubation and mechanical ventilation in some patients with acute exacerbations of COPD. It is indicated in patients with acute exacerbation of COPD and mild to moderate respiratory acidosis (blood pH < 7.35 or P_aCO_2 > 6 kPa) who have failed to respond to initial bronchodilator therapy.

■ The respiratory stimulant, doxapram, 1.5–4.0 mg/min by slow i.v. infusion, may help in the short term to arouse

the patient and to stimulate coughing, with clearance of some secretions. This is rarely used, largely due to the increasing availability of non-invasive ventilatory support.
■ Exacerbations of COPD are occasionally the result of pneumothorax, heart failure or pulmonary embolism, and these must be excluded.

Prognosis

The single best predictor of prognosis in COPD is the initial post-bronchodilator FEV_1, e.g. only about 10% of patients with a $FEV_1 < 20\%$ of that predicted will be alive at 5 years.

Obstructive sleep apnoea (*K&C* 6e p. 907)

Obstructive sleep apnoea (OSA) is characterized by repetitive apnoea (cessation of breathing for 10 seconds or more) as a result of obstruction of the upper airway during sleep.

Epidemiology

OSA affects about 2% of the population and is most common in overweight middle-aged men. It can also occur in children, particularly those with enlarged tonsils.

Aetiology

Apnoea occurs if the upper airway at the back of the throat is sucked closed when the patient breathes in. This occurs during sleep because the muscles that hold the airway open are hypotonic. Airway closure continues until the patient is woken up by the struggle to breathe against a blocked throat. Contributing factors include alcohol ingestion before sleep, obesity and COPD. It is more common in hypothyroidism and acromegaly.

Clinical features

Loud snoring and excessive daytime sleepiness (leading to impairment of work performance and driving) occur in the majority of patients. Apnoeas may be witnessed by bed partners. Other symptoms are irritability, personality change, morning headaches, impotence and nocturnal choking. Patients with sleep apnoea have an increased risk of hypertension, heart failure, myocardial infarction and stroke.

Diagnosis

Arterial oxygen saturation is measured overnight at home by non-invasive ear or finger oximetry and shows frequent falls in oxygen saturation in some, but not all, patients.

Inpatient oximetry supplemented by video recording is performed if home oximetry is negative or equivocal. More detailed sleep studies (polysomnography) are rarely necessary to make the diagnosis.

The diagnosis of sleep apnoea/hypopnoea is confirmed if there are more than 15 apnoeas or hypopnoeas in any 1 hour of sleep.

Management

- Predisposing factors, e.g. obesity, tonsillar hypertrophy and facial deformities, should be corrected. Alcohol and sedatives should be avoided.
- CPAP (continuous positive airway pressure) to the airway via a tight-fitting nasal mask – nasal CPAP – during sleep keeps the pharyngeal walls open and is a very effective treatment.

Bronchiectasis (*K&C* 6e p. 908)

Bronchiectasis is defined as permanent dilatation of the bronchi. It may be localized to a lobe or generalized throughout the bronchial tree. There is impaired clearance of bronchial secretions with secondary bacterial infection.

Aetiology

The causes are shown in Table 10.5. Cystic fibrosis (p. 505) is the most common cause in developed countries.

Epidemiology

Most cases arise in childhood. The incidence has decreased in all age groups with effective antibiotic treatment of pneumonia.

Clinical features

Cough and sputum production are the most common symptoms. In severe bronchiectasis there is production of copious amounts of thick, foul-smelling green sputum. Other symptoms are haemoptysis (which may be massive

Table 10.5 Causes of bronchiectasis

Acquired

Post-infective bronchial damage, e.g. measles, whooping cough, TB

Airway obstruction: inhaled foreign body, tumour, enlarged lymph nodes

Acquired immunodeficiency, e.g. AIDS

Congenital

Ciliary dyskinesia
  Primary ciliary dyskinesia (immotile cilia syndrome)
  Kartagener's syndrome (immotile cilia, situs invertus, chronic sinusitis)
  Young's syndrome (bronchiectasis, absent vas deferens)
Cystic fibrosis
Immunoglobulin deficiencies (due to recurrent infections)

and life-threatening), breathlessness and wheeze. On examination there is clubbing and coarse crackles over the affected area, usually the lung bases.

Investigations

- Chest X-ray may be normal or show dilated bronchi with thickened bronchial walls, and sometimes multiple cysts containing fluid.
- High-resolution CT (p. 491) is the investigation of choice and may show airway dilatation, bronchial wall thickening and bronchial wall cysts that are not shown on a standard chest X-ray.
- Sputum culture is essential during an infective exacerbation. The common organisms are *Staphylococcus aureus*, *Pseudomonas aeruginosa* and *Haemophilus influenzae*.
- Further investigations, e.g. serum immunoglobulins, sweat test, in patients where an underlying cause is suspected.

Management

- Postural drainage is essential. The patient is trained by physiotherapists to do this at least three times daily for 20 minutes.

- Antibiotics. In mild cases intermittent chemotherapy with cefaclor 500 mg three times daily may be the only therapy needed. Flucloxacillin is the best treatment if *Staph. aureus* is isolated on sputum culture. If the sputum remains yellow or green despite regular physiotherapy and antibiotics it is probable that there is infection with *Pseudomonas aeruginosa*, which requires specific antibiotics, e.g. ceftazidime, administered by aerosol or parenterally. Oral ciprofloxacin is an alternative.
- Bronchodilators are used for those with demonstrable airflow limitation.
- Inhaled or oral steroids can decrease the rate of progression.
- Surgery is reserved for the very small minority with localized disease. Severe disease sometimes requires lung or heart–lung transplantation.

Complications

The main complications are pneumonia, haemoptysis which may be life-threatening, and cerebral abscess. Most patients with severe bronchiectasis will eventually develop respiratory failure.

Cystic fibrosis (*K&C* 6e p. 909)

Cystic fibrosis (CF) is an autosomal recessive condition occurring in 1 : 2000 live births. It is characterized by an alteration in the viscosity and tenacity of mucus produced at epithelial surfaces. The classical form of the syndrome includes bronchopulmonary infection and pancreatic insufficiency, with a high sweat sodium and chloride concentration. It is caused by mutations in a single gene on the long arm of chromosome 7 that encodes the cystic fibrosis transmembrane conductance regulator (CFTR). Mutations in the *CFTR* gene result in the production of a defective transmembrane protein which is a critical chloride channel in epithelial cell membranes in the pancreas and respiratory, gastrointestinal and reproductive tracts. The decreased chloride transport is accompanied by decreased transport of sodium and water, resulting in dehydrated viscous secretions that are associated with luminal obstruction and destruction and scarring of exocrine glands. The most common mutation is ΔF_{508} (deletion, phenylalanine at position 508).

505

Clinical features

Although the lungs of babies born with CF are normal at birth, respiratory symptoms are usually the presenting features. Bronchiectasis and obstructive pulmonary disease are the primary causes of morbidity and mortality in patients with CF. Infants with CF have persistent endo-bronchial infections due initially to *Staphylococcus aureus*, *Haemophilus influenzae* and Gram-negative bacilli. By the end of the first decade of life *Pseudomonas aeruginosa* is the predominant pathogen (p. 522). The resultant inflammatory response damages the airway, leading to progressive bronchiectasis and eventually respiratory failure. Finger clubbing is seen in patients with moderate or advanced disease. Sinusitis and nasal polyps occur in most patients. Meconium ileus is the presenting problem in about one-fifth of newborns with CF and is virtually pathognomonic of the diagnosis. Episodes of small bowel obstruction may also occur in later life and have been called the meconium ileus equivalent syndrome. There may be steatorrhoea and diabetes mellitus as a result of pancreatic insufficiency. Males are infertile because of failure of development of the vas deferens. Chronic ill-health in children leads to impaired growth and delayed puberty. Many patients are undernourished.

Investigations

The diagnosis in adults and older children is based on the clinical history and:

- A family history of the disease
- A high sweat sodium > 60 mmol/L – this must be performed in a laboratory regularly undertaking testing
- Blood DNA analysis of the gene defect
- Absent vas deferens and epididymis.

Genetic screening for the carrier state should be offered to persons or couples with a family history of CF, together with counselling.

Management

Management of bronchiectasis and exocrine pancreatic insufficiency is described on pages 504 and 180. Specific treatments are based on an understanding of the basic defect and pathogenesis of cystic fibrosis (Table 10.6). Some

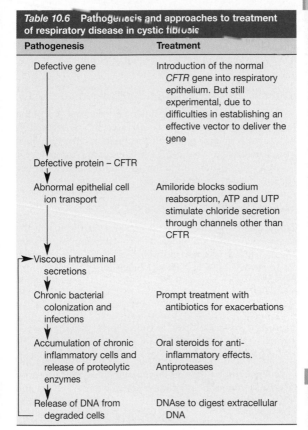

Table 10.6 Pathogenesis and approaches to treatment of respiratory disease in cystic fibrosis

Pathogenesis	Treatment
Defective gene	Introduction of the normal *CFTR* gene into respiratory epithelium. But still experimental, due to difficulties in establishing an effective vector to deliver the gene
Defective protein – CFTR	
Abnormal epithelial cell ion transport	Amiloride blocks sodium reabsorption, ATP and UTP stimulate chloride secretion through channels other than CFTR
Viscous intraluminal secretions	
Chronic bacterial colonization and infections	Prompt treatment with antibiotics for exacerbations
Accumulation of chronic inflammatory cells and release of proteolytic enzymes	Oral steroids for anti-inflammatory effects. Antiproteases
Release of DNA from degraded cells	DNAse to digest extracellular DNA

Amiloride, adenosine or uridine triphosphates (ATP and UTP), DNAse and α_1-antitrypsin are given by aerosol

patients with severe respiratory disease have received lung or heart–lung transplantations (*K&C* 6e p. 911).

The emergence of *Burkholderia cepacia* infection is a problem for patients and doctors alike. It is associated with accelerated lung disease and resistance to antibiotics in some strains. Close contact promotes cross-infection, so siblings and fellow sufferers with cystic fibrosis may pass the organism from one to another.

Prognosis

Ninety per cent of children now survive into their teens, and the median survival for those born after 1990 is estimated at 40 years. Most mortality is the result of pulmonary disease.

ASTHMA (K&C 6e p. 912)

Asthma is a common chronic inflammatory condition of the lung airways, whose cause is incompletely understood. It has three characteristics: airflow limitation, airway hyper-responsiveness to a range of stimuli, and inflammation of the bronchi. Airflow limitation is often reversible, either spontaneously or with treatment.

Epidemiology

The prevalence of asthma is increasing, particularly in the second decade of life, when 10–15% of the population are affected. There is a geographical variation: asthma is more common in New Zealand and much rarer in Far Eastern countries.

Aetiology

There are two major factors involved in the development of asthma:

- *Atopy*. This is the term used in individuals who readily develop antibodies of immunoglobulin E (IgE) class against common environmental antigens such as the house-dust mite, grass pollen and fungal spores from *Aspergillus fumigatus*. Genetic and environmental factors affect serum IgE levels. Included in the genetic influence is the cytokine gene complex on chromosome 5, the interleukin-4 (IL-4) gene cluster, which controls the production of IL-3, IL-4, IL-5 and IL-13. Environmental factors include childhood exposure to respiratory irritants such as tobacco smoke, and intestinal bacterial and child-hood infections. There is evidence that growing up in a relatively clean environment may predispose towards an IgE response to allergens.
- *Increased responsiveness of the airways of the lung* (as measured by a fall in FEV_1) to stimuli such as inhaled histamine and methacholine (bronchial provocation tests, see below).

508

Asthma has traditionally been divided into extrinsic (atopic) and intrinsic (non-atopic) on the basis that in extrinsic asthma allergens can be identified by positive skin-prick reactions to common inhaled allergens. It is now recognized that almost all asthmatic patients show some degree of atopy, and this classification is used less often.

Pathogenesis

The primary abnormality in asthma is narrowing of the airway, which is due to smooth muscle contraction, thickening of the airway wall by cellular infiltration and inflammation, and the presence of secretions within the airway lumen. The pathogenesis of asthma is complex and not fully understood. It involves a number of cells, mediators, nerves and vascular leakage which can be activated by several mechanisms, of which exposure to allergens is the most relevant.

Inflammation The cellular component of the inflammatory response includes eosinophils, T lymphocytes, macrophages and mast cells, which release a number of inflammatory mediators. Macrophages may have a role in the initial uptake and presentation of allergens to lymphocytes. Lymphocytes infiltrating the asthmatic airway primarily bear the T-helper 2 (Th2) phenotype. These lymphocytes, when stimulated by the appropriate antigen, release a restricted panel of cytokines: IL-3, IL-4, IL-5 and GM-CSF which play a part in the migration and activation of mast cells and eosinophils. In addition, production of IL-4 leads to the maintenance of the allergic (Th2) T cell phenotype, favouring switching of antibody production by B lymphocytes to IgE. These IgE molecules attach to mast cells via high-affinity receptors which in turn release a number of powerful mediators acting on smooth muscle and small blood vessels, such as histamine, tryptase, prostaglandin D_2 and leukotriene C_4, which cause the immediate asthmatic reaction. Activation of eosinophils, by IgE binding, leads to release of a variety of mediators, such as eosinophilic cationic protein, which are predominantly toxic to airway cells.

Remodelling Airway smooth muscle undergoes hypertrophy and hyperplasia leading to a larger fraction of the wall being occupied by smooth muscle tissue. The airway wall is further thickened by deposition of repair collagen and matrix proteins below the basement membrane. T airway epithelium is damaged, with loss of the ciliated columnar cells into the lumen. The epithelium undergoes metaplasia with an increase in the number of mucus-secreting goblet cells.

Precipitating factors

The major allergen (Der p1) is contained in the faecal particles of the house-dust mite, *Dermatophagoides pteronnysinus*, which is found in dust throughout the house. Non-specific factors which may cause wheezing are viral infections, cold air, exercise, irritant dusts, vapours and fumes (cigarette smoke, perfume, exhaust fumes), emotion and drugs (NSAIDs, aspirin and β-blockers).

Over 200 materials encountered at the workplace may give rise to wheezing, which typically improves on days away from work and during holidays (occupational asthma). Common occupations associated with asthma are veterinary medicine and animal handling (allergens are mouse, rat and rabbit urine and fur), bakery (wheat, rye) and laundry work (biological enzymes).

A rare cause of asthma is the airborne spores of *Aspergillus fumigatus*, a soil mould. There are fleeting shadows on the chest X-ray and peripheral blood eosinophilia (allergic bronchopulmonary aspergillosis, not to be confused with the severe aspergillus pneumonia occurring in the immuno-compromised).

Clinical features

Patients with asthma suffer from a variety of symptoms none of which are specific for asthma: wheezing, cough, chest tightness and shortness of breath. However, with asthma these symptoms tend to be intermittent, worse at night and provoked by triggers as above. A cough without wheeze may be the only presenting symptom. Some patients have just one or two attacks a year, whereas others have chronic symptoms. On examination, during an attack, there is reduced chest expansion, prolonged expiratory time and bilateral expiratory polyphonic wheezes.

Investigations

The diagnosis of asthma is often made on the history and response to bronchodilators. There is no single satisfactory diagnostic test for all asthmatic patients.

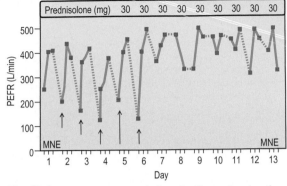

Fig. 10.1 **Classic diurnal variation of asthma, showing the effect of steroids.** The arrows indicate the morning 'dips'. M, morning; N, noon; E, evening.

- Demonstration of variable airflow limitation by measurement of PEFR (looking for a 20% change from baseline and at least 60 L/min) or FEV_1 (15% change and at least 200 mL):
  - Measurement of PEFR by the patient on waking, during the day and before bed – most asthmatic individuals will show obvious diurnal variation, with lowest values occurring in the early morning (the 'morning dip', Fig. 10.1)
  - An increase after inhalation of a bronchodilator, e.g. salbutamol
  - A decrease after 6 minutes of exercise, e.g. running.
- Histamine or methacholine challenge in difficult cases. Bronchial hyperreactivity is demonstrated by asking the patient to inhale gradually increasing doses of histamine or methacholine and demonstrating a fall in FEV_1. The test should not be performed on individuals who have poor lung function ($FEV_1 < 1.5$ L) or a history of 'brittle' asthma.
- Skin-prick tests are used to identify allergens to which the patient is sensitive. A weal develops 15 minutes after allergen injection in the epidermis of the forearm.
- Chest X-ray is performed at diagnosis and usually only repeated in an acute severe asthma attack.

■ *Aspergillus* antibody titres should be measured in those with a marked blood eosinophilia or transient shadowing on the chest X-ray.

■ A trial of steroids (prednisolone 30 mg daily for 2 weeks) should be given to everyone with severe airflow limitation. An improvement in FEV_1 of > 15% confirms some reversibility and indicates that inhaled steroids may prove beneficial.

Management

The effective management of asthma centres on patient and family education, antismoking advice, the avoidance of precipitating factors and specific drug treatment. Self-management programmes have been incorporated into patient care. These programmes involve individualized self-treatment plans based on monitoring of PEFR and symptoms and a written action plan showing patients how to act early in exacerbations. Patients should be offered influenza immunization.

Avoidance of precipitating factors Patients should be discouraged from smoking and avoid allergens, e.g. household pets, which have been shown to provoke attacks. Avoidance of the house-dust mite may be possible with frequent house cleaning and the use of effective covers for bedding. It is necessary to identify occupational asthma because early diagnosis and removal of the patient from exposure may cure the asthma. Continued exposure may lead to severe asthma, which continues even when exposure ceases. β-Blockers in any form are absolutely contraindicated in patients with asthma.

Specific drug treatment Most drugs are delivered directly into the lungs as aerosols (metered-dose inhaler ± spacer) or dry powder inhalers, which means that lower doses can be used and systemic side-effects are reduced compared to oral treatment. Asthma is managed with a stepwise approach which depends partly on repeated measurements of PEFR by the patient (Fig. 10.2). The aim is that the patient starts treatment at the step most appropriate to the initial severity, and when control of symptoms is achieved, treatment is gradually reduced to the previous step over a period of 3–6 months. The aim is to have minimal symptoms with few exacerbations and minimal need for relieving broncho-dilators.

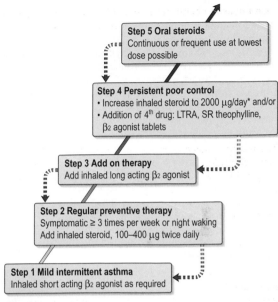

Step 5 Oral steroids
Continuous or frequent use at lowest
dose possible

Step 4 Persistent poor control
• Increase inhaled steroid to 2000 μg/day* and/or
• Addition of 4th drug: LTRA, SR theophylline,
  β2 agonist tablets

Step 3 Add on therapy
Add inhaled long acting β2 agonist

Step 2 Regular preventive therapy
Symptomatic ≥ 3 times per week or night waking
Add inhaled steroid, 100–400 μg twice daily

Step 1 Mild intermittent asthma
Inhaled short acting β2 agonist as required

• Patient measures PEFR at home to guide treatment
• Short-acting inhaled β agonist taken at any step as needed for symptom
  relief
• A rescue of oral steroids may be needed at any time and at any step
• Check inhaler technique and compliance before any increase in treatment
• Decrease treatment after 1-3 months of stability

LTRA = Leukotriene receptor antagonist
SR = Sustained release
* Doses for beclometasone dipropionate, budesonide and fluticasone HFA inhalers

Fig. 10.2 The stepwise management of chronic asthma in
adults.

■ β₂-Adrenoceptor agonists, e.g. salbutamol, terbutaline
   and the longer-acting salmeterol and formoterol
   (eformoterol), relax bronchial smooth muscle and cause
   bronchial dilatation.
■ Antimuscarinic bronchodilators, e.g. ipratropium bromide
   or oxitropium bromide, cause bronchodilatation and
   may be additive to adrenoceptor stimulants.
■ Corticosteroids are powerful anti-inflammatory agents.
   Inhaled steroids, e.g. beclometasone dipropionate,

budesonide and fluticasone propionate, are used as maintenance treatment in all but very mild asthmatic individuals. Side-effects of inhaled steroids are oral candidiasis, hoarseness and rarely cataract formation. Oral steroids are occasionally necessary in those patients not controlled on inhaled steroids. Side-effects are listed on page 625.

■ Anti-inflammatory agents, e.g. sodium cromoglicate, prevent activation of inflammatory cells and may be useful in mild asthma. They are not as effective as inhaled steroids, but are free of side-effects, and thus may have some advantages in children.

■ Leukotriene receptor antagonists (LTRA), e.g. montelukast and zafirlukast, are given orally. Leukotrienes are inflammatory mediators released by mast cells which cause bronchoconstriction and increased production of mucus. LTRA are particularly useful in patients who still have symptoms despite taking high-dose inhaled or oral corticosteroids, and in patients with asthma induced by aspirin.

■ The immunosuppressive drug methotrexate in low doses has been used in severely asthmatic individuals as a steroid-sparing agent.

■ Intravenous aminophylline is occasionally used in acute severe asthma.

Acute severe asthma

Acute severe asthma is diagnosed when a patient has severe progressive asthmatic symptoms over a number of hours or days. It is a medical emergency that must be recognized and treated immediately at home, with subsequent transfer to hospital (Emergency Box 10.1). In the UK, 1500 patients still die annually from this condition.

Clinical features

Features of acute severe asthma are any one of:

■ Inability to complete a sentence in one breath
■ Respiratory rate ≥ 25 breaths/min
■ Tachycardia ≥ 110 beats/min
■ PEFR 33–50% of predicted value or patient's best.

Life-threatening features are any one of the following in a patient with acute severe asthma:

Emergency Box 10.1
Management of acute severe asthma in hospital

- 40–60% oxygen to achieve oxygen saturation of at least 92%
- Salbutamol 5 mg or terbutaline 10 mg via oxygen-driven nebulizer
- Hydrocortisone 100 mg intravenously or 60 mg orally
- No sedatives of any kind
- Antibiotics if definite evidence of infection: focal shadowing on the chest X-ray, purulent sputum
- Chest X-ray to exclude pneumothorax or pneumonia

Monitor in all patients
- Arterial oxygen saturation by pulse oximetry
- Arterial blood gases only if P_aO_2 <92% or life-threatening features
- PEFR 30 min after starting treatment, and then before and after β_2-agonist treatment
- Consider repeat blood gases 2 hours after starting treatment
- Fluid intake, aim for 2.5–3 L/day, intravenously if necessary
- Urea and electrolytes daily – steroids and salbutamol may result in hypokalaemia

If improved – continue
60% oxygen
Prednisolone tablets – reduce from 60 mg to 30 mg daily for at least 5 days until recovery
Nebulized β_2-agonist 4-hourly

After 24 hours – consider
Adding in high-dose inhaled corticosteroid
Change nebulized to inhaled β_2-agonist

Discharge from hospital
When PEFR > 75% predicted or patientís best and diurnal variability < 25%
Whenstable on discharge treatment for 24 hours
Check inhaler technique
Determine reason for exacerbation

Life-threatening features present or poor response to treatment
60% oxygen
Hydrocortisone 100 mg 6-hourly intravenously
Repeat nebulized β_2-agonist every 15–30 min or continuous nebulization at 5–10mg/hour
Add nebulized ipratropium bromide 500 µg 4- to 6-hourly
Single-dose magnesium sulphate 1.2–2gover 20 minutes by intravenous infusion
Consider intravenous:
- Salbutamol: 5 mg in 500mL 0.9% saline or 5% dextrose (i.e.10 mg/mL).Give loading dose of 250µg (25 mL) over 10 min and continue at 10–30 µg/min (1–3 mL/min)
- Aminophylline:loading dose of 5 mg/kg over 20 min;continue at 0.5mg/kg/h.Omit loading dose if patient has been taking oral amino-phylline. Monitor blood concentrationsdaily if continued for 24h, therapeuticrange 10–20 mg/L

If poor response within 1 hour, transfer to ITU for possible intubation and mechanical ventilation

515

- Silent chest, cyanosis or feeble respiratory effort
- Exhaustion, confusion or coma
- Bradycardia or hypotension
- PEFR < 30% of predicted or best (approximately 150 L/min in adults)
- Blood gas markers of a life-threatening attack are P_aO_2 < 8 kPa or S_pO_2 < 92% despite treatment with oxygen.

Near fatal asthma is characterized by a raised P_aCO_2 and/or mechanical ventilation with raised inflation pressures.

The management of acute severe asthma is summarized in Emergency Box 10.1. Patients with moderate asthma (defined as a PEFR 51–75% of predicted and with none of the above features) who present to hospital are treated with a nebulized β-agonist. Provided they improve and are then stable for at least 1 hour, they may be discharged with a tapering dose of prednisolone (e.g. starting at 40 mg daily). Oral prednisolone should be given until the acute attack has completely resolved.

PNEUMONIA (K&C 6e p. 922)

Pneumonia is defined as an inflammation of the substance of the lungs and is usually caused by bacteria. Pneumonia can be classified both anatomically, e.g. lobar (affecting the whole of one lobe) and bronchopneumonia (affecting the lobules and bronchi), or on the basis of aetiology (Table 10.7). *Mycobacterium tuberculosis* is one cause of pneumonia; it is considered separately, as both mode of presentation and treatment are different from the other pneumonias.

Clinical features

Symptoms and signs vary according to the infecting agent and to the immune state of the patient. Most commonly there is pyrexia, combined with respiratory symptoms such as cough, sputum production, pleurisy and dyspnoea. Signs of consolidation and a pleural rub may be present. There may be a pleural effusion. Elderly patients often have fewer symptoms than younger patients or may present with a confusional state. Clinical judgement and CURB-65 criteria (Table 10.8) are used to assess the severity of community-acquired pneumonia. Precipitating factors for pneumonia are underlying lung disease, smoking, alcohol abuse, immunosuppression and other chronic illnesses. The

Table 10.7 The aetiology of pneumonia in the UK

Infecting agent	Frequency as a cause of pneumonia (%)	Clinical circumstances
Streptococcus pneumoniae	50	Community pneumonia. Patients usually previously fit
Mycoplasma pneumoniae	6	As above
Influenza A virus (usually with a bacterial component)	5	As above
Chlamydia pneumoniae	5	As above
Haemophilus influenzae	5	Pre-existing lung disease: COPD
Chlamydia psittaci	3	Contact with birds (though not inevitable)
Staphylococcus aureus	2	Children, intravenous drug abusers, associated with influenza virus infections
Legionella pneumophila	2	Institutional outbreaks (hospitals and hotels), sporadic, endemic
Coxiella burnetii	1	Abattoir and animal-hide workers
Pseudomonas aeruginosa	< 1	Cystic fibrosis and immunocompromised patients
Pneumocystis carinii *Actinomyces israelii* *Nocardia asteroides* Cytomegalovirus *Aspergillus fumigatus*	< 1	Immunosuppressed (AIDS, lymphomas, leukaemias, use of cytotoxic drugs and corticosteroids)
Anaerobic organisms	< 1	Inhalation pneumonia, alcohol abuse, postoperative
None isolated	20	–

Gram-negative organisms, especially *Klebsiella pneumoniae*, *P. aeruginosa* and *Acinetobacter* spp. are an uncommon cause of pneumonia except in patients with severe pneumonia or hospital-acquired (nosocomial) pneumonia

Table 10.8 Severity assessment for community-acquired pneumonia (CURB-65 score): Score ≥ 3 indicates severe pneumonia

Score 1 (maximum score = 6) for each of:
Confusion – new disorientation in person, place or time
Urea > 7 mmol/L
Respiratory rate ≥ 30/min
Blood pressure
    Systolic < 90 mmHg
    Diastolic ≤ 60 mmHg
Age > 65 years

Table 10.9 Prediction (% patients) of mortality and need for hospital admission

CURB-65 Score	Mortality (%)	Hospital admission
0	0.7	Not normally required
1	3.2	Not normally required
2	13	Usually
3	17	Urgent
4	41.5	Urgent, may need ITU admission
5	57	Urgent, may need ITU admission

clinical history should enquire about contact with birds (possible psittacosis), contact with farm animals (*Coxiella burnetii*, causative organism of Q fever), recent stays in large hotels or institutions (*Legionella pneumophila*), chronic alcohol abuse (*Mycobacterium tuberculosis*, anaerobic organisms), intravenous drug abuse (*Staphylococcus aureus*, *Mycobacterium tuberculosis*) and contact with other patients with pneumonia.

Investigations

Many otherwise fit patients with mild (Table 10.9) community-acquired pneumonia are treated as outpatients and the only investigation needed is a chest X-ray, which should be repeated 6–8 weeks after clinical recovery to confirm resolution. Patients admitted to hospital require investigations to identify the cause and severity of the pneumonia.

- Sputum for Gram stain, culture and sensitivity tests.
- Blood count. A white cell count above $15 \times 10^9/L$ suggests bacterial infection. There may be lymphopenia with *Legionella* pneumonia. Marked red cell agglutination on the blood film suggests the presence of cold agglutinins (immunoglobulins that agglutinate reds cells at 4°C), which are raised in 50% of patients with *Mycoplasma* pneumonia.
- Liver biochemistry and serum electrolytes. Liver biochemistry may be non-specifically abnormal.
- Serology. Some organisms, e.g. mycoplasma, causing pneumonia can be diagnosed by detection of a raised IgM antibody by immunofluorescent tests or by a four-fold rise in antibody titre from blood taken early in the clinical course and 10–14 days later.
- Chest X-ray confirms consolidation, but these changes may lag behind the clinical course. A chest X-ray which remains persistently abnormal (> 6 weeks) suggests an underlying abnormality, usually a carcinoma.
- Arterial blood gases. $P_aO_2 < 8$ kPa or rising P_aCO_2 indicates severe pneumonia.
- Patients with severe pneumonia (Table 10.8) should have urine sent for legionella and pneumococcal antigen testing and blood cultures taken.

Differential diagnosis

This includes pulmonary embolism, pulmonary oedema, pulmonary haemorrhage, bronchial carcinoma, acute extrinsic allergic alveolitis and cryptogenic organizing pneumonia (pneumonia of unknown aetiology, no infective agent has been described).

Management

- Mild community-acquired pneumonia is treated with oral amoxicillin, 500 mg 8-hourly for 7 days. Oral clarithromycin or erythromycin is an alternative for patients allergic to penicillin.
- Hospitalized patients without severe pneumonia are treated with a combination of oral amoxicillin and clarithromycin or erythromycin.
- Patients with severe pneumonia (CURB-65 ≥3) are treated with intravenous cefuroxime and clarithromycin or erythromycin. Fluoroquinolones, e.g. ciprofloxacin,

are recommended for those intolerant of penicillins or macrolides. Intravenous antibiotics are switched to oral when the patient has been apyrexial for 24 hours.

If *Staph. aureus* infection is suspected or proven on culture, intravenous flucloxacillin ± sodium fusidate is added. Pleuritic pain requires analgesia, and humidified oxygen is given if there is hypoxaemia. Fluids are encouraged, to avoid dehydration. Physiotherapy is needed to help and encourage the patient to cough. Treatment should be modified in the light of culture and sensitivity results. Patients with severe pneumonia should be assessed for management on the intensive care unit. Hospital-acquired (nosocomial) pneumonia is often due to infection with Gram-negative organisms, and treatment should include ceftazidime and an aminoglycoside (e.g. gentamicin). Metronidazole is added in patients at risk of anaerobic infection, e.g. prolonged ITU stay or aspiration in a comatose patient. Antibiotics are adjusted on the basis of the results of sputum microscopy and culture.

Complications

Complications of pneumonia include lung abscess and empyema.

Specific forms of pneumonia

Mycoplasma pneumoniae (K&C 6e p. 924) *Mycoplasma* pneumonia commonly presents in young adults with generalized features such as headaches and malaise, which may precede chest symptoms by 1–5 days. Physical signs in the chest may be scanty, and chest X-ray appearances frequently do not correlate with the clinical state of the patient. Treatment is with erythromycin or clarithromycin. Extrapulmonary complications (myocarditis, erythema multiforme, haemolytic anaemia and meningoencephalitis) will occasionally dominate the clinical picture.

Haemophilus influenzae (K&C 6e p. 925) This is commonly the cause of pneumonia in patients with COPD. There are no other features to differentiate it from other causes of bacterial pneumonia. Treatment is with oral cefaclor.

Chlamydia (K&C 6e pp. 67 & 925) *Chlamydia pneumoniae* accounts for 5–10% of cases of community-acquired pneumonia. Patients with *C. psittaci* pneumonia may give a history of contact with infected birds, particularly parrots. Symptoms include malaise, fever, cough and muscular pains, which may be low grade and protracted over many months. Occasionally the presentation mimics meningitis, with a high fever, prostration, photophobia and neck stiffness. Diagnosis of *Chlamydia* infection is made by demonstrating a rising serum titre of complement-fixing antibody. *C. pneumoniae* is distinguished from *C. psittaci* infection by type-specific immunofluorescence tests. Treatment of *Chlamydia* infection is with erythromycin or tetracycline.

Staphylococcus aureus (*K&C* 6e p. 925) usually causes pneumonia only after a preceding influenza viral illness, in intravenous drug users or in patients with central venous catheters. It results in patchy areas of consolidation which can break down to form abscesses that appear as cysts on the chest X-ray. Pneumothorax, effusions and empyemas are frequent, and septicaemia may develop with metastatic abscesses in other organs. All patients with this form of pneumonia are extremely ill and the mortality rate is in excess of 25%. Treatment is with intravenous flucloxacillin.

Legionella pneumophila (*K&C* 6e p. 925) is acquired by the inhalation of aerosols or microaspiration of infected water containing legionella. Infection is linked to contamination of water distribution systems in hotels, hospitals and workplaces and may also occur sporadically and in the immunosuppressed. Pneumonia tends to be more severe than with most other pathogens associated with community-acquired pneumonia.

A strong presumptive diagnosis of *L. pneumophila* infection is possible in the majority of patients if they have three of the four following features:

- A prodromal virus-like illness
- A dry cough, confusion or diarrhoea
- Lymphopenia without marked leucocytosis
- Hyponatraemia.

Diagnosis is by specific antigen detection in the urine or by direct fluorescent antibody staining of the organism in the pleural fluid, sputum or bronchial washings. Treatment is with clarithromycin, ciprofloxacin or rifampicin for 14–21 days.

Pseudomonas aeruginosa (*K&C* 6e p. 926) is seen in the immunocompromised and in patients with cystic fibrosis, in whom its presence is associated with a worsening of the clinical condition and increasing mortality. Treatment includes intravenous ceftazidime, ciprofloxacin, tobramycin or ticarcillin. Tobramycin and ticarcillin can be inhaled directly into the lung in patients with CF.

Pneumocystis carinii (*K&C* 6e p. 926) is the most common opportunistic infection in patients with AIDS. The clinical features and treatment of this and other opportunistic infection are described on page 52.

Severe acute respiratory syndrome (SARS) was first recognized as a global threat in early 2003 with an outbreak beginning in East Asia. It is caused by the SARS corona-virus that is believed to be an animal virus that has crossed the species barrier to humans. Spread between humans is by droplet infection. The illness ranges from a mild disease to acute respiratory infection with fever, malaise and headache followed in the second week by cough, breath-lessness and diarrhoea. Some patients develop ARDS.

Aspiration pneumonia (*K&C* 6e p. 927) Aspiration of gastric contents into the lungs can produce a severe destructive pneumonia as a result of the corrosive effect of gastric acid – Mendelson's syndrome. Aspiration usually occurs into the posterior segment of the right lower lobe because of the bronchial anatomy. It is associated with periods of impaired consciousness, structural abnormalities, such as tracheo-oesophageal fistulae or oesophageal strictures, and bulbar palsy. Infection is often due to anaerobes, and treatment must include metronidazole.

Complications of pneumonia: lung abscess and empyema (*K&C* 6e p. 929)

A lung abscess results from localized suppuration of the lung associated with cavity formation, often with a fluid level on the chest X-ray. Empyema means the presence of pus in the pleural cavity, usually from rupture of a lung abscess into the pleural cavity, or from bacterial spread from a severe pneumonia.

A lung abscess develops in the following circumstances:

■ Complicating aspiration pneumonia or bacterial pneumonia caused by *Staphylococcus aureus* or *Klebsiella pneumoniae*

- Secondary to bronchial obstruction by tumour or foreign body
- From septic emboli from a focus elsewhere (usually *Staphylococcus aureus*)
- Secondary to infarction.

Clinical features

Lung abscess presents with persisting or worsening pneumonia, often with the production of copious amounts of foul-smelling sputum. With empyema the patient is usually very ill, with a high fever and neutrophil leucocytosis. There may be malaise, weight loss and clubbing of the digits.

Investigations

Bacteriological investigation is best conducted on specimens obtained by transtracheal aspiration, bronchoscopy or percutaneous transthoracic aspiration. Bronchoscopy is helpful to exclude carcinomas and foreign bodies.

Management

Antibiotics are given to cover both aerobic and anaerobic organisms. Intravenous cefuroxime, and metronidazole are given for 5 days, followed by oral cefaclor and metronidazole for several weeks. Empyemas should be treated by prompt tube drainage or rib resection and drainage of the empyema cavity. Abscesses occasionally require surgery.

523

TUBERCULOSIS nd *(K&C 6e pp. 86 & 930)*

Epidemiology

Tuberculosis (TB) is the most common cause of death world-wide from a single infectious disease, and is on the increase in most parts of the world. This results primarily from inadequate programmes for disease control, multiple drug resistance, co-infection with HIV and a rapid rise in the world population of young adults, the group with the highest mortality from tuberculosis. In the UK the incidence of tuberculosis is highest in Asian and West Indian immigrants, children of these immigrants, the homeless and those with HIV infection. Rates in the otherwise healthy indigenous white population have fallen to very low levels.

Pathology

The initial infection with *Mycobacterium tuberculosis* is known as primary tuberculosis. It usually occurs in the lung but may occur in the gastrointestinal tract, particularly the ileocaecal region. The primary focus in the lung is usually in the upper region producing a subpleural lesion called the Ghon focus (Fig. 10.3), and is characterized by exudation and infiltration with neutrophil granulocytes. These are replaced by macrophages which engulf the bacilli and result in the typical granulomatous lesions, which consist of central areas of caseation surrounded by epithelioid cells and Langhans' giant cells (both derived from the macrophage). The primary focus is almost always accompanied by caseous lesions in the regional lymph nodes (mediastinal and cervical). The early Ghon focus together with the lymph node lesion constitute the Ghon complex. In most people the primary infection and the lymph nodes heal completely and become calcified. Some of these calcified primary lesions harbour tubercle bacilli, which may become reactivated if there is depression of the host defence system. Occasionally there is dissemination of the primary infection, producing miliary tuberculosis.

Reactivation results in typical post-primary tuberculosis. Post-primary tuberculosis refers to all forms of tuberculosis that develop after the first few weeks of the primary infection when immunity to the mycobacteria has developed. Reinfection after successful treatment for TB is very uncommon except in immunocompromised patients such as HIV-infected individuals.

Clinical features

Primary TB is usually symptomless; occasionally there may be erythema nodosum (p. 791), a small pleural effusion or pulmonary collapse caused by compression of a lobar bronchus by enlarged nodes (Fig. 10.3). Most commonly clinical tuberculosis represents delayed reactivation. Symptoms begin insidiously, with malaise, anorexia, weight loss, fever and cough. Sputum is mucoid purulent or blood-stained, but night sweats are uncommon. There are often no physical signs, although occasionally signs of a pneumonia or pleural effusion may be present. Miliary TB is the result of acute dissemination of tubercle bacilli via the blood-stream. Patients especially the elderly may present with

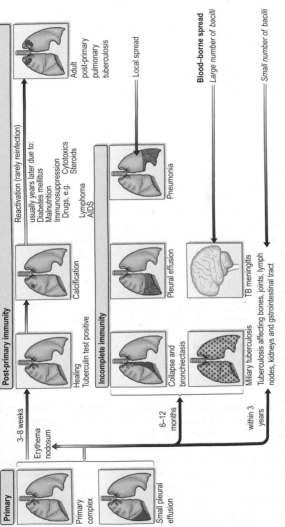

Fig. 10.3 Manifestations of primary and post-primary tuberculosis.

non-specific ill-health, fever of unknown origin, weight loss and few other localizing symptoms. Occasionally the disease presents as tuberculous meningitis, and in the later stages there may be enlargement of the liver and spleen. Choroidal tubercles (yellow/white raised lesions about one-quarter the diameter of the optic disc) are occasionally seen in the eye.

Tuberculous disease (as above) must be differentiated from *latent tuberculous infection*. Infection implies the presence of small numbers of tubercle bacilli in the body; the tuberculin test is positive (as with disease) but the chest X-ray is normal and the patient asymptomatic.

Investigations

In order to minimize the risk of transmission to other people, patients who are suspected of having pulmonary TB should be isolated in a ward side-room until sputum specimens have ruled out TB. This is to minimize the risk of transmission to other patients in a confirmed case. Because of the rising incidence of drug-resistant TB, it is vital to confirm the diagnosis bacteriologically whenever possible and to obtain drug sensitivities.

- Chest X-ray typically shows patchy or nodular shadows in the upper zones, with loss of volume, and fibrosis with or without cavitation. With miliary tuberculosis the chest X-ray may be normal or show miliary shadows 1–2 mm in diameter throughout the lung.
- Sputum is stained with Ziehl–Neelsen (ZN) stain for acid- and alcohol-fast bacilli or auramine-phenol with scanning for fluorescence. The sputum is cultured on Ogana or Lowenstein–Jensen medium for 4–8 weeks. Cultures to determine the sensitivity of the bacillus to antibiotics take a further 3–4 weeks.
- Bronchoscopy with washings of the affected lobes is useful if no sputum is available.
- The diagnosis of extrapulmonary TB depends on a high index of clinical suspicion. Recovery of the organism from specimens is still necessary wherever possible. This may involve lymph node biopsy, bone biopsy, urine testing or aspiration of pericardial fluid.
- Lumbar puncture and CSF examination for evidence of tuberculous infection is indicated in all cases of miliary TB. This is due to the high rate of blood-borne spread

to meninges, and positive CSF will alter the length of treatment.

- Rapid diagnostic tests such as PCR-based testing have been developed in an effort to improve diagnostic accuracy and to speed diagnosis. These tests are not entirely reliable and should not be accepted as a final diagnosis.
- Skin testing for TB (Mantoux test) is rarely of any value in the diagnosis or exclusion of active TB. It is neither sensitive nor specific.
- HIV testing should be considered if risk assessment shows the patient to be from an area or background with increased risk of HIV co-infection. TB is an AIDS-defining illness.

Management

Tuberculosis should be treated by experienced physicians working closely with TB nurse specialists or TB health visitors. The latter have important roles in monitoring patients' compliance with treatment and the accuracy and continuity of prescribing. It is a statutory requirement in the UK that all cases of TB must be notified to the local Public Health Authority so that contact tracing and screening can be arranged.

Patients who are ill, sputum smear positive (patients with three negative smears are considered non-infectious), highly infectious patients (particularly multidrug-resistant TB), and those unlikely to be compliant with treatment should be initially treated in hospital.

A 6-month regimen comprising rifampicin, isoniazid, pyrazinamide and ethambutol for the initial 2 months followed by rifampicin and isoniazid for a further 4 months is recommended as standard therapy for adult TB. Four drugs should be continued for longer than 2 months if susceptibility testing is still outstanding. Ethambutol is omitted in patients with a low risk of resistance to isoniazid – that is, previously untreated white patients who are HIV-negative or thought likely to be HIV-negative on risk assessment and who have not had contact with patients with known drug-resistant organisms. High levels of resistance occur in ethnic minority groups. Pyridoxine 10 mg daily, is given to reduce the risk of isoniazid-induce peripheral neuropathy. Treatment time is extended in meningitis (to 12 months) and bone TB (to 9 mo

Table 10.10	Side-effects of the main antituberculous drugs
Rifampicin	Stains body secretions and urine pink
	Induces liver enzymes – concomitant drug treatment may be less effective
	Elevation of liver enzymes and hepatitis
	Thrombocytopenia (rarely)
Isoniazid	Polyneuropathy (rarely), prevented by co-administration of pyridoxine
	Allergic reactions – skin rash and fever
	Hepatitis
Pyrazinamide	Hepatitis – rarely
	Hyperuricaemia and gout
	Rash and arthralgia
Ethambutol	Optic neuritis – testing of visual acuity (Snellen chart) and red-green colour perception performed before treatment. Patients asked to report visual changes (defects, colour blindness, acuity) during treatment

Streptomycin is now rarely used in the UK, but it may be added if the organism is resistant to isoniazid. Significant side-effects are uncommon and are listed in Table 10.10. A transient asymptomatic rise in the serum aminotransferase level may occur with rifampicin, but treatment is only stopped if hepatitis develops. Multidrug resistance is a major problem and occurs mainly in HIV-infected patients. Three drugs to which the organism is sensitive are used for up to 2 years. A variety of second-line drugs, including capreomycin, clarithromycin, azithromycin and cipro-floxacin, are used for these patients.

The major causes of treatment failure are incorrect prescribing by the doctor and inadequate compliance by the patient. Vagrants, alcoholics, homeless and the mentally ill are most likely to be non-compliant with therapy. In order to improve compliance special clinics are used to supervise treatment regimens where the ingestion of every drug dose is witnessed (directly observed therapy, DOTS). Incentives to attend include free meals and cash payments.

Prevention and chemoprophylaxis

The contacts of a case are screened for evidence of disease with a chest X-ray and a Mantoux test (positive if area of induration ≥ 10 mm 72 hours after intradermal injection of purified protein derivative of *Mycobacterium* TB). Antituberculous treatment is given if the chest X-ray shows evidence of disease, or if the Mantoux test is negative initially but becomes positive on repeat testing 6 weeks later. In adults, an initial positive tuberculin test with a normal chest X-ray is not usually taken as indication of disease.

Vaccination with BCG (bacille Calmette–Guérin) reduces the risk of developing tuberculosis by anywhere between 0–80%. It is a bovine strain of *M. tuberculosis* which has lost its virulence after growth in the laboratory for many years. Immunization produces cellular immunity and a positive Mantoux test. In the UK, BCG vaccination is offered to infants living in areas with a high immigrant population, to previously unvaccinated new immigrants from high-prevalence countries for TB, to persons at occupational risk of TB (healthcare workers, veterinary staff, staff of prisons) and to contacts of known cases. BCG vaccination is given to all persons in developing countries where TB is more prevalent.

Targeted tuberculin testing for latent TB infection is an essential component of TB control and identifies people at high risk for developing clinical disease. High-risk groups for developing TB include recent immigrants from high-prevalence countries, injection drug users and HIV-positive patients. Patients with tuberculous infection identified by tuberculin testing are usually treated with one drug for 6 months (chemoprophylaxis) to prevent progression to disease.

Patients with chest X-ray changes compatible with previous tuberculosis and who are about to undergo treatment with an immunosuppressive agent should also receive chemoprophylaxis with isoniazid.

DIFFUSE DISEASES OF THE LUNG PARENCHYMA (*K&C* 6e p. 934)

A wide variety of diseases can affect the parenchyma of the lung (Table 10.11). They are also referred to as interstitial lung disease and are often classified together because of similar clinical, radiographic, physiological or pathogenic manifestations. Sarcoidosis and cryptogenic fibrosing alveolitis are the commonest forms of diffuse parenchymal

Table 10.11 Some causes of interstitial lung disease
Granulomatous lung disease, e.g. sarcoidosis
Cryptogenic fibrosing alveolitis
Associated with connective tissues diseases
Granulomatous vasculitis
Exposure to organic dusts, farmer's lung, bird fancier's lung
Exposure to inorganic dusts, e.g. silicosis, asbestosis, coal worker's pneumoconiosis
Drug-induced, e.g. amiodarone, methotrexate, bleomycin
Radiation pneumonitis
Pulmonary infiltration with eosinophilia

lung diseases (DPLD) and are of unknown cause. The commonest identifiable causes of DPLD are related to occupational and environmental exposure, often to a variety of dusts. Patients with DPLD commonly present with shortness of breath on exertion, a persistent non-productive cough, with an abnormal chest X-ray, or with pulmonary symptoms associated with another disease such as a connective tissue disease. Pulmonary infection, malignancy, and pulmonary oedema may mimic interstitial lung disease.

Granulomatous lung disease (K&C 6e p. 934)

A granuloma is a mass or nodule of chronic inflammatory tissue formed by the response of macrophages and histiocytes to a slowly soluble antigen or irritant. It is characterized by the presence of epithelioid multinucleate giant cells. Sarcoidosis is the most common cause of lung granulomas.

Sarcoidosis (K&C 6e p. 935)

Sarcoidosis is a multisystem granulomatous disorder of unknown aetiology and is more common in young adults. It usually presents with bilateral hilar lymphadenopathy (BHL), pulmonary infiltrations and skin or eye lesions. In about half of cases, the disease is detected incidentally on a routine chest X-ray in an asymptomatic individual.

Epidemiology

Sarcoidosis occurs in all ethnic groups but is uncommon in Japan. The course of the disease is more severe in African blacks than in whites. The peak incidence is in the third and fourth decades with a female preponderance.

Immunopathology

■ The typical non-caseating (compare with TB) sarcoid granuloma consists of a focal accumulation of epithelioid cells, macrophages and lymphocytes, mainly T cells.
■ There is a depressed cell-mediated reactivity to antigens, such as tuberculin and *Candida albicans*, and an overall lymphopenia with low circulating T cells, as a result of sequestration of lymphocytes within the lung and slightly increased B cells.
■ There is an increased number of cells in the broncho-alveolar lavage, particularly CD4 helper cells.
■ Transbronchial biopsies show infiltration of alveolar walls and interstitial spaces with mononuclear cells before granuloma formation.

Clinical features

The most common presentation is with bilateral hilar lymphadenopathy, which may be found incidentally on a routine chest X-ray or be associated with mild fever, malaise, arthralgia and erythema nodosum (p. 791). Pulmonary infiltration may predominate, and, in a minority of patients there is progressive fibrosis resulting in increasing effort dyspnoea, cor pulmonale and death. The chest X-ray is negative at presentation in up to 20% of non-respiratory cases. Skin and ocular sarcoidosis are the most common extrapulmonary problems (Table 10.12). Hepatitis and

531

Table 10.12	**Extrapulmonary features of sarcoidosis**
Skin	Erythema nodosum, skin papules, lupus pernio (red/blue infiltration of the nose)
Eye	Anterior uveitis, conjunctivitis, keratoconjunctivitis sicca, uveoparotid fever (bilateral uveitis, parotid gland enlargement, facial nerve palsy)
Bone	Arthralgias, bone cysts
Metabolic	Hypercalcaemia (sarcoid macrophages produce 1,25-dihydroxyvitamin D)
Liver	Granulomatous hepatitis, hepatosplenomegaly
CNS	VIIth cranial nerve palsy, hypothalamic involvement, hypopituitarism
Heart	Ventricular arrhythmias, conduction defects, cardiomyopathy with cardiac failure

hepatosplenomegaly are uncommon, but granulomas may often be found if a liver biopsy is performed. Cardiac involvement is rare.

Investigations

Diagnosis depends on a compatible clinical picture, exclusion of other causes of granulomatous diseases, such as tuberculosis and beryllium poisoning, and in some cases histological evidence of non-caseating granulomas.

- Chest X-ray may show typical features (see above). CT scanning is useful for assessment of diffuse lung involvement.
- Transbronchial biopsy is the most useful investigation and gives positive histological evidence in 90% of cases of pulmonary sarcoidosis.
- Lung function tests show a restrictive lung defect in patients with pulmonary infiltration. There is a decrease in total lung capacity, FEV_1, FVC and gas transfer.
- Serum angiotensin-converting enzyme (ACE) is raised in 75% of patients. It is useful in assessing the activity of disease and response to treatment, but is not of diagnostic value because it is also elevated in patients with lymphoma, tuberculosis, asbestosis, silicosis and Gaucher's disease.
- Tuberculin test is negative in 80% of patients. It is of interest but of no diagnostic value.
- Biopsy and histological examination of involved lymph nodes, liver or skin lesions is sometimes necessary for diagnosis.

Differential diagnosis

The differential diagnosis of bilateral hilar lymphadenopathy includes:

- Lymphoma
- Pulmonary tuberculosis
- Bronchial carcinoma with secondary spread.

The combination of symmetrical bilateral hilar lymphadenopathy and erythema nodosum only occurs in sarcoidosis.

Management

The requirement for treatment and the role of steroids are presently contested in many aspects of this disease. Hilar lymphadenopathy with no other evidence of lung involvement on chest X-ray or lung function testing does not require treatment. Infiltration or abnormal lung function tests that persist for 6 months after diagnosis should be treated with 30 mg prednisolone for 6 weeks, reducing to 15 mg on alternate days for 6–12 months. Most patients with hypercalcaemia or other evidence of extrapulmonary sarcoidosis probably require treatment with prednisolone. Topical steroids are used for eye involvement.

Prognosis

In patients of African origin the mortality rate may be up to 10%, but is less than 5% in Caucasians. Death is mainly as a result of respiratory failure or renal damage from hypercalciuria. The prognosis is best in those with BHL and no infiltration on the chest X-ray: the disease remits within 2 years in over two-thirds of patients.

Pulmonary vasculitis and granulomatosis (*K&C* 6e p. 937)

There are two main groups:

- Pulmonary vasculitis associated with systemic connective tissue diseases including rheumatoid arthritis, systemic lupus erythematosus and systemic sclerosis (Ch. 6).
- The vasculitides associated with the presence of antineutrophil cytoplasmic antibodies (ANCAs) including Churg–Strauss syndrome (p. 291), microscopic polyangiitis (p. 291) and Wegener's granulomatosis.

Wegener's granulomatosis is a vasculitis of unknown aetiology characterized by lesions involving the upper respiratory tract, the lungs and the kidneys. The disease often starts with rhinorrhoea, with subsequent nasal mucosal ulceration, cough, haemoptysis and pleuritic pain. Chest X-ray shows nodular masses or pneumonic infiltrates with cavitation which often show a migratory pattern. Antineutrophil cytoplasmic antibodies are found in the serum in over 90% of cases with active disease, and measurement is useful both diagnostically and as a guide to disease activity in the treated patient. Typical histological changes are best shown in the kidney, where there is a necrotizing glomerulonephritis. Treatment is with cyclophosphamide.

Pulmonary fibrosis and honeycomb lung (K&C 6e p. 940)

Pulmonary fibrosis is the end result of many diseases of the respiratory tract. It may be one of the following types:

- Localized, e.g. following unresolved pneumonia
- Bilateral, e.g. in TB
- Widespread, e.g. in cryptogenic fibrosing alveolitis.

Honeycomb lung is the radiological appearance seen with widespread fibrosis. Dilated and thickened terminal and respiratory bronchioles produce cystic airspaces, giving a honeycomb appearance on chest X-ray.

Cryptogenic fibrosing alveolitis (K&C 6e p. 941)
Cryptogenic fibrosing alveolitis (CFA) is a rare disorder of unknown aetiology characterized by sequential acute lung injury with subsequent scarring and end-stage lung disease. It presents in late middle age.

Clinical features

Patients with CFA typically present with exertional dyspnoea and a non-productive cough. Eventually there is respiratory failure, pulmonary hypertension and cor pulmonale. Finger clubbing occurs in two-thirds of cases, and fine inspiratory basal crackles are heard on auscultation. Rarely, an acute form known as the Hamman–Rich syndrome occurs.

Investigations

- Chest X-ray appearances are initially of a ground-glass appearance, progressing to fibrosis and honeycomb lung. These changes are most prominent in the lower lung zones.
- High-resolution CT scan is the most sensitive imaging technique, and shows irregular linear opacities and honeycombing.
- Respiratory function tests show a restrictive defect (p. 490) with reduced lung volumes and impaired gas transfer.
- Blood gases show hypoxaemia with a normal $P_a\text{CO}_2$.

- Histological confirmation with transbronchial or open lung biopsies may be required in younger people.
- Autoantibodies, such as antinuclear factor and rheumatoid factor, are present in one-third of patients.

Differential diagnosis

The diagnosis of CFA is usually made in a patient presenting with the above signs and characteristic CT changes. The differential diagnosis is from other causes of lung fibrosis: rheumatoid arthritis, systemic lupus erythematosus, systemic sclerosis, sarcoidosis, radiation, pneumoconiosis, chronic extrinsic allergic alveolitis and drugs (amiodarone, busulfan, bleomycin, methysergide, cyclophosphamide). A detailed occupational exposure history and drug history are required to exclude other causes of pulmonary fibrosis.

Treatment

Large doses of prednisolone are used (30 mg daily); azathioprine and cyclophosphamide may also be tried. Single lung transplantation is now an established treatment for some individuals.

Prognosis

The median survival without lung transplantation is approximately 5 years.

Extrinsic allergic alveolitis (*K&C* 6e p. 942)

Extrinsic allergic alveolitis is characterized by a widespread diffuse inflammatory reaction in the alveoli and small airways of the lung as a response to inhalation of a range of different antigens (Table 10.13). By far the most common is farmer's lung, which affects up to 1 in 10 of the farming community in poor wet areas around the world.

Clinical features

There is fever, malaise, cough and shortness of breath several hours after exposure to the causative antigen. Physical examination reveals tachypnoea, and coarse end-inspiratory crackles and wheezes. Continuing exposure leads to a chronic illness with weight loss, effort dyspnoea, cough and the features of fibrosing alveolitis.

Diffuse diseases of the lung parenchyma

Table 10.13 Extrinsic allergic bronchiolar alveolitis – some causes

Disease	Situation	Antigens
Farmer's lung	Forking mouldy hay or other vegetable material	*Micropolyspora faeni*
Bird fancier's lung	Handling pigeons, cleaning lofts or budgerigar cages	Proteins present in feathers and excreta
Malt worker's lung	Turning germinating barley	*Aspergillus clavatus*
Humidifier fever	Contaminated humidifying systems in air conditioners or humidifiers	A variety of bacteria or amoebae
Mushroom workers	Turning mushroom compost	Thermophilic actinomycetes
Cheese washer's lung	Mouldy cheese	*Penicillium casei* *Aspergillus clavatus*
Wine maker's lung	Mould on grapes	Botrytis

Investigations

- Chest X-ray shows fluffy nodular shadowing with the subsequent development of streaky shadows, particularly in the upper zones.
- Full blood count shows a raised white cell count in acute cases.
- Lung function tests show a restrictive defect with a decrease in gas transfer.
- Precipitating antibodies to causative antigens are present in the serum (these are evidence of exposure and not disease).
- Bronchoalveolar lavage shows increased T lymphocytes and granulocytes.

Management

Prevention is the aim, with avoidance of exposure to the antigen if possible. Prednisolone in large doses (30–60 mg daily) may be required to cause regression of the disease in the early stages.

OCCUPATIONAL LUNG DISEASE (K&C 6e p. 944)

Exposure to dusts, gases, vapours and fumes at work can lead to the following types of lung disease:

- Acute bronchitis and pulmonary oedema from irritants such as sulphur dioxide, chlorine, ammonia or oxides of nitrogen
- Pulmonary fibrosis due to mineral dust such as coal, silica, asbestos, iron and tin
- Occupational asthma – this is the commonest industrial lung disease in the developed world
- Extrinsic allergic alveolitis (p. 535)
- Bronchial carcinoma due to asbestos, polycyclic hydrocarbons and radon in mines.

Coal worker's pneumoconiosis (K&C 6e p. 945)

Most inhaled particles cause no damage to the lung because they are trapped in the nose, removed by the mucociliary clearance system or destroyed by alveolar macrophages. Small inorganic dust particles that reach the acinus and damage macrophages initiate an inflammatory reaction and subsequent fibrosis. Coal worker's pneumoconiosis is the term used for the accumulation of coal dust in the lungs and the reaction of the lung tissue to its presence. Improved working conditions and reduction in the coal industry has led to a considerable reduction in the number of cases of pneumoconiosis. The disease is subdivided into simple pneumoconiosis and progressive massive fibrosis (PMF). Simple pneumoconiosis produces small (< 1.5 mm) pulmonary nodules on the chest X-ray. The importance of simple pneumoconiosis is that it may lead to the development of PMF with continued exposure. PMF is characterized by large (1–10 cm) fibrotic masses, predominantly in the upper lobes. Unlike simple pneumoconiosis, the disease may progress after exposure to coal dust has ceased. Symptoms are dyspnoea and cough productive of black sputum. Eventually respiratory failure may supervene. There is no specific treatment and further exposure must be prevented. Patients with PMF and some with simple pneumoconiosis (depending on the severity of radiological changes) are eligible for disability benefit in the UK.

Table 10.14 The effects of asbestos on the lung

Disease	Pathology and clinical features
Asbestos bodies	No symptoms or change in lung function
	Serve only as a marker of exposure
Pleural plaques	Fibrotic plaques on parietal and diaphragmatic pleura
	Usually produce no symptoms
Pleural effusion	Recurrent effusions
	Pleuritic pain and dyspnoea
Bilateral diffuse pleural thickening*	Thickening of parietal and visceral pleura
	Effort dyspnoea and restrictive ventilatory defect
Mesothelioma*	Tumour arising from mesothelial cells of pleura, peritoneum and pericardium
	Often presents with a pleural effusion
	Median survival 2 years
Asbestosis*	Progressive dyspnoea, finger clubbing, bilateral basal end-inspiratory crackles
	Restrictive ventilatory defect
Lung cancer, often adenocarcinoma*	Presentation and treatment is that of lung cancer (see below)

*The diseases indicated are all eligible for compensation under the Social Security Act of 1975 (UK)

538

Asbestosis (*K&C* 6e p. 945)

Asbestos is a mixture of fibrous silicates which have the common properties of resistance to heat, acid and alkali, hence their widespread use at one time. Chrysotile or white asbestos constitutes 90% of the world production and is less fibrogenic than the other forms – crocidolite (blue asbestos) and amosite (brown asbestos). The diseases caused by asbestos (Table 10.14) are all characterized by a long latency period (20–40 years) between exposure and disease.

CARCINOMA OF THE LUNG (*K&C* 6e p. 947)

Epidemiology

Bronchial carcinoma accounts for 95% of primary lung tumours. The rest are benign tumours and rarer types of cancers. Bronchial carcinoma is the most common malignant tumour in the western world, and in the UK is the third most common cause of death after heart disease and pneumonia. There is a 3 : 1 male : female ratio, but although the rising mortality of this disease has levelled off in men, it continues to rise in women.

Aetiology

Smoking is by far the most common aetiological factor, although there is a higher incidence in urban areas than in rural areas even when allowances are made for smoking. Other aetiological factors are passive smoking, exposure to asbestos, and possibly also contact with arsenic, chromium, iron oxides and the products of coal combustion.

Pathology

These are broadly divided into small cell and non-small cell cancer (Table 10.15).

Clinical features

Local effects of tumour within a bronchus   Cough, chest pain, haemoptysis and breathlessness are typical symptoms.

Spread within the chest   Tumour may directly involve the pleura and ribs, causing pain and bone fractures. Spread to involve the brachial plexus causes pain in the shoulder and inner arm (Pancoast's tumour), spread to the sympathetic ganglion causes Horner's syndrome (p. 713), and spread to the left recurrent laryngeal nerve causes hoarseness and a bovine cough. In addition, the tumour may directly involve the oesophagus, heart or superior vena cava (causing upper limb oedema, facial congestion and distended neck veins).

Metastatic disease   Metastases present as bone pain, epilepsy or with focal neurological signs.

Non-metastatic manifestations   These are rare apart from finger clubbing (Table 10.16). There may, in addition, be non-specific features such as malaise, lethargy and weight loss.

On examination of the chest there are often no physical signs, although lymphadenopathy, signs of a pleural effusion, lobar collapse or unresolved pneumonia may be present.

Table 10.15 Types of bronchial carcinoma		
Cell type	% Lung carcinomas	Characteristics
Non-small cell		
Squamous	40	Most present as obstructive lesion leading to infection
		Occasionally cavitates
		Local spread common, widespread metastases occur late
Large cell	25	Poorly differentiated tumour
		Metastasizes early
Adenocarcinoma	10	Most common lung cancer associated with asbestos exposure
		Proportionately more common in non-smokers
		Usually occurs peripherally
		Local and distant metastases
Alveolar cell	1–2	Presents as a peripheral solitary nodule or as diffuse nodular lesions of multicentric origin
Small cell (oat cell)	20–30	Arises from endocrine cells (Kulchitsky cells)
		Often secretes polypeptide hormones resulting in paraneoplastic syndromes, e.g. production of ACTH and Cushing's syndrome
		Early development of widespread metastases. Responds to chemotherapy. Poor prognosis

540

Table 10.10 Non-metastatic extrapulmonary manifestations of bronchial carcinoma

Endocrine	Ectopic secretion of:
	ACTH causing Cushing's syndrome
	ADH causing dilutional hyponatraemia
	PTH-like substance causing hypercalcaemia
	HCG or related hormones resulting in gynaecomastia
Neurological	Cerebellar degeneration
	Myopathy, polyneuropathies
	Myasthenic syndrome (Eaton–Lambert syndrome)
Vascular/ haematological (rare)	Thrombophlebitis migrans
	Non-bacterial thrombotic endocarditis
	Anaemia
	Disseminated intravascular coagulation
Skeletal	Clubbing
	Hypertrophic pulmonary osteoarthropathy (clubbing, painful wrists and ankles)
Cutaneous (rare)	Dermatomyositis
	Acanthosis nigricans (pigmented overgrowth of skin in axillae or groin)
	Herpes zoster

Investigations

The aim of investigation is to confirm the diagnosis, determine the histology and assess tumour spread as a guide to treatment.

Confirm the diagnosis Chest X-ray is the most valuable initial test, although tumours need to be between 1 and 2 cm to be recognized reliably. They usually appear as a round shadow, the edge of which often has a fluffy or spiked appearance. There may be evidence of cavitation, lobar collapse, a pleural effusion or secondary pneumonia. Spread through the lymphatic channels gives rise to lymphangitis carcinomatosis, appearing as streaky shadowing throughout the lung.

Determine the histology Sputum is examined by a cytologist for malignant cells. Bronchoscopy is used to obtain biopsies for histological investigation and washings for cytology. Transthoracic fine needle aspiration biopsy under radiographic or CT screening is useful for obtaining tissue diagnosis from peripheral lesions.

Assess spread of the tumour   At bronchoscopy, involvement of the first 2 cm of either main bronchus or of the recurrent laryngeal nerve (vocal cord paresis) indicates inoperability. Patients being considered for surgery should have a CT of the thorax to include the liver and adrenal glands to assess the mediastinum and the extent of tumour spread. PET scanning (p. 961) is the investigation of choice for confirmation or exclusion of intrathoracic lymph nodes metastases and is used when available to assess suitability for surgery. Mediastinoscopy and lymph node biopsy may be necessary before surgery if staging scans shows lymphadenopathy, which can be reactive or involved by tumour. In general, no further staging procedures are necessary unless clinical features or biochemical tests suggest the presence of bony or liver metastases. However, the incidence of subclinical metastatic disease is high in small cell lung cancer and patients considered for surgery should in addition have scanning of bones and brain and iliac crest sampling.

Determine patient suitability for major operation Physical examination and respiratory function tests.

Treatment

Treatment of lung cancer involves several different modalities and is best planned by a multidisciplinary team.

- Surgery with neo-adjuvant chemotherapy is the only treatment of any curative value for non-small cell cancer. In the 20% of cases that are suitable for resection the 5-year survival rate is 25–30%.
- Radiotherapy in high doses can produce results that are equal to surgery in patients with localized tumours but who are otherwise unfit for surgery, e.g. poor lung function testing. Palliative radiotherapy is useful for bone pain, haemoptysis and superior vena cava obstruction.
- Chemotherapy in small cell cancer has resulted in a fivefold increase in median survival, from 2 to 10 months. A small number of patients achieve several years of remission. In non-small cell lung cancer the response is

less satisfactory, though newer agents, e.g. gemcitabine, achieve response rates of greater than 20% and significantly extend median survival.

■ Local treatment. Endoscopic laser therapy, endobronchial irradiation and transbronchial stenting are being increasingly employed to deal with distressing symptoms in inoperable cases. Malignant pleural effusions should be aspirated to dryness and a sclerosing agent (e.g. tetracycline, bleomycin) instilled into the pleural space. In the terminal stages, the quality of life must be maintained as far as possible. In addition to general nursing, counselling and medical care, patients may need oral or intravenous opiates for pain (given with laxatives to prevent constipation), and prednisolone may improve the appetite.

Differential diagnosis

In most cases the diagnosis is straightforward. The differential diagnosis is usually from other solitary nodules on the chest X-ray (Table 10.3).

Metastatic tumours in the lung (*K&C* 6e p. 951)

Metastases in the lung are common, usually presenting as round shadows 1.5–3 cm in diameter. The most common primary sites are the kidney, prostate, breast, bone, gastrointestinal tract, cervix or ovary.

DISEASES OF THE PLEURA

Dry pleurisy (*K&C* 6e p. 952)

Dry pleurisy is the term used to describe inflammation of the pleura when there is no effusion. This results in localized sharp pain made worse on deep inspiration, coughing and bending or twisting movements. Common causes are pneumonia, pulmonary infarct and carcinoma.

Epidemic myalgia (Bornholm disease) is the result of infection with Coxsackie B virus. It is characterized by an upper respiratory tract infection followed by pleuritic pain and abdominal pain with tender muscles. The chest X-ray remains normal and the illness clears in 1 week.

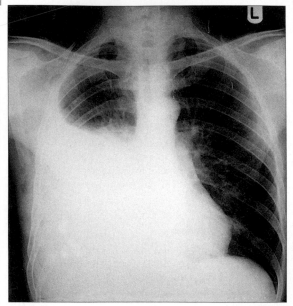

Fig. 10.4 **The chest radiographic appearances of a pleural effusion.** Physical signs on the affected side:
- Reduced chest wall movement
- Dull ('stony dull') to percussion
- Absent breath sounds
- Reduced vocal resonance
- Mediastinum shifted away.

Pleural effusion (*K&C* 6e p. 952)

A pleural effusion is an excessive accumulation of fluid in the pleural space. It can be detected clinically when there is more than 500 mL present, and by X-ray when there is more than 300 mL. Massive effusions are most commonly malignant in origin. A pleural effusion may be asymptomatic (if small) or cause breathlessness. The physical signs and chest X-ray appearances are shown in Figure 10.4.

Aetiology

Serous effusions may be transudates or exudates (Table 10.17). Transudates occur when the balance of hydrostatic

Table 10.17 Causes of a pleural effusion	
Transudate	**Exudate**
	Pleural fluid protein/serum protein > 0.5, and/or Pleural fluid LDH/serum LDH > 0.6
Common	**Common**
Left ventricular failure	Bacterial pneumonia
Cirrhosis	Carcinoma of the bronchus
Hypoalbuminaemia	Pulmonary infarction
Peritoneal dialysis	Tuberculosis
	Connective tissue disease
Others	**Rare**
Constrictive pericarditis	Post-myocardial infarction syndrome
Hypothyroidism	Acute pancreatitis
Nephrotic syndrome	Mesothelioma
Meigs' syndrome (ovarian fibroma, pleural effusion, ascites)	Sarcoidosis
	Drugs, e.g. methotrexate, amiodarone

forces in the chest favour the accumulation of pleural fluid; occasionally they occur because of movement of fluid from the peritoneum or retroperitoneal space. Exudates result from pleural and lung inflammation (resulting in a capillary protein leak) or from impaired lymphatic drainage of the pleural space. More rarely, effusions consist of blood (haemothorax), pus (empyema) or lymph (chylothorax). Chylous effusions are caused by leakage of lymph from the thoracic duct as a result of trauma or infiltration by carcinoma.

Investigations

Pleural fluid aspiration (unless the clinical picture clearly suggests a transudate, e.g. a patient with left ventricular failure) is carried out using a green needle (21G) and 20 mL syringe. Small effusions often require radiological guidance. The appearance of the pleural fluid is noted (bloody, turbid, milky) and the sample analysed for:

- Protein
- Lactic dehydrogenase (LDH)
- pH (< 7.3 suggests bacterial or tumour cell metabolism)

- Microbiological analysis (Gram stain and culture after inoculating into blood culture bottles, acid-fast bacilli stain and culture)
- Cytological analysis (differential white cell count, malignant cells)
- Occasionally: amylase, rheumatoid factor, glucose.

If pleural fluid is non-diagnostic, a contrast-enhanced thoracic CT scan with the pleural fluid still present is performed. This allows identification of pleural nodularity and image-guided needle biopsy of any focal area of abnormality. In the absence of focal areas a blind percutaneous pleural biopsy can be performed. Tissue is sent for TB smear, culture and histology.

Management

This depends on the underlying cause. Exudates are usually drained, and transudates are managed by treatment of the underlying cause. Malignant effusions usually reaccumulate after drainage. They can be treated by aspiration to dryness followed by instillation into the pleural space of a sclerosing agent such as tetracycline or bleomycin.

Pneumothorax (K&C 6e p. 953)

Pneumothorax means the presence of air in the pleural space, and this may occur spontaneously or be secondary to chest trauma. A 'tension pneumothorax' is rare unless the patient is on a mechanical ventilator or nasal non-invasive ventilation. In this situation the pleural tear acts as a one-way valve through which air passes only during inspiration. Positive pressure builds up, causing increasing cardio-respiratory embarrassment and eventually cardiac arrest. Treatment is immediate decompression by needle thoraco-centesis (2nd intercostal space, mid-clavicular line) and then intercostal tube drainage.

Aetiology

Spontaneous primary pneumothorax typically occurs in otherwise healthy tall males between the ages of 10 and 30 years and is the result of rupture of a subpleural bleb (thought to be a congenital defect in the connective tissue of the alveolar wall). Secondary pneumothorax is associated with underlying lung disease (often COPD).

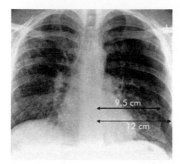

Volume of pneumothorax
$(12^3 - 9.5^3) / 12^3 = 50\%$

Fig. 10.5 The chest radiographic appearances and physical signs of a pneumothorax. The size of a pneumothorax is estimated by measuring the distance from the lateral edge of the lung to the inner wall of the ribs. A distance > 2 cm implies that the pneumothorax is at least 50%, and hence large in size. Sometimes with a large pneumothorax there is a shift of the trachea and mediastinum. (From Henry M, Arnold T, Harvey J on behalf of the BTS Pleural Disease Group. BTS guidelines for the management of spontaneous pneumothorax. *Thorax* 2003; 58 (Suppl ii): ii39–52 with permission of the BMJ Publishing Group & British Thoracic Society.)

Clinical features

There is a sudden onset of pleuritic pain with increasing breathlessness. The physical signs and chest X-ray appearances are shown in Figure 10.5.

Investigations

A standard PA chest X-ray will usually confirm the diagnosis. When a pneumothorax is suspected and not confirmed by standard films, a lateral decubitus film will provide additional information. In patients with severe bullous lung disease CT scanning will differentiate emphysematous bullae from pneumothoraces and save the patient a potentially dangerous needle aspiration.

Management

The management of a spontaneous primary pneumothorax is summarized in Figure 10.6. The management of patients with secondary pneumothoraces differs in four respects:

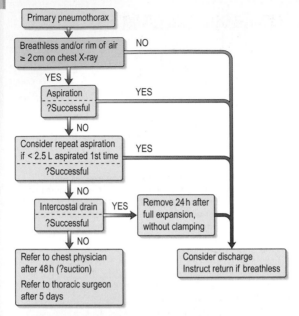

Fig. 10.6 **Treatment of a primary spontaneous pneumothorax.** All patients admitted to hospital should receive high-flow oxygen (10 L/min) to increase absorption of air from the pleural cavity.

548

- All patients should remain in hospital.
- A single attempt at aspiration is recommended only in minimally breathless patients < 50 years with small pneumothoraces (< 2 cm).
- Chest drain insertion is indicated in all other patients.
- Oxygen is given via a fixed-performance mask to patients with COPD (p. 501).

Indications for surgical referral in patients with pneumothorax include persistent air leaks (Fig. 10.6), recurrent pneumothorax and after a first pneumothorax in professions at risk (pilots, divers). Cessation of smoking reduces the recurrence rate.

DISORDERS OF THE DIAPHRAGM (*K&C* 6e p. 954)

The most common cause of unilateral diaphragmatic paralysis is the result of involvement of the phrenic nerve (C2–C4) in the thorax by a bronchial carcinoma. Other common causes of phrenic paralysis are trauma, surgery and motor neurone disease. Unilateral paralysis produces no symptoms.

The characteristic features of bilateral diaphragmatic weakness are orthopnoea, paradoxical (inward) movement of the abdominal wall on inspiration and a large fall in FVC on lying down. It may be the result of trauma or occur as part of a generalized muscular or neurological condition, such as motor neurone disease, muscular dystrophy or Guillain–Barré syndrome. Treatment is either diaphragmatic pacing or night-time assisted ventilation.

Intensive care medicine 11

Intensive care medicine (or 'critical care medicine') is concerned mainly with the management of patients with acute life-threatening conditions ('the critically ill') in a specialized unit. It also encompasses the resuscitation and transport of those who become acutely ill, or are injured, either elsewhere in the hospital or in the community. An intensive care unit (ICU) has the facilities and expertise to provide cardiorespiratory support to these sick patients, some of whom also have kidney or liver failure, and management of this is described in the relevant chapters.

All patients admitted to the ICU require skilled nursing care (patient to nurse ratio of 1 : 1) and physiotherapy. Many require nutritional support; the enteral route should be used where possible (p. 121). General medical management includes management of pain and distress with analgesics and sedation as necessary, the prevention of venous thrombosis (p. 234), pressure sores and constipation, and insulin infusions to normalize blood sugar. H_2-receptor antagonists are indicated in certain high-risk individuals to prevent stress-induced peptic ulceration. A number of scoring systems, such as the APACHE score, are in use to evaluate the severity of the patient's illness and progress.

High dependency units (HDUs) offer a level of care intermediate between that available on the general ward and that provided in an ICU. They provide monitoring and support for patients with acute (or acute on chronic) single organ failure and for those who are at risk of developing organ failure, including facilities for short-term ventilatory support and immediate resuscitation. They can also provide a 'step-down' facility for patients being discharged from intensive care.

Critical care outreach

Within an acute hospital there are patients on general wards who are 'at risk' and deteriorating who may require care above the 'general level'. Prompt recognition of these patients and institution of expert treatment will often prevent their progression to severe illness. Critical care outreach is an organizational approach to ensure high-quality care for these patients. Outreach services have three aims:

- To avert admissions to critical care or to ensure that admissions are timely, by early identification of patients who are deteriorating
- To enable discharges from critical care by supporting the continued recovery of discharged patients, and their relatives, on wards and after discharge from hospital
- To share critical care skills with staff on the ward and in the community.

Terminal cardiovascular, neurological or respiratory collapse is often preceded by a period of abnormal basic physiological observations (heart rate, systolic blood pressure, respiratory rate, urine output, and conscious level) during which time potential life-saving therapeutic interventions may be initiated. Early-warning systems based upon these observations have been developed in order to identify a trigger point at which the critical care outreach team is called. The scoring systems and trigger events vary between hospitals.

ACUTE DISTURBANCES OF HAEMODYNAMIC FUNCTION (SHOCK) (K&C 6e p. 962)

The term 'shock' is used to describe acute circulatory failure with inadequate or inappropriately distributed tissue perfusion resulting in decreased oxygen delivery to the tissues. The effects of inadequate tissue perfusion are initially reversible but prolonged oxygen deprivation leads to critical derangement of cell processes and eventually cell death, end-organ failure, and death. Thus the prompt recognition and treatment of shock is essential. The causes of shock are listed in Table 11.1. Shock is often the result of a combination of these factors.

Pathophysiology

Sympathoadrenal In response to hypotension there is a reflex increase in sympathetic nervous activity and

---

Table 11.1 **Causes of shock**

Hypovolaemic (reduced preload)
Haemorrhage: trauma, gastrointestinal bleeding, fractures, ruptured aortic aneurysm
Fluid loss: burns, severe diarrhoea, intestinal obstruction (fluid accumulates in the intestine)

Cardiogenic (pump failure)
Myocardial infarction
Myocarditis
Atrial and ventricular arrhythmias
Bradycardias
Rupture of a valve cusp

Obstructive
Obstruction to outflow: massive pulmonary embolism, tension pneumothorax
Restricted cardiac filling: cardiac tamponade, constrictive pericarditis

Distributive (decrease in systemic vascular resistance)
Vascular dilatation: drugs, sepsis
Arteriovenous shunting
Maldistribution of flow e.g. sepsis, anaphylaxis

---

catecholamine release from the adrenal medulla. The resulting vasoconstriction, increased myocardial contractility and heart rate help restore blood pressure and cardiac output. Activation of the renin–angiotensin system also leads to vasoconstriction and salt and water retention, which help to restore circulating volume.

Neuroendocrine response There is release of pituitary hormones such as ACTH and vasopressin, cortisol which causes fluid retention and antagonizes insulin, and glucagon, which raises blood sugar.

Release of mediators In severe infection, the presence of large areas of damaged tissue or prolonged episodes of hypoperfusion can trigger a massive inflammatory response with activation of leucocytes, complement, and the coagulation cascade. There is release and activation of pro-inflammatory cytokines (tumour necrosis factor and interleukin-1), platelet-activating factor, prostaglandins and endothelium-derived vasoactive mediators (nitric oxide and endothelin-1). The end result of these processes is vasodilatation, increased vascular permeability, endothelial cell damage and platelet aggregation. Vasodilatation and increased vascular permeability are also seen in shock secondary to anaphylaxis.

Microcirculatory changes In the early stages of septic shock there is vasodilatation, increased capillary permeability with interstitial oedema, and arteriovenous shunting. Vasodilatation and increased capillary permeability also occur in anaphylactic shock. In the initial stages of other forms of shock, and in the later stages of sepsis and anaphylaxis, there is capillary sequestration of blood. Fluid is forced into the extravascular space, causing interstitial oedema, haemoconcentration and an increase in plasma viscosity.

In all forms of shock there may be activation of the coagulation pathway, with the development of disseminated intravascular coagulation (DIC, see p. 231). The disseminated inflammatory response and microcirculatory changes may lead to progressive organ failure (*multiple organ dysfunction syndrome* (MODS), also known as multiple organ failure (MOF)); the lungs are usually affected first, with the development of the *acute respiratory distress syndrome* (ARDS). The mortality in MODS is high and treatment is supportive.

Clinical features

554

The history will often indicate the cause of shock, e.g. a patient with major injuries (often internal and thus concealed) will often develop hypovolaemic shock. A patient with a history of peptic ulceration may now be bleeding into the gastrointestinal tract, and rectal examination will show melaena. Anaphylactic shock may develop in susceptible individuals after insect stings and eating certain foods, e.g. peanuts (Emergency Box 11.1).

Hypovolaemic shock Peripheral vasoconstriction (as blood is redirected from the periphery to vital organs) leads to inadequate tissue perfusion with cold clammy skin and slow capillary refill. The latter allows a simple method to assess peripheral perfusion. The patient's skin (usually a digit) is compressed for 5 seconds with sufficient pressure to cause blanching. After release of pressure the time taken

> **Emergency Box 11.1**
> **Anaphylactic shock**

Pathophysiology

Massive release of mediators from mast cells and basophils induced by cross-linking of surface IgE with trigger antigen (e.g. penicillin, bee sting, radiographic contrast media, eggs, peanuts, shellfish) leads to increase in vascular permeability, vasodilatation and respiratory smooth muscle contraction.

Clinical features

Onset of symptoms usually within 5–60 min of antigen exposure. Urticaria, wheezing, upper airway obstruction, hypotension.

Diagnosis

Clinical – typical symptoms and signs developing after exposure to an agent known to provoke anaphylaxis.

Management

Remove the precipitating cause, e.g. stop administration of the offending drug.

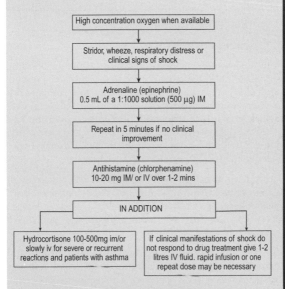

1. An inhaled β_2-agonist, e.g. salbutamol, is used as an adjunctive measure if bronchospasm is severe and does not respond rapidly to other treatment.

2. If profound shock judged **immediately** life-threatening, give CPR/ALS if necessary. Consider **slow** i.v. epinephrine (adrenaline) 1:10 000 solution. This is **hazardous** and is recommended only for an experienced practitioner who can also obtain i.v. access without delay. Note different strength of epinephrine that is required for i.v. use.

3. If adults are treated with an epinephrine autoinjector, 300 µg will usually be sufficient. A second dose may be required. Half doses of epinephrine may be safer for patients on amitriptyline, imipramine, or β-blocker.

4. A crystalloid may be safer than a colloid.

Prevent further attacks

Refer to an immunologist or allergist, identify responsible allergen (careful history, skin testing, serum antibody tests by RAST or ELISA).

Patients who have had an attack of anaphylaxis and who are at risk of developing another should carry a preloaded syringe of epinephrine for subcutaneous self-administration (e.g. Epipen device) and wear an appropriate information bracelet (e.g. Medic Alert).

for the area to return to the same colour as the surrounding skin is normally less than 2 seconds. The blood pressure (particularly when supine) may be maintained initially, but later hypotension supervenes (systolic BP < 100 mmHg) with oliguria (< 30 mL of urine/h), tachypnoea, confusion and restlessness. Increased sympathetic tone causes tachycardia (pulse > 100/min) and sweating, though extreme hypovolaemia may be associated with bradycardia.

Cardiogenic shock Additional clinical features are those of heart failure, e.g. raised jugular venous pressure (JVP), pulsus alternans (alternating strong and weak pulses), a 'gallop' rhythm (p. 432), basal crackles and pulmonary oedema.

Mechanical shock Muffled heart sounds, pulsus paradoxus (pulse fades on inspiration), elevated JVP and Kussmaul's sign (JVP increases on inspiration) occur in cardiac tamponade. In pulmonary embolism there are signs of right heart strain, with a raised JVP with prominent 'a' waves, right ventricular heave and a loud pulmonary second sound.

Anaphylactic shock Profound vasodilatation leads to warm peripheries and low blood pressure. Erythema, urticaria, angio-oedema, bronchospasm, and oedema of the face and larynx may all be present.

Septic shock In the early stages there is vasodilatation, pyrexia and rigors. At a later stage there are features of hypovolaemic shock. Sepsis in elderly people or in the immunosuppressed is common without the classic clinical features.

Management (*K&C* 6e p. 972)

This is summarized in Emergency Box 11.2. The underlying cause must be identified and treated appropriately. What-

> ### *Emergency Box 11.2*
> ### Management of shock
>
> **Ensure adequate oxygenation and ventilation**
> - Maintain patent airway: use oropharyngeal airway or endotracheal tube if necessary.
> - Administer 100% oxygen via tight-fitting face mask.
> - Monitor respiratory rate, blood gases and chest X-ray.
>
> **Restore cardiac output and BP**
> - Lay patient flat or head-down.
> - Expand circulating volume with appropriate fluids given quickly via large-bore cannulae.
> - Monitor skin colour, pulse and blood pressure, peripheral temperature, urine output, ECG.
> - CVP monitoring is required in most cases, Swan–Ganz catheter in selected cases.
>
> **Investigations**
> - FBC, U & E, glucose, liver biochemistry, and blood gases in all cases.
> - Infection screen, lactate levels, fibrinogen degradation products and crossmatch blood in selected cases.
> - Echocardiogram in post-MI patients to identify patients with intra- or extramyocardial rupture.
>
> **Treat underlying cause**
> - Haemorrhage
> - Sepsis
> - Anaphylaxis.
>
> **Treat complications**
> - e.g. Coagulopathy, renal failure.

ever the aetiology of shock, tissue blood flow and blood pressure must be restored as quickly as possible to avoid the development of MOF.

Expansion of the circulating volume Volume replacement is obviously necessary in hypovolaemic shock, but also in anaphylactic and septic shock, where there is vasodilatation, sequestration of blood and loss of circulating volume secondary to capillary leakage. High filling pressures may also be needed in mechanical shock. Care must be taken to prevent volume overload, which leads to a reduction in stroke volume and a rise in left atrial pressure with a risk of pulmonary oedema. The choice of fluid depends on the clinical situation:

- Whole blood is conventionally given for haemorrhage as soon as it is available. In extreme emergencies, cross-match can be performed in about 30 minutes and is as safe as the standard procedure. Complications of massive blood transfusion are hypothermia (minimized by using a blood warmer during infusion), coagulopathy (stored blood has almost no effective platelets and is deficient in clotting factors), hypocalcaemia (citrate anticoagulation in stored blood binds calcium), hyperkalaemia (passive leakage from stored red cells), and acute lung injury due to microaggregates in stored blood. The platelet count, prothrombin time, activated partial thromboplastin time, plasma calcium and potassium should be measured after rapid transfusion of 3–5 units of blood.

- Colloidal solutions increase colloid osmotic pressure and produce a greater and more sustained increase in plasma volume than crystalloid solutions. They are used to replace fluid in hypovolaemic patients and are useful for the maintenance of blood volume, but have no oxygen-carrying capacity. Polygelatin solutions (e.g. Gelofusin and Haemaccel) are the most widely used. Human albumin solution and dextrans are less commonly used because of the expense (albumin) and higher complication rate (dextrans). Colloid solutions are often used for acute blood loss before whole blood becomes available, and for volume replacement in anaphylactic and septic shock.

- Crystalloids, e.g. 5% dextrose, 0.9% saline, are readily available and cheap. Once in the circulation they quickly redistribute into the interstitial fluid; therefore large volumes are needed to restore circulating volume and the excess fluid in the interstitial space may contribute to pulmonary oedema. Large volumes of crystalloid (> 2 litres) as a treatment for shock are best avoided. However, crystalloids are frequently used for volume replacement in diarrhoea and vomiting, and sometimes with burns.

Myocardial contractility and inotropic agents   Myocardial contractility is impaired in cardiogenic shock and at a later stage in other forms of shock as a result of hypoxaemia, acidosis and the release of mediators. It is recommended that the treatment of acidosis should concentrate on correcting the cause; intravenous bicarbonate should only be administered to correct extreme (pH < 7.0) persistent metabolic acidosis. Drugs that impair cardiac performance, e.g. β-blockers, should be stopped. When a patient remains hypotensive despite adequate volume replacement, inotropic agents are administered. This must be via a large central vein and the effects must be carefully monitored. The inotropic agents used and their clinical effects are shown in Table 11.2. Many consider dopamine to be the inotrope of choice in critically ill patients, but dobutamine is a better choice when vasoconstriction caused by dopamine could be dangerous. Norepinephrine (noradrenaline) in combination with dobutamine (depending on the cardiac output) is used for shocked patients with a low peripheral resistance, e.g. septic patients.

Additional treatment   Vasodilators, e.g. sodium nitroprusside and isosorbide dinitrate, may be useful in selected patients who remain vasoconstricted and oliguric despite adequate volume replacement and a satisfactory blood pressure. Finally, in patients with a potentially reversible depression of left ventricular function (e.g. cardiogenic shock secondary to a ruptured interventricular septum), intra-aortic balloon counterpulsation (IABCP) may be used as a temporary measure to maintain life until definitive surgical treatment can be carried out.

Specific treatment of the cause   In all cases the cause of shock must be identified if possible and specific treatment given when indicated.

■ *Septic shock*. Treatment of septicaemia is discussed on page 12. Antibiotic therapy should be directed towards the probable cause. In the absence of helpful clinical

Acute disturbances of haemodynamic function (shock)

Table 11.2 Inotropic agents used in the management of shock: the effect of each inotrope on the adrenergic and dopaminergic receptors is shown

(Dose, µg/kg/min)	Relative α- and β-adrenergic and dopaminergic effects	Comments
Epinephrine (adrenaline) Low dose (0.06–0.1) Moderate dose (0.1–0.18) High dose (> 0.18)	β effects predominate at low dose with increase in cardiac output and fall in systemic vascular resistance (SVR). At high dose, α_1-adrenergic effects predominate with increased SVR. This may increase renal perfusion pressure and urine output but excessive vasoconstriction leads to decreased cardiac output, oliguria and peripheral gangrene	Potent agent and useful in refractory hypotension. Agent of choice in septic shock when haemodynamic monitoring not available
Norepinephrine (noradrenaline)	Predominantly an α-adrenergic agonist. Administration leads to increased inotropy and an increase in SVR	Useful for those patients with hypotension and low SVR, and is used most commonly for treating septic shock, sometimes in combination with dobutamine
Dopamine Low dose (1–3) Moderate dose (3–10) High dose (> 10)	At low doses acts predominantly on D_1 receptor resulting in selective vasodilatation. β_1 receptors also stimulated at moderate doses with increased heart rate, myocardial contractility and cardiac output. At high doses the predominant effect is to stimulate α-adrenergic receptors with an increase in SVR	Often used as a first-line agent for restoring blood pressure at low to moderate doses. High-dose dopamine is best avoided

Continued

Table 11.2 Inotropic agents used in the management of shock: the effect of each inotrope on the adrenergic and dopaminergic receptors is shown—cont'd

(Dose, μg/kg/min)	Relative α- and β-adrenergic and dopaminergic effects	Comments
Dopexamine	Dopamine analogue that activates β2 receptors as well as D1 and D2 receptors. Weakly positive inotrope and powerful splanchnic vasodilator, reducing afterload and improving blood flow to vital organs	Most useful in patient with a low cardiac output and peripheral vasoconstriction. Has been used as an adjunct to the perioperative management of high-risk patients
Dobutamine	Predominantly β1 activity. Minimal α and β2 receptor activity results in vasodilatation. The net effect is increased cardiac output with decreased SVR	Useful in patients with cardiogenic shock. Useful in combination with norepinephrine for the management of patients who are shocked with a low systemic resistance, e.g. septic shock
Phosphodiesterase inhibitors (milrinone, enoximone)	Inotropic and vasodilator effects through non-adrenergic mechanisms	Used to treat patients with impaired cardiac function and medically refractory, heart failure. In vasodilated septic patients they may worsen hypotension
Vasopressin	Increases blood pressure and SVR	Used in refractory septic shock

$α_1$-adrenergic receptors are located in the vascular wall and heart, and mediate vasoconstriction (increase systemic vascular resistance, SVR) and duration of cardiac contraction
$β_1$-adrenergic receptors are located in the heart and have inotropic and chronotropic action resulting in increased cardiac output
$β_2$-adrenergic receptors are located in blood vessels and mediate vasodilatation
Postsynaptic D_1 receptors mediate vasodilatation of mesenteric, renal, coronary and cerebral circulation
Presynaptic D_2 receptors cause vasoconstriction by inducing norepinephrine release

guidelines, 'blind' intravenous antibiotic therapy (e.g. cefuroxime and gentamicin) should be started after performing an infection screen: chest X-ray and culture of blood, urine and sputum. Lumbar puncture, ultrasonography and CT of the chest and abdomen are useful in selected cases. Abscesses require drainage. Steroids have no role in the treatment of septic shock.

■ *Anaphylactic shock* must be identified and treated immediately (Emergency Box 11.1).

Monitoring (*K&C* 6e p. 967)

This is by both clinical and invasive means.

Clinical An assessment of skin perfusion, measurement of pulse, BP, JVP and urinary flow rate will guide treatment in a straightforward case. Additional invasive monitoring will be required in seriously ill patients who do not respond to initial treatment.

Invasive

■ *Blood pressure.* A continuous recording may be made with an intra-arterial cannula, usually in the radial artery.

■ *Central venous pressure* (CVP) is related to right ventricular end-diastolic pressure, which depends on circulating blood volume, venous tone, intrathoracic pressure and right ventricular function. CVP is measured by inserting a catheter percutaneously into the superior vena cava and connecting it to a manometer system (p. 803). The normal range is 0–4 cmH$_2$O above the manubriosternal angle in a supine patient. In shock CVP may be normal, because in spite of hypovolaemia there is increased venous tone. A better guide to circulating volume is the response to a fluid challenge (Fig. 11.1).

■ *Left atrial pressure.* In uncomplicated cases the CVP is an adequate guide to the filling pressures of both sides of the heart. However, if there is disparity in function between the two ventricles (e.g. infarction of the left ventricle), left atrial pressure must be measured. A Swan–Ganz catheter is introduced percutaneously into a central vein and then guided through the chambers of the heart into the pulmonary artery. By inflating a balloon at the tip of the catheter, pulmonary artery occlusion pressure (PAWP) is measured, which is a reflection of left atrial pressure.

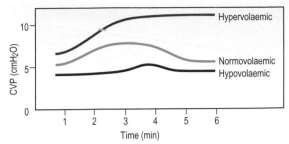

Fig. 11.1 **The effect of rapid administration (200 mL of 0.9% saline over 1–3 minutes) of a fluid challenge to patients with a CVP within the normal range.** (From Sykes MK (1963) Venous pressure as a clinical indication of adequacy of transfusion. *Annals of the Royal College of Surgeons of England* 33: 185–197.)

■ *Cardiac output* is measured, using a modified Swan–Ganz catheter, by recording temperature changes in the pulmonary artery after injecting a bolus of cold dextrose into the right atrium.

RESPIRATORY FAILURE (K&C 6e p. 979)

Respiratory failure occurs when pulmonary gas exchange is sufficiently impaired to cause hypoxaemia with or without hypercapnia. In practical terms, respiratory failure is present when the P_aO_2 is < 8 kPa (60 mmHg) or the P_aCO_2 is > 7 kPa (55 mmHg).

563

It can be divided into two types (Table 11.3):

■ Type 1 respiratory failure in which the P_aO_2 is low and the P_aCO_2 is normal or low. It is most commonly caused by diseases that damage lung tissue. The hypoxaemia is due to ventilation–perfusion mismatch or right-to-left shunts.
■ Type 2 respiratory failure in which the P_aO_2 is low and the P_aCO_2 is high is caused by alveolar hypoventilation.

Monitoring

Clinical Assessment should be made on the following criteria: tachypnoea, tachycardia, sweating, pulsus paradoxus, use of accessory muscles of respiration, intercostal recession

Table 11.3 Causes of respiratory failure	
Type 1	Type 2
Pulmonary oedema	COPD
Pneumonia	Life-threatening acute severe
Acute severe asthma	asthma
Pneumothorax	Respiratory muscle weakness,
COPD	e.g. Guillain–Barré syndrome
Pulmonary embolism	Respiratory centre depression,
Acute respiratory distress	e.g. with sedatives
syndrome	Sleep apnoea
Fibrosing alveolitis	Chest wall deformities
Right-to-left cardiac shunts	Inhaled foreign body

and inability to speak. Signs of carbon dioxide retention may be present, such as asterixis (coarse tremor), bounding pulse, warm peripheries and papilloedema.

Pulse oximetry Lightweight oximeters placed on an earlobe or finger can give a continuous reading of oxygen saturation by measuring the changing amount of light transmitted through arterial blood. The normal range is 95–100%, but in general, if the saturation is greater than 90%, oxygenation can be considered to be adequate. Although simple and reliable, these instruments are not very sensitive to changes in oxygenation. They also give no indication of carbon dioxide retention.

Forced vital capacity (FVC) In patients with acute neuro-muscular problems, e.g. Guillain–Barré syndrome and myasthenia gravis, FVC is used as a guide to deterioration. ITU admission is recommended when the FVC is less than 20 mL/kg, and typically intubation and ventilation are necessary when the FVC is less than 10 mL/kg.

Arterial blood gas analysis Analysis of arterial blood gives definitive measurements of P_aO_2, P_aCO_2, oxygen saturation, pH and bicarbonate (p. 799). In type 2 respiratory failure, retention of carbon dioxide causes P_aCO_2 and [H^+] to rise, resulting in respiratory acidosis. In chronic type 2 failure (COPD, chest wall deformities) the bicarbonate concentration is also raised secondary to renal retention and the pH may partially or completely normalize due to this metabolic compensation. In type 1 respiratory failure or in hyperventilation there may be a fall in P_aCO_2 and [H^+], resulting in respiratory alkalosis. Other abnormalities of acid–base balance are discussed on page 327.

Capnography This allows the continuous breath-by-breath analysis of expired carbon dioxide concentrations, and is mandatory in patients having tracheal intubation outside the ITU.

Management

This includes the administration of supplemental oxygen, control of secretions, treatment of pulmonary infection, control of airway obstruction and limiting pulmonary oedema. Correction of abnormalities which may lead to respiratory muscle weakness, e.g. hypokalaemia, hypo-phosphataemia, and undernutrition, is also necessary. In most patients oxygen is given by a face mask or nasal cannulae. With these devices, inspired oxygen concentration varies from 35–55%, with flow rates between 6 and 10 litres. However, in patients with chronically elevated carbon dioxide (e.g. COPD), hypoxia rather than hypercapnia maintains the respiratory drive, and thus fixed-performance masks (e.g. Venturi masks) should be used, in which the concentration of oxygen can be accurately controlled. Respiratory stimulants such as doxapram have a very limited role in treatment.

Respiratory support Respiratory support should be considered when the above measures are not sufficient. The type depends on the underlying disorder and its clinical severity. Careful consideration should be given to ventilating patients with severe chronic lung disease, as those who are severely incapacitated may be difficult to wean from the ventilator.

- *Continuous positive airway pressure (CPAP)* is used for acute type 1 respiratory failure. Oxygen is delivered to the spontaneously breathing patient under pressure via a tightly fitting face mask (non-invasive positive-pressure ventilation, NIPPV) or endotracheal tube. Oxygenation and vital capacity improve and the lungs become less stiff.
- Bilevel positive airway pressure (BiPAP) has been shown to be of use in patients with hypercapnic respiratory failure secondary to acute exacerbations of COPD who do not require immediate intubation and ventilation. BiPAP should be instituted at an early stage in the

hospital admission when the pH falls below 7.35 and the respiratory rate exceeds 30 breaths per minute. BiPAP is usually given for at least 6 hours a day, and oxygen is administered to maintain arterial oxygen saturation above 90%. BiPAP reduces the need for intubation, complications, mortality and hospital stay.

■ *Intermittent positive-pressure ventilation (IPPV)*. IPPV requires tracheal intubation and therefore anaesthesia if the patient is conscious. The indications for mechanical ventilation are listed in Table 11.4. The beneficial effects include improved carbon dioxide elimination, improved oxygenation, and relief from exhaustion as the work of ventilation is removed. High concentrations of oxygen (up to 100%) may be administered accurately. If adequate oxygenation cannot be achieved, a positive airway

Table 11.4 **Indications for IPPV**

Indication	Comment

Acute respiratory failure	With signs of severe respiratory distress despite maximal therapy:
	    respiratory rate > 40/min
	    inability to speak
	    patient exhausted, confused or agitated
	Rising P_aCO_2 > 8 kPa
	Extreme hypoxaemia < 8 kPa, despite oxygen therapy

Acute ventilatory failure, e.g. myasthenia gravis, Guillain–Barré syndrome	Institute when vital capacity fallen to 10–15 mL/kg High P_aCO_2, particularly if rising, is an indication for urgent mechanical ventilation
Prophylactic postoperative ventilation	In poor-risk patients
Head injury	With acute brain oedema. Intracranial pressure is decreased by elective hyperventilation as this reduces cerebral blood flow
Trauma	e.g. Chest injury and lung contusion
Severe left ventricular failure	
Coma with breathing difficulties	e.g. Following drug overdose

pressure can be maintained at a chosen level throughout expiration by attaching a threshold resistor valve to the expiratory limb of the circuit. This is known as positive end-expiratory pressure (PEEP), and its primary effect is to re-expand underventilated lung areas, thereby reducing shunts and increasing P_aO_2.

■ *Intermittent mandatory ventilation (IMV).* This technique allows the ventilated patient to breathe spontaneously between mandatory tidal volumes delivered by the ventilator. These coincide with the patient's own respiratory effort. It is used as a method of weaning patients from artificial ventilation, or as an alternative to IPPV.

The major complications of intubation and assisted ventilation are:

■ Trauma to the upper respiratory tract from the endo-tracheal tube
■ Secondary pulmonary infection
■ Barotrauma – overdistension of the lungs and alveolar rupture may present with tension pneumothorax (p. 546) and surgical emphysema
■ Reduction in cardiac output – the increase in intrathoracic pressures during controlled ventilation impedes cardiac filling and lowers cardiac output
■ Abdominal distension due to intestinal ileus – cause not known
■ Increased ADH and reduced atrial natriuretic peptide secretion. Together with a fall in cardiac output and reduced renal perfusion this leads to salt and water retention.

ACUTE LUNG INJURY/ACUTE RESPIRATORY DISTRESS SYNDROME *(K&C 6e p. 986)*

Acute lung injury (ALI) and acute respiratory distress syndrome (ARDS) are defined as respiratory distress occurring with stiff lungs, diffuse bilateral pulmonary infiltrates, refractory hypoxaemia, in the presence of a recognized precipitating cause and in the absence of cardiogenic pulmonary oedema (i.e. the pulmonary capillary wedge pressure is less than 16 mmHg).

Aetiology

The commonest precipitating factor is sepsis. Other causes include trauma, burns, pancreatitis, fat or amniotic fluid embolism, aspiration pneumonia or cardiopulmonary bypass.

Pathophysiology

The cardinal feature is pulmonary oedema as a result of increased vascular permeability caused by the release of inflammatory mediators. Oedema may induce vascular compression resulting in pulmonary hypertension, which is later exacerbated by vasoconstriction in response to increased autonomic nervous activity. A haemorrhagic intra-alveolar exudate forms, which is rich in platelets, fibrin and clotting factors. This inactivates surfactant, stimulates inflammation and promotes hyaline membrane formation. These changes may result in progressive pulmonary fibrosis.

Clinical features

Tachypnoea, increasing hypoxia and laboured breathing are the initial features. The chest X-ray shows diffuse bilateral shadowing, which may progress to a complete 'white-out'.

Management

This is based on the treatment of the underlying condition. Pulmonary oedema should be limited with fluid restriction, diuretics, and haemofiltration if these measures fail.

Steroids currently have no role in the prophylaxis of this condition, but may be beneficial when administered during the late fibroproliferative phase. Aerosolized surfactant, inhaled nitric oxide and aerosolized prostacyclin are experimental treatments whose exact role in the management of ARDS is unclear. Repeated positional change, i.e. changing the patient from supine to prone may allow reductions in airway pressures and the inspired oxygen fraction in those with severe hypoxaemia.

Prognosis

Although the mortality has fallen over the last decade, it remains at 30–40%, most patients dying from sepsis. The prognosis is very dependent on the underlying cause, and rises steeply with age and with the development of multiorgan failure.

Poisoning, drug and alcohol abuse

12

In many hospitals in the developed world, acute poisoning is one of the most common reasons for acute admission to a medical ward. Such poisoning may be:

- Deliberate self-administration of an excess quantity of prescribed and over-the-counter medicines, or illicit drugs
- Occupational exposure to chemicals
- Inappropriate prescribing by a doctor, e.g. digoxin toxicity
- In children due to accidental ingestion or Münchausen's syndrome by proxy.

Self-poisoning is the most common way by which people commit or attempt suicide (these categories are encompassed by the term 'deliberate self-harm'); other means are usually by violent methods, e.g. hanging, shooting or drowning. Attempted suicide by a violent method is associated with future suicide and these patients must be assessed by a psychiatrist. In adults with self-poisoning admitted to hospital in the UK the most common drugs taken are paracetamol and benzodiazepines, antidepressants, non-steroidal anti-inflammatory drugs (NSAIDs) and aspirin. In many cases more than one substance is taken; alcohol is frequently a secondary poison. Outside hospital, where most deaths occur, the commonest cause is deliberate carbon monoxide poisoning from inhalation of vehicle exhaust fumes. This is also seen in cases of accidental poisoning with faulty appliances using natural gas. In the developing world ingestion of pesticides, heating fuels, antimalarials and traditional medicines is more common.

The majority of cases (80%) of self-poisoning do not require intensive medical management but all require a sympathetic and caring approach to their problems. Both the patient and the family may require psychiatric help (see p. 574) and the social services should be contacted to help with social and domestic problems.

569

Clinical features (*K&C* 6e p. 1003)

Eighty per cent of adults are conscious on arrival at hospital and the diagnosis of self-poisoning can usually be made easily from the history. In the unconscious patient a history from friends or relatives is helpful, and the diagnosis can often be inferred from tablet bottles or a suicide note brought by the ambulance attendants. Tablet identification may be helped by the use of TICTAC, a visual drug identification database with information and high-quality images on thousands of tablets, capsules and related products (http://www.tictac.org). In any patient with an altered conscious level drug overdose must always be considered in the differential diagnosis.

On arrival at hospital the patient must be assessed urgently in the accident and emergency department. A full physical examination must include an assessment of cardiorespiratory status and conscious level (p. 720).

The physical signs that may aid identification of the agents responsible for poisoning are shown in Table 12.1.

Investigations

Blood and urine samples should always be taken on admission for the determination of drug levels, as these are invaluable for the management of certain poisons (Table 12.2) and are helpful in legal disputes. Drug screens of blood and urine are also occasionally helpful in the seriously ill unconscious patient in whom the cause of coma is unknown. Further investigations depend on the drugs ingested and clinical assessment of the patient, e.g. arterial blood gases in the comatose patient.

Management (*K&C* 6e p. 1004)

Most patients with self-poisoning require only general care and support of the vital systems. However, for a few drugs, additional therapy is required. The online TOXBASE® database (http://www.spib.axl.co.uk) provides up-to-date information about the diagnosis, management and treatment of patients suffering from exposure to a wide range of substances and products. It should be the first point of reference in all cases of poisoning. The management of a patient with overdose is summarized in Table 12.3.

Table 12.1 Some physical signs of poisoning	
Features	**Likely poisons**
Constricted pupils	Opioids
	Organophosphorus insecticides
	Nerve agents
Dilated pupils	Tricyclic antidepressants
	Amfetamines
	Cocaine
	Antimuscarinic drugs
Convulsions	Tricyclic antidepressants
	Theophylline
	Opioids
	Mefanamic acid
	Isoniazid
	Amfetamines
Dystonic reactions	Metoclopramide
	Phenothiazines
Delirium and hallucinations	Antimuscarinic drugs
	Amfetamines
	Cannabis
	Recovery from tricyclic antidepressant overdose
Loss of vision	Methanol
	Quinine
Divergent strabismus	Tricyclic antidepressants
Papilloedema	Carbon monoxide
	Methanol
Nystagmus	Phenytoin
	Carbamazepine
Hypertonia and hyperreflexia	Tricyclic antidepressants
	Antimuscarinic drugs
Tinnitus and deafness	Salicylates
	Quinine
Hyperventilation	Salicylates
	Phenoxyacetate herbicides
	Theophylline
Hyperthermia	MDMA (Ecstasy)
Blisters	Usually occur in comatose patients
Lips and skin 'cherry red'	Carbon monoxide poisoning

Emergency resuscitation (ABCDE, p. 723)

■ Nurse the patient in the lateral position with the lower leg straight and the upper leg flexed; this reduces the risk of aspiration.

■ Clear the airway and intubate if the gag reflex is absent.

Table 12.2 **Agents for which emergency measurement of blood concentrations is appropriate**

Aspirin (salicylate)
Digoxin
Ethanol (ethylene glycol and methanol poisoning)
Ethylene glycol
Iron
Lithium (do not use a lithium heparin tube for blood sampling)
Methanol
Paracetamol
Theophylline

Table 12.3 **Principles of management of patients with self-poisoning**

1. Emergency resuscitation
2. Prevent further drug absorption
3. Increase drug elimination
4. Administration of specific drug antidotes
5. Psychiatric assessment

- Administer 60% oxygen by face mask in patients not intubated.
- Artificial ventilation is sometimes necessary if ventilation is inadequate (p. 564).
- Treat hypotension (p. 556), arrhythmias (p. 408) and convulsions (p. 740).
- Respiratory function (arterial blood gas analysis or pulse oximetry) and ECG monitoring in selected patients.
- Measure temperature with a low-reading rectal thermometer and treat hypothermia (< 35°C) with 'space blankets', warm (37°C) intravenous fluids and inspired gases.

Prevention of further drug absorption Most patients coming to hospital after an overdose are not at serious risk. These measures are usually reserved for those who have taken a potentially serious overdose by mouth.

- *Gastric lavage* is used to remove the drug from the stomach by repeated instillation and aspiration of small amounts of water or saline (200–300 mL, 38°C) via a large-bore orogastric tube. It should only be considered if a patient has ingested a potentially life-threatening amount of a poison and the procedure can be undertaken within 1 hour of ingestion. The main danger of gastric lavage is aspiration. It is performed with the patient in the left lateral decubitus position and the unconscious patient must be intubated with a cuffed endotracheal tube if the gag reflex is absent. Lavage is contraindicated for some poisons, e.g. corrosives, petrol or paraffin, because of the risk of pneumonitis.

- *Whole bowel irrigation* is considered for potentially toxic ingestions of sustained-release or enteric-coated drugs. Polyethylene glycol electrolyte solution (2000 mL/h) is infused via a nasogastric tube until the rectal effluent is clear.
- *Single-dose activated charcoal* (50 g) administered by mouth adsorbs unabsorbed poison still present in the gut. It is considered if a patient has ingested a potentially toxic amount of a drug absorbed by charcoal (e.g. aspirin, digoxin, paracetamol, barbiturates) up to 1 hour previously.
- *Induction of vomiting* with ipecacuanha syrup is no longer used in the management of poisoning.

Increasing drug elimination

- *Multiple-dose activated charcoal* (50 g initially followed by 50 g 4-hourly until charcoal appears in the faeces or recovery occurs) is considered if a patient has ingested a life-threatening amount of carbamazepine, phenobarbital, dapsone, quinine, or theophylline. It increases drug elimination by interrupting the enterohepatic circulation and adsorbing the drug that has diffused into intestinal juices.
- *Urinary alkalinization* depends on the principle that ionization of acid drugs is increased in alkaline urine and thus renal tubular reabsorption is reduced (as only lipophilic non-ionized drugs cross the lipid membrane readily). In practice urine alkalinization is only employed in salicylate (p. 575) and chlorophenoxy herbicide poisoning.
- *Haemodialysis* is used with some drugs in cases of severe poisoning, e.g. lithium, ethanol, methanol, ethylene glycol and salicylate (blood salicylate level > 700 mg/L, or 5.07 mmol/L) refractory to urine alkalization.

573

Table 12.4 SAD PERSONS scale

The presence of each factor is given a point of 1. Total scores range from 0–10. A total score of 0–2 usually indicates that this is not a high-risk situation. A score ≥ 7 indicates a patient at high risk of a subsequent suicide attempt. Patients with a score of 3–6 may be able to go home after a psychiatric assessment

S ex	1 if male
A ge	1 if < 19 or > 45 years
D epression/hopelessness	1 if present
P revious deliberate self-harm	1 if present
E xcessive alcohol or drug abuse	1 if present
R ational thinking, loss of	1 if patient is psychotic (schizophrenia, affective illness, organic brain syndrome)
S ocial supports lacking	1 if these are lacking especially with recent loss of a significant other
O rganized or serious attempt	1 if any of: lethal method, well thought out, suicide note, changed will, affairs in order
N o social supports	1 if divorced, separated, widowed, single, no children
S ickness	1 especially if chronic, severe, debilitating (e.g. cancer, epilepsy, multiple sclerosis)

574 **Antagonizing the effects of poisons** Specific antidotes are available for a small number of drugs; these will be considered under the individual drugs.

Psychiatric assessment All suicide attempts must be taken seriously and an assessment made of suicidal intent. The SAD PERSONS scale (Table 12.4) aims to assess suicide risk and is used to alert the clinician that the patient may be at high risk. In some patients, often young females, the act was not premeditated, they have no wish to die and the tablets were taken in response to an acute situation, e.g. an argument with the boyfriend. The risk of suicide is low and formal psychiatric assessment is not always necessary. In the absence of potential medical problems these patients may not necessarily need to be admitted to hospital, provided there is the necessary social and emotional back-up at home. In other patients there is clear suicidal intent: the act was planned, a suicide note was written and efforts were made not to be discovered. These patients must be assessed by a psychiatrist before they leave hospital.

SPECIFIC DRUG PROBLEMS

In this section only specific treatment regimens will be discussed. The general principles of management of self-poisoning should always be applied.

Aspirin (K&C 6e p. 1009)

Overdosage of aspirin (salicylate) stimulates the respiratory centre, directly increasing the depth and rate of respiration and thereby producing a respiratory alkalosis. Compensatory mechanisms include renal excretion of bicarbonate and potassium, which results in a metabolic acidosis, and a fall in arterial pH indicates serious poisoning. Salicylates also interfere with carbohydrate, fat and protein metabolism, as well as with oxidative phosphorylation. This gives rise to increased lactate, pyruvate and ketone bodies, all of which contribute to the acidosis.

Clinical features

Symptoms and signs of aspirin poisoning include tinnitus, nausea and vomiting, overbreathing, hyperpyrexia and sweating with a tachycardia. Alternatively, the patient may appear completely well, even with high plasma concentrations of salicylate. Ingestion of 10–20 g of aspirin by an adult (or one-tenth of this amount for a child) is likely to cause moderate or severe toxicity.

In severe poisoning (plasma salicylate concentration > 700 mg/L; 5.07 mmol/L) there may be cerebral and pulmonary oedema resulting from increased capillary permeability. Coma and respiratory depression may be seen with severe poisoning, but more frequently are due to the ingestion of a second drug or alcohol.

Investigations

- Plasma salicylate concentration to determine the severity of poisoning. Initial and repeat levels after 2–4 hours should be performed.

Specific drug problems

- Serum urea and electrolytes.
- Blood glucose (hypoglycaemia may occur).
- Prothrombin time (may be prolonged).
- Arterial blood gases.
- Chest X-ray.

Management

- Correct dehydration and hypokalaemia with intravenous fluids.
- Intravenous vitamin K (10 mg) to correct hypoprothrombinaemia.
- Consider gastric lavage or activated charcoal (50 g) in a patient who has taken a large amount of aspirin less than 1 hour previously.
- Urine alkalinization for moderately severe poisoning (plasma salicylate poisoning 500–700 mg/L, 3.62–5.07 mmol/L). Approximately 225 mL of an 8.4% (1 mmol bicarbonate/mL) solution of sodium bicarbonate is infused intravenously over 1 hour to ensure a urinary pH (measured by narrow-range indicator paper or pH meter) of more than 7.5 and preferably close to 8.5.
- Haemodialysis is indicated for severe poisoning (plasma salicylate > 700 mg/L (5.07 mmol/L)).

Paracetamol (acetaminophen) (K&C 6e p. 1017)

Paracetamol in overdose may cause fatal hepatic necrosis and is the commonest form of poisoning encountered in the UK today. Paracetamol is converted to a toxic metabolite, N-acetyl-p-benzoquinoneimine (NAPQI), which is normally inactivated by conjugation with reduced glutathione. After a large overdose, glutathione is depleted and NAPQI binds covalently with sulphydryl groups on liver cell membranes, causing necrosis. Marked liver cell necrosis can occur with as little as 7.5 g (15 tablets), and death with 15 g. The prothrombin time or international normalized ratio (INR) is the best guide to the severity of the liver damage.

Clinical features

The main danger is liver failure, which usually becomes apparent in 72–96 hours after drug ingestion. Initial symptoms include malaise, nausea and vomiting, with

Emergency Box 12.1
Management of paracetamol poisoning

- Take blood for paracetamol levels (at or after 4 h since ingestion), full blood count, INR and ALT/AST, U & E and glucose.
- Gastric lavage or single-dose activated charcoal (50 g) if patient presents within 1 hour of ingestion and potentially serious overdose (ingestion of > 150 mg/kg bodyweight or > 10 g in adults, whichever is the smaller).
- Give intravenous NAC in 5% dextrose immediately if potentially serious overdose (see above):
  150 mg/kg in 200 mL over 15 min, then
  50 mg/kg in 500 mL over 4 h, then
  100 mg/kg in 1 litre over 16 h.
- Make decision to continue treatment based on paracetamol levels and nomogram (Fig. 12.1). Discontinue treatment if the plasma paracetamol concentration is below the relevant treatment line and there is no abnormality of INR, plasma creatinine or ALT.
- In patients presenting more than 24 hours after ingestion, NAC should not be started until results of investigations are available and toxicological advice has been sought.
- Repeat blood investigations (except paracetamol) at the end of NAC treatment. If the patient is asymptomatic and the investigations are normal, there is little risk of serious complications and the patient can be discharged.

NAC, N-acetylcysteine

preserved consciousness unless another drug has also been taken. Acute renal failure may occur in the absence of severe liver failure.

Management

Treatment depends on the interval between overdose and presentation and on the plasma concentrations of paracetamol. The investigation and management of paracetamol poisoning are summarized in Emergency Box 12.1 and Figure 12.1. The two antidotes in use for paracetamol poisoning increase the availability of glutathione. Intravenous N-acetylcysteine (NAC) is the treatment of choice. Anaphylactoid reactions (urticarial rash, angio-oedema, bronchospasm, hypotension) occasionally occur with NAC and are treated by stopping the infusion, giving an antihistamine and usually restarting the infusion once the reaction has

Specific drug problems

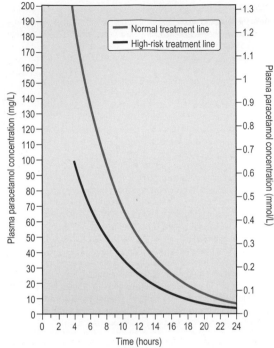

Fig. 12.1 **Nomogram for treatment of paracetamol poisoning.** (From *British National Formulary* (1998) with permission.) Patients whose plasma paracetamol concentrations are above the **normal treatment line** should be treated with acetylcysteine. **The high-risk (lower) treatment line** should be used in patients with:

- Regular alcohol excess
- Poor nutrition
- Anorexia nervosa
- HIV infection
- Pre-existing liver disease
- Recent ingestion of enzyme-inducing drugs (carbamazepine, phenobarbital, phenytoin, rifampicin, St John's wort).

The prognostic accuracy after 15 hours is uncertain but a plasma-paracetamol concentration above the relevant treatment line should be regarded as carrying a serious risk of liver damage and treated with NAC.

settled. Oral methionine (four doses of 2.5 g at 4-hour intervals) is an alternative, but absorption and efficacy are erratic if the patient is vomiting. Patients who develop liver damage with a raised INR should remain in hospital until the values are returning to normal. Fresh frozen plasma should not normally be given to patients with a raised INR, as the trend in the INR is important in assessing prognosis and in determining the need for possible transplantation. A poor prognosis is indicated by an INR value above 3, raised serum creatinine concentration or a blood pH below 7.3 recorded more than 24 hours after the overdose and after correction of hypovolaemia. If any of these abnormalities is present, advice should be sought from a specialist liver unit. Patients with severe hepatic damage may require liver transplantation.

Other drugs (*K&C* 6e p. 1008)

Table 12.5 outlines the clinical features and management of the other drugs that are commonly taken in cases of overdose. For all of those that are taken by mouth the initial management should include gastric lavage and activated charcoal if the patient presents in time.

Carbon monoxide (*K&C* 6e p. 1010)

Carbon monoxide (CO) poisoning is usually the result of inhalation of smoke, car exhaust or fumes from improperly maintained and ventilated heating systems. Methylene chloride, a component of paint remover, is readily absorbed and metabolized to CO by the liver and may lead to poisoning. CO combines readily with haemoglobin to form carboxyhaemoglobin, thus preventing the formation of oxyhaemoglobin. The clinical features include headache, mental impairment and, in severe cases, convulsions, coma and cardiac arrest. In spite of hypoxaemia the skin is pink. Carboxyhaemoglobin (COHb) levels should be measured in a venous blood sample, although they do not correlate precisely with clinical outcome. Treatment consists of removing the patient from the CO source and giving 100% oxygen via a tightly fitting face mask. Referral for hyperbaric oxygen treatment should be considered if the victim is, or has been, unconscious or has a blood carboxyhaemoglobin concentration of more than 40%, or is pregnant with a carboxyhaemoglobin concentration of more than 20%.

Table 12.5 Clinical features and specific management for certain drugs taken in overdose

Drug	Clinical features	Management
Tricyclic antidepressants	Tachycardia, hypotension, fixed dilated pupils, convulsions, urinary retention, arrhythmias, decreased conscious level	Treat convulsions with diazepam. Supraventricular and ventricular tachycardia is treated with intravenous sodium bicarbonate (8.4%) 50 mmol (50 mL) over 20 min, even in the absence of acidosis
Benzodiazepines	Drowsiness, ataxia, dysarthria, respiratory depression and coma. Potentiate the effects of other CNS depressants taken concomitantly	Flumazenil (0.5 mg i.v. and repeated if necessary) a benzodiazepine antagonist is used if respiratory depression is present
Phenothiazines	Hypotension, hypothermia, arrhythmias. Depression of consciousness and respiration. Convulsion and dystonic reactions	Symptomatic treatment of complications, e.g. diazepam for convulsions. Dystonic reactions treated with i.v. benzatropine
NSAIDs	Coma, convulsions, metabolic acidosis and renal failure	Treatment is symptomatic and supportive
β-Blockers	Bradycardia and hypotension. Coma, convulsions and hypoglycaemia with severe overdose	Atropine (0.6–1.2 mg i.v.) for brady-cardia. In resistant cases i.v. glucagon (5–10 mg followed by an infusion of 1–5 mg/h) has a positive inotropic action on the heart

Alcohol

Acute intoxication with alcohol produces severe depression of consciousness and hypoglycaemia, particularly in children. Treatment usually only consists of gastric lavage with an endotracheal tube in position. Blood glucose is measured and glucose given if indicated.

DRUG ABUSE (*K&C* 6e p. 1305)

Under the Misuse of Drugs Regulations of 1985, drugs with a high abuse potential, drugs of addiction and other drugs with non-therapeutic psychotropic activity are categorized as controlled drugs. These include opiates, cocaine, barbiturates, lysergide, amfetamines and related drugs. Any patient who is believed to be dependent on or addicted to controlled drugs must, by law, be notified to the Home Office.

Opioids

Opioid drugs, e.g. diamorphine (heroin), codeine and buprenorphine, produce physical dependency, such that an acute withdrawal syndrome develops ('cold turkey') if the drugs are stopped. These severe symptoms – profuse sweating, tachycardia, dilated pupils, leg cramps, diarrhoea and vomiting – may be reduced by giving methadone, a pharmaceutical preparation of an opioid.

Drug addicts frequently overdose themselves, causing varying degrees of coma, respiratory depression and pinpoint pupils. Treatment is with intravenous naloxone, an opiate antagonist, 1.2 mg i.v. every 2 minutes until breathing is adequate. The drug is short acting and repeated doses or an infusion may be necessary, with the rate titrated according to the clinical response.

581

Management of body packers

Body packers or 'mules' are persons who attempt to smuggle drugs by swallowing drug-filled packets, often containing cocaine or heroin. The packet may rupture in the gut resulting in massive intoxication or cause gastro-intestinal obstruction or perforation. Suspected body packers should have a plain abdominal X-ray and a urine drug screen. Contrast-enhanced CT scan is performed if the plain film is negative and there is a high index of suspicion. Asymptomatic carriers are treated with an oral polyethylene glycol/electrolyte lavage solution at a rate of 2 L per hour to speed passage of packets, with follow-up imaging to document clearance of packets. Packets in the vagina can be removed manually. Immediate surgery is indicated if there is evidence of intestinal obstruction, perforation or systemic toxicity, particularly if the drug involved is cocaine for which there is no antidote.

Cannabis

Cannabis is usually smoked and is often taken casually. It is a mild hallucinogen, seldom accompanied by a desire to increase the dose; withdrawal symptoms are uncommon.

Lysergide

Lysergic acid diethylamine (LSD) is a much more potent hallucinogen; its use can lead to severe psychotic states in which life may be at risk. Even in overdose, severe physiological reactions do not seem to occur. Adverse reactions are treated with repeated reassurance; a sedative, e.g. diazepam, is sometimes necessary. Phenothiazines may be necessary in severe cases.

Cocaine

Cocaine can be taken by injection, inhalation ('crack') or ingestion. It stimulates the central nervous system, producing euphoria, agitation and tachycardia. Convulsions, pyrexia and cardiorespiratory depression may occur in severe cases of overdose and management is supportive with diazepam for agitation and active external cooling for hyperthermia. β-Blockers may worsen hypertension and are contraindicated.

Amfetamines

Amfetamines are taken for their stimulatory effect. In overdose there is confusion, delirium, hallucinations and violent behaviour. Cardiac arrhythmias can be a major problem. Treatment is with sedatives, such as diazepam. Forced acid diuresis may be used but is rarely required.

Ecstasy (MDMA, 3,4-methylenedioxy-methamfetamine) is a synthetic amfetamine derivative taken orally as tablets or capsules. In Britain it is used almost exclusively as a 'dance drug' and the adverse effects are the result of the drug's pharmacological properties compounded by physical exertion. Serious acute complications are convulsions, hyperpyrexia, coagulopathy, rhabdomyolysis, renal and liver failure and death. Treatment is rehydration, diazepam for severe agitation and dantrolene (1 mg/kg bodyweight i.v.) for hyperthermia.

Solvents

The inhalation of organic solvents has become a common problem, particularly in teenagers. The patient presents either in the acute intoxicated state (with euphoria and excitement) or as a chronic abuser with excoriation and rashes over the face and a peripheral neuropathy. Sudden death can occur and is probably the result of cardiac arrhythmias.

Alcohol abuse (*K&C* 6e p. 1302)

Drinking-related problems have increased in recent years. Approximately one in five male admissions to acute medical wards is directly or indirectly the result of alcohol. Over the past 20 years admissions to psychiatric hospitals for the treatment of alcohol-related problems has increased 25-fold.

A number of medical, social and psychiatric problems are related to alcohol abuse (see below) and may be seen in the absence of actual physiological dependence. Alcohol dependence has seven essential elements:

■ A compulsive need to drink
■ A regular (daily) drinking routine to avoid or relieve withdrawal symptoms
■ Drinking takes priority over other activities
■ Increased tolerance to alcohol
■ Repeated withdrawal symptoms often worse on waking in the morning
■ Early-morning drinking to avoid withdrawal symptoms (nausea, sweating, agitation)
■ Reinstatement after abstinence.

Guidelines for safe limits of drinking are 21 units per week in men and 14 units in women (1 unit = a measure of spirits, a glass of wine or half a pint of standard-strength beer). A

Drug abuse

slightly higher intake is probably unlikely to lead to harm, but more than 36 units per week in men and 24 units in women increases the risk to health. An elevated serum γ-GT (γ-glutamyl transpeptidase) (p. 127) and raised red cell mean corpuscular volume (MCV, p. 193) are useful screening tests for alcohol abuse and are helpful in monitoring progress. Blood and urine alcohol levels are sometimes measured to demonstrate high intake.

Consequences of alcohol abuse and dependence

Physical complications

These usually occur after a long period of heavy drinking, e.g. 10 years. Problems are generally seen earlier in women than in men. Damage is the result of direct tissue toxicity and the effects of malnutrition and vitamin deficiency which often accompany alcohol abuse.

- *Cardiovascular.* A direct toxic effect in the heart leads to a cardiomyopathy and arrhythmias.
- *Neurological.* Acute intoxication leads to ataxia, falls and head injury with intracranial bleeds. Long-term complications include polyneuropathy (p. 773), myopathy, cerebellar degeneration (p. 707), dementia (p. 780) and epilepsy.

Wernicke's encephalopathy (WE) is the result of vitamin B_1 deficiency (thiamin) and thus may also be seen in severe starvation and prolonged vomiting. The classic triad of WE (confusion, ataxia and ophthalmoplegia) occurs together in only a minority of patients. Mental changes are the most common (acute confusion, drowsiness, pre-coma, coma) whereas ataxia and ophthalmoplegia occur in less than one-third of patients. The diagnosis is clinical. As in a patient presenting with these features the alcohol history may be unknown, a high index of suspicion and a low threshold for making a presumptive diagnosis are appropriate. Treatment is with an intravenous complex of B vitamins (e.g. two pairs of ampoules of Pabrinex IVHP three times daily for 3 days followed by one pair of ampoules daily for 5 days), which may reverse some of the early changes. Inappropriately managed, WE is fatal in 20% of patients. Of survivors, many will develop long-term brain damage (Korsakoff's syndrome) with a gross defect of short-term memory, associated with confabulation. Patients at risk of WE (significant weight loss, signs of undernutrition, alcohol withdrawal symptoms requiring hospital admission) should be treated prophylactically with one pair of ampoules of Pabrinex IVHP daily for 3–5 days followed with oral B vitamins on discharge. Patients must receive B vitamins before glucose because of a risk of acutely precipitating WE.

- *Gastrointestinal effects.* These include liver damage (p. 163), pancreatitis (p. 175), oesophagitis and an increased incidence of oesophageal carcinoma.
- *Haematological complications.* These include thrombo-cytopenia (alcohol inhibits platelet maturation and release from bone marrow), a raised MCV and anaemia caused by dietary folate deficiency.
- *Psychiatric complications.* There is an increased incidence of depression and deliberate self-harm among alcoholics. In these patients attempted suicide must always be taken seriously and psychiatric referral considered (p. 574).
- *Social complications.* These include marital and sexual difficulties, employment problems, financial difficulties and homelessness.

Alcohol withdrawal
Most heavy drinkers will experience some form of withdrawal symptoms if they attempt to reduce or stop drinking.

- Early mild features occur within 6–12 hours and include tremor, nausea and sweating. Treatment is with a reducing dose of diazepam or alternative drug (see Emergency Box 12.2). In mild cases this can be on an outpatient basis as long as the patient attends daily for medication and monitoring and has good social support.
- Late major features usually occur within 2–3 days but may take up to 2 weeks:
  - Generalized tonic–clonic seizures (p. 737)
  - Delirium tremens with fever, tremor, tachycardia, agitation and visual hallucinations ('pink elephants'). Treatment must be given urgently (see Emergency Box 12.2).

After alcohol withdrawal it is essential that relapse is prevented. This involves local alcohol services, specialist psychiatry and the alcohol nurse specialist. 'Brief interventions' refers to 10–15 minutes of counselling, with feedback about drinking, advice and goal setting, and follow-up

> **Emergency Box 12.2**
> **Management of delirium tremens**
>
> - Admit the patient to a medical bed.
> - Prevent or treat established Wernicke's encephalopathy by administration of intravenous B vitamin complex (see p 584). Give before administration of glucose-containing i.v. fluids.
> - Treat infection.
> - Correct dehydration and electrolyte imbalance.
> - Give prophylactic phenytoin, if previous history of withdrawal fits.
> - Give diazepam 10–20 mg or chlordiazepoxide 30–60 mg *or* lorazepam 2–4 mg and repeat after 1 hour depending on response.
> - Continue maintenance treatment:
>   - Diazepam, 10 mg every 6 hours for 4 doses then 5 mg every 6 hours for 8 doses, *or*
>   - Chlordiazepoxide, 30 mg every 6 hours for 4 doses then 15 mg every 6 hours for 8 doses, *or*
>   - Lorazepam, 2 mg every 6 hours for 4 doses then 1 mg every 6 hours for 8 doses.
> - Further benzodiazepine dosing depends on patient assessment, response and support network if outpatient.

contact (one or more discussions lasting 10–15 minutes with a clinician or specialist nurse). Oral acamprosate, a GABA analogue, reduces relapses by 50%. Naltrexone is a pure opioid receptor antagonist that modifies the effects of alcohol by blunting its pleasurable effects and by reducing the craving. It reduces relapse rate but is not yet licensed in the UK.

Endocrinology 13

Hormones are chemical messengers produced by a variety of specialized secretory cells. They may act:

- At a site distant from their site of secretion into the blood (endocrine effect)
- Directly on nearby cells (paracrine effect)
- On the cell of origin (autocrine effect)
- As neurotransmitters in the brain and gastrointestinal tract.

Hormones act by binding to specific receptors either on the target cell surface or within the cell (e.g. thyroid hormones, cortisol) (*K&C* 6e p. 1036). The result is a cascade of intra-cellular reactions within the target cell which frequently amplifies the original stimulus and leads ultimately to a response by the target cell. Some hormones, e.g. growth hormone and thyroxine, act on most tissues of the body. Others act on only one tissue, e.g. thyroid-stimulating hormone (TSH) and adrenocorticotrophin (ACTH) are secreted by the anterior pituitary and have specific target tissues, namely the thyroid gland and the adrenal cortex.

The hypothalamus and pituitary (*K&C* 6e p. 1041)

The hypothalamus contains many vital centres for functions such as appetite, thirst, thermal regulation and sleep/waking. It also plays a role in circadian rhythm, the menstrual cycle, stress and mood. Releasing factors produced in the hypothalamus reach the pituitary via the portal system, which runs down the pituitary stalk. These releasing factors stimulate or inhibit the production of hormones from distinct cell types (e.g. production of growth hormone by acidophils), each of which secretes a specific hormone in response to unique hypothalamic stimulatory or inhibitory hormones. The anterior pituitary hormones, in turn, stimulate the peripheral glands and tissues. This pattern is illustrated in Figure 13.1. The posterior pituitary acts as a storage organ for antidiuretic hormone (ADH, vasopressin)

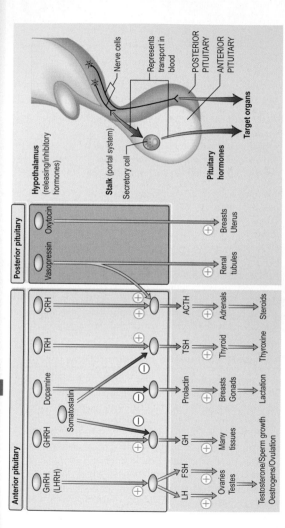

Fig. 13.1 **Hypothalamic releasing hormones and the pituitary trophic hormones.** See the text for abbreviations and explanation.

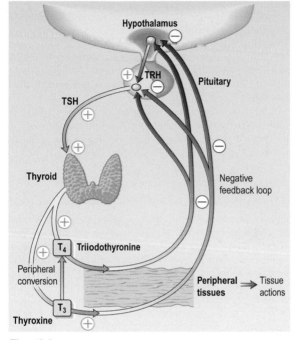

Fig. 13.2 **The hypothalamic–pituitary–thyroid feedback system.**

and oxytocin, which are synthesized in the supraoptic and paraventricular nuclei in the anterior hypothalamus and pass to the posterior pituitary along a single axon in the pituitary stalk. ADH is discussed on page 629; oxytocin produces milk ejection and uterine myometrial contractions.

Control and feedback (*K&C* 6e p. 1037)

Most hormone systems are controlled by some form of feedback; an example is the hypothalamic–pituitary–thyroid axis (Fig. 13.2). Thyrotrophin-releasing hormone (TRH), secreted in the hypothalamus, stimulates TSH secretion from the anterior pituitary which, in turn, stimulates the synthesis and release of thyroid hormones from the thyroid gland. Circulating thyroid hormone feeds back on the pituitary, and possibly the hypothalamus, to suppress the production of TSH and TRH, and hence bring about a fall in thyroid hormone secretion. This is known as a 'negative feedback' system and represents the most common mechanism for regulation of circulating hormone levels. Conversely, a fall in thyroid hormone secretion (e.g. after thyroidectomy) leads to increased secretion of TSH and TRH.

A patient with a hormone-producing tumour fails to show negative feedback and this is useful in diagnosis, e.g. the dexamethasone suppression test in the diagnosis of Cushing's syndrome.

COMMON PRESENTING SYMPTOMS IN ENDOCRINE DISEASE (K&C 6e p. 1040)

Hormonal abnormalities have a wide range of clinical effects and there are many presenting symptoms and signs of endocrine disease, the commonest of which are shown in Table 13.1. Many of these are vague and non-specific, e.g. tiredness in hypothyroidism, weight loss or weight gain, anorexia and malaise in Addison's disease, and the differential diagnosis is often wide. Precocious puberty (< 9 years) or delayed puberty (> 15 years) is often the result of a familial tendency, although hypothalamic–pituitary disease may present in this way, and endocrine investigations are usually undertaken.

Pituitary tumours (K&C 6e p. 1044)

Benign pituitary tumours (adenomas) are the most common form of pituitary disease. Symptoms may arise as a result of inadequate hormone production, excess hormone secretion, or from pressure and local infiltration.

Underproduction
This is the result of disease at either a hypothalamic or a pituitary level, and it results in the clinical features of hypopituitarism (p. 592).

Overproduction
Overproduction of pituitary hormones may cause the following:

- Growth hormone (GH) excess, resulting in acromegaly or gigantism

---

Table 13.1 Common presenting complaints in endocrine disease

Body size and shape	Skin
Short stature	Hirsutism
Tall stature	Hair thinning
Excessive weight or weight gain	Pigmentation
Loss of weight	Dry skin
	Excess sweating
Metabolic effects	
Tiredness	**Reproduction/sex**
Weakness	Loss or absence of libido
Increased appetite	Erectile dysfunction
Decreased appetite	Oligomenorrhoea/
Polydipsia/thirst	amenorrhoea
Polyuria/nocturia	Subfertility
Tremor	Galactorrhoea
Palpitation	Gynaecomastia
Anxiety	Delayed puberty
	Precocious puberty
Local effects	
Swelling in the neck	
Carpal tunnel syndrome	
Bone or muscle pain	
Protrusion of eyes	
Visual loss (acuity and/or fields)	
Headache	

- Prolactin excess, which may be clinically silent or produce galactorrhoea
- Cushing's disease, resulting from excess ACTH production
- Tumours producing luteinizing hormone (LH), follicle-stimulating hormone (FSH) or TSH are very rare.

Local effects

Local infiltration of or pressure on surrounding structures (Fig. 13.3), may result in:

- Visual loss with field defects. This is typically a bitemporal hemianopia caused by pressure on the optic chiasm (p. 710).
- Headache produced by tumour involvement of the meninges and bony structures.
- Obesity and altered appetite and thirst. This is due to involvement of the hypothalamus. In children, hypothalamic involvement may lead to early puberty (precocious puberty).

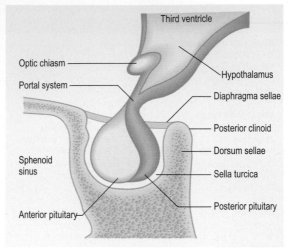

Fig. 13.3 **A sagittal section of the pituitary fossa, showing the important anatomical relationships.** The cavernous sinus lies lateral to the pituitary and is seen on a coronal view.

- Hydrocephalus caused by interruption of cerebrospinal fluid flow.
- Cranial nerve lesions (III, IV and VI) by infiltration of the cavernous sinus.

Hypopituitarism *(K&C 6e p. 1046)*

Deficiency of hypothalamic-releasing hormones or pituitary hormones may be either selective or multiple. Multiple deficiencies usually result from tumour growth or other destructive lesions, and there is usually a progressive loss of function, with GH and gonadotrophins (FSH and LH) being affected first and TSH and ACTH last. Rather than prolactin deficiency, hyperprolactinaemia occurs relatively early because of loss of tonic inhibitory control by dopamine (see Fig. 13.1). Panhypopituitarism is a deficiency of all anterior pituitary hormones. Vasopressin and oxytocin secretion will only be affected if the hypothalamus is involved by either hypothalamic tumour or by extension of a pituitary lesion.

Table 13.2	Causes of hypopituitarism	
Neoplastic	**Traumatic**
Primary tumours	Skull fracture
Secondary deposits	Surgery
Craniopharyngioma	
	Infiltrations
Infective	Sarcoidosis
Meningitis	Haemochromatosis
Encephalitis	
Syphilis	**Others**
	Radiation damage
Vascular	Chemotherapy
Pituitary apoplexy	
Sheehan's syndrome	**Functional**
'Empty sella' syndrome	Anorexia
	Starvation
Immunological	Emotional deprivation
Pituitary antibodies	
Congenital	
Kallmann's syndrome	

Aetiology

The causes of hypopituitarism are listed in Table 13.2. The commonest cause (> 70% of cases) is a pituitary tumour or treatment of the tumour either by surgical removal or radiotherapy.

Clinical features

These depend on the extent of hypothalamic–pituitary deficiencies. Gonadotrophin deficiency results in loss of libido, amenorrhoea (absent menstruation) and erectile dysfunction, whereas hyperprolactinaemia results in galactorrhoea (breast milk secretion unrelated to pregnancy) and hypogonadism. Growth hormone deficiency is usually clinically silent except in children, although it may impair well-being in adults. Secondary hypothyroidism and adrenal failure lead to tiredness, slowness of thought and action, and mild hypotension. Long-standing hypopituitarism may give the classic picture of pallor with hairlessness (alabaster skin). Particular syndromes related to hypopituitarism are:

- *Congenital deficiency of gonadotrophin-releasing hormone (GnRH)* leads to deficiency of FSH and LH with otherwise normal function of the anterior pituitary gland. The presence of anosmia (absent sense of smell) with congenital GnRH deficiency is referred to as Kallmann's syndrome.
- *Sheehan's syndrome.* This situation, now rare, is pituitary infarction following severe postpartum haemorrhage.
- *Pituitary apoplexy.* A pituitary tumour may occasionally enlarge rapidly owing to infarction or haemorrhage within the tumour. This may produce severe headache and sudden severe visual loss, sometimes followed by acute life-threatening hypopituitarism.
- *'Empty sella' syndrome.* The sella turcica appears radiologically devoid of pituitary tissue; the pituitary is actually placed eccentrically and function is usually normal.

Investigation

Each axis of the hypothalamic–pituitary system requires separate investigation. The presence of normal gonadal function (ovulatory menstruation or normal libido/erections) suggests that multiple defects of the anterior pituitary are unlikely. Tests range from measurement of basal hormone levels to stimulatory tests of the pituitary and tests of feedback for the hypothalamus.

Management

Steroid and thyroid hormones are essential for life and are given as oral replacement drugs (e.g. 15–40 mg hydrocortisone daily in divided doses, 100–150 µg thyroxine daily) with the aim of restoring clinical and biochemical normality. Androgens and oestrogens are replaced for symptomatic control. If fertility is desired, LH and FSH analogues are used. GH therapy should be given to the growing child under appropriate specialist supervision and it may also produce substantial benefits to the GH-deficient adult in terms of work capacity and psychological well-being.

Two warnings are necessary:

- Thyroid replacement should not commence until normal glucocorticoid function has been demonstrated or replacement steroid therapy initiated, as an adrenal 'crisis' may otherwise be precipitated.

Table 13.3 **Consequences of androgen deficiency in the male**

Pre-pubertal onset
Increased height and arm span
Lack of adult hair distribution
High-pitched voice
Small penis, testes and scrotum
Decreased muscle mass

Post-pubertal onset
Decreased prostate size
Diminished rate of growth of beard and body hair
Fine feminine skin
Decreased potency and libido
Gynaecomastia

- Glucocorticoid deficiency masks impaired urine concentrating ability. Diabetes insipidus is apparent after steroid replacement, the steroids being necessary for excretion of a water load.

MALE REPRODUCTION AND SEX (K&C 6e p. 1049)

Gonadotrophin-releasing hormone (GnRH, also called luteinizing hormone-RH) is released episodically from the hypothalamus (during and after puberty) and stimulates LH and FSH secretion from the anterior pituitary gland. LH and FSH stimulate the production of testosterone and sperm respectively from the testes.

Male hypogonadism (K&C 6e p. 1054)

Male hypogonadism is a descriptive term for the clinical features associated with androgen deficiency. The presentation depends on the age of onset of hypogonadism (Table 13.3). In prepubertal onset the patient presents with delayed puberty and eunuchoid body proportions resulting from the continued growth of long bones, which occurs because of delayed fusion of the epiphyses. Eunuchoid body proportions include a lower body segment (floor to pubis) more than 2 cm longer than the upper body segment (pubis to crown) and an arm span that is more than 2 cm longer than height.

> ### Table 13.4 Causes of male hypogonadism
>
> **Disease of the pituitary or hypothalamus**
> Congenital GnRH deficiency
> Hypopituitarism
> Severe systemic illness
> Severe malnourishment
> Hyperprolactinaemia (interferes with pulsatile secretion of LH
> and FSH)
>
> **Disease of the testes**
> Congenital: Klinefelter's syndrome, anorchia, Leydig cell
> agenesis, failure of testicular descent
> Acquired: trauma, torsion, chemotherapy, radiation
>
> **Target tissues**
> Androgen-receptor deficiency

A large number of diseases can lead to destruction or malfunction of the hypothalamic–pituitary–testicular axis (Table 13.4).

Klinefelter's syndrome is the most common cause of male hypogonadism, with an incidence of 1 in 1000 live births. It is the result of the presence of an extra X chromosome (47, XXY). Accelerated atrophy of the testicular germ cells gives rise to sterility and small firm testes. The clinical picture varies: in the most severely affected there is complete failure of sexual maturation, eunuchoid body proportions, gynaecomastia and learning difficulties.

Investigations

A low or low-normal serum testosterone confirms the clinical diagnosis of hypogonadism. Supranormal serum concentrations of FSH and LH indicate that the patient has primary hypogonadism (testicular disease), and normal or low levels of FSH/LH indicate disease of the pituitary or hypothalamus (secondary hypogonadism). Further investigations, e.g. serum prolactin, chromosomal analysis, pituitary MRI scan and pituitary function tests, will depend on the likely site of the defect.

Gynaecomastia

Management

The cause can rarely be reversed and the mainstay of treatment is androgen replacement. Although hypogonadotrophic patients have the potential for fertility, LH and FSH or pulsatile GnRH are only used (instead of testosterone) when fertility is desired, as these regimens are expensive and complex.

Loss of libido and erectile dysfunction (*K&C* 6e p. 1055)

Erectile dysfunction is defined as failure to initiate an erection or to maintain an erection until ejaculation. Erection is the result of increased vascularity of the penis controlled via the sacral parasympathetic outflow; it may be impaired by vascular disease, autonomic neuropathy and nerve damage after pelvic surgery. The nervous pathways for ejaculation are centred on the lumbar sympathetics, and abnormalities may occur with autonomic neuropathy (most commonly with diabetes mellitus) and traumatic nerve damage. Psychological factors, endocrine factors (causes of hypogonadism described above), alcohol and drugs, e.g. cannabis, and diuretics, may cause abnormalities of both parasympathetic and sympathetic nerves. A careful history and examination will identify the cause in many patients. The presence of nocturnal emissions and morning erections is suggestive of psychogenic erectile dysfunction.

Offending drugs should be stopped. Phosphodiesterase type-5 inhibitors (sildenafil, tadalafil, vardenafil) which increase penile blood flow are usually first choice for therapy. Other methods of treatment include apomorphine, intracavernosal injections of alprostadil, papaverine or phentolamine, vacuum expanders and penile implants.

Many cases are the result of psychological factors, and the patient may respond to psychosexual counselling.

Gynaecomastia (*K&C* 6e p. 1056)

Gynaecomastia is development of breast tissue in the male. It results from an increase in the oestrogen : androgen ratio (Table 13.5) and is most commonly a result of liver disease or drug side-effects. Gynaecomastia is common in early puberty as a result of relative oestrogen excess, and usually resolves spontaneously. Unexplained gynaecomastia may

Table 13.5 Causes of gynaecomastia

Physiological
Neonatal, resulting from the influence of maternal hormones
Pubertal
Old age

Deficient testosterone secretion
Any cause of hypogonadism (Table 13.4)

Oestrogen-producing tumours
Of the testis or adrenal gland

HCG-producing tumours
Of the testis or the lung

Drugs
Digitalis
Spironolactone
Cyproterone
Cimetidine
Oestrogens
Cannabis
Heroin

Other
Hyperthyroidism
Liver disease

HCG, human chorionic gonadotrophin

occur, especially in elderly people, and is a diagnosis of exclusion after thorough examination and investigation. The treatment is either of the underlying cause or by removal of the drug if possible. Occasionally surgery is needed.

FEMALE REPRODUCTION AND SEX (K&C 6e p. 1056)

In the adult female higher brain centres impose a menstrual cycle of 28 days upon the activity of hypothalamic GnRH. Pulses of GnRH stimulate the release of pituitary LH and FSH. LH stimulates ovarian androgen production and FSH stimulates follicular development and aromatase activity (an enzyme required to convert ovarian androgens to oestrogens). Oestrogens are necessary for normal pubertal development and, together with progesterone, for maintenance of the menstrual cycle; they also have effects on a variety of tissues.

The menopause (K&C 6e p. 1052)

The menopause, or cessation of periods, naturally occurs about the age of 45–55 years. During the late 40s, first FSH and then LH concentrations begin to rise, probably as a result of diminishing follicle supply. Oestrogen levels fall and the cycle becomes disrupted. Menopause may also occur surgically, with radiotherapy to the ovaries and with ovarian disease (e.g. premature menopause in the 20s and 30s). Symptoms of the menopause are hot flushes, vaginal dryness and breast atrophy. There may also be vague symptoms of depression, loss of libido and weight gain. There is loss of bone density (osteoporosis, p. 298) and the premenopausal protection against ischaemic heart disease disappears.

Oestrogen replacement is the most effective treatment available for the relief of menopausal symptoms and also reduces the risk of colorectal cancer and osteoporotic fractures. Oestrogens, when given alone, increase the risk of endometrial cancer and so combination treatment with progestogens is given to women with an intact uterus. Recent studies have shown that women taking combined HRT have an increased risk of breast cancer, coronary heart disease (CHD), stroke and venous thromboembolism. These observations have led to changes in the recommendations for HRT and at present the primary indication for HRT is for control of menopausal symptoms. Furthermore, treatment is given for the shortest time possible rather than long term. HRT is contraindicated in women with a history of thromboembolism, stroke, CHD or breast cancer. HRT is also given to women with premature ovarian failure, and the data regarding adverse effects in menopausal women cannot be extrapolated to this group.

HRT is no longer recommended as treatment for prevention of postmenopausal osteoporosis; bisphosphonates or raloxifene are preferred. Raloxifene is one of the selective oestrogen receptor modulators (SERMs), which have the advantage of positive oestrogen effects on bone with no effect on oestrogen receptors of breast and uterus. Raloxifene has no effect on menopausal symptoms.

Female hypogonadism and amenorrhoea (*K&C* 6e p. 1056)

Amenorrhoea is the absence of menstruation. It is often physiological, e.g. during pregnancy and lactation, and after the menopause. Primary amenorrhoea is failure to start spontaneous menstruation by the age of 16 years. Secondary amenorrhoea is the absence of menstruation for 3 months in a woman who has previously had menstrual cycles. In the female, hypogonadism almost always presents as amenorrhoea or oligomenorrhoea (fewer than nine menses per year). The other features of oestrogen deficiency include atrophy of the breasts and vagina, loss of pubic hair and osteoporosis.

Aetiology

The causes of amenorrhoea are listed in Table 13.6. Polycystic ovary syndrome is the most common cause of oligo-

---

Table 13.6 **Pathological causes of amenorrhoea**

Hypothalamic
GnRH deficiency (isolated or as part of Kallmann's syndrome)*
Weight loss, physical exercise, stress
Post oral contraceptive therapy

Pituitary
Hyperprolactinaemia
Hypopituitarism

Gonadal
Polycystic ovary syndrome
Premature ovarian failure – autoimmune basis
Defective ovarian development (dysgenesis)*
Androgen-secreting ovarian tumours
Radiotherapy

Other diseases
Thyroid dysfunction
Cushing's syndrome
Adrenal tumours
Severe illness

Uterine/vaginal abnormality
Imperforate hymen or absent uterus*

---

*Presents as primary amenorrhoea

menorrhoea and amenorrhoea in clinical practice, though one should always consider pregnancy as a possible cause. Severe weight loss (e.g. anorexia nervosa) has long been associated with amenorrhoea, but it is now recognized that less severe forms of weight loss, produced by dieting and exercise, are a common cause of amenorrhoea caused by abnormal secretion of GnRH.

Investigations

The cause of amenorrhoea may be apparent after a full history and examination. Basal levels of serum FSH, LH, oestrogen and prolactin will allow a distinction between primary gonadal and hypothalamic–pituitary causes. Further investigations, e.g. ultrasonography of the ovaries, laparoscopy and ovarian biopsy, pituitary MRI and measurement of serum testosterone, will depend on the probable site of the defect and the findings on clinical examination.

Management

Treatment is of the cause where possible, e.g. increase weight, treat hypothyroidism and hyperprolactinaemia. In patients where the underlying defect cannot be corrected, cyclical oestrogens are given to reverse the symptoms of oestrogen deficiency and prevent early osteoporosis. Patients with isolated GnRH deficiency or hypopituitarism are treated with human FSH/LH. The management of polycystic ovaries is discussed on page 603.

Hirsutism and polycystic ovary syndrome (PCOS) (*K&C* 6e p. 1058)

Hirsutism is an excess growth of hair in a male pattern (androgen dependent): beard area, abdominal wall, thigh and around the nipples. There is, however, considerable variation in normal hair growth between individuals, families and races, being more extensive in the Mediterranean and some Asian Indian subcontinent populations.

Hirsutism is caused in almost all cases by increased androgen production by the ovaries or adrenal glands. The most common causes of hirsutism are idiopathic and PCOS. 'Idiopathic' hirsutism may well be a mild variant of PCOS. Only about 2% of patients with hirsutism will have an endocrine disorder other than PCOS. These include congenital adrenal hyperplasia, ovarian or adrenal tumour, prolactinoma and acromegaly. The presence of more severe virilization (clitoromegaly, recent-onset frontal balding, male phenotype) implies substantial androgen excess, and usually indicates a rarer cause rather than PCOS.

Hirsutism must be differentiated from *hypertrichosis* which refers to a general increase in body hair caused by drugs (ciclosporin, phenytoin, minoxidil), systemic illness (hypothyroidism, undernutrition) and as a paraneoplastic syndrome in some patients with cancer.

PCOS is one of the most common hormonal disorders affecting women. It is characterized by multiple small cysts within the ovary and by excess androgen production from the ovaries and, to a lesser extent, from the adrenals, although whether the basic defect is in the ovary, adrenal or pituitary remains unknown. The ovarian 'cysts' represent arrested follicular development. PCOS is associated with anovulation and insulin resistance, which may also be associated with hypertension and hyperlipidaemia. The precise mechanisms that link this syndrome remain to be elucidated, but may play a role in the causation of macrovascular disease in women.

Clinical features

Typically, PCOS presents with amenorrhoea/oligomenorrhoea, hirsutism and acne, usually beginning shortly after menarche. It is sometimes associated with marked obesity, but weight may be normal. Mild virilization occurs in severe cases. A short history, accompanying virilization, and severe menstrual disturbance are suggestive of significant androgen secretion with a more serious underlying cause, e.g. adrenal tumour.

Investigations

The diagnosis of PCOS is made on a clinical basis supported by:

- Serum testosterone concentrations are increased. However, values > 150 ng/dL suggest an ovarian or adrenal tumour
- Serum LH concentrations are increased or normal
- Serum FSH concentrations are normal
- Ovarian ultrasound shows a thickened capsule with multiple cysts.

Other investigations in a patient presenting with hirsutism include measurement of serum androgens and CT/MRI of the adrenal glands to exclude other causes of hirsutism. Serum prolactin may be slightly elevated in PCOS but higher values suggest pituitary or hypothalamic disease.

Management

The management is to identify and treat the underlying cause. Excess hair can be removed or disguised by shaving, bleaching and waxing. Other potentially useful treatments for hirsutism include:

- Cyproterone acetate (an *antiandrogen*)
- Oestrogens, which reduce free androgens by increasing levels of the sex hormone-binding globulin
- Spironolactone which has an antiandrogen activity
- Finasteride, a 5α-reductase inhibitor, inhibits dihydro-testosterone formation in skin.

Patients with PCOS who require induction of ovulation are treated with the anti-oestrogen, clomifene. For those not concerned with fertility, menstrual irregularity can be managed with oral contraceptives. Symptoms of hyper-androgenism can be managed by antiandrogens such as cyproterone acetate.

HYPERPROLACTINAEMIA (*K&C* 6e p. 1062)

Unlike other pituitary hormones, prolactin release is tonically inhibited by dopamine from the hypothalamus via the pituitary stalk (Fig. 13.1). There is a physiological increase in serum prolactin during pregnancy and postpartum breast-feeding.

603

Aetiology

The commonest cause of pathological hyperprolactinaemia is a prolactin-secreting pituitary adenoma (prolactinoma). Other pituitary or hypothalamic tumours may also cause hyperprolactinaemia by interfering with dopamine inhibition of prolactin release. Other causes include primary hypo-thyroidism (high TRH levels stimulate prolactin) and drugs, metoclopramide and phenothiazines (caused by inhibition of dopamine), oestrogens and cimetidine. Mildly increased serum prolactin levels (400–600 mU/L) may be physiological and asymptomatic but higher levels require a diagnosis. Levels above 5000 mU/L always imply a prolactin-secreting pituitary tumour.

Clinical features

Prolactinomas are rarely diagnosed in men. The cardinal feature is galactorrhoea. Other features such as oligo- or amenorrhoea, subfertility and erectile dysfunction occur as a result of inhibition of GnRH by high levels of prolactin. If there is a pituitary tumour there may be headache and visual field defects.

Investigations

- Serum prolactin level. At least three measurements should be taken. Further tests are appropriate after physiological and drug causes have been excluded.
- Thyroid function tests, as hypothyroidism is a cause of hyperprolactinaemia.
- MRI of the pituitary.
- Pituitary function should be checked if a pituitary tumour is suspected.
- Visual fields should be checked by clinical assessment and plotted formally by perimetry (p. 709) if a pituitary tumour is the cause.

Management

Causative drugs should be withdrawn if possible and hypothyroidism treated. Hyperprolactinaemia is controlled with a dopamine agonist such as cabergoline 500 µg once or twice a week judged on clinical response and prolactin levels. Bromocriptine has been longer established and is preferred if pregnancy is planned. Definitive therapy is controversial and depends on the size of the tumour, the patient's wish for fertility and the facilities available. Surgical removal of the tumour via a trans-sphenoidal approach, combined with postoperative radiotherapy for large tumours, often restores normoprolactinaemia but there is a high late recurrence rate (50% at 5 years). Small tumours (microadenomas) in asymptomatic patients may only need observation.

THE GROWTH AXIS (K&C 6e p. 1065)

Growth hormone (GH) is secreted from the anterior pituitary in a pulsatile fashion under the regulation of two hypothalamic peptides: GH releasing hormone (GHRH) stimulates growth hormone synthesis and secretion, and somatostatin inhibits GH release. GH exerts its activity indirectly through the induction of insulin-like growth factor (IGF-1) synthesized in the liver and other tissues, or directly on tissues such as liver, muscle, bone or fat to induce metabolic changes. Deficiency of GH produces short stature in children but in adults it is often clinically silent, although it may result in significant impairment in well-being and work capacity. Excessive GH production leads to gigantism in children (if acquired before fusion of the epiphyses of the long bones) and acromegaly in adults.

Acromegaly

Acromegaly is rare and caused by a benign pituitary GH-producing adenoma in almost all cases. Males and females are affected equally and the incidence is highest in middle age.

Clinical features

Symptoms and signs are shown in Figure 13.4. The clinical manifestations of acromegaly can be divided into those due to local tumour expansion with compression of surrounding structures –headaches, visual field loss and hypopituitarism – and those due to the metabolic effects of excess GH and IGF-1 secretion. Old photographs of the patient may be useful to demonstrate a change in appearance and physical features. The onset is insidious with many years between onset of symptoms and diagnosis. Inadequately treated acromegaly is associated with an increased mortality rate, particularly from cardiovascular disease and cancer.

Investigations

- Plasma GH levels may exclude acromegaly if undetectable but a detectable value is non-diagnostic.
- Serum IGF-1 levels are almost always raised in acromegaly, and fluctuate less than those of GH. A normal serum IGF-1 concentration is strong evidence that the patient does not have acromegaly.

Symptoms		Signs
Change in appearance	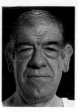	Prominent supraorbital ridge
Increased size of hands/feet		**Prognathism**
Headaches		**Interdental separation**
Excessive sweating		**Large tongue**
Visual deterioration		Hirsutism
Tiredness		Thick greasy skin
Weight gain		**Spade-like hands and feet**
Amenorrhoea oligomenorrhoea in women		**Tight rings**
Galactorrhoea		Carpal tunnel syndrome
Impotence or poor libido		Visual field defects
Deep voice		Galactorrhoea
Goitre		Hypertension
Breathlessness		Oedema
Pain/tingling in hands		Heart failure
Polyuria/polydipsia		Arthropathy
Muscular weakness		Proximal myopathy
Joint pains		Glycosuria (plus possible signs of hypopituitarism)
Old photographs are frequently useful Symptoms of hypopituitarism may also be present		

Fig. 13.4 **The symptoms and signs of acromegaly.** Bold type indicates signs of greater discriminant value.

- Glucose tolerance test is diagnostic. If the serum IGF-1 concentration is high or equivocal, serum GH should be measured 2 hours after an oral glucose load. In a positive test there is failure of the normal suppression of serum GH below 1 mU/L. Some show a paradoxical rise. Twenty-five per cent of individuals with acromegaly have a diabetic glucose tolerance test.
- MRI scan of the pituitary will almost always reveal the adenoma.
- Visual field defects are common and should be plotted by perimetry.
- Pituitary function testing usually shows evidence of hypopituitarism.
- Hyperprolactinaemia occurs in 30%.

Management

Treatment is indicated in all except elderly people or those with minimal abnormalities, because untreated acromegaly is associated with markedly reduced survival. Most deaths result from heart failure, coronary artery disease and hypertension-related causes. The aim of therapy is to reduce the serum IGF-1 concentration to within the age-adjusted reference range and to lower the mean GH level to below 5 mU/L; this has been shown to reduce mortality to normal levels. The preferred treatment is controversial, and complete cure, if possible, is often slow. The choice lies among the following:

Surgery This is the treatment of choice in suitable cases and is usually trans-sphenoidal (via an incision in the nose that is extended through the sphenoid sinus to the floor of the pituitary fossa). Transfrontal surgery is rarely required except for massive macroadenomas. Surgery is often combined with radiotherapy because excision is rarely complete with large tumours (macroadenomas, i.e. > 1 cm in diameter).

External beam radiotherapy is normally used after pituitary surgery fails to normalize GH levels, rather than as primary therapy. It may take 1–10 years to be effective when used alone.

Drugs Octreotide and the long-acting preparation, lanreotide, are analogues of somatostatin (GH release inhibitory hormone) and are given by subcutaneous injection in resistant cases. They are given to shrink tumours before definitive treatment or to control symptoms. Bromocriptine is usually reserved for elderly and frail people. Pegvisomant, a GH-receptor antagonist, is reserved for treatment of patients in whom GH and IGF levels cannot be reduced to safe levels with somatostatin analogues alone.

THE THYROID AXIS (K&C 6e p. 1069)

The thyroid gland secretes predominantly thyroxine (T_4) and only a small amount of the biologically active hormone triiodothyronine (T_3). These hormones control the metabolic rate of many tissues. Most circulating T_3 is produced by peripheral conversion of T_4. Over 99% of T_4 and T_3 circulate bound to plasma proteins, mainly thyroxine-binding globulin

(TBG). The feedback pathway that controls the secretion of TSH is discussed on page 589. Thyroid function is assessed by measurement of:

- Serum TSH concentration
- Serum free T_4 (or T_3) concentration.

Free hormone concentrations are measured in preference to total hormone concentrations (i.e. bound and free) because free hormone is that which is available for uptake by cells and interaction with nuclear receptors. Drugs and illness can alter the concentrations of binding proteins or interaction of the binding hormones with T_4 and T_3. Thus free and total hormone concentrations may not be concordant. For instance, oestrogens (e.g. in pregnancy and in women taking the oral contraceptive pill) increase concentrations of TBG and hence total T_4 but the physiologically important free T_4 concentrations are normal.

Assessment of thyroid function tests (K&C 6e p. 1070)

Measurement of thyroid function is indicated in the following clinical settings:

- Patients with symptoms or signs suggestive of hypo- or hyperthyroidism (Table 13.7). Thyroid function should not be assessed in seriously ill patients unless thyroid disease is strongly suspected since changes in thyroid

Table 13.7 **Characteristics of thyroid function tests in thyroid disease**

	TSH (0.3–3.5 mU/L)	Free T_4 (10–25 pmol/L)	Free T_3 (1.2–3.1 nmol/L)
Hyperthyroid	Undetectable	Increased	Increased
T_3 toxicosis	Undetectable	Normal	Increased
Primary hypo-thyroidism	Increased	Decreased	Normal or low
Secondary hypo-thyroidism	Low or borderline	Low or borderline	Low or borderline
Subclinical hypo-thyroidism	Slightly increased (5–10 mU/L)	Normal	Normal

hormones, TSH and binding proteins occur in severe non-thyroidal illness (the 'sick euthyroid syndrome'). Most will be euthyroid on re-testing after recovery from the acute illness.

- Patients receiving thyroxine treatment for hypothyroidism or a goitre.
- Patients receiving treatment for hyperthyroidism.
- Yearly TSH to monitor for hypothyroidism in patients who have had treatment of thyroid conditions with radio-iodine or surgery.

Hypothyroidism (*K&C* 6e p. 1071)

Underactivity of the thyroid gland may be primary, from disease of the thyroid gland, or, much less commonly, secondary to hypothalamic–pituitary disease.

Aetiology

Hypothyroidism is common, affecting 0.1–2% of the population. It is much more common in women, and the incidence increases with age. The most common cause in iodine-replete areas of the world is chronic autoimmune (Hashimoto's) thyroiditis.

Chronic autoimmune (Hashimoto's) thyroiditis There is cell- and antibody-mediated destruction of thyroid tissue. The condition has two forms, goitrous and atrophic; they differ in the extent of lymphocytic infiltration, fibrosis and thyroid follicular cell regeneration. Almost all patients have serum antibodies to thyroglobulin, thyroid peroxidase enzyme (thyroid microsomal antibodies) and antibodies that block the binding of TSH to its receptor. It is associated with other autoimmune conditions, such as pernicious anaemia and Addison's disease.

Iatrogenic Thyroidectomy (for treatment of hyper-thyroidism or goitre), radioiodine treatment or external radiation therapy for head and neck cancer all cause hypo-thyroidism.

Drugs Lithium, amiodarone and interferon-α can cause hypothyroidism.

Iodine deficiency This still exists in some areas, particularly mountainous areas (Alps, Himalayas, South America). Goitre, occasionally massive, is common. Iodine

Symptoms	Signs
Tiredness/malaise	**Mental slowness**
Weight gain	Ataxia
Anorexia	Poverty of movement
Cold intolerance	Deafness
Poor memory	Psychosis/dementia
Change in appearance	(rare)
Depression	
Poor libido	'Peaches and
Goitre	cream' complexion
Puffy eyes	**Dry thin hair**
Dry, brittle	Loss of eyebrows
unmanageable hair	
Dry, coarse skin	Hypertension
Arthralgia	Hypothermia
Myalgia	Heart failure
Muscle	**Bradycardia**
weakness/Stiffness	Pericardial effusion
Constipation	
Menorrhagia or	Cold peripheries
oligomenorrhoea	Carpal tunnel syndrome
in women	Oedema
Psychosis	Periorbital oedema
Coma	Deep voice
Deafness	Goitre
	Dry skin
	Overweight/obesity
	Myotonia
	Muscular hypertrophy
	Proximal myopathy
	Slow-relaxing reflexes
	Anaemia

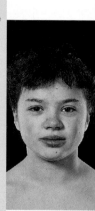

Fig. 13.5 **The symptoms and signs of hypothyroidism.** Bold type indicates signs of greater discriminant value.

excess can also cause hypothyroidism in patients with pre-existing thyroid disease.

Dyshormonogenesis This rare condition is caused by genetic defects in the synthesis of thyroid hormones.

Clinical features

Symptoms and signs of hypothyroidism are illustrated in Figure 13.5. The term myxoedema refers to the accumulation of mucopolysaccharide in subcutaneous tissues. Features are often difficult to distinguish in elderly people and young women. Hypothyroidism should be excluded in all patients with oligomenorrhoea/amenorrhoea, menorrhagia, infertility and hyperprolactinaemia. Many cases are detected on routine biochemical screening.

Investigations

Measurement of serum TSH is the investigation of choice. A high TSH with a compatible clinical picture confirms primary hypothyroidism.

- Serum free T_4 levels are low.
- Thyroid antibodies and other organ-specific antibodies may be present in the serum.
- Other features include anaemia (normocytic or macrocytic), hypercholesterolaemia and hyponatraemia (due to increased antidiuretic hormone and impaired clearance of free water).
- Creatine kinase levels may be increased with associated myopathy.

Management

Replacement therapy with thyroxine (100–200 µg/day) is required for life. The starting dose is 100 µg/day (50 µg/day in elderly people) and the adequacy of replacement is assessed clinically and by thyroid function tests after at least 6 weeks on a steady dose. The aim of treatment is normalization of serum TSH concentrations. In patients with ischaemic heart disease, starting doses should be even lower (25 µg/day) and increased at intervals of 3–4 weeks if ischaemic symptoms and a baseline ECG do not deteriorate.

611

Borderline hypothyroidism or 'compensated euthyroidism' (*K&C* 6e p. 1073)

Borderline hypothyroidism is defined as a normal serum free T_4 concentration and a slightly high serum TSH concentration (Table 13.7). The causes are the same as overt hypothyroidism and many patients will eventually develop overt hypothyroidism if followed up long enough; the risk is greatest in those with high titres of antithyroid antibodies. Treatment with thyroxine is normally recommended where the TSH is consistently above 10 mU/L, or when possible symptoms, high-titre thyroid antibodies or lipid abnormalities are present.

> **Emergency Box 13.1**
> **Management of myxoedema coma**
>
> **Investigations**
> - Serum TSH, T_4 and cortisol before thyroid hormone is given
> - Full blood count, serum urea and electrolytes, blood glucose and blood cultures
> - ECG monitoring for cardiac arrhythmias
>
> **Treatment**
> - Oxygen (by mechanical ventilation if necessary)
> - Gradual rewarming (Emergency Box 13.5)
> - Intravenous T_3 2.5–10 µg 8-hourly, depending on patient's age and coexistent cardiovascular disease
> - Intravenous hydrocortisone 100 mg 8-hourly (in case hypothyroidism is a manifestation of hypopituitarism)
> - Intravenous dextrose to prevent hypoglycaemia
> - Supportive management of the comatose patient (p. 724)
> - Change to oral maintenance thyroxine treatment after clinical improvement and patient stable

Myxoedema coma

Severe hypothyroidism may rarely present with confusion and coma, particularly in elderly people. Typical features include hypothermia (p. 644), cardiac failure, hypoventilation, hypoglycaemia and hyponatraemia. The optimal treatment is controversial and data are lacking, but a summary is given in Emergency Box 13.1. Treatment should be begun on the basis of clinical suspicion without waiting for the results of laboratory tests. Clues to the possible presence of myxoedema coma include a previous history of thyroid disease and a history from family members suggesting antecedent symptoms of thyroid dysfunction.

Myxoedema madness

Depression is common but occasionally, with severe hypothyroidism in elderly people, the patient may become frankly demented or psychotic, sometimes with striking delusions. This may occur shortly after starting thyroxine replacement.

Hyperthyroidism (*K&C* 6e p. 1073)

Hyperthyroidism (thyroid overactivity, thyrotoxicosis) is common, affecting 2–5% of all women at some time, mainly between the ages of 20 and 40 years. Three intrinsic thyroid disorders account for the vast majority of cases of hyper-thyroidism: Graves' disease, toxic adenoma and toxic multinodular goitre. Rarer causes include de Quervain's thyroiditis, thyroiditis factitia (surreptitious T_4 consumption), drugs (amiodarone), metastatic differentiated thyroid carcinoma and TSH-secreting tumours (e.g. of the pituitary).

Graves' disease Graves' disease is the most common cause of hyperthyroidism and is the result of IgG antibodies binding to the TSH receptor and stimulating thyroid hormone production. It is associated with characteristic clinical features (see below) and other autoimmune diseases, such as pernicious anaemia and myasthenia gravis.

Toxic multinodular goitre Many patients with toxic multinodular goitre have been euthyroid for several years before the development of nodular autonomy. Toxic multi-nodular goitre commonly occurs in older women, and drug therapy is rarely successful in inducing a prolonged remission.

Solitary toxic nodule (Plummer's disease) This is responsible for about 5% of cases. Prolonged remission is again rarely induced by drug therapy.

de Quervain's thyroiditis Transient hyperthyroidism sometimes results from acute inflammation of the gland, probably as a result of viral infection. It is usually accompanied by fever, malaise and pain in the neck. Treat-ment is with aspirin, reserving prednisolone for severely symptomatic cases.

Pregnancy Human chorionic gonadotrophin is a weak thyroid stimulator which may cause mild transient hyper-thyroidism during pregnancy.

Clinical features

Typical symptoms and signs of hyperthyroidism are shown in Figure 13.6.

Clinical features vary with age and the underlying aetiology. Ophthalmopathy (see below), pretibial myxo-edema (raised, purple-red symmetrical skin lesions over anterolateral aspects of the shins) and thyroid acropachy (clubbing, swollen fingers and periosteal new bone formation) occur only in Graves' disease. Elderly patients may present with atrial fibrillation and/or heart failure, or

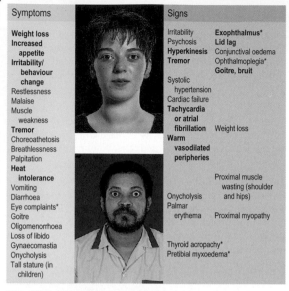

Symptoms		Signs	
Weight loss		Irritability	**Exophthalmus***
Increased		Psychosis	**Lid lag**
appetite		**Hyperkinesis**	Conjunctival oedema
Irritability/		**Tremor**	**Ophthalmoplegia***
behaviour			**Goitre, bruit**
change			
Restlessness		Systolic	
Malaise		hypertension	
Muscle		Cardiac failure	
weakness		**Tachycardia**	
Tremor		**or atrial**	
Choreoathetosis		**fibrillation**	Weight loss
Breathlessness		**Warm**	
Palpitation		**vasodilated**	
Heat		**peripheries**	
intolerance			Proximal muscle
Vomiting			wasting (shoulder
Diarrhoea		Onycholysis	and hips)
Eye complaints*		Palmar	
Goitre		erythema	Proximal myopathy
Oligomenorrhoea			
Loss of libido			
Gynaecomastia		Thyroid acropachy*	
Onycholysis		Pretibial myxoedema*	
Tall stature (in			
children)			

***Fig. 13.6** The symptoms and signs of hyperthyroidism.*
Bold type indicates signs of greater discriminatory value.
* indicates only in Graves' disease. Additional features are
hypercalcaemia and osteoporosis.

with a clinical picture resembling hypothyroidism ('apathetic
thyrotoxicosis').

Investigations

- Serum TSH is suppressed (< 0.05 mU/L).
- Serum free T_4 and T_3 are elevated. Occasionally T_3 alone
  is elevated (T_3 toxicosis).
- Serum microsomal and thyroglobulin antibodies are
  present in most cases of Graves' disease. TSH receptor
  antibodies are not measured routinely.
- Thyroid ultrasound will help differentiate Graves' disease
  from a toxic adenoma.

Management

Antithyroid drugs Carbimazole (10–20 mg 8-hourly)
blocks thyroid hormone biosynthesis and also has immuno-

suppressive effects which will affect the Graves' disease process. As clinical benefit may not be apparent for 10–20 days, β-blockers (usually propranolol) may be used to provide rapid symptomatic control because many manifestations are mediated via the sympathetic system. After 2–3 months at full dose, carbimazole is gradually reduced over the next 12–18 months to 5 mg daily. The aim of treatment during this time is to maintain normal free T_4 and TSH levels. Some physicians prefer the 'block and replace regimen', whereby full doses of carbimazole 30–45 mg/day are given for 18 months to suppress the thyroid completely, while replacing thyroid activity with thyroxine. Claimed advantages are avoidance of under- or overtreatment and better use of the immunosuppressive action. Fifty per cent of patients with Graves' disease will relapse on discontinuation of drug treatment, mostly within the following 2 years. The most severe side-effect of carbimazole is agranulocytosis. All patients starting treatment must be warned to stop carbimazole and seek an urgent blood count if they develop a sore throat or unexplained fever.

Radioactive iodine is widely used for the treatment of hyperthyroidism and in some countries is first-line treatment for Grave's disease. It is contraindicated in pregnancy and while breast-feeding. Radioiodine is administered orally as sodium ^{131}I. It accumulates in the gland and results in local irradiation and tissue damage with return to normal thyroid function over 4–12 weeks. If hyperthyroidism persists, a further dose of ^{131}I can be given, although this increases the rate of subsequent hypothyroidism.

Surgery Subtotal thyroidectomy should only be performed in patients who have been rendered euthyroid. Antithyroid drugs are stopped 10–14 days before the operation and replaced with oral potassium iodide, which inhibits thyroid hormone release and reduces the vascularity of the gland. Complications of surgery include bleeding, hypocalcaemia, hypothyroidism, hypoparathyroidism, recurrent laryngeal nerve palsy and recurrent hyperthyroidism.

The choice of therapy for hyperthyroidism depends on patient preference and local expertise. Radioiodine or surgical treatment is particularly indicated when there are persistent drug side-effects, poor compliance with drug therapy, or recurrent hyperthyroidism following drug treatment. Lifelong measurement of TSH is indicated after

The thyroid axis

> ⚠ *Emergency Box 13.2*
> **Management of thyroid crisis**
>
> **Investigations**
> - Full blood count, blood glucose, serum urea and electrolytes, thyroid function tests, blood cultures
> - Chest X-ray and ECG
>
> **Give antithyroid drugs**
> - Propranolol 5 mg i.v. 6-hourly or 80 mg orally 12-hourly (contraindicated in asthma or heart failure)
> - Carbimazole 20 mg 8-hourly by mouth or nasogastric tube
> - Potassium iodide by mouth or nasogastric tube 15 mg 6-hourly. Give at least 1 hour after carbimazole. Stop after 1 week if clinical improvement
> - Hydrocortisone 100 mg i.v. 6-hourly
>
> **Additional management**
> - Heart failure is usually associated with rapid atrial fibrillation. Treat with intravenous digoxin, diuretics and heparin
> - Supportive treatment, including oxygen, i.v. fluids and management of hyperpyrexia
> - Search for and treat precipitating cause

surgery or radioiodine treatment. Surgical treatment is particularly suited to patients with large goitres which are unlikely to remit after medical treatment.

Thyroid crisis (*K&C* 6e p. 1076)

Thyroid crisis or storm is a rare life-threatening condition in which there is a rapid deterioration of thyrotoxicosis with hyperpyrexia, tachycardia, extreme restlessness and eventually delirium, coma and death. It is most commonly precipitated by infection, stress, and surgery or radioactive iodine therapy in an unprepared patient. Management (Emergency Box 13.2) includes the administration of large doses of carbimazole and propranolol, iodine to block acutely the release of thyroid hormone from the gland, and corticosteroids which inhibit peripheral conversion of T_4 to T_3.

Thyroid eye disease (*K&C* 6e p. 1077)

Lid retraction (white of sclera visible above the cornea as the patient looks forwards) and lid lag are a result of increased catecholamine sensitivity of the levator palpebrae superioris and may occur in any form of hyperthyroidism. Exophthalmos (proptosis, protruding eyeballs) and ophthalmoplegia (limitation of eye movements) only occur in patients with Graves' disease (ophthalmic Graves' disease)

Aetiology

It is thought that an antigen in retro-orbital tissue with similar immunoreactivity to the TSH receptor leads to an autoimmune response causing retro-orbital inflammation, with swelling and oedema of the extraocular muscles leading to limitation of movement. In patients with Graves' disease the major clinical risk factor for developing thyroid eye disease is smoking.

Clinical features

The clinical appearances are characteristic and may be unilateral or bilateral. Exophthalmos and ophthalmoplegia are direct effects of retro-orbital inflammation, whereas conjunctival oedema (chemosis), lid lag and corneal scarring are secondary to the proptosis and lack of eye cover (Fig. 13.7). Eye manifestations do not parallel the clinical

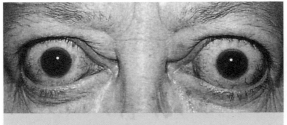

Grade 0	No signs or symptoms
Grade 1	Only signs, no symptoms
Grade 2	Soft tissue involvement
Grade 3	Proptosis (measured with exophthalmometer)
Grade 4	Extraocular muscle involvement
Grade 5	Corneal involvement
Grade 6	Sight loss with optic nerve involvement

Fig. 13.7 **The eye signs of Graves' disease.**

course of Graves' disease and may appear before the onset of hyperthyroidism.

Diagnosis

The diagnosis is usually made clinically by finding typical clinical features on a background of Graves' disease. MRI of the orbits will exclude other causes of proptosis, e.g. retro-orbital tumour, and show enlarged muscles and oedema.

Management

Thyroid status should be normalized and hypothyroidism avoided because this may exacerbate the eye problem. Smokers should be advised to stop. Specific treatment includes methylcellulose eyedrops or, if more severe, high-dose systemic steroids to reduce inflammation. Lateral tarsorrhaphy will protect the cornea if the lids cannot be closed. Occasionally irradiation of the orbits or surgical decompression of the orbit(s) is required.

Goitre (thyroid enlargement) (K&C 6e p. 1078)

Goitre is more common in women than in men and may be physiological or pathological in origin (Table 13.8). The

---

Table 13.8 Causes of goitre

Diffuse
Autoimmune: Graves' disease, Hashimoto's disease
Physiological:* puberty, pregnancy
Acute viral thyroiditis (de Quervain's thyroiditis)*
Iodine deficiency (endemic goitre)
Dyshormonogenesis
Goitrogens, e.g. sulphonylureas

Nodular
Multinodular goitre
Solitary nodule
Fibrotic (Riedel's thyroiditis)
Cysts
Tumours: adenoma, carcinoma, lymphoma
Sarcoidosis
Tuberculosis

---

*Goitre usually resolves spontaneously

presence of a goitre gives no indication about the thyroid status of the patient.

Clinical features

It is usually noticed as a cosmetic defect, although discomfort and pain in the neck can occur, and occasionally tracheal or oesophageal compression produces difficulty in breathing or dysphagia. The gland may be diffusely enlarged, multinodular or possess a solitary nodule. A bruit may be present and occasionally there is lymphadenopathy.

Investigations

- Thyroid function tests: TSH plus T_4 or T_3.
- Ultrasound can delineate nodules and differentiate simple cysts which have a low risk of being malignant, from solid nodules or from mixed solid and cystic nodules, which have a 5% chance of being malignant.
- Fine-needle aspiration for cytology should be performed for solitary nodules or a dominant nodule in a multi-nodular goitre because there is a 5% chance of malignancy.
- Chest and thoracic inlet X-rays where appropriate to detect tracheal compression.
- Other tests are not usually required. Thyroid scan (^{125}I or ^{131}I) distinguishes between a functioning ('hot') or non-functioning ('cold') nodule. Hot nodules are rarely malignant, whereas cold nodules are malignant in up to 10% of cases.

Management

Treatment is usually not required, apart from inducing euthyroidism if necessary. Surgical intervention may be required for cosmetic reasons, pressure effects, or if there is a persisting concern of malignancy.

619

Thyroid carcinoma (K&C 6e p. 1080)

Thyroid cancer is relatively uncommon, being responsible for 400 deaths annually in the UK. Characteristics are listed in Table 13.9. Most differentiated thyroid cancers present as asymptomatic thyroid nodules, but the first sign of disease is occasionally lymph-node metastases or, in rare cases, lung or bone metastases. Features that suggest carcinoma in a patient presenting with a thyroid nodule are a history of

Table 13.9 **Characteristics of thyroid cancer**

Cell type	Frequency (%)	Behaviour	Spread	Prognosis
Papillary	70	Young people, slow growing	Local	Good, most do not die of their disease
Follicular	20	More common in females	Lung/bone	Good if resected
Anaplastic	< 5	Aggressive	Local	Usually rapidly fatal
Lymphoma	2	Variable		Sometimes responds to radio-therapy
Medullary cell – arises from para-follicular (C) cells	5	May be familial and part of MEN syn-drome Secretes calcitonin	Local/meta-stases	Poor

MEN, multiple endocrine neoplasia

progressive increase in size, a hard and irregular nodule, and the presence of enlarged lymph nodes on examination. Fine-needle aspiration cytology is the best test for distinguishing between benign and malignant thyroid nodules. Treatment of follicular and papillary cancers is surgical, with total thyroidectomy. Ablative radioactive iodine is subsequently given which will be taken up by remaining thyroid tissue or metastatic lesions. Treatment of anaplastic carcinoma is largely palliative.

THE GLUCOCORTICOID AXIS (K&C 6e p. 1080)

The adrenal gland consists of an outer cortex producing steroids (cortisol, aldosterone and androgens) and an inner medulla secreting catecholamines. Aldosterone secretion is under the control of the renin–angiotensin system (see later). Corticotrophin-releasing hormone (CRH) from the hypothalamus stimulates ACTH (from the anterior pituitary), which stimulates cortisol production by the adrenal cortex. The cortisol secreted feeds back on the hypothalamus and pituitary to inhibit further CRH/ACTH release. CRH release, and hence cortisol release, is in response to a circadian rhythm (light–dark), stress and other factors. Random 'one-off' serum cortisol measurements may therefore be misleading in the diagnosis of hypoadrenalism or Cushing's syndrome. Cortisol has many effects, particularly on carbohydrate metabolism. It leads to increased protein catabolism, increased deposition of fat and glycogen, sodium retention, increased renal potassium loss and a diminished host response to infection.

Synthetic steroids are widely used in the treatment of a variety of inflammatory disorders and replacement therapy in adrenal insufficiency. They differ in their structure and potency (compared in *K&C* 6e p. 1081, and in the *National Formulary*) and include cortisone, prednisolone, prednisone, methyprednisolone and dexamethasone. Fludrocortisone is produced by modification of hydrocortisone. It has potent mineralocorticoid activity and is used to replace natural aldosterone in patients with primary adrenal insufficiency.

Addison's disease – primary hypoadrenalism (*K&C* 6e p. 1082)

This is an uncommon condition in which there is destruction of the entire adrenal cortex.

Aetiology

More than 90% of cases result from destruction of the entire adrenal cortex by organ-specific autoantibodies. This is associated with other autoimmune conditions, e.g. autoimmune thyroid disease, ovarian failure, pernicious anaemia and type 1 diabetes mellitus. Rarer causes are adrenal gland tuberculosis, surgical removal, haemorrhage (in meningococcal septicaemia), malignant infiltration and secondary adrenocortical failure as a result of pituitary disease (p. 593).

Clinical features

Adrenal insufficiency has an insidious presentation with lethargy, depression, anorexia and weight loss. It may also present as an emergency (Addisonian crisis), with vomiting, abdominal pain, profound weakness and hypovolaemic shock. The important signs are hypotension (which may only be postural) caused by salt and water loss, and hyperpigmentation (buccal mucosa, pressure points, skin creases and recent scars) resulting from stimulation of melanocytes by excess ACTH. There may be vitiligo and loss of body hair in women because of the dependence on adrenal androgens.

Investigations

- Serum urea and electrolytes may be normal but classically there is hyponatraemia, hyperkalaemia, a raised urea and hypoglycaemia.
- Serum calcium may be high.
- Blood count shows a neutrophil leucocytosis and eosinophilia.
- Adrenal antibodies are detected in most cases of autoimmune adrenalitis.
- X-rays of the chest and abdomen may show evidence of tuberculosis, with calcified adrenals.

The diagnosis is usually made using the short tetracosactide (synachen or synthetic ACTH) test (Table 13.10). Addisonian crisis is a life-threatening emergency that requires immediate treatment before full investigation (Emergency Box 13.3). Treatment should be begun on the basis of clinical suspicion without waiting for the results of laboratory tests.

Management

This is with lifelong steroid replacement taken as tablets.

- *Hydrocortisone.* The usual dose is 20 mg on waking and 10 mg in the evening, which mimics the normal diurnal rhythm. The dose is best monitored by measuring a series of cortisol levels throughout the day.
- *Fludrocortisone,* a synthetic mineralocorticoid, 50–300 µg daily. The dose is adequate when serum electrolytes are normal, there is no postural drop in blood pressure and plasma renin levels are suppressed to within the normal range.

Patients should wear a Medic Alert bracelet or necklace and carry the medical information card supplied with it. Both should indicate the diagnosis, daily medications and doses.

Table 13.10 Tetracosactide (synacthen tests)

Short test
1. Take blood for measurement of plasma cortisol and 9.00 a.m, ACTH
2. Administer tetracosactide 250 µg i.m./i.v.
3. Take blood for measurement of cortisol after 30 minutes
4. Interpretation: adrenal failure is excluded if the basal plasma cortisol exceeds 170 nmol/L and exceeds 600 nmol/L at 30 minutes. A subnormal response confirms adrenal insufficiency, and further tests (plasma ACTH and long synacthen test) are needed to establish its type and cause. A high plasma ACTH with low cortisol confirms primary hypoadrenalism

Long test
1. Take blood for measurement of plasma cortisol
2. Administer tetracosactide 1 mg i.m.
3. Take blood for cortisol at hourly intervals for 5 hours, then at 8 and 24 hours
4. Interpretation: patients with normal adrenal glands reach a plasma cortisol concentration of over 1000 nmol/L by 4 hours. In patients with Addison's disease the cortisol response is impaired throughout, and in secondary adrenal insufficiency a delayed but normal response is seen

They should also keep an (up-to-date) ampoule of hydrocortisone at home in case of major illness or if they are unable to take their oral medication due to vomiting. In a normal individual, stress of any type, e.g. infection, trauma and surgery, causes an immediate and marked increase in ACTH and hence in cortisol. This is a necessary response and therefore it is essential in patients on steroid replacement that the dose is increased when they are placed in any of these situations. The usual dose is 100 mg hydrocortisone intramuscularly for minor surgery and, for major surgery, 100 mg hydrocortisone 6-hourly until oral medication is resumed. The dose is doubled during minor illness.

Uses and problems of therapeutic steroid therapy (K&C 6e p. 1088)

In addition to their use as therapeutic replacement for deficiency states, steroids are widely used for a variety of non-endocrine conditions such as inflammatory bowel disease, asthma and rheumatological conditions. Long-term

> **Emergency Box 13.3**
> **Management of Addisonian crisis**
>
> **Investigations**
> - Take blood for plasma cortisol (will be inappropriately low) and ACTH (will be high because of loss of negative feedback) before administration of hydrocortisone
> - Full blood count, urea and electrolytes, blood glucose, serum calcium and blood cultures
>
> **Immediate**
> - Hydrocortisone 100 mg intravenously
> - 0.9% saline, 1 litre over 30–60 minutes
> - 50 mL of 50% dextrose if hypoglycaemic
> - Search for precipitating cause, e.g. infection, gastroenteritis
>
> **Subsequent**
> - Hydrocortisone 100 mg intramuscular 6-hourly until BP stable and vomiting ceased
> - 0.9% saline 2–4 litres intravenously in 12–24 hours; monitor by JVP or CVP
> - Expect recovery, with normal BP, blood glucose and serum sodium, within 12–24 hours
> - When stable, convert to oral maintenance treatment (see p. 622) continued lifelong

steroid use may be associated with significant side-effects (Table 13.11) and may also result in suppression of the adrenal axis if used continually for more than 3–4 weeks. All patients receiving steroids should carry a 'Steroid Card' and should be made aware of the following points:

■ Long-term steroid therapy must never be stopped suddenly.
■ Doses should be reduced very gradually.
■ Doses should be doubled in times of serious intercurrent illness.
■ Other physicians, anaesthetists and dentists must be told about steroid therapy.

Patients should also be informed of potential side-effects and all this information should be documented in the patient records. The clinical need for high-dose steroids should be continually and critically assessed. Steroid-sparing agents (e.g. azathioprine) should always be considered and screening and prophylactic therapy for osteoporosis introduced.

Table 13.11 Adverse effects of corticosteroids

Physiological
Adrenal and/or pituitary
suppression

Pathological

Cardiovascular
Increased blood pressure

Gastrointestinal
Peptic ulceration exacerbation
(possibly)
Acute pancreatitis

Renal
Polyuria
Nocturia

Central nervous
Depression
Euphoria
Psychosis
Insomnia

*Increased susceptibility to
infection*
(signs and fever are frequently
masked)
Septicaemia
Reactivation of tuberculosis
Skin (e.g. fungi)

Endocrine
Weight gain
Glycosuria, hyperglycaemia
(diabetes mellitus)
Impaired growth in children

Bone and muscle
Osteoporosis
Proximal myopathy and
wasting
Aseptic necrosis of the hip
Pathological fractures

Skin
Thinning
Easy bruising

Eyes
Cataracts (including with
inhaled drugs)

Secondary hypoadrenalism (*K&C* 6e p. 1085)

This may arise from hypothalamic–pituitary disease or
from long-term steroid therapy leading to hypothalamic–
pituitary–adrenal suppression. The clinical features are the
same as those of Addison's disease but there is no pigmentation because ACTH levels are low and, in pituitary
disease, there are usually features of failure of other
pituitary hormones. A long tetracosactide (synacthen) test
(see Table 13.10) will differentiate between primary and
secondary adrenal failure. Treatment is with hydrocortisone;
fludrocortisone is unnecessary. If adrenal failure is
secondary to long-term steroid therapy, the adrenals will
recover if steroids are withdrawn very slowly.

Table 13.12	Aetiology of Cushing's syndrome

ACTH-dependent causes
Pituitary disease (Cushing's disease)
Ectopic ACTH-producing tumours (small-cell lung cancer, carcinoid tumours)
ACTH administration

Non-ACTH-dependent causes
Adrenal adenomas
Adrenal carcinomas
Glucocorticoid administration
Alcohol-induced pseudo-Cushing's syndrome

Cushing's syndrome (*K&C* 6e p. 1085)

Cushing's syndrome is caused by persistently and inappropriately elevated glucocorticoid levels. Most cases result from administration of synthetic steroids or ACTH for the treatment of medical conditions, e.g. asthma. Spontaneous Cushing's syndrome is rare and two-thirds of cases result from excess ACTH secretion from the pituitary gland (Table 13.12). Cushing's disease must be distinguished from Cushing's syndrome. The latter is a general term which refers to the abnormalities resulting from a chronic excess of glucocorticoids whatever the cause, whereas Cushing's disease specifically refers to excess glucocorticoids resulting from inappropriate ACTH secretion from the pituitary (usually a microadenoma, less often corticotroph hyperplasia). Alcohol excess mimics Cushing's syndrome clinically and biochemically (pseudo-Cushing's syndrome). The pathogenesis is incompletely understood but the features resolve when alcohol is stopped.

Clinical features

Patients are obese: fat distribution is typically central, affecting the trunk, abdomen and neck (buffalo hump). They have a plethoric complexion with a moon face. Many of the features are the result of the protein-catabolic effects of cortisol: the skin is thin and bruises easily, and there are purple striae on the abdomen, breasts and thighs (Fig. 13.8). Pigmentation occurs with ACTH-dependent cases. Patients with ectopic production of ACTH tend to have rapidly

Symptoms	Signs	
Weight gain (central)	Depression/ psychosis	Frontal balding (female)
Change of appearance	Acne, hirsuties	
Depression	**Thin skin**	Moon face
Psychosis	**Bruising**	**Plethora**
Insomnia	**Hypertension**	'Buffalo hump'
Amenorrhoea/ oligomenorrhoea		Kyphosis
Poor libido	Rib fractures	Centripetal obesity
Thin skin/ easy bruising	Osteoporosis	Pigmentation
Hair growth/acne	**Pathological fractures**	**Striae (purple)**
Muscular weakness		Skin infections
Growth arrest in children	Poor wound healing	
Back pain		Glycosuria
Polyuria/polydipsia		
Old photographs may be useful	Proximal muscle wasting	
Symptoms of hypopituitarism are rare	**Proximal myopathy**	
	Oedema	

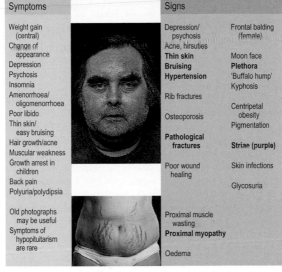

Fig. 13.8 **The symptoms and signs of Cushing's syndrome.**
Bold type indicates signs of most value in discriminating
Cushing's syndrome from simple obesity and hirsutes.

progressive symptoms and signs, and may have evidence
of the primary tumour.

Investigations

In a patient with suspected spontaneous Cushing's syndrome
the purpose of investigation is firstly to confirm the
presence of cortisol excess, and secondly to determine
the cause.

Confirm raised cortisol

- The *48-hour low-dose dexamethasone suppression test* is the
  most reliable screening test. Dexamethasone 0.5 mg
  6-hourly is given orally for 48 hours. Normal individuals
  suppress plasma cortisol to < 50 nmol/L 2 hours after the
  last dose of dexamethasone.
- 24-hour *urinary free cortisol* is raised (normal < 700 nmol/
  24 h) in most cases.

- *Circadian rhythm studies* show loss of the normal circadian fall of plasma cortisol at 24 hours in patients with Cushing's syndrome.

Establishing the cause of Cushing's syndrome

- Adrenal CT or MRI will detect adrenal adenomas and carcinomas, as those which produce Cushing's syndrome are usually large.
- Pituitary MRI and CT will detect some, but not all, pituitary adenomas.
- *Plasma ACTH levels* are low or undetectable in adrenal gland disease (non-ACTH dependent) and should lead to adrenal imaging. High or inappropriately normal values suggest pituitary disease or ectopic production of ACTH.
- *High-dose dexamethasone suppression test*. Dexamethasone 2.0 mg 6-hourly is given orally for 48 hours. Most patients with pituitary-dependent Cushing's disease suppress plasma cortisol by 48 hours. Failure of suppression suggests an ectopic source of ACTH or an adrenal tumour.
- *Corticotrophin-releasing hormone test*. An exaggerated plasma ACTH response to exogenous CRH (bolus given intravenously) suggests pituitary-dependent Cushing's disease.
- *Other tests* will depend on the probable cause of Cushing's syndrome, which has been established from the above tests. Chest X-ray, bronchoscopy and CT of the body may localize ectopic ACTH-producing tumours. Selective venous sampling for ACTH will localize pituitary tumours and an otherwise occult ectopic ACTH-producing tumour.
- *Radiolabelled octreotide* (^{111}In octreotide) is occasionally helpful in locating ectopic ACTH sites.

Management

Surgical removal is indicated for most pituitary (usually a trans-sphenoidal approach) and adrenal tumours and may be appropriate for many cases of ectopic ACTH-producing tumours.

Drugs which inhibit cortisol synthesis (metyrapone, ketoconazole or aminoglutethimide) may be useful in cases not amenable to surgery.

External-beam irradiation of the pituitary produces a very slow response and is restricted to cases where surgery is unsuccessful, contraindicated or unacceptable to the patient.

Iatrogenic Cushing's syndrome responds to a reduction in steroid dosage when possible. Immunosuppressant drugs such as azathioprine may be used in conjunction with steroids to enable lower doses to be used to control the underlying disease.

Incidental adrenal tumours

With the advent of improved abdominal imaging, unsuspected adrenal masses have been discovered in about 1% of scans. These include primary tumours, metastases and cysts. Functional tests to exclude secretory activity (subclinical Cushing's syndrome and phaeochromocytoma) should be performed if a tumour is found. Most authorities recommend surgical removal of large (> 4–5 cm) and functional tumours but observation of smaller hormonally inactive lesions.

THE THIRST AXIS (*K&C* 6e p. 1089)

The secretion of antidiuretic hormone (ADH, vasopressin) from the posterior pituitary gland is determined principally by the plasma osmolality. The major hormonal action is on the collecting tubule of the kidney to cause water reabsorption. At high concentrations vasopressin also causes vasoconstriction. ADH secretion is suppressed at plasma osmolality below 280 mmol/kg, thus allowing maximal water diuresis. Secretion increases to a maximum at a plasma osmolality of 295 mmol/kg. Large falls in blood pressure or volume also stimulate vasopressin secretion.

Syndrome of inappropriate ADH secretion (SIADH) (*K&C* 6e p. 1091)

There is continued ADH secretion in spite of plasma hypotonicity and a normal or expanded plasma volume.

Aetiology

SIADH is caused by disordered hypothalamic–pituitary secretion or ectopic production of ADH, e.g. small-cell lung cancer (Table 13.13).

Clinical features

There is nausea, irritability and headache with mild dilutional hyponatraemia (serum sodium 115–125 mmol/L).

Table 13.13	Causes of syndrome of inappropriate ADH
Cancer	Many tumours, of which the most common is small-cell cancer of the lung
Brain	Meningitis, cerebral abscess, head injury, tumour
Lung	Pneumonia, tuberculosis, lung abscess
Metabolic	Porphyria, alcohol withdrawal
Drugs	Opiates, chlorpropamide, carbamazepine, vincristine

Fits and coma may occur with severe hyponatraemia (< 115 mmol/L).

Investigations

SIADH must be differentiated from other causes of dilutional hyponatraemia (p. 317). The criteria for diagnosis are:

- Low serum sodium (< 125 mmol/L)
- Low plasma osmolality
- Urine osmolality 'inappropriately' higher than plasma osmolality
- Continued urinary sodium excretion (> 30 mmol/L)
- Absence of hypokalaemia, hypotension and hypovolaemia
- Normal renal, adrenal and thyroid function.

Management

Mild asymptomatic cases need no treatment other than that of the underlying cause. For symptomatic cases the options are:

- Water restriction: 500–1000 mL in 24 hours
- Dimethylchlorotetracycline (demeclocycline) inhibits the action of vasopressin on the kidney and may be useful if water restriction is poorly tolerated or ineffective
- Hypertonic saline, with furosemide (frusemide) to prevent circulatory overload, may be necessary in severe cases (Emergency Box 7.1, p. 320).

Diabetes insipidus (K&C 6e p. 1090)

Impaired vasopressin secretion (cranial diabetes insipidus, CDI) or renal resistance to its action (nephrogenic diabetes

Table 13.14 Causes of diabetes insipidus	
Cranial diabetes insipidus	**Nephrogenic diabetes insipidus**
Hypothalamic–pituitary surgery*	Metabolic
	Hypokalaemia*
Head injury*	Hypercalcaemia
Idiopathic*	Drugs*
Hypothalamic–pituitary tumours	Lithium chloride
	Dimethylchlorotetracycline
Granulomas: sarcoidosis, histiocytosis	Glibenclamide
	Renal tubular acidosis
Infections: meningitis, encephalitis	Sickle cell disease
	Prolonged polyuria of any cause
Vascular: haemorrhage, thrombosis	Familial (mutation in ADH receptor)
Familial	

*Indicates the most common causes. Diabetes insipidus after surgery may only be transient

insipidus, NDI) leads to polyuria (dilute urine in excess of 3 L/24 h), nocturia and compensatory polydipsia. It must be distinguished from primary polydipsia, which is a psychiatric disturbance characterized by excessive intake of water, and other causes of polyuria and polydipsia, e.g. hyperglycaemia.

Aetiology

The causes are listed in Table 13.14.

Clinical features

631

There is polyuria (as much as 15 L in 24 h) and polydipsia. Patients depend on a normal thirst mechanism and access to water to maintain normonatraemia.

Investigations

- Urine volume must be measured to confirm polyuria.
- Plasma biochemistry shows high or high-normal sodium concentration and osmolality. Blood glucose, serum potassium and calcium should be measured to exclude common causes of polyuria.
- Urine osmolality is inappropriately low for the high plasma osmolality.

Table 13.15 **Response to fluid deprivation and desmopressin in polyuric patients**

Urine osmolality (mmol/kg)		Diagnosis
After 8 h fluid deprivation	After desmopressin	
< 300	> 800	CDI
< 300	< 300	NDI
> 800	> 800	Primary polydipsia

- A water deprivation test with exogenous desmopressin (a synthetic vasopressin analogue) is the usual investigation for polyuric patients with normal blood glucose and serum electrolytes. It confirms the diagnosis of DI and will usually distinguish between CDI, NDI and primary polydipsia (Table 13.15). Water is restricted for 8 hours, during which time blood and urine osmolality are measured hourly. Patients are weighed hourly and the test stopped if bodyweight drops by 5%, as this indicates significant dehydration. In equivocal cases the measurement of plasma vasopressin during water deprivation provides a definitive diagnosis, but this test is not routinely available.
- MRI of the pituitary and hypothalamus is performed in cases of CDI.

Management

Treatment of the underlying condition seldom improves established CDI. In mild cases (3–4 L urine per day) no specific treatment is necessary. Desmopressin, administered orally, nasally or intramuscularly, is useful for more severe cases. Treatment of the cause will usually improve NDI.

CALCIUM, PHOSPHATE AND THE PARATHYROIDS (*K&C* 6e p. 1091)

The control of calcium and bone metabolism is discussed on page 298. Total plasma calcium is normally 2.2–2.6 mmol/L. Usually only 40% of total plasma calcium is ionized and physiologically relevant; the remainder is bound to albumin and thus unavailable to the tissues. Routine analytical methods measure total plasma calcium and this must be corrected for the serum albumin concentration: add or subtract 0.02 mmol/L for every g/L by which the simultaneous albumin lies below or above 40 g/L. For critical measurements, samples should be taken in the fasting state without the use of an occluding cuff, which may increase the local plasma protein concentration.

Hypercalcaemia (K&C 6e p. 1092)

Mild asymptomatic hypercalcaemia occurs in about 1 in 1000 of the population, especially elderly women, and is usually the result of primary hyperparathyroidism.

Aetiology

Primary hyperparathyroidism and malignancy account for > 90% of cases (Table 13.16). Tumour-related hypercalcaemia is caused by the secretion of a peptide with PTH-like activity, or by direct invasion of bone and production of local factors that mobilize calcium. Ectopic PTH secretion by tumours is very rare.

Hyperparathyroidism may be primary, secondary or tertiary.

Primary hyperparathyroidism affects about 0.1% of the population and is usually caused by a single parathyroid gland adenoma, occasionally hyperplasia, and rarely carcinoma.

Secondary hyperparathyroidism is a physiological response to hypocalcaemia (e.g. in renal failure or vitamin D deficiency). Calcium is low or low-normal.

Tertiary hyperparathyroidism is the development of apparently autonomous parathyroid hyperplasia after long-standing secondary hyperparathyroidism, most often in renal disease. Plasma calcium and PTH are both raised. Treatment is parathyroidectomy.

Clinical features

Mild hypercalcaemia (corrected serum calcium < 3 mmol/L) is often asymptomatic and discovered on biochemical screening. More severe hypercalcaemia produces symptoms such as general malaise and depression, bone pain, abdominal pain, nausea and constipation. Calcium deposition in the renal tubules causes polyuria and nocturia. Renal

Calcium, phosphate and the parathyroids

Table 13.16 Causes of hypercalcaemia

Excess PTH
Primary hyperparathyroidism (commonest cause)*
Tertiary hyperparathyroidism
Ectopic PTH (very rare)

Malignant disease*†

Multiple myeloma	Prostate
Breast cancer	Renal cell
Bronchus	Lymphoma
Thyroid	

Excess action of vitamin D
Self-administered vitamin D†
Sarcoidosis

Excess calcium intake
'Milk–alkali' syndrome

Other endocrine disease
Thyrotoxicosis
Addison's disease

Drugs
Thiazides
Lithium
Vitamin A and retinoic acid

Miscellaneous
Long-term immobility
Familial hypocalciuric hypercalcaemia (rare)

*Indicates commonest causes of hypercalcaemia
†Conditions causing severe hypercalcaemia (> 3.5 mmol/L)

calculi and renal failure may develop. With very high levels (> 3.8 mmol/L) there is dehydration, confusion, clouding of consciousness and a risk of cardiac arrest. Hypercalcaemia is rarely the presenting feature of malignancy and it is rare for the malignancy not to be clinically apparent when the hypercalcaemia is first noted. Thus, hypercalcaemia in an otherwise well outpatient is most likely to be due to primary hyperparathyroidism.

Investigations

- Several fasting serum calcium and phosphate samples should be performed. The serum phosphate is low in primary hyperparathyroidism and some cases of malignancy. It is normal or high in other causes of hypercalcaemia.
- Serum PTH levels. Detectable or elevated levels during hypercalcaemia are inappropriate and imply hyperparathyroidism. When this combination is present in an asymptomatic patient then further investigation is usually unnecessary.
- Radiology. Subperiosteal erosions in the phalanges are seen in hyperparathyroidism.
- If PTH is undetectable or equivocal the following tests should be considered:
  - Protein electrophoresis for myeloma
  - TSH to exclude hyperthyroidism
  - Synacthen test to exclude Addison's disease
  - Hydrocortisone suppression test: hydrocortisone 40 mg orally three times daily for 10 days leads to suppression of plasma calcium in sarcoidosis, vitamin D-mediated hypercalcaemia and some malignancies.

Management

This involves lowering of the calcium levels to near normal and treatment of the underlying cause. Severe hypercalcaemia (> 3.5 mmol/L) is a medical emergency which must be treated aggressively whatever the underlying cause (Emergency Box 13.4). Treatment is based on the corrected calcium value.

Treatment of primary hyperparathyroidism

The treatment of a symptomatic parathyroid adenoma is surgical removal. Conservative therapy may be indicated in asymptomatic patients with mildly raised serum calcium levels (2.65–3 mmol/L). In those with parathyroid hyperplasia all four glands are removed.

> **Emergency Box 13.4**
> **Management of severe hypercalcaemia**

- **Rehydrate with intravenous fluid (0.9% saline)**
  4–6 litres of intravenous saline over 24 h and then
  3–4 litres for several days thereafter
  Amount and rate depend on clinical assessment and
    measurement of serum urea and electrolytes

- **After minimum of 2 litres of intravenous fluids give bisphosphonate infusion**
  Pamidronate disodium 15–60 mg as an intravenous infusion
    in 0.5 litre 0.9% saline over 2–8 h

- **Measure**
  Serum urea and electrolytes at least daily
  Do not measure serum calcium for a least 48 h after
    initiation of treatment, normalization may take 3–5 days

- **Prednisolone (30–60 mg daily)**
  May be useful in some cases (myeloma, sarcoidosis and
    vitamin D excess) but in most cases ineffective

- **Prevent recurrence**
  Treat underlying cause if possible
  With untreatable malignancy consider maintenance
    treatment with bisphosphonates

Hypocalcaemia and hypoparathyroidism (*K&C* 6e p. 1094)

Aetiology

The causes of hypocalcaemia are listed in Table 13.17. Renal failure is the most common cause of hypocalcaemia, which results from the inadequate production of active vitamin D and renal phosphate retention, leading to microprecipitation of calcium phosphate in the tissues. Mild transient hypocalcaemia often occurs after parathyroidectomy, and a few patients develop long-standing hypoparathyroidism.

Clinical features

Hypocalcaemia causes increased excitability of nerves. There is numbness around the mouth and in the extremities, followed by cramps, tetany (carpopedal spasm: opposition of the thumb, extension of the interphalangeal and flexion of the metacarpophalangeal joints), convulsions and death if untreated. Two important physical signs are Chvostek's

Table 13.17 Causes of hypocalcaemia

Increased serum phosphate levels
Chronic renal failure*
Phosphate therapy

Hypoparathyroidism
Post-thyroidectomy and parathyroidectomy (usually transient)*
Congenital deficiency (DiGeorge syndrome)
Idiopathic hypoparathyroidism (autoimmune)
Severe hypomagnesaemia (inhibits PTH release)

Vitamin D deficiency
Osteomalacia
Resistance

End-organ resistance to PTH
Pseudohypoparathyroidism

Drugs
Calcitonin
Bisphosphonates

Miscellaneous
Acute pancreatitis*
Citrated blood in massive transfusion

*Indicates common cause of hypocalcaemia

sign (tapping over the facial nerve in the region of the parotid gland causes twitching of the facial muscles) and Trousseau's sign (carpopedal spasm induced by inflation of the sphygmomanometer cuff to a level above systolic blood pressure). With prolonged hypocalcaemia there may be cataract formation and rarely papilloedema.

Tetany may also develop in the presence of alkalosis, and potassium and magnesium deficiency as well as in hypocalcaemia. Hyperventilation alters the protein binding of calcium such that the ionized fraction is decreased, and may therefore cause hypocalcaemic tetany even with a normal plasma total calcium.

Investigations

The clinical picture is usually diagnostic and is confirmed by a low corrected serum calcium. Additional tests identify the cause:

- Serum urea and creatinine for renal disease
- Serum PTH levels, which are absent or low in hypoparathyroidism and elevated in other causes of hypocalcaemia
- Serum parathyroid antibodies – present in autoimmune disease
- Serum 25-hydroxyvitamin D level
- Serum magnesium.

Management

Acute (e.g. with tetany): 10 mL of 10% calcium gluconate (2.25 mmol) intravenously and repeated as necessary as an infusion over 4 hours. Infusion is over 10 minutes if there is tetany.

Maintenance therapy is with alfacalcidol (1α-OH-D$_3$).

Hypophosphataemia

Hypophosphataemia is common and often unrecognized. There are three major mechanisms by which hypophosphataemia can occur (Table 13.18). Phosphate molecules are critical to many biochemical processes, and deficiency can lead to widespread cell dysfunction (skeletal and respiratory muscle weakness, cardiac arrhythmias, confusion, haemolysis) and death. Oral treatment is preferred (e.g. Phosphate-Sandoz one tablet 4-hourly). Severe deficiency (< 0.4 mmol/L) is treated with intravenous phosphate

Table 13.18 **Causes of hypophosphataemia**

Redistribution of phosphate from extracellular fluid into cell
Treatment of diabetic ketoacidosis
Refeeding syndrome
Acute respiratory alkalosis
Hungry bone syndrome after parathyroidectomy

Decreased intestinal absorption
Poor oral intake
Some antacids
Diarrhoea

Increased urine excretion
Hyperparathyroidism
Vitamin D deficiency
Primary renal abnormality

Table 13.19	Endocrine causes of hypertension
Excessive production of	
Renin	Renal artery stenosis, renin-secreting tumours
Aldosterone	Adrenal adenoma, adrenal hyperplasia
Mineralocorticoids	Cushing's syndrome (cortisol is a weak mineralocorticoid)
Catecholamines	Phaeochromocytoma
Growth hormone	Acromegaly
Oral contraceptive pill (mechanism unclear)	

(9–18 mmol/24 h). Plasma concentrations of calcium, phosphate, magnesium and potassium should be monitored during treatment.

ENDOCRINOLOGY OF BLOOD PRESSURE CONTROL (*K&C* 6e p. 1095)

Blood pressure is determined by cardiac output and peripheral resistance, and thus an increase in blood pressure may be due to an increase in one or both of these. In approximately 90% of cases no cause can be found (p. 476) and patients are said to have essential hypertension. In the remaining minority an underlying cause can be identified, and these include endocrine causes (Table 13.19). Young patients (< 35 years), those with an abnormal baseline screening test (p. 478) or patients with hypertension resistant to treatment should be screened for secondary causes.

The renin–angiotensin system

The renin–angiotensin–aldosterone system is illustrated in Figure 13.9. *Angiotensin*, an α_2-globulin of hepatic origin, circulates in plasma. The enzyme *renin* is secreted by the kidney in response to decreased renal perfusion pressure or flow; it cleaves the decapeptide *angiotensin I* from angiotensinogen. Angiotensin I is inactive but is further cleaved by converting enzyme (present in lung and vascular endothelium) into the active peptide, *angiotensin II*, which has two major actions:

- It causes powerful vasoconstriction (within seconds)
- It stimulates the adrenal zona glomerulosa to increase aldosterone production.

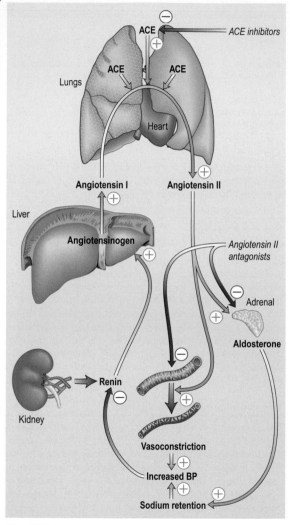

Fig. 13.9 **The renin–angiotensin–aldosterone system.** ACE, angiotensin-converting enzyme. Angiotensin II antagonists act on the adrenals and blood vessels.

Aldosterone causes sodium retention and urinary potassium loss (hours to days). This combination of changes leads to an increase in blood pressure, and the stimulus to renin production is reduced. Sodium deprivation or urinary loss also increases renin production, whereas dietary sodium excess will suppress production.

Primary hyperaldosteronism (K&C 6e p. 1097)

This is a rare condition (<1% of all hypertension) where high aldosterone levels exist independently of the renin–angiotensin system. It is caused by an adrenal adenoma secreting aldosterone (Conn's syndrome, 60% of cases) or by bilateral adrenal hyperplasia.

Clinical features

The major function of aldosterone is to cause an exchange transport of sodium and potassium in the distal renal tubule; that is, absorption of sodium (and hence water) and excretion of potassium. Therefore, hyperaldosteronism causes hypertension, resulting from expansion of intravascular volume, and hypokalaemia, which is rarely low enough to produce symptoms.

Investigations

- Urea and electrolytes show a low serum potassium and normal or high sodium.
- The diagnosis is made by demonstrating increased plasma aldosterone levels that are not suppressed with saline infusion (300 mmol over 4 h) or fludrocortisone (a mineralocorticoid), associated with suppressed plasma renin levels.
- Antihypertensives, except bethanidine and prazosin, interfere with renin activity and should be stopped before these investigations.
- CT or MRI of the adrenals is used to differentiate adenomas from hyperplasia.

Management

An adenoma is removed surgically. Hypertension resulting from hyperplasia is treated with the aldosterone antagonist spironolactone.

Phaeochromocytoma (K&C 6e p. 1098)

This is a rare (0.1% of hypertension) catecholamine-producing tumour of the sympathetic nervous system; 10% are malignant and 10% occur outside the adrenal gland. Some are associated with multiple endocrine neoplasia (see below).

Clinical features

Symptoms may be episodic and include headache, palpitations, sweating, anxiety, nausea and weight loss. The signs, which may also be intermittent, include hypertension, tachycardia and pallor. There may be hyperglycaemia.

Investigations

- A 24-hour urine collection for urinary metanephrines (degradation products of epinephrine (adrenaline)) is a useful screening test; normal levels on three separate collections virtually exclude the diagnosis.
- Raised levels of plasma catecholamines confirm the diagnosis.
- Plasma chromogranin A (a storage vesicle protein) is raised.
- CT/MRI is useful to localize the tumour.
- Scintigraphy using meta-[^{131}I]iodobenzylguanidine (mIBG), which is selectively taken up by adrenergic cells, is useful with extra-adrenal tumours.

Management

The treatment of choice is surgical excision of the tumour under α- and β-blockade using phenoxybenzamine and propranolol, which is started before the operation. These drugs can also be used long term where operation is not possible.

Multiple endocrine neoplasia (K&C 6e p. 1099)

The multiple endocrine neoplasia syndromes (MEN) are rare, but recognition is important both for treatment and for evaluation of family members. MEN is the name given to the synchronous or metachronous (i.e. occurring at different times) occurrence of tumours involving a number of endocrine glands (Table 13.20). MEN is subdivided into

Table 13.20 Multiple endocrine neoplasia (MEN) syndrome

Organ	Frequency	Tumours/clinical manifestations
Type 1		
Functioning adenomas in:		
Parathyroid	95%	Hypercalcaemia
Pituitary	30%	Prolactinoma, acromegaly, Cushing's disease
Enteropancreatic tumours	60%	Gastrinoma, insulinoma, glucagonoma, VIPoma
Other:		
Foregut carcinoids	10%	Thymic, bronchial gastric
Adrenal cortex adenomas	25%	Non-functional tumours
Cutaneous tumours	60%	Angiofibromas, collagenomas, lipomas
Type 2A		
Medullary thyroid carcinoma	95%	Thyroid mass, diarrhoea, raised plasma calcitonin
Adrenal medulla	40%	Phaeochromocytoma
Parathyroid hyperplasia	10%	Hypercalcaemia
Type 2B		
Like type 2A (but not parathyroid disease) with a typical phenotypic appearance: slim body habitus and neuromas of lips, tongue, and gastrointestinal tract		

VIP, vasoactive intestinal polypeptide

type 1, type 2a and type 2b. They are inherited in an autosomal dominant manner. MEN type 1 is due to a mutation in the *menin* gene on chromosome 11; the normal protein product of this gene acts as a tumour suppressor. The genetic abnormality in MEN 2 lies within the *Ret* proto-oncogene on chromosome 10; the gene product plays an important role in central and peripheral nerve development and function. Management involves surgical excision of the tumours if possible. Asymptomatic family members should be screened by measurement of serum calcium in MEN 1 (due to the high penetrance of hyperparathyroidism) and by genetic testing for *Ret* mutations in MEN 2 families. In a patient known to have MEN, constant surveillance is required for additional features of the syndrome, which may develop many years after the initial presentation.

DISORDERS OF TEMPERATURE REGULATION

Normal body temperature is 36.5–37.5°C and is controlled by temperature-sensitive cells within the hypothalamus which control heat generation and loss. Fever during an infection is due to cytokines, particularly interleukin-1, released from inflammatory cells acting in the hypothalamus affecting the thermoregulatory set-point.

Hypothermia (K&C 6e p. 1026)

Hypothermia is defined as a drop in core (i.e. rectal) temperature to below 35°C. It is frequently fatal when the temperature falls below 28°C.

Aetiology

Very young and elderly individuals are particularly prone to hypothermia, the latter having a reduced ability to feel the cold. Hypothyroidism, hypnotics, alcohol or intercurrent illness may contribute. In healthy individuals, prolonged exposure to extremes of temperature or prolonged immersion in cold water are the most common underlying causes.

Clinical features

Mild hypothermia (32–35°C) causes shivering and a feeling of intense cold. More severe hypothermia leads progressively to altered consciousness and coma. This is usually associated with a fall in pulse rate and blood pressure, muscle stiffness and depressed reflexes. As coma ensues, the pupillary and other brainstem reflexes are lost. Ventricular arrhythmias or asystole are the usual causes of death.

Diagnosis

Measurement of core temperature with a low-reading thermometer (oesophageal, rectal or tympanic) makes the diagnosis. Alteration in consciousness usually indicates a core temperature of below 32°C; this is a medical emergency. With severe hypothermia there are ECG changes, including an increase in the PR interval, widening of the QRS

> **Emergency Box 13.5**
> **Management of hypothermia**
>
> **Investigations**
> ● Arterial blood gases
> ● Full blood count, urea and electrolytes, blood glucose, thyroid function tests, blood cultures
> ● Chest X-ray, ECG
>
> **Management**
> ● Give oxygen by face mask and attach an ECG monitor
> ● Search for and treat infection, pneumonia is common
> ● Intubate and ventilate patients who are comatose or in respiratory failure
> ● Warmed (37°C) intravenous fluids to achieve urine output 30–40 mL/h
> ● Passive external warming if core temperature > 32°C
> – Place patient in a warm room (27–29°C)
> – 'Space' blankets
> – Warm bath water
> ● Active external rewarming if core temperature 28–32°C
> – Warm blankets, heating pads or forced warm air
> – Rewarm trunk *before* extremities to minimize peripheral vasodilatation
> – Warm bath water
> ● Active internal rewarming if core temperature < 28°C
> – Humidified and warmed (40–46°C) oxygen
> – Lavage (gastric, peritoneal, bladder) with warm fluids (40°C)
> – Extracorporeal shunt (haemodialysis, arteriovenous or venovenous) rewarming
> – Cardiopulmonary bypass – treatment of choice for arrested hypothermic patients
> ● Monitor core temperature, oxygen saturation by pulse oximetry, urine output and central venous pressure

complex and 'J' waves (prominent convex deflections at the junction of the QRS complex and ST segment, best seen in the precordial leads).

Management

The principles of treatment are to rewarm the patient gradually while correcting metabolic abnormalities (if severe) and treating cardiac arrhythmias (Emergency Box 13.5). Hypothyroidism should always be looked for and, if suspected, should be treated with intravenous triiodothyronine. Clues to the presence of hypothyroidism include previous radioiodine treatment or surgery for thyrotoxicosis, and preceding symptoms of hypothyroidism (p. 610). Hypothermia may protect organs from ischaemia in patients with prolonged hypothermia-induced cardiopulmonary arrest. Therefore, resuscitation should be continued (maybe for some hours) until arrest persists after rewarming or until attempts to raise the core temperature have failed. Drugs used in the usual arrest situation, e.g. epinephrine (adrenaline), have reduced efficacy at low temperatures and are withheld until the temperature is greater than 30°C.

Hyperthermia (hyperpyrexia) (*K&C* 6e p. 1025)

Hyperpyrexia is a body temperature above 41°C. Causes include:

- Injury to the hypothalamus (trauma, surgery, infection)
- Malignant hyperpyrexia – rare autosomal dominant condition in which skeletal muscle generates heat in the presence of certain anaesthetic drugs, e.g. suxamethonium
- Ingestion of 3,4-methylenedioxy-methamfetamine (Ecstasy)
- Neuroleptic malignant syndrome: idiosyncratic reaction to therapeutic dose of neuroleptic medication, e.g. phenothiazines.

Treatment includes stopping the offending drug, cooling, and the administration of dantrolene sodium.

Diabetes mellitus and other disorders of metabolism

14

DIABETES MELLITUS

Glucose metabolism (K&C 6e p. 1101)

Blood glucose levels are closely regulated in health and rarely stray outside the range of 3.5–8.0 mmol/L (63–144 mg/dL), despite the varying demands of food, fasting and exercise. Whole blood values are about 10–15% lower than *plasma values*, and *capillary values* are about 7% higher than plasma values The principal organ of glucose homeostasis is the liver, which absorbs and stores glucose (as glycogen) in the post-absorptive state and releases it into the circulation between meals to match the rate of glucose utilization by peripheral tissues. The liver also combines 3-carbon molecules derived from breakdown of fat (glycerol), muscle glycogen (lactate) and protein (e.g. alanine) into the 6-carbon glucose molecule by the process of gluconeogenesis. Insulin is the key hormone involved in the storage of nutrients in the form of glycogen in liver and muscle, and triglyceride in fat. During a meal insulin is released from the beta (β) cells of the pancreatic islets and facilitates glucose uptake by fat and muscle. In the fasting state the main action of insulin is to regulate glucose release by the liver. The counter-regulatory hormones, glucagon, epinephrine (adrenaline), cortisol and growth hormone, oppose the actions of insulin and cause greater production of glucose from the liver and less utilization of glucose in fat and muscle for a given plasma level of insulin.

Types of diabetes (K&C 6e p. 1103)

Diabetes mellitus is a common group of metabolic disorders that are characterized by chronic hyperglycaemia resulting from relative insulin deficiency, insulin resistance or both. Diabetes is usually primary but may be secondary to other conditions, which include pancreatic (e.g. total pancreatectomy, chronic pancreatitis, haemochromatosis)

Table 14.1 The spectrum of diabetes: a comparison of type 1 and type 2 diabetes

	Type 1	Type 2
Epidemiology	Peak incidence around puberty, can present at any age	Usually presents after age 40
	Usually lean	Often overweight
	European extraction (usually)	All racial groups, commoner in African/Asian
Inheritance	HLA-DR3 and/or DR4 in > 90%	No HLA links
	30–50% concordance in identical twins	50% concordance in identical twins
Pathogenesis	Autoimmune beta-cell destruction	No evidence of immune disturbance
Clinical picture	Complete insulin deficiency	Relative insulin deficiency, and insulin resistance
	May develop ketoacidosis	May develop non-ketotic hyperosmolar state
	Always need insulin treatment	Sometimes need insulin

and endocrine diseases (e.g. acromegaly and Cushing's syndrome). It may also be drug induced, most commonly by thiazide diuretics and corticosteroids.

Primary diabetes is divided into type 1 diabetes (insulin-dependent diabetes mellitus, IDDM) and the much more prevalent type 2 diabetes (non-insulin-dependent diabetes, NIDDM). Type 1 diabetes is most prevalent in Northern European countries, particularly Finland, and the incidence is increasing in most populations, particularly in young children. Type 2 diabetes is common in all populations enjoying an affluent lifestyle and, like type 1 diabetes, is increasing in frequency, particularly in adolescents.

Clinical distinction between the two forms can sometimes be difficult and they should be considered to represent two ends of a spectrum with a degree of overlap (Table 14.1).

Aetiology and pathogenesis

Type 1 diabetes mellitus is thought to be a polygenic disorder and the genes (as yet unknown) causing diabetes are transmitted along with particular HLA types (Table 14.1). An autoimmune aetiology is suggested by:

- Antibodies directed against insulin and several islet cell antigens (e.g. glutamic acid decarboxylase) predating clinical onset by many years
- Infiltration of pancreatic islets by mononuclear cells (insulitis) resembling that in other autoimmune diseases, e.g. thyroiditis
- Association with other organ-specific autoimmune diseases, e.g. autoimmune thyroid disease, Addison's disease and pernicious anaemia.

Type 2 diabetes mellitus is a polygenic disorder and the genes responsible for the majority of cases have yet to be identified. However, the genetic causes of some of the rare forms of type 2 diabetes have been identified and include mutations of the insulin receptor and structural alterations of the insulin molecule. Environmental factors, notably central obesity, appear to trigger the disease in genetically susceptible individuals. The beta-cell mass is reduced to about 50% of normal at the time of diagnosis in type 2 diabetes. Hyperglycaemia is the result of reduced insulin secretion (inappropriately low for the glucose level) and peripheral insulin resistance.

Clinical features (*K&C* 6e p. 1108)

- *Acute presentation.* Young people present with a brief history (2–4 weeks) of thirst, polyuria, weight loss and lethargy. Polyuria is the result of an osmotic diuresis that results when blood glucose levels exceed the renal tubular reabsorptive capacity (the renal threshold). Fluid and electrolyte losses stimulate thirst. Weight loss is caused by fluid depletion and breakdown of fat and muscle as a result of insulin deficiency. Ketoacidosis (see later) is the presenting feature if these early symptoms are not recognized and treated.
- *Subacute presentation.* Older patients may present with the same symptoms, although less marked and extending over several months. They may also complain of lack of

649

Table 14.2 The oral glucose tolerance test		
	Fasting venous plasma glucose (mmol/L)	**2-Hour plasma glucose (mmol/L)**
Normal	< 7.0	< 7.8
Diabetes mellitus	> 7.0	≥ 11.1
Impaired glucose tolerance (IGT)	< 7.0	7.8–11.0

After an overnight fast 75 g of glucose is taken in 250–350 mL of water. Blood samples are taken before and 2 hours after the glucose has been given. Individuals with IGT have an increased risk of cardiovascular disease compared to the normal population and 2–4% yearly will go on to develop diabetes. Results are for venous plasma – whole blood values are lower

energy, visual problems and pruritus vulvae or balanitis due to *Candida* infection.

■ *With complications* (see later).
■ *In asymptomatic individuals* diagnosed at routine medical examinations, e.g. for insurance purposes.

Investigations (*K&C* 6e p. 1108)

The diagnosis of diabetes mellitus is made by demonstrating:

■ Fasting (no calorie intake for at least 8 hours) plasma glucose ≥ 7.0 mmol/L
■ Random (without regard to time since last meal) plasma glucose ≥ 11.1 mmol/L
■ One abnormal laboratory value is diagnostic in a patient with typical hyperglycaemic symptoms; two values are needed in asymptomatic people.

A glucose tolerance test (Table 14.2) is only used for borderline cases and for the diagnosis of gestational diabetes. Glycosuria does not necessarily indicate diabetes and may be found in normoglycaemic subjects who have a low renal threshold for glucose excretion.

Other routine investigations at diagnosis include screening the urine for proteinuria (p. 337), full blood count, serum urea and electrolytes, liver biochemistry, and a fasting blood sample for cholesterol and triglyceride levels.

Management

Impaired glucose tolerance

This is not a clinical entity but a risk factor for future diabetes and cardiovascular disease. Obesity and lack of regular physical exercise make progression to frank diabetes more likely. The classification is complicated by the poor reproducibility of the oral glucose tolerance test. The group is heterogeneous; some patients are obese, some have liver disease, and others are on medication that impairs glucose tolerance. Individuals with IGT have the same risk of cardiovascular disease as in frank diabetes but do not develop the specific microvascular complications.

Impaired fasting glucose

This diagnostic category (fasting plasma glucose 6.1–6.9 mmol/L) is not a clinical entity, but does predict future risk of frank diabetes and cardiovascular disease. This category only overlaps with IGT to a limited extent, and therefore the associated risks of cardiovascular disease and future diabetes are not directly comparable.

Management (*K&C* 6e p. 1109)

A multidisciplinary approach involving, among others, the hospital doctor, the general practitioner, nurse specialists, dieticians and chiropodists is important in the management of this condition. It is essential that the patient understands the risks of diabetes, the potential benefits of good glycaemic control and the importance of maintaining a lean weight, stopping smoking and taking care of the feet. Patients requiring insulin or oral hypoglycaemic drugs should be offered influenza immunization (p. 495).

651

Management involves:

- Achieving good glycaemic control. In young patients with type 1 diabetes the aim is to maintain blood glucose concentrations as near normal as possible to minimize long-term complications.
- Advice regarding regular physical activity and reduction of bodyweight in the obese, both of which improve glycaemic control in type 2 diabetes.
- Aggressive treatment of hypertension and hyper-lipidaemia, both of which are additional risk factors for long-term complications of diabetes.

Table 14.3   Regular checks for patients with diabetes

Checked each visit
Review of monitoring results and current treatment
Talk about targets and change where necessary
Talk about any general or specific problems
Continued education

Checked at least once a year
Biochemical assessment of metabolic control (e.g. glycosylated haemoglobin test)
Measure bodyweight
Measure blood pressure
Measure plasma lipids (except in extreme old age)
Measure visual acuity
Examine state of retina (ophthalmoscope or retinal photo)
Test urine for proteinuria
Test blood for renal function (creatinine)
Check condition of feet, pulses and neurology
Review cardiovascular risk factors
Review self-monitoring and injection techniques
Review eating habits

■ Regular checks of metabolic control and physical examination for evidence of diabetic complications (Table 14.3).

Principles of treatment

All patients with diabetes require diet therapy. Regular exercise is encouraged to control weight and reduce cardiovascular risk. Insulin is always indicated in a patient who presents in ketoacidosis, and is usually indicated in those under 40 years of age. Insulin is also indicated in other patients who do not achieve satisfactory control with oral hypoglycaemics. Treatment of type 2 diabetes is summarized in Figure 14.1.

Diet   The diet for people with diabetes is no different from the normal healthy diet recommended for the rest of the population. Recommended food should:

■ Be low in sugar (though not sugar-free)
■ Be high in starchy carbohydrate (especially foods with a low glycaemic index such as pasta which is slowly absorbed and thus prevents rapid fluctuations in blood glucose). Carbohydrate should represent about 40–60% of total energy intake

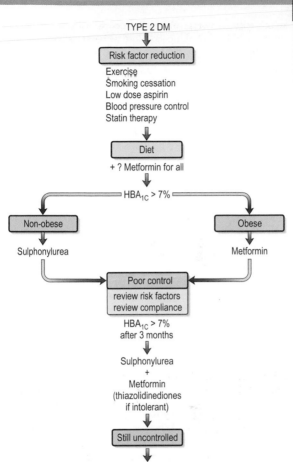

Fig. 14.1 Treatment of type 2 diabetes.

- Be high in fibre
- Be low in fat (especially saturated fat) which should represent less than 35% of total energy intake
- Include protein representing about 15% of total energy intake (1 g per kg ideal bodyweight).

The nutrient load should be spread throughout the day (three main meals with snacks in between and at bedtime), which reduces swings in blood glucose. The overweight or obese should be encouraged to lose weight by a combination of changes in food intake and physical activity.

Tablet treatments for type 2 diabetes These are used in association with dietary treatment when this alone has failed to control hyperglycaemia.

- *Biguanides*. Metformin reduces glucose production by the liver and sensitizes target tissues to insulin. It is used as first-line monotherapy in overweight patients who have not achieved optimal glucose control with a diet. Metformin is preferred in this situation because, unlike the sulphonylureas, appetite is not increased. It is also used in combination with sulphonylureas when a single agent has failed to control diabetes. Side-effects include anorexia and diarrhoea. Lactic acidosis has occurred in patients with severe heart failure, liver disease or renal disease (serum creatinine > 150 μmol/L), in whom its use is contraindicated.
- *Sulphonylureas* promote insulin secretion. Glibenclamide is the most popular choice, but is best avoided in elderly people and in those with renal failure because of its relatively long duration of action (12–20 hours) and renal excretion. Tolbutamide, which is shorter acting and metabolized by the liver, is a better choice in these patient groups. The most common side-effect of this group of drugs is hypoglycaemia, which may be prolonged.
- *Meglitinides* such as repaglinide and nateglinide are insulin secretagogues that promote insulin secretion in response to meals, and which might thus reduce between-meal hypoglycaemia. Whether they have advantages over established short-acting sulphonylureas such as tolbutamide has not been addressed by clinical trials.
- *Thiazolidinediones* (glitazones), e.g. rosiglitazone and pioglitazone, bind to and activate a transcription factor called nuclear peroxisome proliferator-activated receptor-gamma (PPAR-gamma), which is a nuclear receptor expressed predominantly in adipose tissue. It is thought to be involved in the transcription of insulin-responsive genes that are involved in lipid metabolism and insulin action. Their place in the initial therapy of type 2 diabetes remains unclear but they may be an appropriate monotherapy choice in patients intolerant of metformin. They are also licensed for use in combination with metformin

in obese patients with insufficient glycaemic control and in combination with sulphonylureas if metformin is either not tolerated or contraindicated. They are contraindicated in patients with hepatic impairment or cardiac failure (past or present).

- *Intestinal enzyme inhibitors.*
  - Alpha-glucosidase inhibitors such as acarbose inhibit intestinal α-glucosidases, thus impairing carbohydrate digestion and slowing glucose absorption. Postprandial glucose peaks are reduced. Gastrointestinal side-effects, e.g. flatulence, bloating and diarrhoea, are common and limit the dose and acceptability of this treatment.
  - Lipase inhibitors such as orlistat cause fat malabsorption by rendering intestinal lipase enzymes less effective, and therefore reducing the absorption of fat from the diet. It can contribute to weight loss in patients who are already under careful dietary supervision because it has the effect of inducing unpleasant steatorrhoea, and patients therefore reduce their fat intake and lose weight. Its place in diabetes management remains unclear.

Insulin Almost all insulin now used in developed countries is synthetic (recombinant) human insulin.

There are three main types of insulin:

1. *Short-acting insulins.* These insulins start working within 30–60 minutes and last for 4–6 hours. They are the only insulins to be used in emergencies such as ketoacidosis, or for surgical operations.
2. *Short-acting insulin analogues.* Modifications have been made to the insulin molecule to prevent it from forming dimers and other complexes (in contrast to regular insulin). As a result, the onset of action of these monomeric insulins (insulin lispro and insulin aspart) is quicker (within 15 minutes) and they have a shorter duration of action (2–4 hours) than regular soluble insulin. They are the preferred insulin preparation for pre-meal bolus doses for patients who experience hypoglycaemia between meals on multiple injection regimens.
3. *Longer-acting insulins.* Insulins premixed with retarding agents (either protamine or zinc) that precipitate crystals of varying size according to the conditions employed. These insulins are intermediate (12–24 hours) or long acting (more than 24 hours). The protamine insulins are

655

also known as isophane or NPH insulins, and the zinc insulins as lente insulins. Insulin glargine is a structurally modified insulin that precipitates in tissues and is then slowly released from the injection site.

In young patients a reasonable starting regimen is subcutaneous injection of an intermediate-acting insulin, 8–10 units administered half an hour before breakfast and before the evening meal. In many patients who present acutely with diabetes there is some recovery of endogenous insulin secretion soon after diagnosis ('the honeymoon period') and the insulin dose may need to be reduced. Requirements rise thereafter, and a multiple injection regimen (often using a 'pen injector' device), which may improve control and allows greater meal flexibility, is then appropriate for most younger patients. An example of this is soluble insulin administered before each meal and an intermediate-acting insulin given at bedtime. Target blood values should normally be 4–7 mmol/L before meals and 4–10 mmol/L after meals. An alternative to multiple injections is to use a small pump strapped to the waist, which delivers a continuous subcutaneous insulin infusion (CSII). Meal-time doses are delivered when the patient presses a button on the side of the pump. This should only be used under the guidance of specialized centres.

In many patients with type 2 diabetes who eventually require insulin, a twice-daily regimen of premixed soluble and isophane insulin (e.g. Mixtard) is suitable.

The most common complications of insulin therapy are hypoglycaemia and weight gain.

Measuring control (*K&C* 6e p. 1116)

Patients may feel very well and be asymptomatic even if their blood glucose is consistently above the normal range. Self-monitoring at home is therefore necessary because of the immediate risks of hyper- and hypoglycaemia, and because it has been shown that persistently good control (i.e. near normoglycaemia) reduces the risk of progression to retinopathy, nephropathy and neuropathy in both type 1 and type 2 diabetes.

Home testing

- Most patients, especially those on insulin, are taught to monitor control by testing finger-prick blood samples with enzyme-impregnated reagent strips, which change colour according to the capillary blood glucose level. Patients are asked to take regular profiles (e.g. four times daily samples on 2 days each week) and to note these in a diary or record book.

■ Urine testing for glucose (using Stix) is a crude measure of glycaemic control because glycosuria only appears above the renal threshold for glucose (which varies between a blood glucose of 7 and 13 mmol/L) and because urine glucose lags behind blood glucose. It is usually reserved for the elderly patient in whom tight control is unnecessary.

■ Urine ketones, also measured with Stix (Ketostix), are useful if the patient is unwell, because ketonuria indicates potentially serious metabolic derangement.

Hospital testing   Single random blood glucose measurements, obtained at clinic visits, are of limited value.

■ Glycosylated haemoglobin (HbA_{1c}) is produced by the attachment of glucose to Hb and measurement of this Hb fraction (normally 4–8%) is a useful measure of the average glucose concentration over the life of the Hb molecule (approximately 6 weeks). Good control is indicated by a $HbA_{1c} < 7.0\%$.

■ Glycosylated plasma proteins (fructosamine) are less reliable than HbA_{1c} but may be useful in certain situations, e.g. thalassaemia where haemoglobin is abnormal.

Whole pancreas and pancreatic islet transplantation

Whole pancreas transplantation is sometimes performed, usually in diabetic patients who require immunosuppression for a kidney transplant. Lasting graft function can be achieved, but the procedure adds to the risks of renal transplantation.

More recently, islet transplantation has been performed by harvesting pancreatic islets from cadavers, which are then injected into the portal vein. These then seed themselves into the liver. While results are improving, this form of treatment remains experimental.

DIABETIC METABOLIC EMERGENCIES

Hypoglycaemia

This is the most common complication of insulin treatment and may also occur in patients taking sulphonylureas.

Clinical features

Symptoms of sympathetic overactivity usually develop when blood glucose levels fall below 3.0 mmol/L and include hunger, sweating, pallor and tachycardia. Untreated, the symptoms of neuroglycopenia develop and later there is personality change, fits, occasionally hemiparesis, and finally coma. In patients with long-standing diabetes and autonomic neuropathy the early 'adrenergic features' may be absent.

Investigations

Immediate diagnosis and treatment are essential. A blood glucose confirms the diagnosis but treatment should begin immediately (while waiting for the result) if hypoglycaemia is suspected on clinical grounds.

Management

A rapidly absorbed carbohydrate, e.g. sugary water, should be given orally if possible. In unconscious patients, treatment is with intravenous dextrose (50 mL of 50% dextrose into a large vein though a large-gauge needle) followed by a flush of normal saline, as concentrated dextrose is highly irritant. Intramuscular glucagon (1 mg) acts rapidly by mobilizing hepatic glycogen and is particularly useful where intravenous access is difficult. Oral glucose is given to replenish glycogen reserves once the patient revives. Hypoglycaemia may recur after treatment, particularly if it is a result of treatment with long-acting insulin preparations or oral hypoglycaemics. These patients should be monitored with hourly (4-hourly when stable) blood glucose readings and may require a 10% dextrose drip to prevent recurrent hypoglycaemia.

Diabetic ketoacidosis (K&C 6e p. 1119)

Diabetic ketoacidosis results from insulin deficiency and is the result of previously undiagnosed diabetes, or the stress of intercurrent illness (e.g. infection or surgery) or interruption of insulin therapy in a known diabetic. A common error is for insulin to be reduced or stopped if the patient is ill and feels unable to eat. Insulin should never be stopped and most patients need a larger dose when ill.

Pathogenesis

Ketoacidosis is a state of uncontrolled catabolism associated with insulin deficiency. In the absence of insulin there is an unrestrained increase in hepatic gluconeogenesis. High circulating glucose levels result in an osmotic diuresis by the kidneys and consequent dehydration. In addition, peripheral lipolysis leads to an increase in circulating free fatty acids, which are converted within the liver to acidic ketones, leading to a metabolic acidosis. These processes are accelerated by the 'stress hormones' – catecholamines, glucagon and cortisol – which are secreted in response to dehydration and intercurrent illness.

Clinical features

There is profound dehydration secondary to water and electrolyte loss from the kidney. The eyes are sunken, tissue turgor is reduced, the tongue is dry and, in severe cases, the blood pressure is low. Kussmaul's respiration (deep rapid breathing) may be present, as a sign of respiratory compensation for metabolic acidosis, and the breath smells of ketones. Some disturbance of consciousness is common, but only 5% present in coma. Body temperature is often subnormal despite intercurrent infection. A few patients have abdominal pain and rarely this may cause confusion with a surgical acute abdomen.

Investigations

The diagnosis is based on the demonstration of hyper-glycaemia in combination with acidosis and ketosis.

- Blood glucose is elevated, usually > 20 mmol/L.
- Plasma ketones are easily detected by centrifuging a blood sample and diluting the plasma obtained 1 : 1 with 0.9% saline before testing with a dipstick that measures ketones, which will usually show +++.
- Urine Stix testing shows heavy glycosuria and ketonuria.
- Arterial blood gases show a metabolic acidosis. Calculation shows a high anion gap (p. 329).
- Serum urea and electrolytes. Urea and creatinine are often raised as a result of dehydration. The total body potassium is low as a result of osmotic diuresis, but the serum potassium concentration is often raised because of the absence of the action of insulin, which allows potassium to shift out of cells. Serum bicarbonate is low.

Table 14.4 Average loss of fluid and electrolytes in an adult with ketoacidosis

Water	6 L
Sodium	500 mmol
Potassium	400 mmol

- Full blood count may show an elevated white cell count even in the absence of infection.
- Further investigations are directed towards identifying a precipitating cause: blood cultures, chest radiograph and urine microscopy and culture to look for evidence of infection, and an ECG to look for evidence of myocardial infarction.

Management

Admission to the intensive care unit is recommended in the seriously ill. The aims of treatment are to replace fluid and electrolyte loss (Table 14.4), replace insulin, and restore acid–base balance over a period of about 24 hours. Therapy of diabetic ketoacidosis shifts potassium into cells, which may lead to profound hypokalaemia and death if not treated prospectively. A treatment regimen for a patient with severe ketoacidosis is set out in Emergency Box 14.1. Cerebral oedema (presenting with headache and reduced conscious level) may complicate therapy in some patients and results from rapid lowering of blood glucose and osmolality. When the patient has recovered, it is necessary to determine the cause of the episode and provide advice and information to prevent recurrence.

Non-ketotic hyperosmolar state (*K&C* 6e p. 1122)

This condition, in which severe hyperglycaemia develops without significant ketosis, is the metabolic emergency characteristic of uncontrolled type 2 diabetes mellitus. It is often precipitated by consumption of glucose-rich fluids, concomitant medication such as thiazides or steroids or by intercurrent illness.

Clinical features

Endogenous insulin levels are reduced but are still sufficient to inhibit hepatic ketogenesis, whereas glucose production

> ### Emergency Box 14.1
> **Management of diabetic ketoacidosis**

Phase I management

- Insulin: soluble Insulin I.v. 6 units/h by infusion, or 20 units i.m. stat. followed by 6 units i.m. hourly. Aim for fall in blood glucose of approx. 5 mmol per hour. Adjust infusion rate by 50% to achieve this.
- Fluid replacement: 0.9% sodium chloride with 20 mmol KCl per litre. An average regimen would be 1 litre in 30 minutes, then 1 litre in 1 hour, then 1 litre in 2 hours, then 1 litre in 4 hours, then 1 litre in 6 hours.
- Adjust KCl concentration depending on results of 2 hours' blood K measurement. Temporarily delay if serum potassium > 5.0 mmol/L. Increase to 30–40 mmol/L if serum potassium is low, e.g. < 3.5 mmol/L.

IF:

- Blood pressure below 90 mmHg, give plasma expander
- pH below 7.0 give 500 mL of sodium bicarbonate 1.26% plus 10 mmol KCl over 1 hour. Repeat if necessary to bring pH up to 7.0.

Phase 2 management

- When blood glucose falls to 10–12 mmol/L swap infusion fluid to 1 litre 5% dextrose plus 20 mmol KCl 6-hourly. Continue insulin with dose adjusted according to hourly blood glucose test results.

Phase 3 management

- Once stable and able to eat and drink normally, transfer patient to four-times-daily subcutaneous insulin regimen (based on previous 24 hours insulin consumption, and trend in consumption).

Special measures

- Broad-spectrum antibiotic if infection likely.
- Bladder catheter if no urine passed in 2 hours.
- Nasogastric tube if drowsy.
- Consider CVP pressure monitoring if shocked or if previous cardiac or renal impairment.
- Consider s.c. prophylactic heparin in comatose, elderly or obese patients.

Subsequent management

- Monitor glucose hourly for 8 hours.
- Monitor electrolytes 2-hourly for 8 hours.
- Adjust K replacement according to results.

Note: The regimen of fluid replacement set out above is a guide for patients with severe ketoacidosis. Excessive fluid can precipitate pulmonary and cerebral oedema; adequate replacement must therefore be tailored to the individual and monitored carefully throughout treatment.

Table 14.5 The main biochemical differences between diabetic ketoacidosis and non-ketotic hyperosmolar coma

Examples of blood values	Severe ketoacidosis	Non-ketotic hyperosmolar coma
Na^+ (mmol/L)	140	155
K^+ (mmol/L)	5	5
Cl^- (mmol/L)	100	110
HCO_3^- (mmol/L)	5	30
Urea (mmol/L)	8	15
Glucose (mmol/L)	30	50
Serum osmolality (mOsm/kg)*	328	385
Arterial pH	7.0	7.35

*See page 316 for definition and discussion of plasma osmolality

is unrestrained. Patients present with profound dehydration (secondary to an osmotic diuresis) and a decreased level of consciousness, which is directly related to the elevation of plasma osmolality. The main biochemical differences between ketoacidosis and hyperosmolar coma are illustrated in Table 14.5.

Management

Investigations and treatment are the same as for ketoacidosis with the exception that a lower rate of insulin infusion (3 U/h) is often sufficient, as these patients are extremely sensitive to insulin. The rate may be doubled after 2–3 h if glucose is falling too slowly. The hyperosmolar state predisposes to stroke, myocardial infarction, or arterial thrombosis, and prophylactic subcutaneous heparin is given.

Prognosis

Mortality rate is around 20–30%, mainly because of the advanced age of the patients and the frequency of inter-current illness. Unlike ketoacidosis, non-ketotic hyper-glycaemia is not an absolute indication for subsequent insulin therapy, and survivors may do well on diet and oral agents.

Lactic acidosis (K&C 6e p. 1122)

Lactic acidosis is a rare complication in patients taking metformin. Patients present with severe metabolic acidosis without significant hyperglycaemia or ketosis. Treatment is rehydration with intravenous saline. Intravenous bicarbonate is used only in severe acidosis (pH < 7).

COMPLICATIONS OF DIABETES

Patients with diabetes have a reduced life expectancy. Cardiovascular problems (70%) followed by renal failure (10%) and infections (6%) are the most common cause of premature death in treated patients. Complications are directly related to the degree and duration of hyper-glycaemia and can be reduced by improved diabetic control.

Vascular

Macrovascular complications (*K&C* 6e p. 1123)
Diabetes is a risk factor for atherosclerosis and this is additive with other risk factors for large vessel disease, e.g. smoking, hypertension and hyperlipidaemia. Atherosclerosis results in stroke, ischaemic heart disease and peripheral vascular disease. The risk is reduced not only by good diabetic control but also modification of other risk factors. This includes aggressive control of blood pressure (target <130/80 mmHg), cessation of smoking, treatment with a statin for most type 2 diabetics irrespective of serum cholesterol and treatment with an ACE inihibitor for patients with one other major cardiovascular risk factor. Some patients depending on age and other cardiovascular risk factors are also treated with aspirin.

Microvascular complications (*K&C* 6e p. 1124)
In contrast to macrovascular disease, microvascular disease is specific to diabetes. Small vessels throughout the body are affected, but the disease process is of particular danger in three sites: the retina, the renal glomerulus and the nerve sheath. Diabetic retinopathy, nephropathy and neuropathy tend to manifest 10–20 years after diagnosis in young patients. They present earlier in older patients, probably because they have had unrecognized diabetes for months or even years before diagnosis.

Diabetic eye disease (*K&C* 6e p. 1124)

About one-third of young diabetics develop visual problems, and in the UK 5% have become blind after 30 years of diabetes. However, the prevalence is falling.

Complications of diabetes

Retinopathy

Background retinopathy is the earliest feature of retinopathy. Capillary microaneurysms appear on ophthalmoscopy as tiny red dots, haemorrhages are seen as larger red spots (blot haemorrhages), and capillary leaks of fluid rich in lipid and protein give rise to hard exudates (yellow-white discrete patches). There is no specific treatment for background retinopathy, but patients should undergo regular eye examination by an ophthalmologist to look for any deterioration. Background retinopathy does not itself constitute a threat to vision, but may progress to two other distinct forms of retinopathy: maculopathy or proliferative retinopathy. Both are the consequence of damage to retinal blood vessels and resultant retinal ischaemia.

Maculopathy Macular oedema is the first feature of maculopathy and will result in permanent damage if not treated early. It cannot be detected by standard ophthalmoscopy and the only sign may be deteriorating visual acuity detected by Snellen chart testing. At a later stage there are perimacular haemorrhages and hard exudates.

Pre-proliferative retinopathy is characterized by 'cotton-wool spots', which are indistinct pale lesions and represent oedema from retinal infarcts. Venous beading and/or venous loops are other pre-proliferative changes.

Proliferative retinopathy Hypoxia is thought to be the signal for new vessel formation. These are fragile and bleed easily, resulting in loss of vision because of vitreous haemorrhage. Fibrous tissue associated with new vessels may shrink and cause retinal detachment.

Maculopathy and proliferative retinopathy are indications for urgent referral to an ophthalmologist and are treated by laser photocoagulation of the retina. Effective early therapy of proliferative retinopathy reduces the risk of visual loss by about 50%.

Other eye complications

- Blurred vision (caused by reversible osmotic changes in the lens in patients with acute hyperglycaemia)
- Cataracts
- Glaucoma
- External ocular palsies, especially of the VIth nerve, can occur (a mononeuritis).

The diabetic kidney (K&C 6e p. 1126)

The kidney may be damaged by diabetes as a result of:

- Glomerular disease
- Ischaemic renal lesions
- Ascending urinary tract infection.

Diabetic nephropathies   Clinical nephropathy secondary to glomerular disease usually manifests 15–25 years after diagnosis and affects 25–30% of patients diagnosed under the age of 30 years. On histological investigation there is thickening of the glomerular basement membrane and later glomerulosclerosis, which may be a diffuse or nodular form (Kimmelstiel–Wilson lesion). The earliest clinical evidence of glomerular damage is 'microalbuminuria' (defined as an increase above the normal range in urinary albumin excretion but undetectable by conventional dipsticks) which in turn may, after some years, progress to intermittent albuminuria followed by persistent proteinuria, sometimes with a frank nephrotic syndrome. At the stage of persistent proteinuria the plasma creatinine is normal but the average patient is only some 5–10 years from end-stage renal failure.

The urine of all patients should be checked regularly by dipsticks for the presence of protein. Most centres also screen for microalbuminuria, because meticulous glycaemic control and treatment with angiotensin-converting enzyme (ACE) inhibitors at this stage (even in the absence of hypertension) may delay the onset of frank proteinuria. Aggressive control of blood pressure (target below 130/80 mmHg) is the most important factor to reduce disease progression in those with established proteinuria, and ACE inhibitors or angiotensin receptor II antagonists are the treatment of choice. Many will develop end-stage renal failure and need dialysis and eventually renal transplantation. A segmental pancreatic graft is sometimes performed at the same time as a renal graft.

Ischaemic lesions   Arteriolar lesions with hypertrophy and hyalinization of the vessels affect both afferent and efferent arterioles. The appearances are similar to those of hypertensive disease but are not necessarily related to the blood pressure in patients with diabetes.

Infective lesions   Urinary tract infections are common (p. 354). A rare complication is renal papillary necrosis, in

665

Complications of diabetes

Table 14.6	Diabetic neuropathies
Progressive	Symmetrical sensory polyneuropathy
	Autonomic neuropathy
Reversible	Acute painful neuropathy
	Mononeuropathy and mononeuritis multiplex
	Cranial nerve lesions
	Isolated peripheral nerve lesions
	Diabetic amyotrophy

which renal papillae are shed in the urine and may cause ureteral obstruction.

Diabetic neuropathy (Table 14.6) (*K&C* 6e p. 1128)

Diabetic neuropathy is thought to result from nerve ischaemia from occlusion of the vasa vasorum, or the accumulation of fructose and sorbitol (metabolized from glucose in peripheral nerves), which disrupts the structure and function of the nerve.

Symmetrical mainly sensory neuropathy This is the most common form of neuropathy and first affects the most distal parts of the longest nerves, i.e. the toes and the soles of the feet. Symptoms consist of numbness, tingling and pain, which is typically worse at night. Involvement of the hands is less common and results in a 'stocking and glove' sensory loss. Complications include unrecognized trauma, beginning as blistering caused by an ill-fitting shoe or a hot-water bottle, and leading to ulceration. Abnormal mechanical stress and repeated minor trauma, usually prevented by pain, may lead to the development of a neuropathic arthropathy (Charcot's joints) in the ankle and knee, where the joint is grossly deformed and swollen. All patients with diabetic sensory neuropathy are at risk of insensitive foot ulceration. They should learn the principles of foot care (p. 667) and visit a chiropodist regularly.

Autonomic neuropathy may present with erectile dysfunction (p. 597), postural hypotension, diarrhoea, and nausea and vomiting as a consequence of gastroparesis. In addition, bladder involvement may result in a neuropathic bladder with painless urinary retention.

Acute painful neuropathy   The patient describes burning or crawling pains in the lower limbs. Symptoms are typically worse at night, and pressure from bedclothes may be intolerable. Treatment is with good diabetic control, tricyclic antidepressants, gabapentin and carbamazepine.

Diabetic mononeuropathy   Individual nerves are affected. In some instances this relates to local pressure, e.g. carpal tunnel syndrome. In others it results from a localized nerve infarction: commonly the IIIrd and VIth cranial nerves are affected, resulting in diplopia (p. 713). More than one nerve may be affected (mononeuritis multiplex).

Diabetic amyotrophy   presents with painful wasting, usually asymmetrical, of the quadriceps muscles. The wasting may be marked and knee reflexes are diminished or absent.

The diabetic foot *(K&C 6e p. 1130)*

Foot problems are a major cause of morbidity and mortality in patients with diabetes mellitus, with infection, ischaemia and neuropathy all contributing to produce tissue necrosis. On physical examination evidence of a neuropathy is demonstrated by reduced sensation to vibration, temperature and pin-prick. There may be evidence of Charcot arthropathy. Signs of vascular disease in the lower leg include thin skin and absence of hair, bluish discoloration of the skin, reduced skin temperature and absent foot pulses. Many diabetic foot ulcers are avoidable, so patients need to learn the principles of foot care: well-fitting lace-up shoes, regular chiropody, no 'bathroom' surgery, daily inspection of feet and early advice for any damage, and finally avoiding sources of heat, such as radiators and hot bath water. Management of foot lesions involves:

- Swabbing of ulcers for bacterial culture and early antibiotic treatment
- Good local wound care and, if necessary, surgical debridement of ulcers
- Evaluation for peripheral vascular disease by clinical examination, measurement of blood flow (by Doppler probe) and femoral angiography if clinically indicated
- Reconstructive vascular surgery for localized areas of arterial occlusion.

Infections (*K&C* 6e p. 1130)

Poorly controlled diabetes impairs the function of poly-morphonuclear leucocytes and confers an increased risk of infection, particularly of the urinary tract and skin, e.g. cellulitis, boils and abscesses. Tuberculosis and muco-cutaneous candidiasis are more common in diabetic individuals. Infections may lead to loss of glycaemic control and are a common cause of ketoacidosis. Insulin-treated patients may need to increase their insulin therapy even if they feel nauseated and unable to eat. Non-insulin-treated patients may need insulin for the same reasons.

The skin (*K&C* 6e pp. 1131 & 1345)

- Lipohypertrophy is where fat lumps develop at frequently used insulin injection sites, and may be avoided by varying the injection site from day to day.
- Necrobiosis lipoidica diabeticorum is an unusual compli-cation of diabetes characterized by erythematous plaques, often over the shins, which gradually develop a brown waxy discoloration.
- Vitiligo is symmetrical white patches seen in diabetes mellitus and other organ-specific autoimmune diseases.
- Granuloma annulare, which presents as flesh-coloured rings and nodules, principally over the extensor surfaces of the fingers.

SPECIAL SITUATIONS

Surgery (*K&C* 6e p. 1131)

Smooth control of diabetes minimizes the risk of infection and balances the catabolic response to anaesthesia and surgery. If possible, diabetic patients should be admitted 1 or 2 days before major surgery and glucose control optimized. They should be first on the operating list and a blood glucose of 6–11 mmol/L maintained during the perioperative period.

Insulin-treated patients

- Stop long-acting insulins the day before surgery; substitute with soluble insulin.
- Start glucose/potassium/insulin infusion (GKI: 500 mL 10% glucose + 10 mmol KCl + 16 U soluble insulin over 5 hours) on the morning of surgery and continue until first meal.

- Check blood glucose levels 2-hourly and serum potass... every 4–6 hours.
- Increase or decrease insulin in GKI by 5 U if blood glucose > 11 or < 6 mmol/L respectively.
- Postoperatively, continue infusion until patient is able to eat.

Non-insulin-treated patients
- Omit oral hypoglycaemics 2 days before operation.
- Check blood glucose 4-hourly.
- Patients with fasting blood glucose > 8 mmol/L: treat as for insulin-treated.
- Patients with fasting blood glucose < 8 mmol/L: treat as non-diabetic.
- Restart oral hypoglycaemics with first meal.

Pregnancy and diabetes (*K&C* 6e p. 1132)

Poorly controlled diabetes is associated with congenital malformations, macrosomia (large babies), hydramnios, pre-eclampsia and intrauterine death. In the neonatal period there is an increased risk of hyaline membrane disease and neonatal hypoglycaemia (unlike insulin, maternal glucose crosses the placenta and causes hypersecretion of insulin from the fetal islets, which continues when the umbilical cord is cut). Meticulous control of blood glucose levels achieves results comparable to those with non-diabetic pregnancies.

Gestational diabetes is diabetes that develops in the course of pregnancy and remits following delivery. Treatment is with diet in the first instance, but most patients require insulin cover during pregnancy. It is likely to recur in subsequent pregnancies, and diabetes may develop later in life.

Acutely ill hospital inpatients

Acutely ill diabetic patients are susceptible to hyperglycaemia because of increased release of counter-regulatory stress hormones (epinephrine (adrenaline), cortisol and growth hormone), physical inactivity and possibly an alteration in diet. Good glucose control reduces mortality in acute myocardial infarction, stroke and critically ill patients on ITU. Metformin should not be given to an ill patient in hospital because of the risk of lactic acidosis.

Table 14.7   A sliding scale to maintain good glucose control in acutely ill hospital inpatients

Blood glucose concentration (mmol/L)	Insulin infusion rate (unit/hour)
0–3.9	0
4–6.9	1
7–8.9	2
9–10.9	3
11–12.9	4
13+	6

A patient whose usual insulin dose is more than 100 units per day may require an additional 1 unit per hour

Patient who are not eating are managed with intravenous fluids with added potassium and a sliding scale of intravenous soluble insulin administered by a syringe pump (Table 14.7). The dose of insulin is decided by hourly blood glucose measurements (BM stix) with a target blood glucose of 4–9 mmol/L (4–7 in stroke and MI).

Patients who are eating or who are coming off a sliding scale are managed with a short-acting insulin analogue before breakfast, dinner and tea, and a long-acting insulin before bed. The usual insulin dose is divided into four to decide the amount given at each of these four time points. Blood glucose is measured before and 2 hours after meals and before bed to decide if the dose should be increased. The first dose is given 30 minutes before stopping a sliding scale and the last dose given at lunchtime before resuming normal insulin therapy at teatime.

670

Unstable diabetes (K&C 6e p. 1132)

This is used to describe patients with recurrent ketoacidosis and/or recurrent hypoglycaemic coma. Of these, the largest group is made up of those who experience recurrent severe hypoglycaemia.

HYPOGLYCAEMIA (K&C 6e pp. 1115 & 1133)

The causes and mechanism of hypoglycaemia are listed in Table 14.8. Insulin or sulphonylurea therapy for diabetes accounts for the vast majority of cases of severe hypo-

Table 14.8   Causes of hypoglycaemia

Cause	Mechanism of hypoglycaemia
Drug induced: insulin, sulphonylureas, quinine, pentamidine and salicylates in overdose	Variety of mechanisms
Islet cell tumour of the pancreas (insulinoma)	Inappropriately high circulating insulin levels
Non-pancreatic tumours, e.g. sarcoma, hepatoma	Secretion of IGF-1 by some tumours
Endocrine causes: Addison's disease	Impaired counter-regulation to the action of insulin
Fulminant liver failure	Failure of hepatic gluconeogenesis
End-stage renal failure	Failure of renal cortical gluconeogenesis
Excess alcohol	Enhanced insulin response to carbohydrate Inhibition of hepatic gluconeogenesis
After gastric surgery	Rapid gastric emptying, mismatch of food and insulin
Factitious hypoglycaemia	Surreptitious self-administration of insulin or sulphonylureas, often in a non-diabetic

IGF-1, insulin-like growth factor: normally mainly produced by the liver, primarily a growth factor in physiological concentrations

glycaemia encountered in an accident and emergency department.

Insulinomas

671

These are rare pancreatic islet cell tumours (usually benign) that secrete insulin. They may be part of the multiple endocrine neoplasia syndrome (p. 642).

Clinical features

The classic presentation is with fasting hypoglycaemia. Hypoglycaemia produces symptoms as a result of neuroglycopenia and stimulation of the sympathetic nervous system. These include sweating, palpitations, diplopia and weakness, progressing to confusion, abnormal behaviour, fits and coma.

stigations

e diagnosis is made by demonstrating hypoglycaemia in association with inappropriate or excessive insulin secretion:

- Measurement of overnight fasting plasma glucose and insulin levels on three occasions
- Performing a prolonged 72-hour supervised fast if overnight testing is inconclusive and symptoms persist. Blood is taken at intervals for measurement of glucose, insulin and C-peptide.

A plasma insulin concentration of $3\,\mu U/mL$ or more when the plasma glucose is below 3.0 mmol/L indicates an excess of insulin. C-peptide is co-secreted from the pancreas with insulin and is used to distinguish endogenous hyperinsulinaemia (e.g. as a result of an insulinoma when C-peptide levels are detectable) from exogenous hyperinsulinaemia (e.g. due to factitious insulin administration when C-peptide levels are undetectable).

Further investigations are usually necessary to localize tumours before surgery as they are often very small. These include highly selective angiography, high-resolution CT scanning, scanning with radiolabelled somatostatin (some tumours express somatostatin receptors) and endoscopic ultrasound.

Treatment

The treatment of choice is surgical excision of the tumour. Diazoxide, which inhibits insulin release from islet cells, is useful when the tumour is malignant, in patients in whom a tumour is very small and cannot be located, or in elderly patients with mild symptoms. Symptoms may also remit using a somatostatin analogue (octreotide or lanreotide).

DISORDERS OF LIPID METABOLISM (K&C 6e p. 1135)

Fats are transported in the bloodstream as lipoprotein particles composed of lipids (principally triglycerides, cholesterol and cholesterol esters), phospholipids and proteins, called apoproteins. These proteins exert a stabilizing function and allow the particles to be recognized by receptors in the liver and peripheral tissues.

Disorders o.

There are five principal types of lipoprotein particles:

- *Chylomicrons* are synthesized in the small intestine postprandially and serve to transport exogenous dietary fat (mainly triglycerides, small amounts of cholesterol) to the liver and peripheral tissues.
- *Very-low-density lipoproteins (VLDLs)* are synthesized and secreted by the liver and transport endogenous triglycerides (formed in the liver from plasma free fatty acids) to the periphery. In fat and muscle, triglycerides are removed from chylomicrons and VLDLs by the tissue enzyme lipoprotein lipase and the essential cofactor apoprotein C-II.
- *Intermediate-density lipoproteins (IDLs)*, derived from the peripheral breakdown of VLDLs, are transported back to the liver and metabolized to yield the cholesterol-rich particles – low-density lipoproteins (LDLs).
- *Low-density lipoproteins (LDLs)* deliver most cholesterol to the periphery and liver with subsequent binding to LDL receptors in these tissues.
- *High-density lipoproteins (HDLs)* transport cholesterol from peripheral tissues to the liver. HDL particles carry 20–30% of the total quantity of cholesterol in the blood.

The major clinical significance of hypercholesterolaemia (both total plasma and LDL concentration) is as a risk factor for atheroma and hence ischaemic heart disease. The risk is greatest in those with other risk factors, e.g. smoking and hypertension. There is a weak independent link between raised concentrations of (triglyceride-rich) VLDL particles and cardiovascular risk. More than half of all patients aged under 60 with angiographically confirmed coronary heart disease have a lipoprotein disorder. In addition, severe hypertriglyceridaemia (> 6 mmol/L) may induce acute pancreatitis and retinal vein thrombosis. In contrast, HDL particles, which transport cholesterol away from the periphery, appear to protect against atheroma.

Measurement of plasma lipids

Most patients with hyperlipidaemia are asymptomatic, with no clinical signs, and they are discovered through routine screening (Table 14.9). A single fasting blood sample is necessary for the measurement of total plasma cholesterol, total triglyceride and HDL cholesterol levels. Specific diag-

673

Table 14.9	Indications for measurement of plasma lipids

Coronary heart disease or other major atherosclerotic disease

Family history of coronary heart disease (especially below 50 years of age)

First-degree relative with a lipid disorder

Presence of a xanthoma

Presence of xanthelasma or corneal arcus before age 40 years

Obesity

Diabetes mellitus

Hypertension

Acute pancreatitis

Patients undergoing renal replacement therapy

Table 14.10	Causes of secondary hyperlipidaemia

Hypothyroidism

Poorly controlled diabetes mellitus

Obesity

Renal impairment

Nephrotic syndrome

Dysglobulinaemia

Hepatic dysfunction

Alcohol

Drugs: oral contraceptives in susceptible individuals, thiazide diuretics, corticosteroids

nosis of the defect (see below) requires the measurement of individual lipoproteins by electrophoresis, but this is not usually necessary. If a lipid disorder has been detected it is vital to carry out a clinical history, examination and simple special investigations (i.e. plasma glucose, urea and electrolytes, liver biochemistry and thyroid function tests) to detect the causes of secondary hyperlipidaemia (Table 14.10).

The primary hyperlipidaemias (K&C 6e p. 1137)

Disorders of VLDL and chylomicrons – hypertriglyceridaemia alone

- Polygenic hypertriglyceridaemia accounts for most cases, in which there are many genes both acting together and interacting with environmental factors to produce a modest elevation in serum triglyceride levels.
- Familial hypertriglyceridaemia is inherited in an autosomal dominant fashion. The exact defect is not known

and the only clinical feature is a history of pancreatitis or retinal vein thrombosis in some individuals.

■ Lipoprotein lipase deficiency and apoprotein C-II deficiency are rare diseases which usually present in childhood with severe hypertriglyceridaemia complicated by pancreatitis, retinal vein thrombosis and eruptive xanthomas – crops of small yellow lipid deposits in the skin.

Disorders of LDL – hypercholesterolaemia alone

■ Familial hypercholesterolaemia is the result of under-production of the LDL cholesterol receptor in the liver, which results in high plasma concentrations of LDL cholesterol. Heterozygotes may be asymptomatic or develop coronary artery disease in their 40s. Typical clinical features include tendon xanthomas (lipid nodules in the tendons, especially the extensor tendons of the fingers and the Achilles tendon) and xanthelasmas. Homozygotes have a total absence of LDL receptors in the liver. They have grossly elevated plasma cholesterol levels (> 16 mmol/L) and, without treatment, die in their teens from coronary artery disease.

■ Mutations in the apoprotein B-100 gene result in a clinical picture resembling heterozygous familial hypercholesterolaemia. LDL particles normally bind to their clearance receptor in the liver through apoprotein B-100, and the mutation results in high LDL concentrations in the blood.

■ Polygenic hypercholesterolaemia accounts for those patients with a raised serum cholesterol concentration, but without one of the monogenic disorders above. The precise nature of the polygenic variation in plasma cholesterol remains unknown.

Combined hyperlipidaemia (hypercholesterolaemia and hyperlipidaemia)

Polygenic combined hyperlipidaemia and familial combined hyperlipidaemia account for the vast majority of patients in this group. A small minority is the result of the rare condition, remnant hyperlipidaemia.

Management of hyperlipidaemia (*K&C* 6e p. 1139)

Guidelines to therapy

The initial treatment in all cases of hyperlipidaemia is dietary modification, but additional measures are usually necessary.

Patients with familial hypercholesterolaemia will probably need drug treatment. Secondary hyperlipidaemia should be managed by treatment of the underlying condition wherever possible. In all patients, other treatable cardiovascular risk factors, including smoking, hypertension and excess weight should also be addressed in tandem with treatment of hyperlipidaemia.

Lipid-lowering diet

- Dairy products and meat are the principal sources of fat in the diet. Chicken and poultry should be substituted for red meats and the food grilled rather than fried. Low-fat cheeses and skimmed milk should be substituted for the full-fat varieties.
- Polyunsaturated fats, e.g. corn and soya oil, should be used instead of saturated fats.
- Reduction of cholesterol intake from liver, offal and fish roe.
- Increased intake of soluble fibres, e.g. pulses and legumes, which reduce circulating cholesterol.
- Avoid excess alcohol and obesity, both causes of secondary hyperlipidaemias.

Lipid-lowering drugs (Table 14.11)

- HMG-CoA reductase inhibitors (statins), e.g. atorvastatin, pravastatin, simvastatin, inhibit the enzyme hydroxy-methylglutaryl-coenzyme A (HMG-CoA) reductase, an enzyme involved in cholesterol synthesis in the liver. They are more effective than other classes of drugs in lowering LDL cholesterol. Side-effects of statins include hepatitis, muscle injury (myalgia, myositis, and rhabdo-myolysis); and gastrointestinal problems (abdominal

Table 14.11 **Drugs used in the management of hyperlipidaemias (listed in the order in which they are usually selected for treatment)**

Hypertriglyceridaemia	Hypercholesterolaemia	Combined
Fibrates	Statins	Fibrates
Nicotinic acid	Ezetimibe/fibrates	Nicotinic acid
Fish oil capsules	Bile acid-binding resins (ω-3 marine triglycerides)	

pain, diarrhoea, flatulence). Liver biochemistry should be measured before and within 1–3 months of starting treatment and thereafter at intervals of 6 months for 1 year, unless indicated earlier by symptoms or signs suggestive of hepatotoxicity. Treatment is discontinued if serum transaminases rise to and persist at three times the upper limit of normal. Patients should be asked to report unexplained muscle pain, and treatment is stopped if the serum creatine kinase is greater than five times the upper limit of normal.

- Cholesterol absorption inhibitors. e.g. ezetimibe, inhibit gut absorption of cholesterol from food and also from bile. The mechanism of this inhibition is currently unclear. They mostly act in the gut and little is absorbed. Thus short-term safety is good. They may be used when a second drug in addition to a statin is required.
- Fibrates, e.g. gemfibrozil and bezafibrate, are regarded as broad-spectrum lipid-modulating agents. They decrease serum triglycerides, raise HDL cholesterol and reduce LDL cholesterol concentrations. They are the drugs of first choice for treating hypertriglyceridaemia and are also used in patients with modest hypercholesterolaemia. The exact mechanism of action is not known. A rare but serious side-effect is muscle toxicity (myositis, rhabdomyolysis).
- Bile acid-binding resins, e.g. colestyramine and colestipol, bind bile acids in the intestine, preventing their reabsorption and thus lowering the cholesterol pool. They reduce LDL cholesterol and have a synergistic effect when given with a statin.
- Fish-oils, rich in omega-3 marine triglycerides, reduce plasma triglycerides.
- Nicotinic acid reduces total and LDL cholesterol levels and can reduce triglyceride levels. It is not widely used because of side-effects.

Whom to treat

Primary prevention for people at risk of cardiovascular disease Lipid-lowering therapy using a statin, or alternatives as above, should be considered in asymptomatic individuals irrespective of the total or LDL cholesterol level in type 2 diabetes alone, or with two or more of: positive family history of cardiovascular disease, albuminuria, hypertension, smoking.

Primary prevention for people without risk factors In the absence of risk factors, lipid-lowering therapy should be considered in asymptomatic men with total cholesterol levels persistently above 6.5 mmol/L despite dietary change. Many would use lipid-lowering therapy in an asymptomatic man with this level of total cholesterol if he had a positive family history of cardiovascular disease and no other risk factors. The situation for women is less clear.

Secondary prevention In general, statin treatment is warranted for any patient with known macrovascular disease (coronary artery disease, TIA or stroke, peripheral artery disease), irrespective of the total or LDL cholesterol level. If a statin is not tolerated, a fibrate or fibrate/cholesterol absorption inhibitor combination is an alternative.

Aims of treatment

Statins reduce cardiovascular events and all-cause mortality. Treatment should be adjusted to achieve a target total cholesterol of less than 5 mmol/L or a reduction of 20–25% from baseline if that produces a lower concentration. In terms of LDL-cholesterol, the target should be below 3.0 mmol/L or a reduction of about 30% if that produces a lower concentration.

THE PORPHYRIAS (K&C 6e p. 1148)

The porphyrias form a rare heterogeneous group of inherited disorders of haem synthesis. This leads to an overproduction of the intermediate compounds called porphyrins (Fig. 14.2). In porphyrias the excess production of porphyrins occurs within the liver (hepatic porphyria) or in the bone marrow (erythropoietic porphyria), but porphyrias can also

be classified in terms of clinical presentation as acute or non-acute (Table 14.12). Acute porphyrias usually produce neuropsychiatric problems and are associated with excess production and urinary excretion of δ-aminolaevulinic acid (δ-ALA) and porphobilinogen. These metabolites are not increased in the non-acute porphyrias.

Acute intermittent porphyria

This is an autosomal dominant disorder caused by a defect at the level of porphobilinogen deaminase. It is the commonest of the acute porphyrias. Presentation is in early adult life, and women are affected more than men.

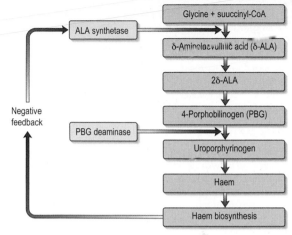

Fig. 14.2 Pathways in porphyrin metabolism.

Table 14.12	The classification of the porphyrias	
	Hepatic	**Erythropoietic**
Acute	Acute intermittent porphyria	
	Variegate porphyria	
	Hereditary coproporphyria	
Non-acute	Porphyria cutanea tarda	Congenital porphyria
		Erythropoietic protoporphyria

Clinical features

Abdominal pain, vomiting and constipation are the most common presenting features, occurring in 90% of patients (mimicking an acute abdomen, especially as there may be fever and leucocytosis). Additional features include poly-neuropathy (especially motor), hypertension, tachycardia and neuropsychiatric disorder (fits, depression, anxiety and frank psychosis). The urine may turn red or brown on standing. Attacks may be precipitated by alcohol and a variety of drugs, especially those such as barbiturates, which are enzyme-inducing drugs and increase δ-ALA synthetase activity.

Investigations

During an attack there may be a neutrophil leucocytosis, abnormal liver biochemistry and a raised urea.

The diagnosis is made during an attack by demonstrating increased urinary excretion of porphobilinogen. Erythrocyte porphobilinogen deaminase may be measured between attacks or, in some cases, urinary porphobilinogen remains high.

Management

Abdominal pain is severe and may require opiate analgesia. A high carbohydrate intake (oral or intravenous glucose) must be maintained because this depresses δ-ALA synthetase activity. Haem arginate is a stable preparation of haem and is given intravenously during an acute attack. Haem inhibits ALA synthetase (Fig. 14.2) and hence reduces levels of the intermediate precursors.

Other porphyrias

Porphyria cutanea tarda (PCT) has both sporadic and inherited forms (autosomal dominant) that are indistinguishable clinically. It presents with a bullous skin eruption on exposure to light or minor trauma. The eruption heals with scarring. Many patients with sporadic PCT have underlying chronic liver disease (particularly due to alcohol or hepatitis C infection).

Variegate porphyria and hereditary coproporphyria present with features similar to those of acute intermittent porphyria, together with the cutaneous features of PCT.

The erythropoietic porphyrias are very rare and present with photosensitive skin lesions.

AMYLOIDOSIS (K&C 6e p. 1147)

This is a heterogeneous group of disorders characterized by extracellular deposition of an insoluble fibrillar protein called amyloid. Amyloidosis is acquired or hereditary, and may be localized or systemic. Clinical features are the result of amyloid deposits affecting the normal structure and function of the affected tissue. The diagnosis of amyloidosis is usually made with Congo red staining of a biopsy of affected tissues. In systemic amyloid a simple rectal biopsy may be used for histological diagnosis. Amyloid deposits

Table 14.13 Classification of the more common types of amyloid and amyloidosis

Type	Fibril protein precursor	Clinical syndrome
AI	Monoclonal immunoglobulin light chains	Associated with myeloma, Waldenström's macroglobulinaemia and non-Hodgkin lymphoma. Presents with cardiac failure, nephrotic syndrome, carpal tunnel syndrome and macroglossia (large tongue)
ATTR (familial)	Abnormal transthyretin (plasma carrier protein)	Neuropathy and cardiomyopathy
AA	Protein A, a precursor of serum amyloid A (an acute-phase reactant)	Occurs with chronic infections (e.g. TB), inflammation (e.g. rheumatoid arthritis) and malignancy (e.g. Hodgkin's disease). Presents with proteinuria and hepatosplenomegaly

stain red and show green fluorescence in polarized light. Scintigraphy using ^{123}I-labelled serum amyloid P component is being increasingly employed for assessment.

The features of some systemic amyloid types are shown in Table 14.13.

Localized amyloid deposits occur in the brain of patients with Alzheimer's disease and in the joints of patients on long-term dialysis.

Inborn errors of metabolism

Most of the inborn errors of metabolism are rare and tend to present early in childhood. They are described in detail in *Clinical Medicine* (*K&C* 6e p. 1144).

The special senses 15

Some disorders of the eye, ear, nose and throat will be discussed in this chapter. Many conditions will be managed in specialized clinics, and the purpose of this chapter is to describe common conditions or those which need an urgent referral for further specialist management.

THE EAR

Hearing loss (K&C 6e p. 1154)

The ear is divided into three parts: an external ear, a middle ear and an inner ear (Fig. 15.1). Each part performs an important function in the process of hearing. Normal hearing requires that sound waves are transmitted through the external auditory canal to the tympanic membrane, which separates the outer from the middle ear. The bony ossicles (stapes, incus and malleus) transmit sound waves from the tympanic membrane to the fluid-filled cochlea in the inner ear. Hair cells in the basilar membrane of the

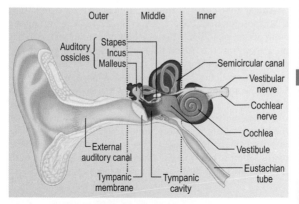

Fig. 15.1 The anatomy of the ear.

cochlea detect the vibrations and transduce these into nerve impulses which pass to the cochlear nucleus and then to the superior olivary nuclei.

The Eustachian tube connects the middle ear with the nasopharynx. It functions as a pressure-equalizing valve for the middle ear, which is normally filled with air. The Eustachian tube normally opens for a fraction of a second periodically in response to swallowing or yawning. It allows air into the middle ear to replace air that has been absorbed by the middle ear lining (mucous membrane) or to equalize pressure changes occurring on changes in altitude. Anything that interferes with this periodic opening and closing or blocks the Eustachian tube may result in hearing impairment or other ear symptoms.

Hearing loss is a common problem that affects many people at least on a temporary basis. Short-lived hearing loss occurs when flying or during an ear infection. In contrast is the permanent sensorineural hearing loss that often occurs with ageing. Deafness can be conductive or sensorineural, and these can be differentiated by the Rinne and the Weber tests (see below). Conductive hearing loss is usually related to abnormalities of the outer or middle ear. The outer ear is examined with an auroscope which may show wax or a foreign body in the external canal or abnormalities of the tympanic membrane such as perforation or loss of the normal light reflex. Sensorineural hearing loss is due to a disorder of the inner ear, cochlea, or the auditory nerve (Table 15.1).

An ear that hears normally should have air conduction that is louder than bone conduction. The Rinne test allows comparison of sound when a vibrating tuning fork, 512 Hz, is placed on the mastoid bone behind the ear (bone conduction) versus when the tuning fork is held next to the ear (air conduction). The Rinne test is normal or positive when the tuning fork placed near the ear is louder than when placed on the mastoid bone. The opposite is the case in a negative test. The Weber test is performed by placing the handle of the vibrating tuning fork on the bridge of the nose and asking the patient if the sound is louder in one ear or the other. The sound is heard equally in patients with normal hearing or with symmetrical hearing loss.

Table 15.1 Causes of deafness

Conductive	Sensorineural
Congenital – atresia	End organ
	Advancing age
External auditory canal	Noise trauma, e.g. shooting
Wax	without ear protectors
Foreign body	Ménière's disease
Canal infection (otitis	Drugs (gentamycin,
externa)	furosemide (frusemide))
Chronic suppuration	
Malignant tumours	
Benign bony growths	Eighth nerve lesions
	Acoustic neuroma
	Cranial trauma
	Inflammatory lesions:
	tuberculous meningitis
Ear drum	sarcoidosis
Perforation/trauma	neurosyphilis
	carcinomatous meningitis
Middle ear	
Otosclerosis (bony	
outgrowth of footplate	
of stapes)	
Disorders of the bony	Brainstem lesions (rare)
ossicles	Multiple sclerosis
Otitis media	Infarction

Vertigo (*K&C* 6e p. 1155)

The inner ear holds the vestibular apparatus as well as the cochlea. The vestibular apparatus provides information to the brainstem (via the eighth cranial nerve) and cerebellum regarding the static head position and turning of the head. Vertigo can arise from peripheral lesions (disorders of the vestibular apparatus or vestibular nerve) or central lesions (e.g. of the brainstem or cerebellum). Benign positional vertigo accounts for about half of cases with peripheral vestibular dysfunction. In this condition calcium debris in one of the semicircular canals (part of the vestibular apparatus) leads to recurrent episodes of vertigo lasting seconds to minutes. Episodes are provoked by specific types of head movements, e.g. turning in bed or sitting up. There is no serious underlying cause and the condition may resolve spontaneously.

Ménière's disease is due to a build-up of endolymphatic fluid in the inner ear. It is characterized by recurrent episodes of vertigo lasting 30 minutes to a few hours. It is associated with a sensation of ear fullness, sensorineural hearing loss, tinnitus and vomiting. Treatment involves the use of vestibular sedatives, e.g. cinnarizine in the acute phase, low-salt diet, betahistine, and avoidance of caffeine.

Central causes of vertigo are often vascular and may also be due to multiple sclerosis or drug-induced (e.g. anticonvulsants, alcohol or hypnotics).

THE NOSE AND THROAT

Common conditions of the nose and throat are epistaxis, nasal obstruction, rhinitis (p. 493), sinusitis (p. 493), nasal fracture, hoarse voice and dysphagia (p. 61).

Epistaxis (*K&C* 6e p. 1157)

Nose bleeds usually occur from Little's area on the septum of the nose. Local causes of nose bleeds include local trauma, nasal fractures, iatrogenic (surgery, intranasal steroids) or tumours of the nose, paranasal sinuses, or nasopharynx. General causes include anticoagulants, bleeding disorders (p. 225), hypertension and in the Osler–Weber–Rendu syndrome (familial haemorrhagic telangiectasia). Initial treatment of epistaxis is with fluid resuscitation and oxygen if necessary, compression of the anterior portion of the external nose, ice packs and leaning the patient forward. Further management includes intranasal packing or cautery of the bleeding vessel and a search for an underlying cause.

Hoarseness (dysphonia) (*K&C* 6e p. 1159)

Most cases of a hoarse voice are due to laryngeal pathology and include inflammation of the vocal cords, nodules on the vocal cords and Reinke's oedema. The latter is due to a collection of tissue fluid in the subepithelial layer of the vocal cord associated with irritation of the cords due to smoking, voice abuse, acid reflux or rarely hypothyroidism. Acute onset of hoarseness, particularly in a smoker, is a worrying symptom and is an indication for urgent referral to an ENT surgeon. It can be due to a paralysed left vocal cord secondary to mediastinal disease, e.g. bronchial carcinoma, or a carcinoma of the larynx.

Stridor (K&C 6e p. 1160)

Stridor or noisy breathing can be divided into inspiratory noise (generated by collapse of the extrathoracic airway during inspiration) or expiratory (intrathoracic trachea or below). It is a medical emergency and the help of an ENT surgeon and senior anaesthetist may be needed urgently. The causes of stridor include inhalation of a foreign body (may be sudden onset of inspiratory stridor), infections (epiglottitis, diphtheria, tonsillitis), tumour of the trachea or larynx, and trauma. If an infection is suspected, examination of the oropharynx should only be undertaken in an area where immediate intubation can take place. Severe stridor due to any cause may be an indication for either intubation or tracheostomy.

THE EYE

The red eye

Many patients with a red eye will have simple benign conditions that do not need specialist referral (Table 15.2). However, some patients will have conditions which can rapidly lead to loss of vision which may be permanent (Table 15.3). This section will discuss the differential diagnosis of a red eye based on the initial history and examination. Many patients will also require a slit lamp examination and measurement of intraocular pressures; these tests will usually be performed under specialist care once clues in the history and examination suggest the need for urgent referral (Table 15.3). The management of a patient presenting with a red eye and a history of trauma or foreign body hitting the eye is beyond the scope of this chapter and is not discussed further.

Conjunctivitis does not usually need referral for a specialist opinion unless the symptoms continue for more than 2 weeks or the eye becomes painful or vision decreases at any stage. Bacterial conjunctivitis is treated with a topical broad-spectrum antibiotic such as chloramphenicol. Conjunctival swabs for Gram stain should be taken if there is no response to treatment or in suspected gonococccal conjunctivitis (rapid onset of symptoms, copious discharge, chemosis, and lid oedema). Viral conjunctivitis is usually self-limiting. The patient is highly contagious while the eye is red, and strict hygiene and keeping towels separate from

Table 15.2 Causes of a red eye that do not need urgent referral

	Causes/definition	History	Visual acuity	Site of redness	Pupil	Cornea
Conjunctivitis	Bacterial, viral, allergic, chlamydial	Often bilateral, itching, gritty but not painful eye. Purulent discharge with bacterial infection	Normal	Diffuse ('conjunctival') redness of ocular surface	Normal	Normal
Subconjunctival haemorrhage	Spontaneous appearance of blood between the sclera (white of the eye) and conjunctiva	May occur after eye rubbing, severe coughing, rarely hypertension or blood clotting disorder	Normal	Diffuse area of bright red blood under the conjunctiva of one eye	Normal	Normal
Episcleritis	Inflammation of the episclera (thin membrane that covers the sclera). Usually idiopathic	Mild eye irritation and redness. There is no pain	Normal	Diffuse or localized injection of the visible conjunctiva	Normal	Normal

Table 15.3 Causes of a red eye requiring urgent (same day) referral to an ophthalmologist

	Causes/definition	History	Visual acuity	Site of redness	Pupil	Cornea
Corneal ulcer	Infections, autoimmune disease, exposure keratopathy, contact lens related	Pain, foreign body sensation, blurred vision, photophobia (bright light hurts the eye)	Reduced	Often 'ciliary injection': redness maximal around the edge of the cornea	Normal	Defect in corneal epithelium. More easily visible with fluorescein drops and a blue light (Fig. 15.2)
Acute glaucoma	Sudden severe rise in intraocular pressure due to reduced aqueous fluid drainage	Sudden onset of severe eye pain, blurred vision, rainbow-like 'haloes' around lights ± nausea, vomiting	Reduced	Diffuse	Semi-dilated and not reactive to light	Cloudy
Anterior uveitis (iritis)	Associated with autoimmune diseases, sometimes infectious	Blurred vision, photophobia, pain if severe	Normal or reduced	Diffuse or localized to the limbus (junction between the cornea and sclera)	Small and fixed	Normal
Scleritis	Inflammation of the sclera. Most patients have underlying vasculitis	Mild to severe eye pain	Normal or decreased	Diffuse or localized injection of the visible conjunctiva	Normal	Normal
Endophthalmitis	Infection of the eyeball after eye surgery, injury or spread via the bloodstream	Blurred vision, painful eye, photophobia, 'floaters'	Decreased	Diffuse or localized	Small and fixed	Cloudy

(a)   (b)

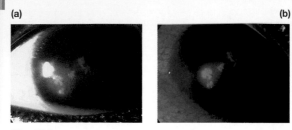

Fig. 15.2 **Dendritic ulcers on the cornea. (a)** Stained with fluorescein. **(b)** Stained with fluorescein and viewed with blue light.

other family members is necessary to reduce the chance of transmission.

Visual loss (*K&C* 6e p. 1171)

Every patient with unexplained visual loss requires ophthalmic referral. A careful history will determine if the visual loss is transient or persistent. Temporary blurring in one or both eyes or seeing 'zig-zag' lines is most commonly due to migraine (p. 760). However, these symptoms can also occur with cerebral vascular lesions or tumours and should not automatically be attributed to migraine unless there is a history of typical migraine headache, the patient is under 50 years and has no other neurological symptoms or signs. Severe temporary visual loss (amaurosis fugax) is due to a transient lack of blood supply to the retina or visual cortex and may occur with a transient ischaemic attack (p. 732) or temporal arteritis (p. 762). Urgent assessment and treatment is necessary as amaurosis fugax is a warning sign of impending blindness or stroke. Rarely, papilloedema due to raised intracranial pressure can cause transient (lasting seconds) loss of vision in one or both eyes.

The causes of sudden severe visual loss and the associated clinical features are summarized in Table 15.4. Acute uveitis and acute glaucoma present with the combination of a red eye (p. 689) and sudden or rapidly progressive visual loss; both conditions are indications for urgent referral to an ophthalmologist, as also are the conditions listed in Table 15.4. Central retinal artery occlusion is an indication for very urgent referral to an ophthalmic

Table 15.4 Causes of sudden or rapidly progressive visual loss

	History	Visual acuity	Pupils	Ophthalmoscopy
Acute retinal detachment	Flashing lights, floating spots (black or red), field loss (like a curtain coming in from the periphery)	Decreased but may be normal if macula is still unaffected. Usually a field defect	Pupil in affected eye dilates in response to light rather than constricting (relative afferent pupillary defect)	Abnormal red reflex. Detached retina looks grey and wrinkled. Normal examination does not exclude diagnosis
Retinal vein occlusion	Sudden loss of vision in all (central vein) or part (branch of retinal vein) of visual field	Acuity decreased, with visual field defect	Relative afferent pupillary defect (RAPD) if severe	Retinal haemorrhages, tortuous dilated retinal veins, macular oedema, cotton wool spots (Fig. 15.3)
Retinal artery occlusion	Sudden painless loss of vision due to clotting of the retinal artery (usually due to atherosclerosis)	Markedly reduced	Relative afferent pupillary defect	Pale retina with central macular 'cherry red spot'

Continued

Table 15.4 Causes of sudden or rapidly progressive visual loss—cont'd

	History	Visual acuity	Pupils	Ophthalmoscopy
Acute optic neuropathy	Rapidly progressive loss of vision, maybe decreased colour vision. Symptoms of underlying disease (usually multiple sclerosis or nerve ischaemia due to atherosclerosis)	Decreased	Relative afferent pupillary defect	Normal or swollen optic disc
Vitreous haemorrhage	Severe visual loss if a major bleed, floating blobs or spots if mild/moderate	Normal or reduced	No relative afferent pupillary defect	Decreased red reflex
'Wet' age-related macular degeneration	Occurs in the elderly. Sudden distortion (straight lines seem curved, central blank patch of vision) or blurring of vision	Decreased acuity with central scotoma (the macula lies in the centre of the retina and disease causes a central blank patch on field testing)	Usually no relative afferent pupillary defect	Macular oedema (swelling) and/or subretinal haemorrhages and hard exudates – due to abnormal new vessels under the macula leaking fluid or bleeding

(a)

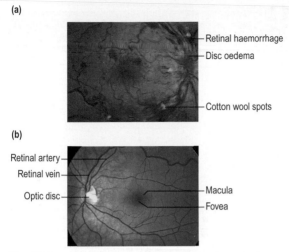

— Retinal haemorrhage
— Disc oedema

— Cotton wool spots

(b)

Retinal artery—
Retinal vein—
Optic disc—

— Macula
— Fovea

Fig. 15.3 (a) The fundus in central retinal vein occlusion compared with (b) the normal appearance of the fundus.

centre (within 1 hour). The initial history and examination of a patient presenting with sudden loss of vision is summarized in Emergency Box 15.1.

Gradual visual loss includes slowly progressive optic atrophy, chronic glaucoma, cataracts, diabetic retinopathy (p. 663), macular degeneration and chronic retinal detachment. In developing countries trachoma due to *Chlamydia trachomatis* and onchocerciasis (river blindness) due to *Onchocerca volvulus* are also causes of visual loss.

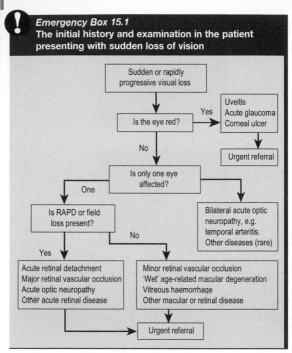

Emergency Box 15.1
The initial history and examination in the patient presenting with sudden loss of vision

RAPD, relative afferent pupillary defect
After Pane A, Simcock P (2005) *Practical Ophthalmology*. Edinburgh, Elsevier Churchill Livingstone.

Neurology 16

COMMON NEUROLOGICAL SYMPTOMS

Headache

Headache is a common complaint and does not usually indicate serious disease. In most patients presenting with headache there are no abnormal physical signs, so the diagnosis may depend entirely upon an accurate history. The causes of headache can be broadly divided according to their onset and subsequent course (Table 16.1). The underlying causes of acute or subacute onset of headache are all

Table 16.1 **Causes of headache**

Acute severe (onset in minutes or hours)
Intracranial haemorrhage
Cerebral venous thrombosis
Dissection of carotid/vertebrobasilar arteries
Meningitis
Head injury
Migraine
Drugs, e.g. glyceryl trinitrate
Alcohol
Infections, e.g. malaria

Subacute onset (onset in days to weeks)
Intracranial mass lesion
Encephalitis
Meningitis
Giant cell arteritis
Sinusitis
Acute glaucoma
Malignant hypertension

Recurrent/chronic
Migraine
Tension headache
Sinusitis
Cluster headaches

potentially serious and require urgent investigation and assessment. In a patient with acute onset of headache the following features in the history suggest a subarachnoid haemorrhage (p. 733):

- Reaches maximum intensity within seconds to minutes after onset
- Rapid onset with strenuous exercise
- The 'worst ever' headache
- Absence of similar headaches in the past
- A change in the level of consciousness.

Neck stiffness and a positive Kernig's sign indicate meningeal irritation, which usually occurs because of bacterial or viral meningitis, or subarachnoid haemorrhage. Fever may also occur with these conditions. The history and physical examination are the keys to distinguishing serious from benign causes of headache in patients with chronic or recurrent headache; most are due to tension-type headache (p. 760) and do not require further investigation. Progressively worsening headaches, or chronic headaches that change in character, may be caused by raised intracranial pressure, e.g. due to a space-occupying lesion, and require imaging by CT scan or MRI. Other features which suggest raised intracranial pressure include headache upon waking in the morning that improves with sitting up, and headache associated with nausea and vomiting (which may also occur with migraine). Ataxia, neurological deficit, papilloedema and altered mental status also indicate a potentially serious underlying cause and require brain imaging. Headache with generalized aches and pains in the elderly suggests giant cell arteritis (p. 762) and requires urgent treatment with steroids to prevent blindness.

Dizziness, faints and 'funny turns' (*K&C* 6e p. 1175)

Episodes of transient disturbance of consciousness are common clinical problems (Table 16.2). Differentiation of seizures from other disorders often depends entirely on the medical history. An eye-witness account is invaluable.

Dizziness and syncope

Syncope describes a temporary impairment of consciousness caused by a reduction in cerebral blood flow. There is usually a rapid and complete recovery.

Table 16.2 Common causes of attacks of altered consciousness and falls in adults

Syncope
  'Simple faint'
  Cough
  Effort
  Micturition
Carotid sinus
Cardiac arrhythmias
Postural hypotension
Epilepsy
Hypoglycaemia
Transient ischaemic attacks
Psychogenic attacks
  Panic attacks
  Hyperventilation
Narcolepsy and cataplexy

Dizziness or faintness precedes syncope, and represents an incomplete form in which cerebral perfusion has not fallen sufficiently to cause loss of consciousness. Dizziness should be differentiated from *vertigo* (p. 685), which is an illusion of rotary movement where the patient feels that the surroundings are spinning. It results from disease of the inner ear, the eighth cranial nerve, or its central connections.

The most frequent cause of dizziness is vasovagal syncope (a simple faint), which occurs as a result of reflex bradycardia and peripheral and splanchnic vasodilatation. Fear, pain and prolonged standing are the principal causes. Fainting almost never occurs in the recumbent position. A prodrome of nausea, pallor, lightheadedness and sweating usually precede a faint. Rapid recovery from the attack and the absence of jerking movements or incontinence of urine suggest a faint as opposed to a fit. Loss of consciousness due to an arrhythmia occurs without warning and may occur in the supine position. Syncope may occur after micturition in men (particularly at night), and when the venous return to the heart is obstructed by breath-holding and severe coughing. Effort syncope occurs on exercise and occurs in patients with aortic stenosis and hypertrophic obstructive cardiomyopathy. Carotid sinus syncope is thought to be the result of excessive sensitivity of the sinus to external pressure. It may occur in elderly patients who lose consciousness following pressure on the sinus (e.g. turning the head). Postural hypotension (drop in systolic BP ≥ 20 mmHg from sitting to standing position after 2 minutes) occurs on standing in those with impaired autonomic reflexes, e.g. elderly people, in autonomic neuropathy and with some drugs (phenothiazines, tricyclic antidepressants). Tilt table testing is performed to investigate patients with unexplained syncope in whom cardiac causes or epilepsy have been excluded. Blood pressure, heart rate, symptoms and ECG are recorded after head-up tilt for 10–60 minutes. Reproduction of symptoms and hypotension indicate a positive test.

Narcolepsy is a rare disorder characterized by periods of irresistible sleep in inappropriate circumstances. *Cataplexy* is a related condition in which sudden loss of tone develops in the lower limbs, with preservation of consciousness. Attacks are set off by sudden surprise or emotion (*K&C* 6e p. 1227).

Weakness (*K&C* 6e p. 1191)

Skeletal muscle contraction is controlled by the motor axis of the central nervous system. Muscle weakness may be due to a defect or damage in one or more components of this system, i.e. the motor cortex, corticospinal tracts, anterior horn cells, spinal nerve roots, peripheral nerves, the neuromuscular junction and muscle fibres. It is necessary to determine whether there is true weakness rather than 'tiredness' or 'slowness', as in Parkinson's disease. The site of the lesion causing true muscle weakness is often identifiable from a detailed neurological examination. The distribution of weakness, the presence or absence of deep tendon reflexes, the plantar response (Table 16.3) and related sensory defects are all helpful in localizing the lesion in the nervous system. Lesions that affect the upper motor neurone and peripheral nerve will also often involve the sensory system because of the proximity of sensory to motor nerves in these areas.

The corticospinal tracts

The upper motor neurone The corticospinal tracts originate from neurones of the motor cortex and terminate on the motor nuclei of the cranial nerves and the anterior spinal horn cells. The pathways cross over in the medulla

Table 16.3 Comparison of the clinical features of upper and lower motor neurone lesions

Upper motor neurone lesion*	Lower motor neurone lesion
Signs are on the opposite side to the lesion	Signs are on the same side as the lesion
No fasciculation	Fasciculation (visible contraction of single motor units)
No muscle wasting	Wasting
Spasticity ± clonus	Hypotonia
Weakness predominantly extensors in the arms, flexors in the legs	Weakness
Exaggerated tendon reflexes	Loss of tendon reflexes
Extensor plantar response	
Drift of the outstretched hand (downwards, medially with a tendency to pronate)	

*Acute injury to the UMN can, however, be manifested by transient flaccid weakness and hyporeflexia

and pass to the contralateral halves of the spinal cord as the crossed lateral corticospinal tracts (Fig. 16.1), which then synapse with the anterior horn cells. This is known as the pyramidal system, disease of which results in upper motor neurone (UMN) lesions with characteristic clinical features (Table 16.3). Appropriate imaging studies of the central nervous system and spine such as MRI or CT scan may be necessary to identify the primary disease.

Two main patterns of clinical features occur in UMN disorders: hemiparesis and paraparesis:

- Hemiparesis means weakness of the limbs of one side, and is usually caused by a lesion within the brain or brainstem, e.g. a stroke.

- Paraparesis (weak legs) indicates bilateral damage to the corticospinal tracts and is most often caused by lesions in the spinal cord below T1 (p. 764). Tetraparesis (quadriplegic, weakness of the arms and legs) indicates high cervical cord damage, most commonly resulting from trauma. Cord lesions result in UMN signs below the lesion, LMN signs at the level of the lesion and unaffected muscles above the lesion.

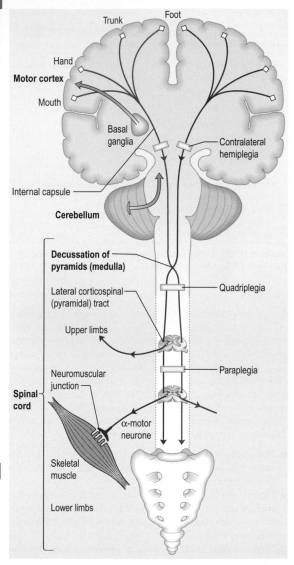

Trunk

Foot

Hand

Motor cortex

Mouth

Basal ganglia

Contralateral hemiplegia

Internal capsule

Cerebellum

Decussation of pyramids (medulla)

Quadriplegia

Lateral corticospinal (pyramidal) tract

Upper limbs

Neuromuscular junction

Paraplegia

α-motor neurone

Spinal cord

Skeletal muscle

Lower limbs

Fig. 16.1 The crossed corticospinal ('pyramidal') tracts showing cortical representation of various parts of the body.

The lower motor neurone   The lower motor neurone
(LMN) is the motor pathway from the anterior horn cell or
cranial nerve via a peripheral nerve to the motor endplate.
Physical signs (Table 16.3) follow rapidly if the LMN is
interrupted at any point in its course. Muscle disease
may give a similar clinical picture, but reflexes are usually
preserved.

LMN lesions are most commonly caused by the following:

- Anterior horn cell lesions, e.g. motor neurone disease,
  poliomyelitis
- Spinal root lesions, e.g. cervical and lumbar disc
  lesions
- Peripheral nerve lesions, e.g. trauma, compression or
  polyneuropathy.

The commonest disease of the neuromuscular junction is
myasthenia gravis, which characteristically produces
weakness of skeletal muscle and is rarely associated with
wasting. Myopathies are discussed on page 776. Weakness
of the proximal muscles, e.g. quadriceps, is typically seen
with the various myopathies. Elevation of plasma muscle
enzymes such as creatine kinase is highly suggestive of
muscle diseases. Muscle biopsy may be necessary to
determine the precise form of myopathy.

Numbness (*K&C* 6e p. 1197)

The sensory system
The peripheral nerves carry all the modalities of sensation
from nerve endings to the dorsal root ganglia and thence to
the cord. These then ascend to the thalamus and cerebral
cortex in two principal pathways (Fig. 16.2):

- Posterior columns, which carry sensory modalities for
  vibration, joint position sense (proprioception), two-
  point discrimination and light touch. These fibres ascend
  uncrossed to the gracile and cuneate nuclei in the
  medulla. Axons from the second-order neurones cross
  the midline to form the medial lemniscus and pass to the
  thalamus.
- Spinothalamic tracts, which carry sensations of pain and
  temperature. These fibres synapse in the dorsal horn of
  the cord, cross the midline and ascend as the spinothalamic tracts to the thalamus.

Common neurological symptoms

702

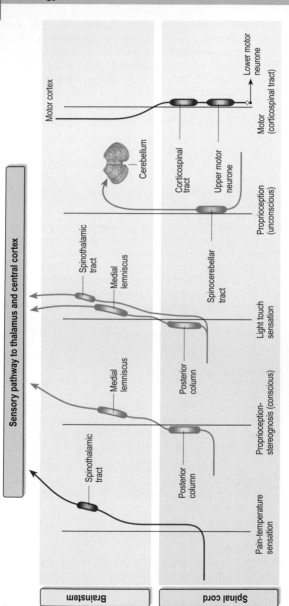

Fig. 16.2 A schematic outline of the major motor and sensory pathways.

Paraesthesiae (pins and needles), numbness and pain are the principal symptoms of lesions of the sensory pathways below the level of the thalamus. The quality and distribution of the symptoms may suggest the site of the lesion

Peripheral nerve lesions Symptoms are felt in the distribution of the affected peripheral nerve, e.g. the ulnar or median nerve. Polyneuropathy is a subset of the peripheral nerve disorders characterized by bilateral symmetrical, distal sensory loss and burning (p. 773).

Spinal root lesions Symptoms are referred to the dermatome supplied by that root, often with a tingling discomfort in that dermatome (Fig. 16.3). This is in contrast to lesions of sensory tracts within the central nervous system, which characteristically present as general defects in an extremity rather than specific dermatome defects.

Spinal cord lesions Symptoms (e.g. loss of sensation) are usually evident below the level of the lesion. A lesion of the pain–temperature pathway (spinothalamic tract), whether within the brainstem or the spinal cord, will result in loss of pain–temperature sensation contralaterally, below the level of the lesion. A lesion at the spinal level of the pathway for proprioception will result in loss of these senses ipsilaterally below the level of the lesion. Dissociated sensory loss suggests a spinal cord lesion, for instance loss of pain–temperature sensation in the right leg and loss of proprioception in the left leg.

Pontine lesions The pons lies above the decussation of the posterior columns. As the medial lemniscus and spinothalamic tracts are close together, pontine lesions result in the loss of all forms of sensation on the side opposite the lesion.

Thalamic lesions A thalamic lesion is a rare cause of complete contralateral sensory loss. Spontaneous pain may also occur, most commonly as the result of a thalamic infarct.

Cortical lesions Sensory loss, neglect of one side of the body and subtle disorders of sensation may occur with lesions of the parietal cortex. Pain is not a feature of cortical lesions.

Common neurological symptoms

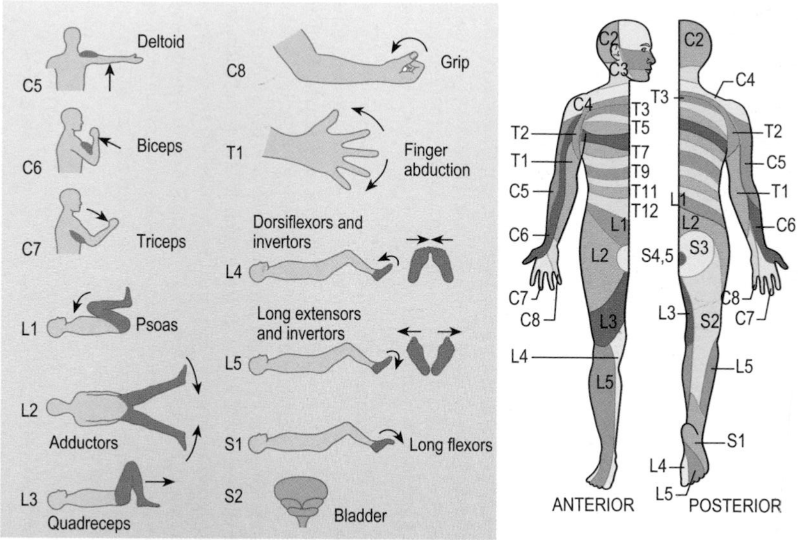

Fig. 16.3 **Simple scheme depicting motor and sensory innervation of arms and legs and root values for reflexes.** (Part of figure adapted from Parsons M (1993) *A Colour Atlas of Clinical Neurology*. London, Mosby Wolfe.)

Reflexes	Root values
Ankle jerks	S1
Knee jerks	L2, 3, 4
Biceps jerks	C5
Supinator jerks	C6
Triceps jerks	C7
Abdominals	T8–11

Tremor

Tremor is a rhythmic involuntary muscular contraction characterized by oscillations of a part of the body. A *resting tremor* is seen in Parkinson's disease, parkinsonism and Wilson's disease. *Postural tremor* occurs when a patient attempts to maintain a posture such as holding the arms outstretched. Causes include physiological (due to any increase in sympathetic activity), essential (p. 745), and in some cases of Parkinson's disease and cerebellar disease. *Intention tremor* occurs during voluntary movement and gets worse when approaching the target, e.g. during finger to nose testing, and occurs with cerebellar disease. *Task-specific tremor* appears when performing goal-orientated tasks such as handwriting, speaking or standing. In many cases the cause of a tremor will be apparent from the history and examination. Investigations include thyroid function tests, testing for Wilson's disease (in anyone under 40 years) and brain imaging in selected cases.

COMMON INVESTIGATIONS IN NEUROLOGICAL DISEASE

Blood tests

An elevated ESR or CRP may point to inflammatory conditions such as vasculitis. Comatose patients may be hypoglycaemic or hyponatraemic, and hypocalcaemia may lead to spasms and tetany.

Imaging

Skull and spinal X-rays are used to identify fractures, metastases, enlargement of the pituitary fossa or intracranial calcification.

Computed tomography (CT) is of value in identifying cerebral tumours, intracerebral haemorrhage and infarction, subdural and extradural haematoma, midline shift of intracranial structures and cerebral atrophy. However, small lesions (< 1 cm) or lesions with the same attenuation as bone or brain (e.g. plaques of multiple sclerosis) are poorly seen. In addition lesions in the posterior fossa are sometimes missed.

Magnetic resonance imaging (MRI) (p. 959) is of particular value in imaging tumours, infarction, haemorrhage, clot, multiple sclerosis plaques, the posterior fossa, the foramen magnum and the spinal cord.

Doppler studies B-mode and colour ultrasound are valuable in the detection of stenosis of the carotid arteries.

Electroencephalography (EEG) The EEG measures brain electrical activity and is recorded from scalp electrodes on 16 channels simultaneously. Its main value is in diagnosing epilepsy and it is a sensitive test for encephalopathies; different patterns are seen with different encephalopathies. Patients with epilepsy often have a normal EEG between seizures. Evoked potentials record brain responses to sound (auditory evoked potentials), touch (somatosensory) and visual stimuli (visual evoked potentials).

Examination of the cerebrospinal fluid (CSF) (See Practical procedures p. 817.) Lumbar puncture (LP) is central to the diagnosis of meningitis and encephalitis, but is also helpful in the diagnosis of other miscellaneous conditions, such as MS, neurosyphilis, sarcoidosis and Behçet's disease. It can also be used therapeutically for intrathecal injection of drugs or for removal of CSF in idiopathic intracranial hypertension. Composition of CSF in normal and diseased states is shown in Table 16.16.

Electromyography (EMG) records the electrical activity of muscles at rest and during voluntary contraction. Recordings are made by placing a small electrode needle into the muscle. EMG is usually performed in conjunction with *nerve conduction studies*, which measure the speed of conduction of impulses through a nerve. These tests are used to investigate disease of the muscles, nerves or neuro-muscular junction.

Investigation of suspected muscle disease

Measurement of serum creatine phosphokinase (CK) and aldose, EMG, and muscle biopsy for histology and immuno-histochemical staining are the three main investigations used in the diagnosis of muscle disease. Muscle biopsy is performed under local anaesthetic with a small skin incision and muscle biopsy needle. MR imaging demonstrates areas of muscle inflammation, oedema and fibrosis. It can image a large bulk of muscle and avoids the sampling error associated with muscle biopsy. Serial images can be used to assess the response to treatment. Currently it is used as well as and not in place of biopsy.

Table 16.4 Some causes of cerebellar lesions

Multiple sclerosis
Space-occupying lesions
  Primary tumour, e.g. medulloblastoma
  Secondary tumour
  Abscess
  Haemorrhage
Chronic alcohol abuse
Anticonvulsant drugs
Non-metastatic manifestation of malignancy
Spinocerebellar ataxia (rare, dominantly inherited)

COORDINATION OF MOVEMENT (K&C 6e p. 1193)

The extrapyramidal system (p. 742) and the cerebellum
coordinate movement. Disorders of these systems will not
produce muscular weakness but may produce incoordination.

The cerebellum

Each lateral lobe of the cerebellum is responsible for
coordinating movement of the ipsilateral limb. The midline
vermis is concerned with maintenance of axial (midline)
balance and posture. Causes of cerebellar lesions are listed
in Table 16.4.

A lesion within one cerebellar lobe causes one or all of the
following:

- An ataxic gait with a broad base; the patient falters to the
  side of the lesion
- An 'intention tremor' (compare Parkinson's disease)
  with past-pointing
- Clumsy rapid alternating movements, e.g. tapping one
  hand on the back of the other (dysdiadochokinesis)
- Horizontal nystagmus with the fast component towards
  the side of the lesion (p. 719)
- Dysarthria, usually with bilateral lesions. The speech has
  a halting jerking quality – 'scanning speech'
- Titubation (rhythmic tremor of the head), hypotonia and
  depressed reflexes. There is no muscle weakness.

Lesions of the cerebellar vermis cause a characteristic ataxia
of the trunk, so that the patient has difficulty sitting up or
standing.

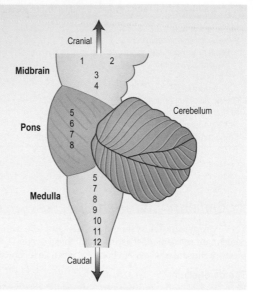

Fig. 16.4 The location of the cranial nerves and their nuclei within the midbrain, pons and medulla as seen laterally.

THE CRANIAL NERVES (*K&C* 6e p. 1179)

The 12 cranial nerves and their nuclei are distributed approximately equally between the three brainstem segments (Fig. 16.4). The exceptions are the first and second cranial nerves (nerves I and II), whose neurones project to the cerebral cortex. In addition, the sensory nucleus of nerve V extends from the midbrain to the spinal cord, and the nuclei of nerves VII and VIII lie not only in the pons but also in the medulla.

The olfactory nerve (first cranial nerve)

The olfactory nerve subserves the sense of smell. The most common cause of anosmia (loss of the sense of smell) is simply nasal congestion. Neurological causes include tumours on the floor of the anterior fossa and head injury.

The optic nerve (second cranial nerve) and the visual system (K&C 6e p. 1179)

The optic nerves enter the cranial cavity through the optic foramina and unite to form the optic chiasm, beyond which they are continued as the optic tracts. Fibres of the optic tract project to the visual cortex (via the lateral geniculate body) and the third nerve nucleus for pupillary light reflexes (Figs 16.5 and 16.6).

The assessment of optic nerve function includes measurement of visual acuity (using a Snellen test chart), colour vision (using Ishihara colour plates) and the visual fields (by confrontation and perimetry), and examination of the fundi with the ophthalmoscope. In addition the pupillary responses, mediated by both the optic and the oculomotor nerve (third cranial nerve), must be tested.

Visual field defects

There are three main types of visual field defects (Fig. 16.5):

- Monocular, caused by damage to the eye or nerve
- Bitemporal, resulting from lesions at the chiasm
- Homonymous hemianopia, caused by lesions in the tract, radiation, or a lesion in the visual cortex.

Optic nerve lesions Unilateral visual loss, starting as a central or paracentral scotoma (an area of depressed vision within the visual field), is characteristic of optic nerve lesions. Complete destruction of one optic nerve results in blindness in that eye and loss of the pupillary light reflex (direct and consensual). Optic nerve lesions result from demyelination (e.g. multiple sclerosis), nerve compression and occlusion of the retinal artery (e.g. in giant cell arteritis). Other causes include trauma, papilloedema, severe anaemia and drugs or toxins, e.g. ethambutol, quinine, tobacco and methyl alcohol.

Defects of the optic chiasm The most common cause of bitemporal hemianopia (i.e. blindness in the outer half of each visual field) is a pituitary adenoma, which compresses the decussating fibres from the nasal half of each eye. Other causes are craniopharyngioma and secondary neoplasm.

Defects of the optic tract and radiation Damage to the tracts or radiation, usually by tumour or a vascular accident, produces a homonymous hemianopia (blindness affecting either the right or the left half of each visual field) in one half of the visual field contralateral to the lesion.

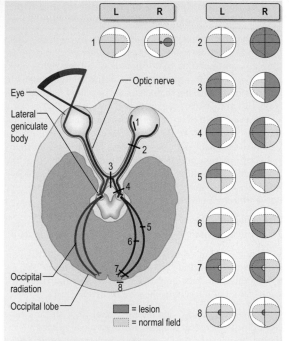

1, Paracentral scotoma – retinal lesion.
2, Mononuclear field loss – optic nerve lesion.
3, Bitemporal hemianopia – chiasmal lesion.
4, Homonymous hemianopia – optic tract lesion.
5, Homonymous quadrantanopia – temporal lesion.
6, Homonymous quadrantanopia – parietal lesion.
7, Homonymous hemianopia – occipital cortex or optic radiation.
8, Homonymous hemianopia – occipital pole lesion.

Fig. 16.5 **Diagram of the visual pathways demonstrating the main field defects.** At the optic chiasm (3), fibres derived from the nasal half of the retina (the temporal visual field) decussate, whereas the fibres from the temporal half of the retina remain uncrossed. Thus the right optic tract (4) is composed of fibres from the right half of each retina which 'see' the left half of both visual fields. Lesions of the retina (1) produce scotoma (small areas of visual loss) or quadrantanopia. Lesion at 2 produces blindness in the right eye with loss of direct light reflex. Lesion at 3 produces bitemporal hemianopia. Lesions at 4, 5 and 6 produce homonymous hemianopia with macular involvement. Lesions at 7 and 8 produce homonymous hemianopia with macular sparing at 7. (Adapted from Swash (1989) Hutchison's Clinical Methods, 19th edn. London, Baillière Tindal)

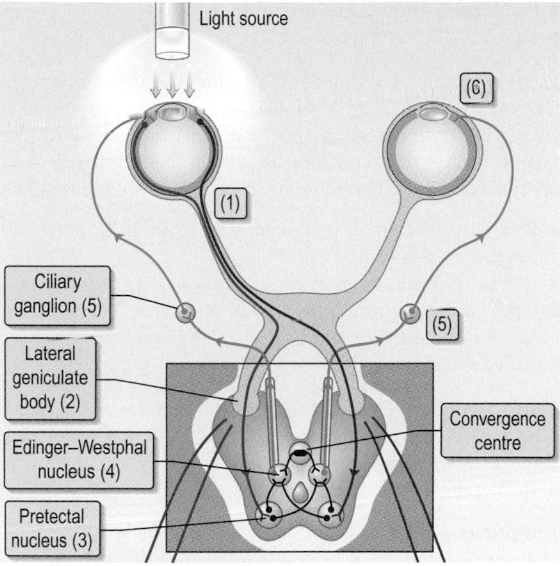

Fig. 16.6 **Pupillary light reflex.**
Afferent pathway
(1) A retinal image generates action potentials in the optic nerve.
(2) These travel via axons, some of which decussate at the chiasm and pass through the lateral geniculate bodies.
(3) Synapse at each pretectal nucleus.

Efferent pathway
(4) Action potentials then pass to each Edinger–Westphal nucleus of III,
(5) then, to the ciliary ganglion via the third nerve,
(6) leading to constriction of the pupil being illuminated (direct reflex) and, by the consensual reflex, the contralateral pupil.

711

Defects of the occipital cortex Homonymous hemianopic defects are caused by unilateral posterior cerebral artery infarction. The macular region may be spared in ischaemic lesions as a result of the dual blood supply to this area from the middle and posterior cerebral arteries. In contrast, injury to one occipital pole produces a bilateral macular (central) field defect.

Optic disc oedema (papilloedema) and optic atrophy
The principal pathological appearances of the visible part of the nerve, the disc, are:

- Swelling (papilloedema)
- Pallor (optic atrophy).

Papilloedema Papilloedema produces few visual symptoms in the early stages. As disc oedema develops there is enlargement of the blind spot and blurring of vision. The exception is optic neuritis, in which there is early and severe visual loss. The common causes of papilloedema are:

- Raised intracranial pressure, e.g. from a tumour, an abscess or meningitis
- Retinal vein obstruction (thrombosis or compression)
- Optic neuritis (inflammation of the optic nerve, often caused by demyelination)
- Accelerated hypertension.

Optic atrophy Optic atrophy is the end result of many processes that damage the nerve (see Optic nerve lesions, above). The degree of visual loss depends upon the underlying cause.

The pupils

The pupils constrict in response to bright light and convergence (when the centre of focus shifts from a distant to a near object). The parasympathetic efferents that control the constrictor muscle of the pupil arise in the Edinger–Westphal nucleus in the midbrain, and run with the oculomotor (third) nerve to the eye. The Edinger–Westphal nucleus receives afferents from the optic nerve (for the light reflex) and from the convergence centre in the midbrain (Fig. 16.6).

Sympathetic fibres which arise in the hypothalamus produce pupillary dilatation. They run from the hypothalamus through the brainstem and cervical cord and emerge from the spinal cord at T1. They then ascend in the neck as the cervical sympathetic chain, and travel with the carotid artery into the head.

The main causes of persistent pupillary dilatation are:

- A third cranial nerve palsy (see later).
- Antimuscarinic eyedrops (instilled to facilitate examination of the fundus).
- The myotonic pupil (Holmes–Adie pupil): this is a dilated pupil seen most commonly in young women. There is absent (or much delayed) reaction to light and convergence. It is of no pathological significance and may be associated with absent tendon reflexes.

The main causes of persistent pupillary constriction are:

- Parasympatheticomimetic eyedrops used in the treatment of glaucoma.
- Horner's syndrome, resulting from the interruption of sympathetic fibres to one eye. There is unilateral pupillary constriction, slight ptosis (sympathetic fibres innervate the levator palpebrae superioris), enophthalmos (backward displacement of the eyeball in the orbit) and loss of sweating on the ipsilateral side of the face. A lesion affecting any part of the sympathetic pathway to the eye results in a Horner's syndrome. Causes include diseases of the cervical cord, e.g. syringomyelia, involvement of the T1 root by apical lung cancer (Pancoast's tumour), and lesions in the neck, such as trauma, surgical resection or malignant lymph nodes.
- The Argyll Robertson pupil: this is the pupillary abnormality seen mainly in neurosyphilis and diabetes mellitus. There is a small irregular pupil which is fixed to light but which constricts on convergence.
- Opiate addiction.

Cranial nerves III–XII

The cranial nerves III–XII may be damaged by lesions in the brainstem or during their intracranial and extracranial course. The causes are listed in Table 16.5. The site of a lesion may be suggested if clinical examination shows the involvement of other cranial nerves at that site, e.g. a seventh-nerve palsy, together with cerebellar signs and involvement of the fifth, sixth and eighth cranial nerves, suggests a lesion of the cerebellopontine angle, commonly a meningioma or acoustic neuroma. In contrast, an isolated seventh-nerve palsy in a patient with a parotid tumour suggests involvement during its extracranial course in the parotid.

The ocular movements and the third, fourth and sixth cranial nerves (K&C 6e p. 1183)

These three cranial nerves supply the six external ocular muscles, which move the eye in the orbit (Fig. 16.7). The abducens nerve (sixth cranial nerve) supplies the lateral rectus muscle and the trochlear (fourth cranial nerve) supplies the superior oblique muscle. All the other extraocular muscles, the sphincter pupillae (parasympathetic fibres) and the

Table 16.5 Some structural causes of lesions of cranial nerves III–XII – according to the site of the lesion

Nerve	Brainstem (UMNL)	Intracranial course (LMNL)	Extracranial course (LMNL)
III	Infarction	Posterior communicating artery aneurysm (III)	
IV	Tumour	'Coning' of the temporal lobe (III)	
	MS	Cavernous sinus lesions, e.g. internal carotid artery aneurysm	Orbital trauma
V	Infarction	Cerebellopontine angle tumours	Neoplastic infiltration of skull base
VI	Tumour	Cavernous sinus lesions (V and VI)	Parotid gland tumour (VII)
VII	MS	Petrous temporal bone lesions (VII and VIII)	
VIII	MND		
IX	Infarction	Infiltrating nasopharyngeal carcinoma	Tumours and trauma in the neck
X	Tumour	Skull-base trauma	
XI	MS		
XII	MND		
	Syringobulbia		

MS, multiple sclerosis; MND, motor neurone disease; UMNL, upper motor neurone lesion; LMNL, lower motor neurone lesion
The nerves may also be involved by any of the causes of mononeuritis multiplex (p. 772). Diabetes mellitus particularly affects the third and sixth nerves

levator palpebrae superioris are supplied by the oculomotor nerve (third cranial nerve). Normally the brainstem (with input from the cortex, cerebellum and vestibular nucleus) coordinates the functions of these three cranial nerves, so that eye movement is symmetrical (conjugate gaze). Thus *infranuclear* (*lower motor neurone*) lesions of the third, fourth and sixth cranial nerves lead to paralysis of individual muscles or muscle groups. *Supranuclear* (*upper motor neurone*)

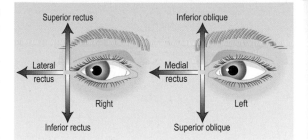

Fig. 16.7 The action of the external ocular muscles.
(Adapted from Swash (1989) *Hutchison's Clinical Methods.*
London, Baillière Tindall.)

lesions, e.g. brainstem involvement by multiple sclerosis, lead to paralysis of conjugate movements of the eyes.

A lesion of the oculomotor (third) nerve causes unilateral complete ptosis, the eye faces 'down and out', and the pupil is dilated and fixed to light and convergence. This is the picture of a complete third-nerve palsy, of which the most common cause is a 'berry' aneurysm arising in the posterior communicating artery, which runs alongside the nerve. Frequently the lesion is partial, particularly in diabetes mellitus, when parasympathetic fibres are spared and the pupil reacts normally. Less common causes are listed in Table 16.5.

In a sixth-nerve lesion the eye cannot be abducted beyond the midline. The unopposed pull of the medial rectus muscle causes the eye to turn inward, thereby producing a squint (squint, or *strabismus*, is the appearance of the eyes when the visual axes do not meet at the point of fixation). Patients complain of diplopia or double vision, which worsens when they attempt to gaze to the side of the lesion.

Isolated lesions of the trochlear nerve are rare. The patient complains of diplopia when attempting to look down and away from the affected side.

Disordered ocular movements may also result from disease of the ocular muscles (e.g. muscular dystrophy, dystrophia myotonica) or of the neuromuscular junction (e.g. myasthenia gravis). In these conditions all the muscles tend to be affected equally, presenting a generalized restriction of eye movements.

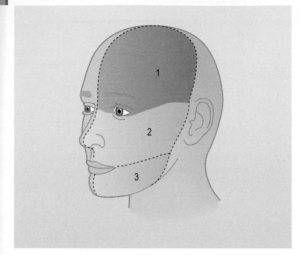

Fig. 16.8 **Cutaneous distribution of the trigeminal nerve.** 1, ophthalmic or first division; 2, maxillary or second division; 3, mandibular or third division.

The trigeminal nerve (fifth cranial nerve) (*K&C* 6e p. 1185)

The trigeminal nerve, through its three divisions, supplies sensation to the face and scalp as far back as the vertex (Fig. 16.8). It also supplies the mucous membranes of the sinuses, the nose, mouth, tongue and teeth. The motor root travels with the mandibular division and supplies the muscles of mastication.

Diminution of the corneal reflex is often the first sign of a fifth-nerve lesion. A complete fifth-nerve lesion on one side causes unilateral sensory loss on the face, tongue and buccal mucosa. The jaw deviates to the side of the lesion when the mouth is opened. A brisk jaw jerk is seen with upper motor neurone lesions, i.e. above the motor nucleus in the pons.

The facial nerve (seventh cranial nerve) (*K&C* 6e p. 1186)

The facial nerve is largely motor in function, supplying the muscles of facial expression. It has, in addition, two major branches: the chorda tympani, which carries taste from the anterior two-thirds of the tongue, and the nerve to the stapedius muscle (this has a damping effect to protect the ear from loud noise). These two branches arise from the facial nerve during its intracranial course through the facial canal of the petrous temporal bone. Therefore, damage to the facial nerve in the temporal bone (e.g. Bell's palsy, trauma, herpes zoster, middle-ear infection) may be associated with undue sensitivity to sounds (hyperacusis) and loss of taste to the anterior two-thirds of the tongue.

Lower motor neurone (LMN) lesions

A unilateral LMN lesion causes weakness of all the muscles of facial expression (cf. UMN, see below) on the same side as the lesion. The face, especially the angle of the mouth, falls and dribbling occurs from the corner of the mouth. There is weakness of frontalis, the eye will not close and the exposed cornea is at risk of ulceration. In adults, Bell's palsy accounts for about 75% of all acute LMN facial palsies (see below). Other structural causes are outlined in Table 16.5. In addition, the nerve may also be affected in polyneuritis (e.g. Guillain–Barré syndrome), when there may be bilateral involvement.

Bell's palsy Bell's palsy is a common, acute, isolated unilateral facial nerve palsy that is probably the result of a viral infection (often herpes simplex) that causes swelling of the nerve within the petrous temporal bone.

Clinical features

There is lower motor neurone weakness of the facial muscles, sometimes with loss of taste on the anterior two-thirds of the tongue. There may be hyperacusis and decreased production of tears.

Investigations

The diagnosis is clinical. The differential diagnosis of LMN facial weakness includes the Ramsay Hunt syndrome (see below) and parotid gland tumour. In addition, the facial nerve is the commonest cranial nerve lesion in meningitis associated with Lyme disease (erythema migrans on the limbs and trunk in a patient with a history of tick bite) and in sarcoidosis (often bilateral).

Management

The eyelid must be closed to protect the cornea from ulceration (either adhesive tape or, in prolonged cases, surgery). Treatment should begin immediately and is with oral prednisolone (60 mg/day reducing to zero over 10 days) and oral aciclovir (400 mg five times daily) for patients seen within 1 week of the onset of symptoms.

Prognosis

Most patients recover completely, although 15% are left with a severe permanent weakness.

Ramsay Hunt syndrome This is herpes zoster (shingles) of the geniculate ganglion (the sensory ganglion for taste fibres) situated in the facial canal. There is an LMN facial palsy, with herpetic vesicles in the external auditory meatus and sometimes in the soft palate. Deafness may occur as a result of involvement of the eighth nerve in the facial canal. Treatment is with aciclovir.

Upper motor neurone (UMN) lesions

An upper motor neurone lesion causes weakness of the lower part of the face on the side opposite the lesion. Upper facial muscles are spared because of the bilateral cortical innervation of neurones supplying the upper face. Wrinkling of the forehead (frontalis muscle) and eye closure are normal. The most common cause is a stroke, when there is an associated hemiparesis.

The vestibulocochlear nerve (eighth cranial nerve) (K&C 6e p. 1188)

The eighth cranial nerve has two components: cochlear and vestibular, subserving hearing and equilibrium respectively. The clinical features of a cochlear nerve lesion are sensorineural deafness and tinnitus. The causes of a cochlear nerve lesion are outlined in Table 16.5; however, deafness is very rare in pontine lesions. Sensorineural deafness may also be the result of disease of the cochlea itself: Ménière's disease (see below), drugs (e.g. gentamicin) and presbyacusis (deafness of old age).

The main symptom of a vestibular nerve lesion is vertigo, which may be accompanied by vomiting. Nystagmus is the principal physical sign, often with ataxia (loss of balance).

Table 16.6	Principal causes of vertigo
Labyrinth	Ménière's disease, vestibular neuronitis, benign positional vertigo
Eighth nerve	Cerebellopontine angle lesions, drugs (e.g. gentamicin)
Brainstem	Tumours, ischaemia/infarction, multiple sclerosis, migraine
Cerebellum	Acute cerebellar lesions

Vertigo

Vertigo is the definite illusion of movement – a sensation as if the external world were revolving around the patient. It results from disease of the inner ear, the eighth nerve or its central connections (Table 16.6).

Nystagmus

Nystagmus is a rhythmic oscillation of the eyes, which must be sustained for more than a few beats to be significant. It is a sign of disease of either the ocular or the vestibular system and its connections. Nystagmus is described as either pendular or jerk.

Pendular nystagmus A pendular movement of the eye occurs; there is no rapid phase. It occurs where there is poor visual fixation (i.e. long-standing severe visual impairment) or a congenital lesion.

Jerk nystagmus Jerk nystagmus has a fast and a slow component to the rhythmic movement.

- Horizontal or rotary nystagmus may be either peripheral (middle ear) or central (brainstem and cerebellum) in origin. In peripheral lesions it is usually transient (minutes or hours); in central lesions it is long lasting (weeks, months or more).
- Vertical nystagmus is caused only by central lesions.

Ménière's disease

Ménière's disease is a disorder of the inner ear in which there is dilatation of the membranous labyrinth because of the accumulation of endolymph. The aetiology is unknown and symptoms rarely start before middle age. It is characterized by recurrent attacks, lasting minutes to hours, of vertigo, tinnitus and deafness. Vomiting and nystagmus may accompany an attack. Ultimately deafness develops and the vertigo ceases. Betahistine, a histamine analogue, is useful in some cases. Recurrent severe attacks may require surgery (ultrasonic destruction of the labyrinth or vestibular nerve section).

Vestibular neuronitis

Vestibular neuronitis is believed to be caused by a viral infection affecting the labyrinth. There is a sudden onset of severe vertigo, nystagmus and vomiting, but no deafness. The attack lasts several days or weeks, and treatment is symptomatic with vestibular sedatives (e.g. prochlorperazine).

Benign positional vertigo

Vertigo occurs with turning and moving. It may follow vestibular neuronitis, head injury or ear infection, and usually lasts for some months; treatment is with vestibular sedatives.

Glossopharyngeal, vagus, accessory and hypoglossal nerves (ninth to twelfth cranial nerves) (*K&C* 6e p. 1190)

The lower four cranial nerves (ninth to twelfth) which lie in the medulla (the 'bulb') are usually affected together; isolated lesions are rare. A *bulbar palsy* is a weakness of the lower motor neurone type, of the muscles supplied by these cranial nerves. There is dysarthria, dysphagia and nasal regurgitation. The tongue is weak, wasted and fasciculating. The most common causes of a bulbar palsy are motor neurone disease (p. 770), syringobulbia (p. 767) and Guillain–Barré syndrome (p. 774). Poliomyelitis is now rare. *Pseudobulbar palsy* is an upper motor neurone weakness of the same muscle groups. There is also dysarthria, dysphagia and nasal regurgitation, but the tongue is small and spastic and there is no fasciculation. The jaw jerk is exaggerated and the patient is emotionally labile. In many patients there is a partial palsy with only some of these features. The most common cause of pseudobulbar palsy is a stroke, but it may also occur in motor neurone disease and multiple sclerosis.

UNCONSCIOUSNESS AND COMA (*K&C* 6e p. 1205)

The central reticular formation, which extends from the brainstem to the thalamus, influences the state of arousal. It consists of clusters of interconnected neurones throughout the brainstem, with projections to the spinal cord, the hypothalamus, the cerebellum and the cerebral cortex.

Table 16.7 Glasgow Coma Scale

Category	Score
Eye opening (**E**)	
Spontaneous	4
To speech	3
To pain	2
None	1
Best verbal response (**V**)	
Orientated	5
Confused	4
Inappropriate	3
Incomprehensible	2
None	1
Best motor response (**M**)	
Obeying commands	6
Localizing – use limb to resist a painful stimulus	5
Limb withdrawing	4
Limb flexing	3
Limb extending	2
None	1

The scores in each category are added up to give an overall score, which may vary from 3 (in the deeply comatose patient) to 15

Coma is a state of unconsciousness from which the patient cannot be roused. A *stuporous* patient is sleepy but will respond to vigorous stimulation. The Glasgow Coma Scale (GCS; Table 16.7) is a simple grading system used to assess the level of consciousness. It is easy to perform and provides an objective assessment of the patient. Serial measurements are particularly useful to monitor the conscious level and thus detect a deterioration which may indicate the need for further investigation or treatment. A very rapid assessment in an unstable patient is obtained using the AVPU score: **A**lert, responds to **V**oice, responds to **P**ain, **U**nresponsive. A patient responding to pain only, broadly corresponds to a GCS of less than 8.

Coma must be differentiated from persistent vegetative state (PVS; p. 961) in which sleep–wake cycles persist, brain death (p. 725) in which there is no possibility of recovery, and the locked-in syndrome in which all voluntary muscles are paralysed except for those that control eye movement. Patients in coma may progress to a PVS.

Table 16.8	Causes of coma and stupor
Toxins	Drug overdose, alcohol, anaesthetic gases, carbon monoxide poisoning
Metabolic	Hypo- or hyperglycaemia
	Hypo- or hypercalcaemia – if severe
	Hypo- or hypernatraemia – if severe
	Hypoxic/ischaemic brain injury
	Hypoadrenalism
	Renal failure
	Hepatic failure
	Respiratory failure with CO_2 retention
Diffuse neurological disease	Subarachnoid haemorrhage
	Hypertensive encephalopathy
	Encephalitis, cerebral malaria
Brainstem lesions	Tumour
	Haemorrhage/infarction
	Demyelination, e.g. multiple sclerosis
	Trauma
	Wernicke–Korsakoff syndrome
Cortical/cerebellar lesions	Tumour
	Haemorrhage/infarction
	Abscess
	Encephalitis

Aetiology

Altered consciousness is produced by three types of processes:

- Diffuse brain dysfunction due to severe metabolic, toxic or neurological disorders
- Brainstem lesions which damage the reticular formation
- Pressure effect on the brainstem such as a cortical or cerebellar lesion which compresses the brainstem, inhibiting the ascending reticular activating system.

722

The principal causes of coma and stupor are shown in Table 16.8. A common cause of coma in young adults is self-poisoning (p. 569).

Assessment

In all patients presenting in coma a history should be obtained from any witnesses and relatives (e.g. speed of onset of coma, diabetes, drug or alcohol abuse, past medical history and medication).

Immediate assessment, which takes only seconds, is essential:

- **A**irway. Clear the airway of vomit, secretions and foreign bodies. A patient not protecting their airway may need intubating.
- **B**reathing. Assess for cyanosis, respiratory rate (normal 12–20), use of accessory muscles of respiration (p. 486), chest auscultation, oxygen saturation by pulse oximetry. Consider intubation and ventilation.
- **C**irculation. Assess pulse, blood pressure and capillary refill (p. 554).
- **D**isability. Conscious level using the Glasgow coma score or AVPU.
- **E**xposure. Full examination of the patient, e.g. head injury, abdominal examination.

Further assessment The depth of coma should be noted (Table 16.7) and a full general examination carried out. Clues to the cause of coma should be looked for, e.g. the smell of alcohol or ketones (in diabetic ketoacidosis) on the breath, needle-track marks in a drug abuser, or a Medic-Alert bracelet, as carried by some diabetic people and patients on steroid-replacement therapy.

The neurological examination must include:

- Head and neck. Look for evidence of trauma, bruits and neck stiffness (indicating meningitis or subarachnoid haemorrhage).
- Pupils. Record size and reaction to light:
  - *A unilateral fixed dilated pupil* indicates herniation of the temporal lobe ('coning') through the tentorial hiatus and compression of the third cranial nerve (p. 715). This indicates the need for urgent neurosurgical intervention.
  - *Bilateral fixed dilated pupils* are a cardinal sign of brain death. They also occur in deep coma of any cause, but particularly coma caused by barbiturate intoxication or hypothermia.
  - *Pinpoint pupils* are seen with opiate overdose or with pontine lesions that interrupt the sympathetic pathways to the dilator muscle of the pupil.
  - *Midpoint pupils* that react to light are characteristic in coma of metabolic origin and coma caused by most CNS-depressant drugs.
- Fundi. Look for papilloedema, which indicates raised intracranial pressure.

- Eye movements. *Conjugate lateral deviation of the eyes* indicates ipsilateral cerebral haemorrhage or infarction (the eyes look away from the paralysed limbs), or a contralateral pontine lesion (towards the paralysed limbs). Passive head rotation normally causes conjugate ocular deviation in the direction opposite to the induced head movement (doll's head reflex). This reflex is lost in very deep coma and is absent in brainstem lesions.
- Motor responses. Asymmetry of spontaneous limb movements, tone and reflexes indicates a unilateral cerebral hemisphere or brainstem lesion. The plantar responses are often both extensor in coma of any cause.

Investigations

In many cases the cause of coma will be evident from the history and examination, and appropriate investigations should then be carried out. However, if the cause is still unclear, further investigations will be necessary.

Blood and urine tests
- Serum and urine for drug analysis, e.g. salicylates
- Serum for urea and electrolytes, liver biochemistry and calcium
- Blood glucose by immediate Stix testing and then formal laboratory testing
- Arterial blood gases
- Thyroid function tests and serum cortisol
- Blood cultures.

Radiology CT of the head may indicate an otherwise unsuspected mass lesion or intracranial haemorrhage.

CSF examination If a mass lesion is excluded on CT, lumbar puncture (p. 817) is performed if subarachnoid haemorrhage or meningoencephalitis is suspected.

Management

The immediate management consists of treatment of the cause, careful nursing, meticulous attention to the airway and frequent observation to detect any change in vital function. Naloxone (400 µg i.v., p. 581) is given if opiate poisoning (pinpoint pupils, hypoventilation, drug addict) is suspected. Flumazenil (p. 580) is given if coma is a complication of benzodiazepines. Give thiamine 100 mg i.v. to alcoholics or malnourished patients.

Prognosis

The outlook depends upon the cause of coma. A cause must be established before decisions are made about withdrawing supportive care.

Brain death

Brain death means the irreversible loss of the capacity for consciousness, combined with the irreversible loss of the capacity to breathe. Two independent senior medical opinions are required for the diagnosis to be made. The three main criteria for diagnosis are as follows:

- Irremediable structural brain damage. A disorder that can cause brainstem death, e.g. intracranial haemorrhage, must have been diagnosed with certainty. Patients with hypothermia, significant electrolyte imbalance or drug overdose are excluded, but may be reassessed when these are corrected.
- Absent motor responses to any stimulus. Spinal reflexes may be present.
- Absent brainstem function, demonstrated by:
  - Pupils fixed and unresponsive to light
  - Absent corneal, gag and cough reflexes
  - Absent doll's head reflex (p. 724)
  - Absent caloric responses: ice-cold water run into the external auditory meatus causes nystagmus when brainstem function is normal
  - Lack of spontaneous respiration.

In suitable cases, and provided the patient was carrying a donor card and/or the consent of relatives has been obtained, the organs of those in whom brainstem death has been established may be used for transplantation.

CEREBROVASCULAR DISEASE (*K&C* 6e p. 1209)

Stroke

Definitions (*K&C* 6e p. 1209)

Stroke is a focal neurological deficit (e.g. hemiplegia) lasting longer than 24 hours which is the result of a vascular lesion. Onset is usually rapid. A completed stroke is when the neurological deficit has reached its maximum (usually within 6 hours).

Stroke in evolution is when the symptoms and signs are getting worse (usually within 24 hours of onset).

A minor stroke is one in which the patient recovers without a significant neurological deficit, usually within 1 week.

Transient ischaemic attack is a focal deficit lasting less than 24 hours and from which there is complete neurological recovery.

Epidemiology

Stroke is the third most common cause of death in the UK and the most common cause of serious long-term physical disability in adults. The incidence rises steeply with age; it is uncommon in those under 40 years. It is slightly more common in men.

Pathogenesis

A stroke is caused by cerebral infarction (due to arterial embolism or thrombosis) or cerebral haemorrhage. The clinical picture of 'stroke' may also be caused by venous thrombosis, multiple sclerosis relapse and a space-occupying lesion in the brain, e.g. a tumour or abscess. In the latter the onset of symptoms and signs is usually much slower than in a stroke. In young adults one-fifth of strokes are caused by carotid or vertebral artery dissection allowing blood to track within the wall of the artery and occlude the lumen. Consider in those with recent neck pain, trauma, or manipulation of the neck. Diagnosis is by MR angiography.

Cerebral infarction (85% of strokes) may be the result of:

- Thrombosis at the site of an atheromatous plaque in a major cerebral vessel or from small vessel disease deep within the brain
- Emboli arising from atheromatous plaques in the carotid/vertebrobasilar arteries, or from cardiac mural thrombi (e.g. following myocardial infarction), or from the left atrium in atrial fibrillation.

Rarely cerebral infarction is the result of severe hypotension (e.g. systolic blood pressure < 75 mmHg), vasculitis, meningovascular syphilis, or emboli from vegetations in infective endocarditis.

Cerebral haemorrhage (15% of strokes) In most cases this is the result of rupture of an intracranial microaneurysm (Charcot–Bouchard aneurysms) in a hypertensive patient.

Risk factors

The major risk factors for thromboembolic stroke are those for atheroma, i.e. hypertension, diabetes mellitus, cigarette smoking and hyperlipidaemia. Others are obesity, oestrogen-containing oral contraceptives, excessive alcohol consumption and polycythaemia (hyperviscosity syndromes). Atrial fibrillation is a major risk factor for embolic stroke (rate 1–5% per year depending on age).

Clinical features

The history and physical examination in all stroke patients must include a search for risk factors (see above) and source of emboli (? atrial fibrillation, valve lesion, carotid bruits in the neck).

In most patients symptoms and signs develop over a few minutes and reach maximum disability within 1–2 hours. Severe headache, vomiting and coma at onset are more common in cerebral haemorrhage than infarction but accurate differentiation requires brain CT or MRI.

The neurological deficit produced by the occlusion of a vessel may be predicted by a knowledge of neuroanatomy and vascular supply (Figs 16.1, 16.9). In practice it is less clear-cut because of collateral supply to brain areas.

Cerebral hemisphere infarcts The most common stroke is the hemiplegia caused by infarction of the internal capsule (the narrow zone of motor and sensory fibres that converges on the brainstem from the cerebral cortex; Fig. 16.1) following occlusion of a branch of the middle cerebral artery. The signs are contralateral to the lesion: hemiplegia (arm > leg), hemisensory loss, upper motor neurone facial weakness and hemianopia. Initially the patient has a hypotonic hemiplegia with decreased reflexes; within days this develops into a spastic hemiplegia with increased reflexes and an extensor plantar response, i.e. an upper motor neurone lesion (Table 16.3). Weakness may recover gradually over days or months.

Occlusion of the main trunk of the middle cerebral artery produces contralateral hemiplegia, hemisensory loss and

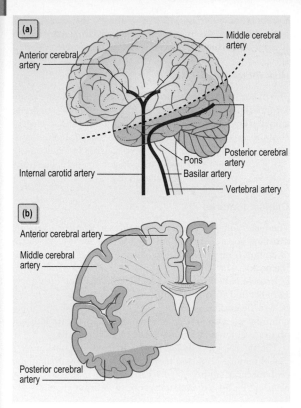

Fig. 16.9 **The arterial supply to the brain. (a)** The area above the dotted line is supplied by the internal carotid artery and the area below the line is supplied by the vertebral artery. **(b)** A coronal section through the brain. The anterior cerebral artery supplies the medial surface of the hemisphere and the middle cerebral artery supplies the lateral surface of the hemisphere, including the internal capsule.

aphasia (if located in the dominant hemisphere). Lacunar infarcts are small infarcts that produce localized deficits, e.g. pure motor stroke, pure sensory stroke.

Brainstem infarction   Brainstem infarction causes complex patterns of dysfunction depending on the sites involved:

- The lateral medullary syndrome, the most common of the brainstem vascular syndromes, is caused by occlusion of the posterior inferior cerebellar artery. It presents with sudden vomiting and vertigo, ipsilateral Horner's syndrome, facial numbness, cerebellar signs and palatal paralysis with a diminished gag reflex. On the side opposite the lesion there is loss of pain and temperature sensation.
- Coma as a result of involvement of the reticular formation.
- Pseudobulbar palsy (p. 720) is caused by lower brainstem infarction.

Multi-infarct dementia is a syndrome caused by multiple small cortical infarcts, resulting in generalized intellectual loss; there is a stepwise progression with each infarct. The final picture is of dementia, pseudobulbar palsy and a shuffling gait resembling Parkinson's disease.

Management

The first stage in management is to make the correct diagnosis through careful history taking, examination and investigation. Subsequent management is summarized in Emergency Box 16.1. Patients with a large intracerebral haematoma causing deepening coma or patients with a cerebellar infarct or bleed causing hydrocephalus should be referred for immediate neurosurgical evaluation.

> *Emergency Box 16.1*
> **Emergency management of acute stroke**
>
> **Investigations**
> - *Brain CT (or MRI).* Demonstrates the site of the lesion; distinguishes between ischaemic/haemorrhagic stroke; identifies conditions mimicking stroke, e.g. cerebral tumour or abscess. Imaging is performed within 24 hours of admission, more urgently if thrombolysis is being considered, there is a recent history of head injury, severe headache at onset, the patient is taking anticoagulant treatment or has a known bleeding tendency or the conscious level is deteriorating. If the underlying pathology is uncertain, the diagnosis is in doubt, or imaging delayed for more than 10 days after stroke, MRI is indicated.
> - *Blood glucose:* to exclude hyper- or hypoglycaemia.
> - *Urea and electrolytes.*

Continued

- *Full blood count:* to identify polycythaemia.
- *INR:* if taking warfarin.
- *ESR:* raised in the few cases of endocarditis and vasculitis.
- *ECG:* to look for atrial fibrillation, myocardial infarction.

Treatment
- *Aspirin.* Aspirin 300 mg daily should be given as soon as possible after the onset of stroke symptoms once a diagnosis of primary haemorrhage has been excluded (orally, via nasogastric tube or rectally).
- *Thrombolysis.* Intravenous tPA (alteplase) improves functional outcome if given within 3 hours of the onset of symptoms in acute *ischaemic stroke*. In the UK most patients would not reach hospital and have a CT scan within this time frame. The dose is 0.9 mg/kg over 60 min with 10% of dose within first minute. Contraindications to thrombolysis are listed on page 234.
- *Hypertension.* Blood pressure should only be lowered in the acute phase where there are likely to be complications of hypertension such as hypertensive encephalopathy, heart failure, or aortic dissection.
- *Heparin.* Low-dose subcutaneous heparin is indicated in patients with acute ischaemic stroke and at high risk of DVT (p. 235), but full anticoagulation is not indicated routinely in acute ischaemic stroke.

Supportive care
- *Stroke unit.* Dedicated stroke units improve outcome compared to management on a general ward.
- *Swallowing and feeding.* Dysphagia is common and may cause aspiration pneumonia and nutritional deficit. Formal assessment of swallowing by trained staff is essential. Feeding by fine-bore nasogastric tube or percutaneous gastrostomy may be necessary.
- *Unconscious patient.* Maintenance of hydration, frequent turning to avoid pressure sores and other measures (p. 724).

National Clinical Guidelines for Stroke (http://www.rcplondon.ac.uk/pubs/books/stroke)

Further management of the stroke patient centres on identification and treatment of risk factors and rehabilitation to restore function. Optimal care is on a stroke rehabilitation unit that provides multidisciplinary services, coordinates disability-related medical care and trains caregivers. Physiotherapy is particularly useful in the first few months in reducing spasticity, relieving contractures and teaching patients to use walking aids. Following recovery, the occupational therapist plays a valuable role in assessing the requirement for and arranging the provision of various aids and modifications in the home, such as stair rails, hoists, or wheelchairs. Patients and relatives may gain useful information and support from the UK Stroke Association (http://www.stroke.org.uk).

Carotid Doppler and duplex ultrasound scanning are indicated in patients with a cerebral infarct who may be suitable for carotid endarterectomy (see below), to look for carotid atheroma and stenosis. Magnetic resonance angiography or digital subtraction angiography should be performed if ultrasound suggests carotid stenosis. Detailed clotting studies and autoantibody screen to look for evidence of conditions associated with thrombophilia (Table 5.17) are indicated in younger patients with unexplained stroke. Echocardiography (in suspected cardioembolic stroke) and syphilis serology are performed in selected patients.

Secondary prevention This involves advice and treatment to reverse risk factors (p. 727). Control of hypertension is the single most important factor in the prevention of stroke.

- Aspirin started for the treatment of acute ischaemic stroke should be continued indefinitely at 75 mg daily. Where patients are aspirin intolerant, an alternative antiplatelet agent, e.g. clopidogrel 75 mg daily or dipyridamole MR 200 mg twice daily, is used.
- Treatment with a statin (e.g. simvastatin 40 mg daily) should be given to patients with ischaemic stroke and total cholesterol of > 3.5 mmol/L.
- Long-term anticoagulation with warfarin is indicated in cerebral infarction when there is atrial fibrillation, with some valvular lesions (uninfected) or dilated cardiomyopathy. Anticoagulation should not be started until 14 days after the onset of ischaemic stroke as bleeding may occur into the infarcted area.
- Internal carotid endarterectomy reduces the risk of recurrent stroke (by 75%) in patients who have had an infarct and who have internal carotid artery stenosis which narrows the arterial lumen by more than 70%. It is considered in patients with a non-disabling stroke who are likely to have some recoverable function.

Prognosis

About one-quarter of patients will die in the first 2 years following a stroke; the prognosis is worse for bleeds than for infarction. Gradual improvement usually follows stroke, with a plateau reached 3–4 months after stroke onset, although one-third of long-term survivors are permanently dependent on the help of others. Only 25% of patients return to a level of everyday participation and physical functioning of community-matched persons who have not had a stroke. About 10% of all patients will suffer a recurrent stroke within 1 year.

Transient ischaemic attacks (*K&C* 6e p. 1211)

Transient ischaemic attacks (TIAs) are less common than strokes but are an important predictive factor for stroke (greatest risk is within the first 72 hours) and myocardial infarction.

Aetiology

TIAs are usually the result of passage of microemboli (which subsequently lyse) arising from atheromatous plaques or from cardiac mural thrombi. The risk factors and causes of TIAs are the same as those for thromboembolic stroke.

Clinical features

There is a sudden loss of function in one region of the brain which, by definition, resolves in 24 hours. Symptoms and signs depend on the site of the brain involved (Table 16.9). The history and physical examination must include a search for risk factors and possible sources of emboli.

Table 16.9 Features of TIAs in different arterial territories

Carotid system	Vertebrobasilar system
Amaurosis fugax	Diplopia, vertigo, vomiting
Aphasia	Choking and dysarthria
Hemiparesis	Ataxia
Hemisensory loss	Hemisensory loss
Hemianopic visual loss	Hemianopic visual loss
	Transient global amnesia
	Loss of consciousness (rare)

Amaurosis fugax is a sudden loss of vision in one eye as a result of the passage of emboli through the retinal arteries. Transient global amnesia is a condition in which there are sudden episodes of amnesia associated with confusion, probably caused by ischaemia in the posterior circulation.

The investigation and management of TIAs is similar to that of stroke. Aspirin (75 mg daily) reduces the incidence of subsequent stroke and is given to most patients. Ideally patients should be assessed and investigated in a specialist service (e.g. a neurovascular clinic) as soon as possible and within 7 days of the event. Patients with more than one TIA in a week should be investigated in hospital.

Primary intracranial haemorrhage (K&C 6e p. 1216)

Intracerebral haemorrhage
This is discussed under Stroke, above.

Subarachnoid haemorrhage (SAH)
Subarachnoid haemorrhage means spontaneous rather than traumatic arterial bleeding into the subarachnoid space.

Incidence

SAH accounts for 5% of strokes and has an annual incidence of 6 per 100 000. The mean age of patients at presentation is 50 years.

Aetiology

SAH is caused by rupture of:

■ Saccular ('berry') aneurysms in 70% of cases. These are acquired lesions that are most commonly located at the branching points (Fig. 16.10) of the major arteries coursing through the subarachnoid space at the base of the brain (the circle of Willis).
■ Congenital arteriovenous malformations in 10%.

In 20% of cases no lesion can be found.

Clinical features

Most intracranial aneurysms remain asymptomatic until they rupture and cause an SAH. Some, however, become symptomatic because of a mass effect, and the most common symptom is a painful third-nerve palsy (p. 715).

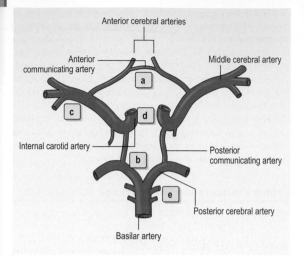

Fig. 16.10 **The main cerebral arteries showing the circle of Willis and the most common sites for berry aneurysms.** Frequency of occurrence, a–e (decreasing order): a, anterior communicating artery; b, origin of the posterior communicating artery; c, trifurcation of the middle cerebral artery; d, termination of the internal carotid artery; e, basilar artery.

The typical presentation of SAH is the sudden onset of severe headache, often occipital, that reaches maximum intensity immediately or within minutes. It is often accompanied by nausea and vomiting, and sometimes loss of consciousness. On examination there may be signs of meningeal irritation (neck stiffness and a positive Kernig's sign), focal neurological signs and subhyaloid haemorrhages (between the retina and vitreous membrane) with or without papilloedema. Some patients have experienced small warning headaches a few days before the major bleed.

Investigation

■ CT scan is the investigation of choice and should be undertaken within 12 hours, or immediately if the conscious level is impaired. It shows subarachnoid or intraventricular blood in 95% of cases undergoing scanning within 24 hours of the haemorrhage.

- Lumbar puncture (LP) is only indicated if there is a strong clinical suspicion of an SAH but the CT scan is normal. It must be performed at least 12 hours after symptom onset. An increase in pigments (bilirubin and/or oxyhaemoglobin released from lysis and phagocytosis of red blood cells) is the key finding which supports the diagnosis of SAH. Detection of oxyhaemoglobin without bilirubin makes SAH less likely. Pigments in the CSF are detected by spectrophotometry of the supernatant after centrifugation of the last fraction of CSF taken at lumbar puncture. The specimen should be protected from light.
- MR angiography is usually performed to establish the source of bleeding in all patients potentially fit for surgery.

Management

Immediate management consists of bed rest and supportive measures with cautious control of hypertension. Nimodipine, a calcium-channel blocker, is given by mouth (60 mg 4-hourly) or by intravenous infusion (1–2 mg per hour via a central line) to reduce cerebral artery spasm, a cause of ischaemia and further neurological deterioration. All patients should be discussed with a neurosurgeon. Obliteration of the aneurysm by surgical clipping or insertion of a fine wire coil under radiological guidance prevents rebleeding. Surviving patients should be advised on secondary prevention, especially on treatment of hypertension and need to stop smoking.

Prognosis

Approximately 50% of patients die suddenly or soon after the haemorrhage. A further 10–20% die in the early weeks in hospital from further bleeding. The outcome is variable in the survivors; some patients are left with major neurological deficits.

Subdural haematoma (SDH)

SDH means accumulation of blood in the subdural space following the rupture of a vein running from the hemisphere to the sagittal sinus. It is almost always the result of head injury, often minor, and the latent interval between injury and symptoms may be weeks or months. Elderly patients and alcoholics are particularly susceptible because they are accident prone and their atrophic brains make the connecting veins more susceptible to rupture. The main clinical symptoms are headache, drowsiness and confusion, which may fluctuate. The diagnosis is usually made on CT, and treatment is by surgical removal of the haematoma.

Extradural haemorrhage

Extradural haematomas are caused by injuries that fracture the temporal bone and rupture the underlying middle meningeal artery. Clinically there is the picture of a head injury with a brief period of unconsciousness followed by a lucid interval of recovery. This is then followed by rapid deterioration with focal neurological signs and deterioration in conscious level if surgical drainage is not carried out.

EPILEPSY AND OTHER CAUSES OF LOSS OF CONSCIOUSNESS (*K&C* 6e p. 1219)

Epilepsy

A seizure is a convulsion or transient abnormal event resulting from a paroxysmal discharge of cerebral neurones. Epilepsy is the continuing tendency to have such seizures.

Epidemiology

Epilepsy is a common condition, with 2% of the UK population having two or more seizures during their lives, and in 0.5% epilepsy is an active problem.

Classification

Seizures are classified clinically as partial or generalized (Table 16.10). Partial seizures involve only a portion of the brain at their onset (e.g. temporal lobe), although these may later become generalized (secondarily generalized tonic–clonic seizures).

- *Tonic–clonic.* There is a sudden onset of a rigid tonic phase followed by a convulsion (clonic phase) in which the muscles jerk rhythmically. The episode lasts typically for seconds to minutes, may be associated with tongue biting and incontinence of urine, and is followed by a period of drowsiness or coma for several hours.
- *Typical absences (petit mal).* This is usually a disorder of childhood in which the child ceases activity, stares and

---

Epilepsy

Table 16.10 **The classification of epilepsy**

Generalized seizures
Tonic–clonic (grand mal)
Absence seizures (petit mal)
Myoclonic seizures (rare form of epilepsy with involuntary
muscle jerks)

Partial seizures
Simple partial seizures (no impairment of consciousness), e.g.
Jacksonian seizures
Complex partial seizures (with impairment of consciousness),
e.g. temporal lobe epilepsy

---

pales for a few seconds only. It is characterized by 3-Hz
spike and wave activity on the electroencephalogram
(EEG).

■ *Jacksonian (motor) seizures.* These simple partial seizures
originate in the motor cortex and result in jerking movements, typically beginning in the corner of the mouth or
thumb and index finger, and spreading to involve the
limbs on the opposite side of the epileptic focus. Paralysis
of the involved limbs may follow for several hours
(Todd's paralysis).

■ *Temporal lobe seizures.* These complex partial seizures are
associated with olfactory and visual hallucinations,
feelings of unreality (jamais-vu) or undue familiarity
(déjà-vu) with the surroundings.

Precipitating factors

Flashing lights or a flickering television screen may
provoke an attack in susceptible patients.

Aetiology

No cause for epilepsy is found in over two thirds of patients.
Known causes include:

■ Cerebrovascular disease (15%)
■ Cerebral tumours (6%)
■ Alcohol-related seizures (6%)
■ Post-traumatic epilepsy (2%).

Rarer causes are hippocampal sclerosis (resection may be
possible), malformations of cortical development, vascular

malformations, hamartomas, brain abscesses, encephalitis and tuberculomas. Occasionally, metabolic disturbances such as hypoglycaemia, hypoxia, hypocalcaemia and hyponatraemia present with convulsions.

About 30% of patients have a first-degree relative with epilepsy, although the exact mode of inheritance is unknown. Primary epilepsies are due to complex developmental abnormalities of neuronal control; there are abnormalities in synaptic connections and distribution and release of neurotransmitters.

Evaluation and investigation

There are three steps in the evaluation of a patient with possible epilepsy:

1. Confirm if the patient has epilepsy. The diagnosis is often made clinically; a detailed description of the attack from an eye-witness is invaluable. Disorders causing attacks of altered consciousness must be differentiated from epilepsy (Table 16.2).
2. Determine the patient's seizure type (see classification).
3. Identify any underlying cause for epilepsy.

- The electroencephalogram (EEG) is the single most useful test in the diagnosis of epilepsy, but the recording is frequently normal between attacks. During a seizure the EEG is almost always abnormal and is shown typically by a cortical spike focus (e.g. in a temporal lobe) or by generalized spike and wave activity.
- CT or MRI should be performed in all patients other than children to exclude an underlying lesion. Even in adults, however, the pick-up rate for treatable lesions is very low.

Management

The emergency treatment is to ensure that patients harm themselves as little as possible and that the airway remains patent.

Drugs are indicated when there is a firm clinical diagnosis of recurrent seizures or a substantial risk of recurrence. Treatment is started with a single first-line antiepileptic drug (Table 16.11). The dose is increased until seizure control is achieved or tolerance exceeded. The therapeutic range of plasma drug concentrations has been established for some antiepileptic drugs and can be used together with the

Table 16.11 Recommended initial treatment depending on seizure type

Seizure type	Drug	Major side-effects of drug treatment
Generalized tonic–clonic	Phenytoin	Rashes, blood dyscrasias, lymphadenopathy
	Carbamazepine	Rashes, leucopenia
	Sodium valproate	Anorexia, hair loss, liver damage
Generalized absence	Sodium valproate	
	Ethosuximide	Rashes, blood dyscrasias, night terrors
Partial seizures	Carbamazepine	
	Phenytoin	
	Sodium valproate	

Table 16.12 Newer antiepileptic drugs and common seizure types

Drug	Partial	2° Generalized	Tonic–clonic	3 Hz absence	Myo-clonic
Felbamate	+	+	?+	?+	?
Gabapentin	+	+	?+	0	?–
Lamotrigine	+	+	+	?	+
Levetiracetam	+	+	+	0	0
Oxcarbazepine	+	+	+	+	+
Tiagabine	+	+	?	?	?
Topiramate	+	+	+	?	+
Vigabatrin	+	+	?+	–	–

+, efficacy proven/probable; 0, ineffective; –, *worsens* seizures; ?, unknown

clinical response as a guide to dosing. Idiosyncratic side-effects (i.e. non-dose related), which tend to be more common than dose-related effects, are listed in Table 16.11. Intoxication with all anticonvulsants causes a syndrome of ataxia, nystagmus and dysarthria. Side-effects of chronic administration of phenytoin (gum hypertrophy, hypertrichosis, osteomalacia and folate deficiency) are reduced by maintaining serum levels within the therapeutic range. Phenytoin is a potent hepatic enzyme inducer and will reduce the efficacy of the contraceptive pill. Many new drugs have been developed and are shown in Table 16.12.

However, there remain different views about the most appropriate drugs for each seizure type.

Gradual withdrawal of drugs should only be considered when the patient has been seizure-free for at least 2 years, and is only achieved successfully in less than 50%. Many patients will have further fits, resulting in a threat to employment and driving (see below).

Neurosurgical treatment (e.g. amputation of the anterior temporal lobe) cures epilepsy in 50% of patients with poorly controlled epilepsy and a clearly defined focus of abnormal electrical activity (< 1% of all patients with epilepsy).

Advice to patients

Patients should restrict their lives as little as possible but follow simple advice, e.g. avoid swimming alone, avoid dangerous sports, such as rock climbing, leave the door open when taking a bath. In the UK patients with epilepsy (whether on or off treatment) may drive a motor vehicle (but not a heavy goods or public service vehicle), provided that they have been seizure-free for 1 year or seizures have only occurred at night for the last 3 years. The British Epilepsy Association (http://www.epilepsy.org.uk) provides information about epilepsy for patients and relatives.

Status epilepticus (*K&C* 6e p. 1223)

Status epilepticus is a medical emergency which exists when two or more seizures follow each other without recovery of consciousness. When grand mal seizures follow one another, there is a risk of death from cardiorespiratory failure. Precipitating factors in a known epileptic include abruptly stopping antiepileptic treatment, intercurrent illness, alcohol abuse and poor compliance with therapy; 60% of all episodes occur in patients without any history of epilepsy. The initial treatment of generalized convulsive status epilepticus is with intravenous lorazepam or rectal diazepam (Emergency Box 16.2). Lorazepam may cause respiratory depression and hypotension, and facilities for resuscitation should be available. If lorazepam fails to control the seizures, an infusion of phenytoin or phenobarbital should be started. Rapid infusion of phenytoin may cause cardiac dysrhythmias, and ECG monitoring is necessary during the infusion. Paraldehyde, given rectally or by

> ## *Emergency Box 16.2*
> ## Management and investigation of status epilepticus
>
> ### General measures
> - Secure the airway: remove false teeth and insert oropharyngeal tube.
> - Administer oxygen by nasal cannula or face mask.
> - Secure venous access: many anticonvulsants cause phlebitis, so choose a large vein.
> - Glucose, 50 mL of 50% intravenously (i.v.) if hypoglycaemia is a possibility.
> - Thiamine, 250 mg i.v. over 10 minutes, if nutrition poor or alcohol abuse suspected.
> - Cardiorespiratory monitoring and pulse oximetry. EEG monitoring in refractory status or diagnosis in doubt (? *pseudostatus*).
>
> ### Control of seizures
> *First line.* Lorazepam 4 mg i.v. at 2 mg/min, repeated after 20 min. Give rectal diazepam (10–20 mg) if intravenous access difficult.
>
> *Second line.* If seizures continue, give phenytoin 15 mg/kg i.v. diluted to 10 mg/mL in 0.9% sodium chloride at a rate not exceeding 50 mg/min (average-sized adult 1000 mg over 20 min). Give a further bolus up to a total loading dose of 30 mg/kg if seizures persist. Maintenance dose 100 mg i.v. at intervals of 6–8 hours. Fosphenytoin, a prodrug of phenytoin, may be given faster and causes fewer infusion site reactions.
>
> *Third line.* Phenobarbital 10 mg/kg at a rate not exceeding 100 mg/min and repeated at intervals of 6–8 hours if necessary. Intravenous clonazepam, paraldehyde and chlomethiazole are also used in refractory cases.
>
> *Refractory status.* If seizures continue despite these measures, use tiopental or propofol general anaesthesia with assisted ventilation.
>
> ### Investigations
> - Urgent: blood glucose, serum electrolytes including calcium and magnesium.
> - Consider brain CT scan, lumbar puncture and blood cultures, depending on clinical circumstances. Serum anticonvulsant levels.

741

intramuscular injection, is occasionally used if intravenous access is difficult or where facilities for resuscitation are poor (it causes little respiratory depression). Once status is controlled, all of these drug treatments must be followed by regular anticonvulsant therapy to prevent subsequent fits. Intravenous treatment is withdrawn when anticonvulsant therapy is established.

EXTRAPYRAMIDAL DISEASE – PARKINSON'S DISEASE AND OTHER MOVEMENT DISORDERS (*K&C* 6e p. 1227)

The extrapyramidal system is a general term for the basal ganglia and their connections with other brain areas, particularly those concerned with movement. The overall function of this system is the initiation and modulation of movement. Clinically, extrapyramidal disorders are broadly classified into the akinetic–rigid syndromes, where there is loss of movement with increase in muscle tone, and dyskinesias, where there are added uncontrollable movements (Table 16.13). Parkinson's disease and essential tremor are the most common of these movement disorders.

Table 16.13 **A classification of movement disorders**

Akinetic–rigid syndromes
Idiopathic Parkinson's disease
Drug-induced parkinsonism, e.g. phenothiazines
MPTP-induced parkinsonism
Postencephalitic parkinsonism
'Parkinsonism plus'
Childhood akinetic–rigid syndromes, e.g. Wilson's disease and
    athetoid cerebral palsy
Dyskinesias

Benign essential tremor
Chorea
Hemiballismus
Myoclonus
Tic or habit spasms
Torsion dystonias

MPTP, methylphenyltetrahydropyridine

Akinetic–rigid syndromes

Idiopathic Parkinson's disease (*K&C* 6e p. 1227)

The clinical features of Parkinson's disease principally result from the depletion of dopamine-containing neurones in the substantia nigra of the basal ganglia and a relative excess of acetylcholine stimulation.

Epidemiology

The disease usually presents in elderly people, the prevalence rising to 1 in 200 in those over 70.

Aetiology

The cause of the disease is unknown. MPTP (methylphenyl-tetrahydropyridine, an impurity produced during illegal synthesis of opiates) produces severe and irreversible parkinsonism. Survivors of an encephalitis epidemic (encephalitis lethargica 1918–1930), which was presumed to be a viral disease, developed parkinsonism. There is no evidence, however, that idiopathic Parkinson's disease is caused by an environmental toxin or an infective agent, though interestingly the disease is less prevalent in tobacco smokers than in lifelong abstainers. The role of genetic factors in sporadic Parkinson's disease of older people is unclear. However, in cases with onset below the age of 40, mutations of the parkin gene on chromosome 6 are commonly present.

Clinical features

There is a combination of tremor, rigidity and akinesia (slow movements), together with changes in posture. The features of Parkinson's disease may be unilateral initially, but the disease subsequently progresses to involve both sides of the body.

- *Tremor*. This is a characteristic 4–7 Hz resting tremor (cf. cerebellar disease), usually most obvious in the hands ('pill-rolling' of the thumb and fingers), improved by voluntary movement and made worse by anxiety.
- *Rigidity* refers to the increase in tone in the limbs and trunk. The limbs resist passive extension throughout movement (lead pipe rigidity, or cogwheel when combined with tremor), in contrast to the hypertonia of an upper motor neurone lesion (p. 699), where resistance falls away as the movement continues (clasp-knife).

- *Akinesia.* There is difficulty in initiating movement (starting to walk, or rising from a chair). The face is expressionless and unblinking and may give the appearance of depression. Speech is slow and monotonous. The writing becomes small (micrographia) and tends to tail off at the end of a line.
- *Postural changes.* A stoop is characteristic and the gait is shuffling, festinant and with poor arm swinging. The posture is sometimes called 'simian', to describe the forward flexion, immobility of the arms and lack of facial expression. Balance is poor, with a tendency to fall.

Other features include dribbling of saliva, dysphagia, constipation, depression and dementia in the later stages. There is gradual progression of the disease over 10–15 years, with death resulting most commonly from broncho-pneumonia.

Investigations

The diagnosis is clinical. Investigations for other akinetic–rigid syndromes are only necessary in an atypical case, e.g. a young patient.

Management

The decision to start treatment is determined by the degree to which the patient is functionally impaired and does not alter the natural history.

Levodopa The treatment of choice is the dopamine precursor levodopa (L-dopa), in combination with a peripheral decarboxylase inhibitor, e.g. Madopar (L-dopa plus benserazide) or Sinemet (L-dopa plus carbidopa). This combined therapy reduces the peripheral side-effects, principally nausea, of L-dopa and its metabolites. Over the years, therapy may become less effective, even with increasing doses. Patients may also switch between periods of dopamine-induced dyskinesias (choreas and dystonic movements) and periods of immobility ('on–off' syndrome). This problem may be ameliorated by slow-release L-dopa; frequent small doses of L-dopa, or the addition of other antiparkinsonian drugs.

Other treatments
- Dopamine agonist, e.g. bromocriptine, lisuride, pergolide.

- Selegiline – a type B monoamine oxidase inhibitor – inhibits the catabolism of dopamine in the brain and sometimes smoothes out the effect of levodopa.
- Amantadine increases the synthesis and release of dopamine and has a weak antiparkinsonian effect.

Additional treatment Physiotherapy can improve gait and help to prevent falls. Selective serotonin reuptake inhibitors are the treatment of choice for depression. Surgery to transplant dopamine-producing cells (fetal or autologous adrenal medulla) has not produced significant clinical improvement. Information and support for patients and relatives is provided by the Parkinson's Disease Society (http://www.parkinsons.org.uk).

Other akinetic–rigid syndromes

Drug-induced parkinsonism (*K&C* 6e p. 1230)
Reserpine, phenothiazines and butyrophenones block dopamine receptors and may induce a parkinsonian syndrome with slowness and rigidity, but usually with little tremor. These syndromes tend not to progress, they respond poorly to L-dopa, and the correct management is to stop the drug.

'Parkinsonism plus'
This describes rare disorders in which there is parkinsonism and evidence of a separate pathology. Progressive supranuclear palsy (Steele–Richardson–Olzewski syndrome) is the most common disorder and consists of axial rigidity, dementia and signs of parkinsonism, together with a striking inability to move the eyes vertically or laterally. Other examples are multiple system atrophies, such as olivo-ponto-cerebellar degeneration and primary autonomic failure (Shy–Drager syndrome). There is a poor response to L-dopa.

Dyskinesias (*K&C* 6e p. 1231)

745

Benign essential tremor
This is usually a familial (autosomal dominant) tremor of the arms and head (titubation) which occurs most frequently in elderly people. Unlike the tremor of Parkinson's disease it is not usually present at rest, but is most obvious when the hands adopt a posture such as holding a glass or a spoon (p. 705). It is made worse by anxiety and improved by alcohol, propranolol, primadone (an anticonvulsant), and mirtazapine (an antidepressant).

Table 16.14	Causes of chorea
Huntington's disease	
Sydenham's chorea (see Rheumatic fever)	
Benign hereditary chorea in elderly people	
Drug induced	
Phenytoin	
L-Dopa	
Alcohol	
Systemic disease	
Thyrotoxicosis	
Systemic lupus erythematosus	
Pregnancy (chorea gravidarum)	
Other CNS disease	
Stroke	
Trauma	
Tumour	

Chorea

Chorea is a continuous flow of jerky, quasi-purposive movements, flitting from one part of the body to another. They may interfere with voluntary movements but cease during sleep. The causes of chorea are listed in Table 16.14. Treatment is with phenothiazines or tetrabenazine.

Huntington's disease

Huntington's disease is a rare autosomal dominant condition with full penetrance. Expansion of CAG repeats in the Huntington's disease gene on chromosome 4 leads to production of mutant *huntingtin* protein. It is not known how the mutant protein causes disease. There is loss of neurones within the basal ganglia, leading to depletion of GABA (γ-aminobutyric acid) and acetylcholine but sparing dopamine. Symptoms begin in middle age and there is then a relentlessly progressive course, with chorea and personality change preceding dementia and death. No treatment arrests the disease, and the management is symptomatic treatment of chorea and genetic counselling of family members.

Hemiballismus

Hemiballismus (also called hemiballism) describes violent swinging movements of one side of the body, usually caused by infarction or haemorrhage in the contralateral subthalamic nucleus.

Myoclonus

Myoclonus is the sudden, involuntary jerking of a single muscle or group of muscles. The most common example is benign essential myoclonus, which is the sudden jerking of a limb or the body on falling asleep. Myoclonus may also occur with epilepsy and some encephalopathies.

Tics

Tics are brief, repeated stereotypical movements, usually involving the face and shoulders. Unlike other involuntary movements it is usually possible for the patient to control tics.

Dystonias

Dystonias are prolonged spasms of muscle contraction. They may occasionally occur as a symptom of neurological disease, e.g. Wilson's disease, but are usually of unknown cause and occur without other neurological problems, e.g. blepharospasm (spasms of forced blinking) or spasmodic torticollis (the head is turned and held to one side or drawn backwards or forwards). The treatment of choice for many dystonias is the injection of minute amounts of botulinum toxin (which inhibits the release of acetylcholine from nerve endings) into the muscle. Acute dystonic reactions are seen with phenothiazines, butyrophenones and metoclopramide, and can occur after a single dose of the drug. Spasmodic torticollis, trismus and oculogyric crises (i.e. episodes of sustained upward gaze) may occur. Acute dystonias respond promptly to an anticholinergic drug administered by intravenous or intramuscular injection, e.g. benzatropine (1–2 mg) or procyclidine (5 mg).

Multiple sclerosis (*K&C* 6e p. 1233)

Multiple sclerosis (MS) is a chronic inflammatory, auto-immune disorder of the central nervous system in which there are multiple areas of demyelination within the brain and spinal cord. These are 'disseminated in time and place' (hence the old name 'disseminated sclerosis').

Epidemiology

MS typically begins in early adulthood and the disease is more common in women. The prevalence varies widely (6 per 10 000 in England); it is rare in tropical countries.

Aetiology

Although the precise aetiology is unknown, there is an inflammatory process against self molecules in the white matter of the brain and spinal cord mediated by CD4 T cells. Genetic factors, viruses and autoimmune mechanisms have all been implicated. However, there are no known links between MS and any infection, and whilst the disease is more common in family members, there is no clear-cut pattern of inheritance.

Pathology

The essential features are perivenular plaques of demyelination which have a predilection for the following sites within the brain and spinal cord:

- Optic nerves
- Periventricular white matter
- Brainstem and cerebellar connections
- Cervical spinal cord – corticospinal tracts and posterior columns.

The peripheral nerves are never affected.

Clinical features

The commonest age of onset is between 20 and 45 years; a diagnosis before puberty or after 60 years is rare. No single group of signs or symptoms is absolutely diagnostic. Despite this, MS is often recognizable clinically by different patterns:

- Relapsing and remitting MS (80–90%)
- Primary progressive MS (10–20% of cases)
- Secondary progressive MS – this follows on from relapsing/remitting disease
- Occasionally (< 10%) MS runs a fulminating course over some months (fulminant MS).

In the most common relapsing and remitting form, symptoms are variable and characteristically evolve over a period of days, before resolving either partially or completely within weeks. Symptoms result from axonal demyelination, which leads to slowing or blockade of conduction. The regression of symptoms is attributed to the resolution of inflammatory oedema and to partial remyelination. When damage is severe, permanent secondary axonal destruction occurs.

Inflammation of the optic nerve produces blurred vision and unilateral eye pain. A lesion in the optic nerve head produces disc swelling (optic neuritis) and pallor (optic atrophy) following the attack. When inflammation occurs in the optic nerve further away from the eye (retrobulbar neuritis) examination of the fundus is normal. Brainstem demyelination produces diplopia, vertigo, dysphagia and nystagmus. Sensory symptoms including numbness and pins and needles are common in MS and reflect spino-thalamic and posterior column lesions. Spastic paraparesis is the result of plaques of demyelination in the cervical or thoracic cord.

In some patients there will only be one or two attacks with little residual neurological deficit, and they remain very well for years. At the other extreme, in some patients an increasing neurological deficit accumulates and spastic tetraparesis, ataxia, brainstem signs, blindness, incontinence and dementia characterize the final stages. Death follows from recurrent urinary tract infection, uraemia and bronchopneumonia.

Differential diagnosis

Initially, individual plaques (e.g. in the optic nerve, brainstem or cord) may cause diagnostic difficulty and must be distinguished from inflammatory (Behçet's disease, systemic lupus erythematosus, sarcoid), mass or vascular lesions. In young patients with a relapsing and remitting course the diagnosis is straightforward, as few other diseases produce this clinical picture.

Investigations

- MRI of brain and spinal cord is the definitive investigation and shows plaques (discrete areas of demyelination and oedema), particularly in the periventricular area and brainstem. Lesions are rarely visible on CT scanning.
- Electrophysiological tests. Visual, auditory and somato-sensory evoked potentials may be prolonged, even in the absence of any past or present visual symptoms.
- CSF examination is usually unnecessary as the diagnosis is made with MRI or evoked potentials and a compatible clinical picture. Protein concentration and white cell count are raised. The IgG portion of the total protein is increased and electrophoresis reveals the non-specific finding of

oligoclonal bands, which indicate the production of immunoglobulin (to unknown antigens) within the CNS.

Management

- Short courses of ACTH or corticosteroids (e.g. i.v. methyl-prednisolone 1000 mg/day for 3 days) may promote remission in relapse, but do not influence the outlook in the long term.
- Subcutaneous administration of β-interferon reduces the relapse rate by a third in relapsing/remitting disease and may delay the time to severe debility. Treatment is prolonged, expensive and associated with side-effects, such as 'flu-like symptoms'.
- Physiotherapy and occupational therapy maintain the mobility of joints, and muscle relaxants (e.g. baclofen, dantrolene and benzodiazepines) reduce the discomfort and pain of spasticity. Multidisciplinary team liaison between patient, carers, medical practitioners and therapists is essential for any patient with chronic disabling disease. Urinary catheterization is eventually needed for those with bladder involvement. The Multiple Sclerosis Society provides information and support for patients and relatives (http://www.mssociety.org.uk).

INFECTIVE AND INFLAMMATORY DISEASE (K&C 6e p. 1236)

Meningitis nd (K&C 6e p. 1236)

Meningitis (inflammation of the meninges) can be caused by infection, drugs and contrast media, malignant cells and blood (following subarachnoid haemorrhage). The term is, however, usually reserved for inflammation caused by infective agents (Table 16.15).

Clinical features

There is usually a rapid onset of severe headache, photophobia (intolerance of light) and vomiting with malaise, fever and rigors. Neck stiffness and Kernig's sign (inability to allow full extension of the knee when the hip is flexed 90°) are usually present. Consciousness is usually not impaired, although the patient may be delirious with a high fever. Papilloedema may occur. The presence of drowsiness, lateralizing signs and cranial nerve lesions indicates the

Table 16.15 Infective causes of meningitis in the UK

Bacteria	*Neisseria meningitidis**
	Streptococcus pneumoniae*
	Staphylococcus aureus
	Streptococcus group B
	Listeria monocytogenes
	Gram-negative bacilli
	Mycobacterium tuberculosis[†]
	Treponema pallidum[†]
	Leptospira spp.
Viruses	Enterovirus (ECHO, Coxsackie, polio)
	Mumps
	Herpes simplex virus
	HIV
	Epstein–Barr virus
Fungi	*Cryptococcus neoformans*[†]
	Candida spp.

*These organisms account for most cases of pyogenic meningitis in otherwise healthy adults
[†]May cause chronic meningitis with symptoms-onset over weeks

existence of a complication, e.g. venous sinus thrombosis, severe cerebral oedema or cerebral abscess.

Acute bacterial meningitis Most cases in adults are caused by meningococci. The organism is carried asymptomatically in the nasopharynx and spread from person to person by respiratory droplets or direct spread. Meningitis occurs after the organism invades the bloodstream from the nasopharynx, to reach the meninges. Characteristically there is a sudden onset of the disease with high fever, and a petechial/purpuric skin rash is often present. In patients with fulminant meningococcal septicaemia there are often large ecchymoses and gangrenous skin lesions.

Pneumococcus is the most common cause of meningitis in elderly people, and may complicate pneumonia or other respiratory tract infections. Direct spread of the organism may occur from an infected middle ear or via a skull fracture. The features of meningitis appear rapidly and the mortality rate may be as high as 30%.

Viral meningitis is usually a benign self-limiting condition lasting for about 4–10 days. There are no serious sequelae.

Chronic meningitis presents with a long history and vague symptoms of headache, lassitude, anorexia and vomiting. Signs of meningism may be absent or appear late in the course of the disease. There is a wide range of infective and non-infective conditions including tuberculosis, *Cryptococcus neoformans*, Behçet's disease, malignancy, sarcoid and SLE.

Differential diagnosis

Conditions which can mimic meningitis include subarachnoid haemorrhage, migraine, viral encephalitis and cerebral malaria.

Management

Suspected bacterial meningitis is a medical emergency with a high mortality rate and requires urgent investigation and treatment (Emergency Box 16.3).

Notification

All cases of meningitis must (by law) be notified to the local Public Health Authority; this allows contact tracing and provides data for epidemiological studies.

Meningococcal prophylaxis

Oral rifampicin or ciprofloxacin is given to patients and close (usually household) contacts to eradicate naso-pharyngeal carriage of the organism. A vaccine for meningococcal group C and *Haemophilus influenzae* is part of routine childhood UK immunization.

Encephalitis (*K&C* 6e p. 1239)

Encephalitis is inflammation of the brain parenchyma. It is caused by a wide variety of viruses and may also occur in bacterial and other infections. In certain groups (e.g. homo-sexuals, intravenous drug abusers), HIV infection and opportunistic organisms (e.g. *Toxoplasma gondii* in patients with full-blown AIDS) are causes.

Acute viral encephalitis

A viral aetiology is often presumed, although not con-firmed serologically or by culture. In the UK the common organisms are ECHO, Coxsackie, mumps and herpes simplex viruses.

> **Emergency Box 16.3**
> **Investigation and treatment of suspected bacterial meningitis**

Note: A petechial or ecchymotic skin rash suggests meningococcal infection and is an indication for immediate treatment with benzylpenicillin: 1200 mg by slow i.v. or i.m. injection in adults. If penicillin allergic, cefotaxime 1 g or chloramphenicol 25 mg/kg i.v. Lumbar puncture should not be performed if meningococcal sepsis is suspected because coning of the cerebellar tonsils may follow – the organism is confirmed by blood culture.

Investigations

- *Head CT scan* should be performed if there is any suspicion of an intracranial mass lesion such as focal neurological signs, papilloedema, loss of consciousness or seizure.
- *Lumbar puncture (LP).* Urgent CSF microscopy, white cell count and differential, and analysis for protein and glucose concentration (Table 16.16). Ziehl–Neelsen (tuberculous) and Indian ink stain (cryptococcal infection) in immunocompromised or other at-risk individual.
- *Other.* Blood cultures, blood glucose, viral and syphilis serology.

Treatment
Note: Antimicrobial therapy should not be delayed if there is a contraindication or inability to perform immediate LP.

- Close liaison between clinician and microbiologist is essential.
- Cefotaxime 2 g 6-hourly i.v. for the initial treatment of bacterial meningitis. Add ampicillin 2 g 4-hourly or co-trimoxazole if risk of *Listeria* (elderly, immunosuppressed).
- Subsequent treatment given depending on the results of Gram stain, culture and the antibiotic sensitivities of the organism (Table 16.17).
- Tuberculous meningitis is treated for at least 9 months with antituberculous therapy (p. 527).

Clinical features

Many of these infections cause a mild self-limiting illness with headache and drowsiness. Less commonly the illness is severe, with focal signs (e.g. hemiparesis, dysphasia), seizures and coma. Severe encephalitis, which has a mortality rate of about 20% even with treatment, is most commonly caused by herpes simplex virus (HSV-1).

Table 16.16	Typical changes in the CSF in meningitis			
	Normal	Pyogenic	Viral	Tuberculous
Appearance	Clear	Turbid/ purulent	Clear/ turbid	Turbid/ viscous
Mononuclear cells/mm³	< 5	< 50	10–100	100–300
Polymorphs/mm³	Nil	200–3000	Nil	0–200
Protein (g/L)	0.2–0.4	0.4–2.0	0.4–0.8	0.5–3.0
Glucose (% blood glucose)	> 50	< 50	> 50	< 30

NB: Malignant meningitis, e.g. with lymphoma, may give similar changes to TB

Table 16.17	Appropriate antibiotics in acute bacterial meningitis	
Organism	Antibiotic	Alternative
Unknown pyogenic	Cefotaxime	Benzylpenicillin plus chloramphenicol
Meningococcus	Benzylpenicillin	Cefotaxime
Pneumococcus	Cefotaxime	Penicillin
Haemophilus	Cefotaxime	Chloramphenicol

Investigations

- CT and MR imaging show diffuse areas of oedema.
- CSF analysis shows a moderate increase in mononuclear cells (5–500 cells/mm³). Protein may also be increased.
- Viral serology of blood and CSF may identify the causative virus.
- EEG often shows non-specific slow-wave activity.

Treatment

Suspected herpes simplex encephalitis is immediately treated with intravenous aciclovir (10 mg/kg every 8 hours). If the patient is in a coma the prognosis is poor, whether or not treatment is given.

Intracranial abscesses (*K&C* 6e p. 1243)

An abscess may develop in the epidural, subdural or intracerebral sites. Epidural abscesses are uncommon; subdural abscess presents similarly to intracerebral abscess (see below).

Cerebral abscess

Cerebral abscess may follow the direct spread of organisms from a skull fracture or a focus of infection in the paranasal sinuses or middle ear. Alternatively, haematogenous spread of infection may occur from the lung (e.g. bronchiectasis), heart (e.g. endocarditis) or bone (e.g. osteomyelitis). Frequently no cause is found. The most common organisms are streptococci, *Bacteroides* spp., staphylococci and enterobacteria. Infection with tubercle bacilli may result in chronic caseating granulomata (tuberculomas) presenting as intracranial mass lesions.

Clinical features

Presenting features include fever, seizures, focal neurological signs, and symptoms and signs of raised intracranial pressure (p. 758).

Investigations

CT or MRI will usually outline the abscess. Lumbar puncture is not performed if an abscess is suspected because of the danger of coning in the presence of raised intracranial pressure (p. 818).

Management

Treatment involves a combination of intravenous antibiotics and surgical drainage.

Neurosyphilis (*K&C* 6e p. 1240)

Syphilis is described on page 46. Neurosyphilis occurs late in the course of untreated infection. It is now rarely seen in the UK because most cases of syphilis are recognized in the early stages and treated with penicillin. The different clinical syndromes (summarized in Table 16.18) may occur alone or in combination.

Management

Treatment is with parenteral benzylpenicillin for 3 weeks, which may arrest (but not reverse) the neurological disease.

Table 16.18	The clinical syndromes of neurosyphilis
Asymptomatic neurosyphilis	Positive CSF serology without symptoms or signs
Meningovascular syphilis 3–4 years after primary infection	Subacute meningitis with cranial nerve palsies and papilloedema. Raised intracranial pressure and focal deficits caused by an expanding intracranial mass (gumma). Paraparesis caused by spinal meningovasculitis
General paralysis of the insane 10–15 years after primary infection	Progressive dementia Brisk reflexes Extensor plantar responses Tremor
Tabes dorsalis 10–35 years after primary infection (caused by demyelination in the dorsal roots)	Lightning pains: short, sharp, stabbing pains in the legs. Ataxia loss of reflexes and sensory loss. Neuropathic joints (Charcot's joints), Argyll Robertson pupils (p. 713), ptosis and optic atrophy

Transmissible spongiform encephalopathy (Creutzfeldt–Jakob disease (CJD)) (*K&C* 6e p. 1242)

This is a progressive dementia, usually developing after 50 years of age, characterized pathologically by spongiform changes in the brain. It is one example of a prion (a proteinaceous infectious particle) disease and the pathology is similar to bovine spongiform encephalopathy (BSE) of cattle. The transmissible agent is resistant to many of the usual processes that destroy proteins. CJD occurs as a sporadic form or an iatrogenic form as a result of contaminated material such as corneal grafts or human growth hormone. There is no known treatment and death is invariable, usually within 6 months of onset.

Variant CJD (vCJD) presents with neuropsychiatric symptoms, followed by ataxia and dementia, and affects a younger age group. Diagnosis can be confirmed by tonsillar biopsy and CSF gel electrophoresis. vCJD and BSE are caused by the same prion strain as a result of transmission

Table 16.19 Relative frequency of the most common intracranial tumours in adults

Tumour	Relative frequency (%)
Primary malignant	35
Glioma	
Embryonal tumours, e.g. medulloblastoma	
Lymphoma	
Benign	15
Meningioma	
Neurofibroma	
Metastases	50
Bronchus	
Breast	
Stomach	
Prostate	
Thyroid	
Kidney	

Gliomas, meningiomas and embryonal tumours account for 95% of primary brain tumours

from the animal to the human food chain, with infection from BSE-infected cattle to humans.

INTRACRANIAL TUMOURS (*K&C* 6e p. 1243)

Primary intracranial tumours account for 10% of all neoplasms, and in the UK about half of all intracranial tumours are metastatic. Primary intracranial tumours may be derived from the skull itself, from any of the structures lying within it, or from their tissue precursors. They may be malignant on histological investigation but rarely metastasize outside the brain. The most common intracranial tumours occurring in adults are listed in Table 16.19. Pituitary tumours are discussed separately on page 590.

757

Clinical features

The clinical features of a cerebral tumour are the result of the following:

- Progressive focal neurological deficit
- Raised intracranial pressure
- Focal or generalized epilepsy.

Neurological deficit is the result of a mass effect of the tumour and surrounding cerebral oedema. The deficit depends on the site of the tumour, e.g. a frontal lobe tumour will initially cause personality change, apathy and intellectual deterioration. Subsequent involvement of the frontal speech area and motor cortex produces expressive aphasia and hemiparesis. Rapidly growing tumours destroy cerebral tissue, and loss of function is an early feature.

Raised intracranial pressure produces headache, vomiting and papilloedema. The headache is typically most severe on waking and decreases as the patient stands up, thereby lowering intracranial pressure. It is made worse by coughing, straining and sneezing.

As the tumour grows there is downward displacement of the brain and pressure on the brainstem, causing drowsiness, which progresses eventually to respiratory depression, bradycardia, coma and death.

Distortion of normal structures at a distance from the growing tumour leads to focal neurological signs (false localizing signs). The most common are a third and sixth cranial nerve palsy (p. 715) resulting from stretching of the nerves by downward displacement of the temporal lobes.

Epilepsy Fits may be generalized or partial in nature. The site of origin of a partial seizure is frequently of value in localization.

Differential diagnosis

The main differential is from other intracranial mass lesions (cerebral abscess, tuberculoma, subdural haematoma and intracranial haematoma) and a stroke, which may have an identical clinical presentation. Benign (idiopathic) intracranial hypertension presents with headache and papilloedema in young obese females. Neuroimaging is normal but at lumbar puncture shows there is raised CSF pressure.

Investigations

■ Radiology. CT with contrast enhancement is the investigation of choice when a tumour is suspected. MRI is of particular value in investigation of tumours of the posterior fossa and brainstem. MR angiography is sometimes necessary to define the site or blood supply of a mass, particularly if surgery is planned. Positron emission tomography (PET) is helpful in grading gliomas Plain skull X-rays are rarely of diagnostic value, with the exception of pituitary tumours.

■ Other investigations. These include routine tests, e.g. chest X-ray if metastatic disease is suspected. Lumbar puncture and examination of the CSF is contraindicated with the possibility of an intracranial mass lesion because of danger of immediate herniation of the cerebellar tonsils, impaction within the foramen magnum and compression of the brainstem ('coning').

Management

■ Surgery. Surgical exploration, and either biopsy or removal of the mass, is usually carried out to ascertain its nature. Some benign tumours, e.g. meningiomas, can be removed in their entirety without unacceptable damage to surrounding structures.

■ Radiotherapy is usually recommended for gliomas and radiosensitive metastases.

■ Medical treatment. Cerebral oedema surrounding a tumour is rapidly reduced by corticosteroids; i.v. or oral dexamethasone is given. Epilepsy is treated with anti-convulsants. Chemotherapy has little real value in the majority of primary or secondary brain tumours though vincristine, procarbazine and temozolamide are used The prognosis is very poor in patients with malignant tumours, with only 50% survival at 2 years for high-grade gliomas.

HYDROCEPHALUS (K&C 6e p. 1246)

Hydrocephalus is a condition marked by an excessive amount of CSF within the cranium. CSF is produced in the cerebral ventricles and normally flows downward into the central canal of the spinal cord and then out into the subarachnoid space, from where it is reabsorbed. Hydro-cephalus occurs when there is obstruction to the outflow of CSF; rarely it is the result of increased production of CSF.

Aetiology

In children, hydrocephalus may be caused by a congenital malformation of the brain (e.g. Arnold–Chiari malformation), meningitis or haemorrhage causing obstruction to the flow of CSF. In adults hydrocephalus is caused by:

- A late presentation of a congenital malformation
- Cerebral tumours in the posterior fossa or brainstem which obstruct the aqueduct or fourth-ventricle outflow
- Subarachnoid haemorrhage, head injury and meningitis
- Normal-pressure hydrocephalus, in which there is dilatation of the cerebral ventricles without signs of raised intracranial pressure. It presents in elderly people with dementia, urinary incontinence and ataxia.

Clinical features

The features are of headache, vomiting and papilloedema caused by raised intracranial pressure. There may be ataxia and bilateral pyramidal signs.

Management

Treatment is by the surgical insertion of a shunt between the ventricles and the right atrium or peritoneum (ventriculoatrial or ventriculoperitoneal).

HEADACHE, MIGRAINE AND FACIAL PAIN (*K&C* 6e p. 1247)

Tension headache (*K&C* 6e p. 1247)

Tension headaches feel like pressure or tightness all around the head and there are no associated features of migraine (aura, nausea, photophobia). The precise pathophysiology is not known. Treatment consists of reassurance, simple analgesia such as paracetamol, and tricyclic antidepressants for patients with chronic headaches requiring daily analgesics.

Migraine (*K&C* 6e p. 1247)

Migraine is recurrent headache associated with both visual and gastrointestinal disturbance; in spite of the origin of the word, it does not invariably mean unilateral headache.

Epidemiology

The prevalence of migraine is approximately 10%; some patients have a strong family history. Onset is usually before the age of 30 years.

Pathogenesis

The cause of migraine remains controversial. The headache is due to vasodilatation or oedema of blood vessels, with stimulation of the nerve endings near affected extracranial meningeal arteries. Release of vasoactive substances such as nitric oxide, 5-hydroxytryptamine, and the neuropeptide calcitonin-gene-related peptide (CGRP) are all thought to play a role in the pathogenesis.

Clinical features

The diagnosis of migraine is clinical. The headache is throbbing and often unilateral and accompanied by nausea, vomiting and photophobia It may last for some days and is made worse by physical exertion. Auras represent progressive neurological deficits or disturbances with usually complete recovery in less than 1 hour. They are usually visual: scotomata, unilateral blindness, hemianopic field loss, flashes and fortification spectra. Other aura include aphasia, tingling, numbness and weakness of one side of the body. Typically headache follows the aura; occasionally they occur together. Migraine may also occur without an aura. The prodrome of migraine should be differentiated from the aura. A prodrome can last from hours to days and is usually associated with changes in mood and appetite and with fluid retention. The most common way in which a migraine attack resolves is through sleep.

Differential diagnosis

The sudden onset of headache may be similar to meningitis or subarachnoid haemorrhage. The hemiplegic, visual and hemisensory symptoms must be distinguished from thromboembolic TIAs. In TIAs the maximum deficit is present immediately and headache is unusual (p. 732).

Management

General measures Patients should avoid precipitating factors (chocolate, cheese, too much or too little sleep). Women taking the oral contraceptive pill may be helped by stopping the drug or changing the brand.

Treatment of the acute attack

■ Simple analgesia, e.g. paracetamol, and an antiemetic, e.g. metoclopramide, may be all that is necessary for many patients.
■ Triptans, e.g. sumatriptan, naratriptan, zolmitriptan and rizatriptan, are 5-HT$_1$ agonists and constrict the cranial arteries. They are used in patients not responding to simple analgesia and may be given orally, by subcutaneous injection or intranasal spray.
■ Ergotamine is less commonly used since the introduction of triptans. It may be given orally, rectally, intravenously or by nasal inhalation. Triptans and ergotamine are contraindicated in patients with ischaemic heart disease and peripheral vascular disease.

Prophylaxis   Prophylaxis is indicated for frequent attacks (more than two per month) which do not respond rapidly to treatment. The options are:

■ β-Blockers, e.g. propranolol
■ Serotonin antagonists: pizotifen and methysergide
■ Amitriptyline at night is sometimes helpful.

An occasional side-effect of methysergide is retroperitoneal fibrosis, which precludes its use for more than 6 months.

Giant cell arteritis (cranial or temporal arteritis) (*K&C* 6e p. 1249)

This is a granulomatous arteritis of unknown aetiology occurring chiefly in those over the age of 60 and affecting in particular the extradural arteries. Giant cell arteritis is closely related to polymyalgia rheumatica (p. 289) and these can occur in the same patient.

Clinical features

There is headache, scalp tenderness (e.g. on combing the hair) and occasionally pain in the jaw and mouth which is characteristically worse on eating (jaw claudication). The superficial temporal artery may become tender, firm and pulseless. Visual loss, caused by inflammation and occlusion of the ciliary and/or central retinal artery, occurs in 25% of untreated cases. Systemic features include weight loss, malaise and a low-grade fever.

Investigations

■ ESR is always elevated > 50 mm/h.
■ Full blood count may show a normochromic, normocytic anaemia
■ Histology. A temporal artery biopsy, which can be performed under local anaesthetic, usually confirms the diagnosis. However, the granulomatous changes may be patchy and therefore missed.

Management

High doses of steroids (oral prednisolone, initially 60–100 mg daily) should be started immediately in a patient with typical features, and a temporal artery biopsy obtained as soon as possible (the histological changes remain for up to a week after starting treatment). The steroid dose is gradually reduced, guided by symptoms and the ESR. Long-term steroids may be needed because the risk of visual loss persists.

Facial pain (*K&C* 6e p. 1248)

The face is richly supplied with pain-sensitive structures – the teeth, gums, sinuses, temporomandibular joints, jaws and eyes – disease of which causes facial pain. Trigeminal (fifth) nerve lesions (Table 16.5) may also present with facial pain, and this is suggested by the presence of trigeminal sensory or motor loss on physical examination.

Cluster headaches (migrainous neuralgia) (*K&C* 6e p. 1248)

Cluster headaches are characterized by recurrent headaches that occur for weeks or months at a time followed by periods of remission. Men are affected more commonly than women with a peak age of onset of 20–50 years. There is a rapid onset of severe unilateral headache which often begins around the eye or temple and usually lasts less than 1–2 hours. Cluster headaches are associated with ipsilateral lacrimation and redness of the eye, rhinorrhoea, and Horner's syndrome. Treatment of an acute attack is with triptans or inhalation of 100% oxygen. Verapamil, topiramate and lithium sometimes prevent attacks.

Trigeminal neuralgia

Trigeminal neuralgia (tic douloureux) is of unknown cause, seen most commonly in old age, and is almost always unilateral.

Clinical features

Severe paroxysms of knife-like pain occur in one or more divisions of the trigeminal nerve (p. 716), although rarely in the ophthalmic division. Each paroxysm is stereotyped, brought on by stimulation of a specific 'trigger zone' in the face. The stimuli may be minimal, and include washing, shaving and eating. There are no objective physical signs and the diagnosis is based on the history.

Management

The anticonvulsant carbamazepine suppresses attacks in most patients. If this fails, thermocoagulation of the trigeminal ganglion or section of the sensory division may be necessary.

Differential diagnosis

Similar pain may occur with structural lesions involving the trigeminal nerve. These lesions are often accompanied by physical signs, e.g. a depressed corneal reflex.

DISEASES OF THE SPINAL CORD (K&C 6e p. 1250)

The spinal cord extends from C1 (its junction with the medulla) to the vertebral body of L1. The spinal canal below L1 is occupied by lumbar and sacral nerve roots, which group together to form the cauda equina and ultimately extend into the pelvis and thigh (Fig. 16.11). Paraplegia (weakness of both legs) is almost always caused by a spinal cord lesion, as opposed to hemiplegia (weakness of one side of the body), which is usually the result of a lesion in the brain.

Spinal cord compression (K&C 6e p. 1250)

This is a medical emergency.

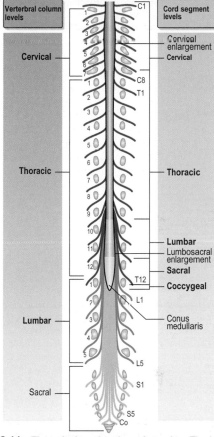

Fig. 16.11 **The spinal cord and cauda equina.** The bony vertebrae are indicated on the left-hand side (7 cervical, 12 thoracic, 5 lumbar and 5 sacral). The spinal cord extends from C1 (its junction with the medulla) to the vertebral body of L1. The spinal cord segments indicated on the right are not necessarily situated at the same vertebral levels as the bony vertebra. For instance the lumbar cord is situated between T9 and T11 vertebrae. A T8 vertebral injury will result in a T12 cord or neurological level (i.e. sensation is diminished below the T12 dermatome, and motor function is reduced in muscles innervated by T12 and below). The *cord* segmental levels are indicated for cervical (blue), thoracic (red), lumbar (green) and sacral (yellow). The spray of spinal roots below the conus is called the cauda equina and is damaged by lesions below the L2 vertebra.

Table 16.20 Causes of spinal cord compression	
Vertebral body neoplasms	Metastases, e.g. from lung, breast, prostate
	Myeloma
	Lymphoma
Disc and vertebral lesions	Trauma
	Chronic degenerative disease
Inflammatory	Epidural abscess
	Tuberculosis (Pott's paraplegia)
Spinal cord neoplasms	Primary cord neoplasm, e.g. glioma, neurofibroma
	Metastases
Rarities	Paget's disease, bone cysts, osteoporotic vertebral collapse
	Epidural haemorrhage, e.g. patients on warfarin

Clinical features

Back pain is usually the first symptom. There is progressive weakness of the legs with upper motor neurone pattern (Table 16.3) and eventual paralysis. The arms are affected if the lesion is above the thoracic spine. There is sensory loss below the level of the lesion. Sometimes there is loss of sphincter control with urinary incontinence. There may be painless urinary retention and constipation in the later stages. The onset may be acute (hours to days) or chronic (weeks to months), depending on the cause.

Aetiology

The causes of spinal cord compression are listed in Table 16.20; vertebral body neoplasms and disc and vertebral lesions are the commonest causes in developed countries. Spinal tuberculosis is a frequent cause in endemic areas (p. 523).

Investigations

Urgent investigation is essential in a patient with suspected cord compression, especially with acute or subacute onset, because irreversible paraplegia may follow if the cord is not decompressed.

- X-ray of the spine may show degenerative bone disease and destruction of vertebrae by infection or neoplasm.
- MRI identifies the cause and site of cord compression.

Management

The treatment depends on the cause, but in most cases the initial treatment involves surgical decompression of the cord and stabilization of the spine. Dexamethasone improves outcome in patients with cord compression due to malignancy.

Differential diagnosis

The differential diagnosis is from intrinsic lesions of the cord causing paraparesis. Transverse myelitis (acute inflammation of the cord resulting from viral infection, syphilis or radiation therapy), anterior spinal artery occlusion and multiple sclerosis may present with a rapid onset of paraparesis. A more insidious onset of weakness occurs with motor neurone disease, subacute combined degeneration of the cord, and as a non-metastatic manifestation of malignancy. MRI should always be performed in a patient with a sensory or motor level. A sensory level is when sensation abruptly diminishes one to two spinal cord segments below the level of the actual anatomical level of spinal cord compression.

Very rarely a parasagittal cortical lesion, e.g. meningioma, may cause paraplegia.

Syringomyelia and syringobulbia (*K&C* 6e p. 1251)

Fluid-filled cavities within the spinal cord (myelia) and brainstem (bulbia) are the essential features of these conditions.

Aetiology

The most frequent cause is blockage of CSF flow from the fourth ventricle in association with an Arnold–Chiari malformation (congenital herniation of the cerebellar tonsils through the foramen magnum). The normal pulsatile CSF pressure waves are transmitted to the delicate tissues of the cervical cord and brainstem, with secondary cavity formation. Hydrocephalus may also occur as a result of disturbed CSF flow.

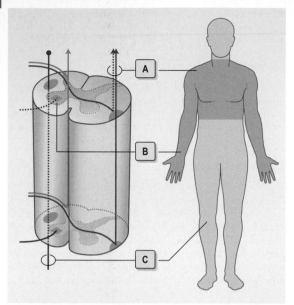

Fig. 16.12 **Production of physical signs in syringomyelia.**
Expanding cavities distend the cord. Pain and temperature (A)
fibres crossing at that level are destroyed, but sensory fibres in
the posterior columns (other sensory modalities) and those that
enter the spinothalamic tract at a lower level are spared. Sensory
loss is therefore 'dissociated' and confined to the upper trunk
and limbs. Further extension damages the anterior horn cells (B),
the pyramidal tracts (C) and the medulla, causing wasting in the
hands, a spastic paraplegia, nystagmus and a bulbar palsy.
(From Parsons M (1993) *A Colour Atlas of Clinical Neurology*.
London, Mosby Wolfe.)

Clinical features

Patients usually present in the third or fourth decade with
pain and sensory loss (pain and temperature) in the upper
limbs. The clinical features are demonstrated in Figure 16.12.

Investigation

MRI is the investigation of choice and demonstrates the
intrinsic cavities.

Treatment

Surgical decompression of the foramen magnum sometimes reduces the rate of deterioration.

Friedreich's ataxia (*K&C* 6e p. 1258)

Friedreich's ataxia is an autosomal recessive disorder and is the most common of the hereditary spinocerebellar degenerations. There is a progressive degeneration of the spinocerebellar tracts and cerebellum causing cerebellar ataxia, dysarthria and nystagmus. Degeneration of the corticospinal tracts causes weakness and an extensor plantar response. The tendon reflexes are absent as a result of peripheral nerve damage. Loss of the dorsal columns causes absent joint position and vibration sense. Other features are pes cavus, optic atrophy, cardiomyopathy, and death by middle age.

Cauda equina lesion (*K&C* 6e p. 1265)

Spinal damage at or distal to L1 (a common cause is central prolapse of an intervertebral disc at the lumbosacral junction) injures the cauda equina, which is formed by the lumbar and sacral nerve roots. This produces various mixtures of flaccid paralysis (compare spastic paralysis of a cord lesion above L1), sacral numbness, urinary retention and impotence.

Management of the paraplegic patient (*K&C* 6e p. 1252)

The paraplegic patient requires skilled and prolonged nursing care. A pressure-relieving mattress and turning the patient every 2 hours will help to prevent pressure sores. Bladder catheterization (sometimes intermittent self-catheterization) is necessary to prevent urinary stasis and infection. Patients may need manual evacuation of faeces. This may become unnecessary as reflex emptying of the bladder and rectum develops. Passive physiotherapy helps to prevent contractures in paralysed limbs. Severe spasticity may be helped by dantrolene sodium, baclofen or diazepam. Many patients graduate to a wheelchair and maintain some degree of independence.

DEGENERATIVE DISEASES (K&C 6e p. 1253)

Motor neurone disease (K&C 6e p. 1253)

In motor neurone disease (MND), there is relentless and unexplained destruction of upper motor neurones and anterior horn cells in the brain and spinal cord. Most patients die within 3 years from respiratory failure as a result of bulbar palsy and pneumonia. It presents in middle age and is more common in men. Motor neurone injury is thought to reflect a complex interplay between genetic factors, oxidative stress, and imbalance of the glutamatergic excitatory control of motor neurones, which may result in damage to critical target proteins and organelles.

Clinical features

One of four clinical patterns may be identified at diagnosis; however, as the disease progresses most patients develop a mixed picture.

- *Progressive muscular atrophy* is a predominantly lower motor neurone lesion of the cord causing weakness, wasting and fasciculation (spontaneous, irregular and brief contractions of part of a muscle) in the hands and arms.
- *Amyotrophic lateral sclerosis* is a combination of disease of the lateral corticospinal tracts and anterior horn cells producing a progressive spastic tetraparesis or paraparesis with added lower motor neurone signs (wasting and fasciculation).
- *Progressive bulbar palsy* results from destruction of upper (pseudobulbar palsy) and lower (bulbar palsy) motor neurones in the lower cranial nerves. There is dysarthria, dysphagia with wasting, and fasciculation of the tongue.
- *Primary lateral sclerosis* is rare. There is a progressive tetraparesis.

There is no involvement of the sensory system or motor nerves to the eyes and sphincters in any of the clinical types.

Investigations

The diagnosis is clinical. An EMG shows muscle denervation, but this is not a specific finding.

Differential diagnosis

The differential diagnosis is a cervical spine lesion, which may present with upper and lower motor neurone signs in the arms and legs. It is often distinguished by the presence of sensory signs. Idiopathic multifocal motor neuropathy (Table 16.21) presents with weakness predominantly in the hands and profuse fasciculation.

Management

Riluzole, a sodium-channel blocker that inhibits glutamate release, slows progression slightly. Ventilatory support and feeding via a PEG (p. 121) helps prolong survival for some months.

Spinal muscular atrophies (*K&C* 6e p. 1254)

This is a group of rare disorders which destroy the anterior horn cells of the spinal cord. Two forms present in adult life, causing a slowly progressive wasting and weakness of the limbs.

DISEASES OF THE PERIPHERAL NERVES (*K&C* 6e p. 1258)

Six principal mechanisms cause nerve malfunction: demyelination, axonal degeneration, e.g. due to a toxin, Wallerian degeneration following nerve section, compression, infarction (in arteritis) and infiltration by inflammatory cells, e.g. sarcoid.

Mononeuropathies (*K&C* 6e p. 1259)

Mononeuropathy is a process affecting a single nerve, and multiple mononeuropathy (or mononeuritis multiplex) is a process affecting several or multiple nerves. Mononeuropathy may be the result of acute compression, particularly where the nerves are exposed anatomically (e.g. the common peroneal nerve at the head of the fibula), or entrapment, where the nerve passes through a relatively tight anatomical passage (e.g. the carpal tunnel). It may also be caused by direct damage, e.g. major trauma, surgery or penetrating injuries.

Carpal tunnel syndrome

Carpal tunnel syndrome is the most common entrapment neuropathy. It results from pressure on the median nerve as it passes through the carpal tunnel.

Aetiology

It is usually idiopathic but may be associated with hypo-thyroidism, diabetes mellitus, pregnancy, obesity, rheumatoid arthritis and acromegaly.

Clinical features

The history is of pain and paraesthesiae in the hand, typically worse at night, when it may wake the patient. On examination there may be no physical signs; or weakness and wasting of the thenar muscles and sensory loss of the palm and palmar aspects of the radial three and a half fingers. Tapping on the carpal tunnel may reproduce the pain (Tinnel's sign).

Management

Treatment with nocturnal splints or local steroid injections gives temporary relief. Surgical decompression is the definitive treatment unless the condition is likely to resolve (e.g. with pregnancy, obesity).

Compression neuropathies may also affect the ulnar nerve (at the elbow), the radial nerve (caused by pressure against the humerus) and the common peroneal nerve (resulting from pressure at the head of the fibula).

Mononeuritis multiplex

Mononeuritis multiplex often indicates a systemic disorder (Table 16.21); treatment is that of the underlying disease.

Table 16.21 Causes of mononeuritis multiplex
Diabetes mellitus
Leprosy (the most common cause world-wide)
Vasculitis
Sarcoidosis
Amyloidosis
Malignancy
Neurofibromatosis
HIV infection
Guillain–Barré syndrome
Idiopathic multifocal motor neuropathy (distal motor, unknown cause)

Acute presentation is most commonly due to vasculitis when prompt treatment with steroids may prevent irreversible nerve damage.

Polyneuropathy (*K&C* 6e p. 1260)

Polyneuropathy describes a diffuse, usually symmetrical, disease process that may be acute or chronic and may involve motor, sensory and autonomic nerves, either alone or in combination. Sensory symptoms include numbness, tingling, 'pins and needles', pain in the extremities and unsteadiness on the feet. Numbness typically affects the distal arms and legs in a 'glove and stocking' distribution. Motor symptoms are usually those of weakness. Autonomic neuropathy causes postural hypotension, urinary retention, impotence, diarrhoea (or occasionally constipation), diminished sweating, impaired pupillary responses and cardiac arrhythmias.

Many varieties of neuropathy affect autonomic function to some degree, but occasionally autonomic features predominate. This occurs in diabetes mellitus, amyloidosis and the Guillain–Barré syndrome. A classification of polyneuropathy is given in Table 16.22. In Europe diabetes mellitus is the commonest cause. First-line investigations in a patient presenting with polyneuropathy include full blood count and erythrocyte sedimentation rate, serum vitamin B_{12}, blood glucose urea and electrolytes and liver biochemistry.

Table 16.22 Classification of polyneuropathy	
Idiopathic (the majority of cases)	
Postinfective (Guillain–Barré syndrome)	
Drugs	Isoniazid, nitrofurantoin, metronidazole, vincristine, antiretrovirals
Toxins	Excess alcohol, lead poisoning
Metabolic	Diabetes mellitus, uraemia, amyloidosis
Vitamin deficiency	B_1, B_6, B_{12}
Non-metastatic manifestation of malignancy	
HIV-associated polyneuropathy	
Autonomic neuropathies	
Neuropathies in connective tissue disease	
Hereditary sensorimotor neuropathy	

Peroneal muscular atrophy (Charcot–Marie–Tooth disease) (K&C 6e p. 1263)

There is distal limb wasting and weakness that progress over many years, mostly in the legs, with variable loss of sensation and reflexes. In advanced cases the distal wasting below the knees is so marked that the legs resemble 'inverted champagne bottles'. The most common form is inherited in an autosomal dominant fashion.

Postinfective polyneuropathy (Guillain–Barré syndrome) (K&C 6e p. 1260)

Guillain-Barré syndrome is an acute inflammatory demyelinating polyneuropathy characterized by progressive muscle weakness and areflexia with recovery being the rule. It is the most common acute neuropathy.

Pathogenesis

It is thought to be caused by a cell-mediated immune response directed at normal peripheral myelin, and this may be provoked in some cases by preceding infection. *Campylobacter jejuni* (p. 34) and cytomegalovirus (p. 18) are well-recognized causes.

Clinical features

There is weakness and areflexia (usually symmetrical) in the distal limbs which ascends over days or weeks. The patient complains of paraesthesias but there is minimal loss of sensation on examination. Disability ranges from mild to very severe, with involvement of the respiratory and facial muscles. Autonomic features, such as postural hypotension, cardiac arrhythmias, ileus and bladder atony, are sometimes seen.

Investigations

The diagnosis is established on clinical grounds and confirmed by nerve conduction studies; these show slowing of motor conduction consistent with segmental demyelination. CSF protein is typically elevated, with a normal sugar and cell count.

Differential diagnosis

Other causes of neuromuscular paralysis (botulism, poliomyelitis, primary muscle diseases, hypokalaemia) are rare and can usually be excluded on clinical grounds and investigation. MRI of the spine may be needed to exclude spinal cord compression.

Management

Monitor:

1. Vital capacity 4-hourly, to recognize respiratory muscle weakness. A fall below 80% of predicted or 20 mL/kg is an indication for transfer to ITU and possible mechanical ventilation.
2. ECG to document cardiac dysrhythmias associated with autonomic dysfunction.

Intravenous immunoglobulin and plasma exchange improve outcome in severe disease (unable to walk unaided, worsening vital capacity, significant bulbar weakness). Supportive treatment includes heparin to prevent thrombosis, physiotherapy to prevent contractures and nasogastric or PEG feeding for patients with swallowing problems. Visiting and counselling services are offered by past patients through the Guillain–Barré Syndrome Support Group (http://www.gbs.org.uk).

Recovery begins (with or without treatment) between several days and 6 weeks from the outset. Prolonged ventilation may be necessary. Improvement towards independent mobility is gradual over many months but may be incomplete. Fifteen per cent of patients die or are left disabled; fatigue is common.

Vitamin deficiency neuropathies (K&C 6e p. 1262)

Thiamin (vitamin B₁)

Alcohol abuse is the most common cause of thiamin deficiency in the West. Presentation is with the Wernicke–Korsakoff syndrome (p. 584). Severe deficiency causes the clinical syndrome of beriberi (polyneuropathy, Wernicke's encephalopathy and cardiac failure), rarely seen in western countries. Treatment is with intravenous or oral thiamine (200 mg daily).

Pyridoxine (vitamin B₆)

Deficiency causes mainly a sensory neuropathy. It may be precipitated during isoniazid therapy (which complexes with pyridoxal phosphate) for tuberculosis in those who acetylate the drug slowly, and prophylactic pyridoxine (10 mg daily) is given with isoniazid.

Vitamin B_{12}

Deficiency causes the syndrome of *subacute combined degeneration of the cord*. This comprises distal sensory loss (particularly the posterior column), absent ankle jerks (as a result of the neuropathy) and evidence of cord disease (exaggerated knee jerk reflexes, extensor plantar responses). Treatment is with intramuscular vitamin B_{12} (p. 841), which reverses the peripheral nerve damage but has little effect on the CNS (cord and brain signs).

DISEASES OF VOLUNTARY MUSCLE (K&C 6e p. 1266)

Myopathies

Weakness is the predominant feature of a myopathy. The myopathies are divided into those that are inherited (muscular dystrophies), inflammatory lesions (the most common is polymyositis, p. 287) and those associated with drugs, toxins and endocrine disease. The latter group usually produces weakness of the limb girdles (proximal myopathy, Table 16.23) and typically the patient is unable to rise from a seated position without the use of their arms. Severe hypokalaemia may produce a generalized flaccid weakness.

Muscular dystrophies (K&C 6e p. 1269)

Muscular dystrophies are an inherited group of progressive myopathic disorders resulting from defects in a number of genes needed for normal muscle function. The Duchenne

Table 16.23 Causes of a proximal myopathy
Prolonged high-dose steroid therapy
Cushing's syndrome
Thyrotoxicosis
Hypothyroidism (occasionally)
Osteomalacia
Hypokalaemia
Prolonged alcohol abuse
Other drugs, e.g. diamorphine, lithium, quinine, chloroquine

Table 16.24 Limb girdle and facioscapulohumeral dystrophies

	Limb girdle	Facioscapulohumeral
Inheritance	Autosomal recessive	Autosomal dominant
Onset	10–20 years	10–40 years
Muscle affected	Shoulder and pelvic girdle	Face, shoulder and pelvic girdle
Progress	Severe disability in 20–25 years	Normal life expectancy
Pseudohypertrophy	Rare	Very rare
Serum CPK levels	Slightly raised	Slightly raised or normal

CPK, creatine phosphokinase

and Becker muscular dystrophies are inherited as X-linked recessive traits caused by a mutation in the dystrophin gene on chromosome 21. Patients with Duchenne muscular dystrophy present in early childhood with weakness in the proximal muscles of the leg. There is progression to other muscle groups with severe disability and death in the late teens. There is no curative treatment. Patients with Becker muscle dystrophy present later and the degree of clinical involvement is milder. Other dystrophies present later in life and are summarized in Table 16.24.

Myasthenia gravis (*K&C* 6e p. 1268)

Myasthenia gravis is an acquired condition characterized by weakness and fatiguability of proximal limb, ocular and bulbar muscles. The heart is not affected. It occurs most commonly in the third decade and is twice as common in women as in men.

Aetiology

The cause is unknown. Serum IgG antibodies to acetylcholine receptors, in the postsynaptic membrane of the neuromuscular junction, cause receptor loss. Myasthenia gravis is associated with thymic hyperplasia in about 70% of patients under 40 years of age, and in about 10% a thymic tumour is found.

Clinical features

Fatiguability is the most marked feature, with the proximal limb muscles, extraocular muscles and muscles of mastication, speech and facial expression being most commonly involved. Fatigue can be demonstrated by ptosis on sustained upward gaze or asking the patient to sit with the arms outstretched and looking for a slow downward drift. The ocular muscles are the first to be involved in about 65% of patients, resulting in ptosis and complex ocular palsies.

Investigations

- Acetylcholine receptor antibodies are specific for myasthenia gravis and are found in the serum in 90% of cases of generalized myasthenia gravis.
- The Tensilon test is positive. (Injection of 10 mg edrophonium, an anticholinesterase, results in rapid temporary improvement in weakness.)
- Nerve stimulation tests show a characteristic decrement in evoked potential following stimulation of the motor nerve.
- Mediastinal imaging with CT or MRI to look for a thymoma.

Management

Anticholinesterases (pyridostigmine, neostigmine) form the mainstay of treatment and the dose is determined by the patient's response.

In patients without thymoma Anticholinesterase medication alone is given in mild disease. In patients under 45 with more severe disease thymectomy is usually

indicated. This results in improvement in about 65% of cases. Immunosuppressive treatment with steroids and/or azathioprine should be considered in those who fail to respond to thymectomy.

In patients with thymoma Thymectomy is indicated in these patients because of the ability of the tumour to invade locally. It is unusual for myasthenia to improve following surgery, and immunosuppressive treatment is usually required.

These conditions are characterized by myotonia (delayed muscle relaxation after contraction) which can be demonstrated by difficulty releasing the grasp after shaking hands. Patients tolerate general anaesthetics poorly. The two most common forms are dystrophia myotonica and myotonia congenita, described below.

Dystrophia myotonica

Dystrophia myotonica is an autosomal dominant condition characterized by progressive distal muscle weakness with myotonia, ptosis, facial muscle weakness and wasting. Other features commonly present are cataracts, frontal baldness, cardiomyopathy, mild mental handicap, glucose intolerance and hypogonadism.

Myotonia congenita

Myotonia congenita is also an autosomal dominant disorder characterized by mild isolated myotonia occurring in childhood and persisting throughout life. The myotonia is often accentuated by rest and cold.

DEMENTIA AND DELIRIUM

Delirium (toxic confusional state) (*K&C* 6e p. 1309)

Delirium is an acute or subacute condition in which impairment of consciousness is accompanied by abnormalities of perception and mood. Impairment of consciousness can vary in severity and often fluctuates (compare with dementia). Confusion is usually worse at night and may be accompanied by hallucinations, delusions, restlessness and aggression. Many diseases (Table 16.25) can be accompanied by delirium, particularly in the elderly. Infection and drugs are the most common causes.

Management

Investigation and treatment of the underlying disease should be undertaken. General measures include withdrawing all drugs where possible, rehydration, and adequate pain relief and sedation. The patient should be nursed in a quiet area of the ward. Sedation should only be used if the patient is

Dementia and delirium

Table 16.25 Causes of delirium

Systemic infection	
Drugs	Tricyclic antidepressants
	Benzodiazepines
	Opiates
	Anticonvulsants
Drug/alcohol withdrawal	
Metabolic disturbance	Hepatic failure
	Renal failure
	Disorders of electrolyte balance
	Hypoxia
	Hypoglycaemia
Vitamin deficiency	Vitamin B_{12}
	Vitamin B_1 (Wernicke–Korsakoff syndrome)
Brain damage	Trauma
	Tumour
	Abscess
	Subarachnoid haemorrhage

at risk of self-injury or aggressive behaviour interferes with management. Benzodiazepines are usually the drugs of choice, although in severe delirium intramuscular haloperidol (2.5–5 mg) may be preferred. Management of alcohol withdrawal is summarized on page 585.

Dementia (*K&C* 6e p. 1254)

Dementia is characterized by a progressive decline of cognitive function, i.e. loss of mind, usually affecting the cerebral cortex as a whole, though sometimes patchily. Consciousness is not, however, clouded. Dementia affects about 10% of those aged 65 years and over, and 20% of those over 80. There are numerous causes of dementia (Table 16.26), although by far the most common is Alzheimer's disease, which accounts for 70%.

Alzheimer's disease

Alzheimer's disease is a primary degenerative cerebral disease of unknown aetiology.

Clinical features

There is an insidious onset with steady progression over years. Short-term memory loss is usually the most prominent early symptom, but subsequently there is slow

---

Table 16.26   Causes of dementia*

Alzheimer's disease
Multiple cerebral infarction
Dementia with Lewy bodies
Excess alcohol (Wernicke–Korsakoff syndrome)
Hypothyroidism
Intracranial mass: subdural haematoma, hydrocephalus
Chronic traumatic encephalopathy, e.g. punch drunkenness
Vitamin B_{12} deficiency
Syphilis
Creutzfeldt–Jakob disease
Huntington's chorea
Late Parkinson's disease

*Commonest causes are in bold

Table 16.27   Simple clinical assessment of the mental state

Age
Time to nearest hour
Address for recall at the end of the test (house number and street name)
Year
Place – name of hospital
Recognition of two people (e.g. doctor, nurse)
Date of birth
Year of 1st World War
Name of present monarch
Count backwards 20 to 1

Each correct answer scores one mark. Healthy patients score > 8

---

disintegration of the personality and intellect, eventually affecting all aspects of cortical function. There are characteristic pathological features, which include neuronal reduction in several areas of the brain, neurofibrillary tangles, argentophile plaques, consisting largely of amyloid protein, and granulovacuolar bodies.

Investigations

The presence of dementia is usually diagnosed clinically by a simple assessment of the mental state (Table 16.27). Exclusion of rare treatable causes of dementia (Table 16.26)

781

should also be considered and blood taken for a full blood count, liver biochemistry, thyroid function tests and measurement of vitamin B_{12} and folate. A brain CT scan should be performed in younger patients or those with an atypical presentation. A social and family history will help to assess how vulnerable the person is in the community and what plans for support will need to be made.

Management

In most cases there is no specific therapy although the associated anxiety and depression often need treatment. Attempts to therapeutically augment cholinergic activity have been based on the observations that there is impaired cortical cholinergic function as a result of reduced cerebral production of choline acetyl transferase and a decrease in acetylcholine synthesis. Acetylcholinesterase inhibitors (donepezil, rivastigmine and galantamine) increase cholinergic transmission by inhibiting cholinesterase at the synaptic cleft. They have a modest benefit and slow intellectual deterioration in patients with mild to moderate Alzheimer's disease. Patients should be managed in the community as much as possible. A whole range of supportive interventions for both patient and carers is needed. Home care, day care, respite care and sitter services are all needed at various points during the progression of the disease. At some point long-term institutional care in a residential or nursing home may be required.

Prognosis

The typical course is one of progressive decline. The average survival is 8–10 years.

Vascular (multi-infarct) dementia

This is the second most common cause of dementia and can be distinguished by its history of onset, clinical features and subsequent course. Features that suggest the diagnosis include a stepwise deterioration with declines followed by short periods of stability. There is usually a history of transient ischaemic attacks, although the dementia may follow a succession of acute cerebrovascular accidents or, less commonly, a single major stroke. There may be other evidence of arteriopathy.

Dementia with Lewy bodies

This is characterized by fluctuating cognition with pronounced variation in attention and alertness. Prominent or persistent memory loss may not occur in the early stages. Impairment in attention, frontal, subcortical and visuospatial ability is often prominent. Depression and sleep disorders occur. Recurrent formed visual hallucinations (e.g. strange faces, frightening creatures) are a feature. Parkinsonism (e.g. slowing, rigidity) is common, with repeated falls. Delusions and transient loss of consciousness occur. Cortical Lewy bodies are prominent at autopsy. These inclusions were first described in idiopathic Parkinson's disease, but are a hallmark of this clinical pattern of dementia. Neuroleptic drugs should not be used.

Dermatology 17

INTRODUCTION

Skin diseases are extremely common, although their exact prevalence is unknown. There are over 1000 different entities described, but two-thirds of all cases are the result of fewer than 10 conditions. The most common include acne, eczema, psoriasis, warts and infections caused by bacteria (*K&C* 6e p. 1318), fungi (*K&C* 6e p. 1322) and viruses (*K&C* p. 1321). Some conditions may be part of normal development, e.g. acne; others may be inherited, e.g. Ehlers–Danlos syndrome; still others are part of a systemic disease, e.g. the rash of systemic lupus erythematosus.

Only the most common skin conditions will be described in the following sections.

COMMON SKIN CONDITIONS

Acne vulgaris (*K&C* 6e p. 1337)

Acne vulgaris is a common condition occurring in adolescence and rarely in early and middle adult life. It is thought to result from hyperactivity of the sebaceous glands leading to increased production of sebum with blockage of the follicular openings and the formation of comedones (blackheads), inflammatory papules, nodules and cysts. Normal skin bacteria, principally *Propionibacterium acnes*, within the blocked follicle are capable of producing pro-inflammatory mediators and lipolytic enzymes, which may be responsible for producing the clinical lesions.

Clinical features

Non-inflammatory lesions include open and closed comedones. Closed comedones (whiteheads) are flesh-coloured papules with an apparently closed overlying surface. Open comedones (blackheads) appear as black plugs which distend the follicular orifice, the pigmentation

785

being provided by oxidation of melanin pigment. These are often the forerunners of the more severe inflammatory lesions, such as papules, pustules, nodules and cysts. Other features that may be present include hypertrophic or keloidal scarring, and hyperpigmentation, which occurs predominantly in patients with darker complexions. There is a tendency for spontaneous improvement over a number of years but acne can persist unabated into adult life.

Management

Acne should be actively treated to avoid unnecessary scarring and psychological distress. The aims of treatment are to decrease sebum production, reduce bacteria, normalize duct keratinization and decrease inflammation. There are a variety of approaches, the choice of which depends on the severity of the disease.

First-line therapy   Local applications such as abrasives, astringents or exfoliatives are useful in mild disease. Topical agents such as antibiotics (tetracycline, clindamycin), keratolytics (benzoyl peroxide), topical retinoids (tretinoin) or retinoid-like agents (adapalene) should be used in mild disease but if these fail second-line agents should be added.

Second-line therapy   Low-dose oral antibiotics, e.g. tetracycline or erythromycin, often help but treatment must be continued over several months.

Hormonal treatment with cyproterone acetate 2 mg/ ethinylestradiol 35 µg (co-cyprindol) may be useful in women if there is no contraindication to oral contraception.

Third-line therapy   Third-line treatment with a retinoid drug (isotretinoin) should be given if:

- The above measures fail
- There is nodulocystic acne with scarring
- There is severe psychological disturbance.

Isotretinoin is a vitamin A analogue that affects cell growth and differentiation. Although highly effective it is also highly teratogenic and is absolutely contraindicated during pregnancy. All women of childbearing age should have a pregnancy test and contraceptive advice prior to treatment and this must now be done monthly during the 4-month course. Over 90% of individuals will respond to this therapy and 65% of people will obtain a long-term 'cure'.

Psoriasis (K&C 6e p. 1331)

Psoriasis is a chronic hyperproliferative disorder characterized by the presence of well-demarcated silvery-scaled plaques over extensor surfaces such as the elbows and knees, and in the scalp. It can affect any group with equal sex incidence, and occurs in about 2% of people in temperate zones.

Aetiology

The cause of the condition is unknown, although genetic factors are felt to be important. It is associated with several HLA-specific antigens, particularly HLA-CW6. It is likely that psoriasis is a T-lymphocyte driven disorder to an unidentified antigen(s) with a possible altered response from the keratinocyte. Trigger factors in genetically susceptible individuals include infections (particularly streptococcal), local trauma, drugs such as lithium carbonate and β-blockers, and probably also stress.

Clinical features

Several clinical patterns are recognized:

- Plaque psoriasis is the most common, occurring as well-demarcated, salmon-pink silvery scaling lesions on the extensor surfaces of the limbs, particularly the elbows and knees (Fig. 17.1). Scalp involvement is common and is most often seen at the hair margin or over the occiput. Nail involvement, which can occur alone or in association with psoriasis elsewhere, is manifest as pitting and onycholysis (separation of the nail from the underlying vascular bed). The arthropathy associated with psoriasis is described on page 271.
- Flexural psoriasis presents as pinkish glazed lesions that are well demarcated and non-scaly. The groin, perianal and sub-mammary areas are most commonly involved. The rash is sometimes misdiagnosed as candida intertrigo but the latter will normally show satellite lesions.
- Guttate psoriasis or 'raindrop-like' psoriasis is a variant most commonly seen in children and young adults An explosive eruption of very small circular or oval plaques appears over the trunk about 2 weeks after a streptococcal sore throat.

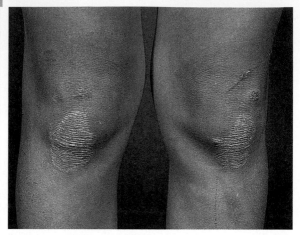

Fig. 17.1 Psoriasis of the knees.

■ Pustular psoriasis most commonly affects the palms or soles. There are areas of well-demarcated scaling and erythema associated with white, yellow or green pustule formation. Identical features are seen as one of the cutaneous features of reactive arthritis (keratoderma blenorrhagica, p. 272).

■ Erythrodermic psoriasis is a severe and potentially life-threatening condition. The trunk and limbs may be involved by an almost universal scaling, sometimes associated with generalized pustule formation. This disease occurs classically following corticosteroid therapy.

Management

The approach depends on the severity of the disease. As no treatment is universally effective, simple local treatment is used for mild disease, with systemic therapy reserved for severe or pustular psoriasis. Treatment should be tailored to the patient's wishes and not just to the doctor's assessment of disease severity.

Local therapy Emollients should always be used to hydrate the skin. Topical steroids, topical vitamin D_3 analogues (e.g. calcipotriol, calcitriol, tacalcitol), 0.05% tazarotene (a vitamin A antagonist, i.e. a retinoid) and occasionally purified coal tar may all be useful for relatively mild disease, and are suitable for use on an outpatient basis. Dithranol which inhibits DNA synthesis can also be helpful but it causes staining of the skin and clothing and it may prove difficult to use at home on a regular basis.

Phototherapy (*K&C* 6e pp. 1333 & 1339)   High-intensity ultraviolet A light (UVA) in conjunction with a photo-sensitizing agent taken by mouth (psoralen) is known as PUVA and is usually highly effective for treating extensive psoriasis. Repeated treatments, however, carry the risk of UV-induced skin cancer.

Systemic therapy   Oral retinoic acid derivatives, e.g. acitretin or etretinate, are useful in severe erythrodermic or pustular psoriasis. Although effective, these agents are potentially toxic and also teratogenic. They should not therefore be used in women of childbearing age.

Low-dose oral methotrexate (7.5–20 mg once a week) can be highly effective, particularly in psoriatic arthritis. Other immunosuppressive agents, such as ciclosporin and tacrolimus, are sometimes useful in severe intractable disease, although toxicity often limits their long-term use.

Biological agents such as infliximab and etanercept are being increasingly employed in resistant disease and in patients who cannot tolerate the conventional systemic treatments. Approximately 60–80% of patients show at least a 75% improvement within 12 weeks, though long-term side-effects of these new biological agents are unknown.

Eczema (*K&C* 6e p. 1326)

Eczema is characterized by superficial skin inflammation with vesicles (when acute), redness, oedema, oozing, scaling and usually pruritus. The terms 'dermatitis' and 'eczema' are usually used interchangeably, as both conditions show similar inflammatory changes in the skin.

Eczema may arise from several different stimuli, but most commonly it is classified as:

■ Endogenous (atopic)
■ Exogenous due to allergy or chemical irritation.

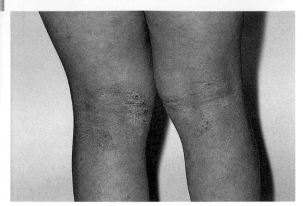

Fig. 17.2 **Atopic eczema behind the knees.**

Endogenous (atopic) eczema

Aetiology

The cause of this condition is not fully understood but there is a selective activation of TH2-type CD4 lymphocytes in the skin which drives the inflammatory process, resulting in a capacity to hyperreact to many environmental factors. There are high levels of serum IgE antibodies, although their significance in contributing to the pathogenesis is unclear. There is also a significant hereditary predisposition.

Clinical features

The disease may start in the first few weeks of life with erythema, weeping, itching and scaling. In adults the flexures at the neck, elbow, wrist and knee are commonly involved (Fig. 17.2).

Management

The offending agents should be removed if possible. Regular use of emollients, such as aqueous cream or emulsifying ointments, is useful in hydrating the skin. Corticosteroid creams form the mainstay of treatment. In general, mild steroids (e.g. 1% hydrocortisone) should be used for the face, whereas more potent steroids (e.g. betamethasone, fluocinolone) are used on the body and soles. Topical immunomodulators such as tacrolimus and pimecrolimus have recently been licensed for use and are particularly helpful for treatment in sensitive areas such as the face and eyelids. Antibiotics are indicated for bacterial superinfection and bandaging helps absorption of treatment and acts as a barrier to prevent scratching.

Second-line treatments in severe non-responsive cases include oral prednisolone, azathioprine and ciclosporin.

Exogenous eczema (contact dermatitis)

In this condition there is acute or chronic skin inflammation, often sharply demarcated, produced by substances in contact with the skin. It may be caused by a primary chemical irritant, or may be the result of a type IV hypersensitivity reaction. Common chemical irritants are industrial solvents used in the workplace, or cleaning and detergent solutions used in the home. With allergic dermatitis there is sensitization of T lymphocytes over a period of time, which results in itching and dermatitis upon re-exposure to the antigen.

Clinical features

An unusual pattern of rash with clear-cut demarcation or odd-shaped areas of erythema and scaling should arouse suspicion and, in combination with a careful history, should indicate a cause. Patch testing, where the suspected allergen is placed in contact with the skin, is often useful in identifying a suspected allergen.

Management

Causative agents should be removed where possible. Steroid creams are useful for short periods in severe disease. Antipruritic agents are used for symptomatic relief of itching.

Erythema nodosum (*K&C* 6e p. 1341)

Erythema nodosum is an acute and sometimes recurrent paniculitis which produces painful nodules or plaques on the shins, with occasional spread to the thighs or arms. Adult females are most commonly affected. Histological features suggest that this is an immunological reaction with immune complex deposition within dermal vessels. In 50% of cases no obvious cause is found. Other causes are listed in Table 17.1.

Table 17.1	Some causes of erythema nodosum
Drugs	Oral contraceptive pill
	Penicillin
	Sulphonamides
Systemic diseases	Sarcoidosis*
	Inflammatory bowel disease*
Infection	Bacteria and viruses*
	Streptococcal*
	Tuberculosis
	Leprosy
	Chlamydia spp.
	Fungal infection (histoplasmosis, blastomycosis)
Pregnancy	

*The most common causes

Clinical features

Painful nodules or plaques up to 5 cm in diameter appear in crops over 2 weeks, and slowly fade to leave bruising and staining of the skin. Systemic upset is common, with malaise, fever and arthralgia.

Management

Symptoms should be treated with NSAIDs, light compression bandaging and bed rest. Recovery may take weeks, and recurrent attacks can occur. Dapsone, colchicine or oral prednisolone may be useful in resistant cases.

Erythema multiforme (*K&C* 6e p. 1342)

This is an acute self-limiting condition affecting the skin and mucosal surfaces which is probably related to the deposition of immune complexes. Children and young adults are most commonly affected. The cause is unknown in 50% of cases but the following should be considered:

- Herpes simplex infection
- *Mycoplasma pneumoniae*
- Drugs, e.g. sulphonamides, sulphonylureas and barbiturates
- Connective tissue diseases
- Wegener's granulomatosis
- Carcinoma, lymphoma.

Clinical features

Symmetrically distributed erythematous papules occur most commonly on the back of the hands, the palms and the forearms. The lesions may show central pallor associated with oedema, bulla formation and peripheral erythema. Severe mucosal disease may predominate in, for example, infection with *Mycoplasma pneumoniae*. Eye changes include conjunctivitis, corneal ulceration and uveitis.

Occasionally there is severe mucosal involvement, oral and genital ulceration, conjunctivitis, and marked constitutional symptoms ('EM major' – previously called Stevens–Johnson syndrome). The term 'EM minor' may be used for cases without mucosal involvement.

Management

The disease usually resolves in 2–4 weeks. Treatment is symptomatic and involves treating the underlying cause. Rarely, recurrent erythema multiforme can occur. This is triggered by herpes simplex infection in 80% of cases, and oral aciclovir can be helpful. In resistant cases, azathioprine (1–2 mg/kg daily) is used.

Pyoderma gangrenosum (*K&C* 6e p. 1342)

This condition presents with erythematous nodules or pustules which frequently ulcerate. The ulcers, which are often large, have a classical bluish black undermined edge and a purulent surface. The disease is idiopathic in 20% of cases but it is associated with several conditions such as:

- Inflammatory bowel disease
- Rheumatoid arthritis
- Myeloma, lymphoma
- Primary biliary cirrhosis.

Management

793

The underlying condition should be treated appropriately. High-dose topical and/or oral steroids are used to prevent progressive ulceration. Other immunosuppressants such as ciclosporin are sometimes used.

OTHER DISEASES AFFECTING THE SKIN

Marfan's syndrome *(K&C 6e pp. 839 & 1356)*

Marfan's syndrome is an autosomal dominant disorder of collagen synthesis. Fragility of the skin may lead to bruising. The most obvious abnormalities are skeletal: tall stature, arm span greater than height, arachnodactyly (long spidery fingers), sternal depression, lax joints and a high arched palate. There is often upward dislocation of the lens as a result of weakness of the suspensory ligament. Cardiovascular complications (ascending aortic aneurysm formation, aortic dissection and aortic valve incompetence) are responsible for a greatly reduced life span.

Ehlers–Danlos syndrome *(K&C 6e pp. 602 & 1356)*

Inherited defects of collagen lead to fragility and hyperelasticity of the skin, with easy bruising, 'paper-thin' scars and hypermobility of the joints. The walls of the aorta and gut are weak and may rarely rupture with catastrophic results.

Neurofibromatosis *(K&C 6e pp. 1257 & 1345)*

Neurofibromatosis is an autosomal dominant disease with distinctive clinical features.

■ Type 1 (von Recklinghausen's disease), with mutations in the *NF1* gene on chromosome 17. Clinical features include multiple cutaneous neurofibromas, multiple 'café-au-lait' spots (light-brown macules of varying size), axillary freckling, scoliosis, and an increased incidence of a variety of neural tumours, e.g. meningioma, eighth-nerve tumours and gliomas.
■ Type 2, with the abnormal gene on chromosome 22. Typically bilateral acoustic neuromas and other neural tumours occur.

Practical procedures 18

The purpose of this chapter is to describe some of the common practical procedures you may have to undertake as a house officer or, for a few of them, as a medical student. Before attempting them alone you should first perform them with a more experienced colleague. Because of space restrictions only a limited number of procedures have been listed as they are the ones that are carried out on a daily basis or which may have to be performed as an emergency. Elective procedures and those usually performed by more senior colleagues are not discussed.

GENERAL PRINCIPLES FOR ALL PROCEDURES

A simple and concise explanation of the procedure must be given to the patient, and feedback obtained from the patient to make sure the procedure has been understood. In some cases, e.g. liver biopsy, written informed consent is obtained, after an explanation to the patient of the risks associated with the procedure. At the end of a procedure all needles, syringes and trocars should be disposed of in a sharps bin, and clinical waste, e.g. blood-soaked swabs, disposed of in appropriate disposal bags.

Sterile procedures

Some procedures are performed under strict aseptic conditions to minimize the risks to the patient of introducing infection. The equipment and methods are similar in each case. The operator washes his or her hands thoroughly with a disinfecting agent such as povidone–iodine (Betadine) or chlorhexidine (Hibiscrub), and wears sterile gloves for the procedure. For chest drain and central line insertion the operator wears a sterile gown and sterile drapes are used to isolate the working area. An assistant, who maintains a no-touch technique, helps to open dressing packs and gives needles and syringes to the operator. The operative field is cleaned with aqueous Betadine or 0.5% chlorhexidine in alcohol, and the skin of the selected entry site is isolated with sterile towels.

Local anaesthesia

A preparation of 1% lidocaine (lignocaine) is usually used for local anaesthesia. The maximum amount used in an adult should be less than 20 mL, although usually much less is necessary. After cleaning the skin a 25 gauge (orange) needle is inserted intradermally and a small bleb raised before infiltrating the deeper tissues with a 23 gauge (blue) needle. Before each injection the plunger of the syringe should be pulled back to ensure that a blood vessel has not been entered.

SPECIFIC PROCEDURES

Venepuncture

Equipment

- Syringe (size will vary according to the amount of blood needed)
- 21 gauge (green) needle
- Tourniquet
- Alcohol swab
- Blood sample tubes as appropriate; label the sample tubes with the patient details after the blood is in them
- Gauze swabs or cotton wool balls.

Many hospitals employ a vacutainer system where the tubes contain a vacuum and are attached to the needle while it is in the vein. This reduces the chances of a needle-stick injury to the operator.

Methods

The antecubital vein in the forearm is an ideal site and, if unsuccessful, more distal sites are attempted. Palpate the vein to locate its position and make sure it is not an artery (which will pulsate). The tourniquet is applied proximally and the skin over the venepuncture site cleaned with a swab. Allow the skin to dry before proceeding. The skin over the vein is rendered tense with the operator's non-dominant hand, thus immobilizing the vein. The syringe with the needle attached is held in the dominant hand and the needle, with the bevel upwards, is passed at an angle of about 15° through the skin and pointed in the direction of blood flow. Loss of resistance is felt when the vein is entered, and blood will appear at the end of the syringe. The required amount of blood is drawn slowly (to prevent both the vein collapsing and red cell haemolysis) up into the syringe. With a vacuum system blood will only appear when the sample tube is pushed onto the needle attachment inside the holder. At the end of the procedure the tourniquet is removed, a dry swab is applied to the venepuncture site and the needle removed from the vein while applying pressure on the swab. Using the non-touch needle-removing device on the sharps bin the needle is removed from the syringe before expelling the blood into the tubes. A butterfly cannula which can be left in situ is used for repeated sampling over a short time period, e.g. a glucose tolerance test.

If you fail…

It is often easier to palpate a suitable vein than to see it. Vasodilatation may be achieved by exercising the arm (clenching and unclenching the fist), placing it in warm water or gently tapping over the vein. Try other sites, e.g. a vein in the foot.

Setting up an intravenous (i.v.) cannula

Indications

- Fluid replacement
- Administration of intravenous drugs (e.g. antibiotics)
- To ensure i.v. access in case of emergency (e.g. coronary care)
- Short-term feeding via a peripheral vein.

Equipment

- Cannula. The size is determined by the type of fluid to be infused and the size and condition of the patient's veins. Table 18.1 provides information on cannula sizes, colours and flow rates
- Alcohol swab
- Adhesive tape
- Tourniquet

Practical procedures

Table 18.1 Types of intravenous cannulas		
Cannula colour	Size	Maximum flow rate for crystalloid (mL/min)
Brown	14G	240
Grey	16G	180
Green	18G	80
Pink	20G	54
Blue	22G	31

- 10 mL of 0.9% sodium chloride to flush the cannula
- Infusion fluid (if necessary) already run through a giving set. All i.v. fluids must be checked by a registered nurse. For some fluids, two nurses are required to check the i.v. fluid. Syringe drivers or pumps are needed to control infusion rate of many solutions
- Sharps bin.

Procedure

Read the protocol for taking venous blood as the methods are similar. Place the tourniquet around the upper arm and search carefully for a vein. Asking the patient to lower the arm and clench/release their fist will maximize venous distension. Aim for a palpable vein, preferably away from joints and in the non-dominant arm. Place a towel or pad under the arm. Clean the skin with an alcohol swab and, if a large-bore cannula is being inserted (e.g. 14–16 gauge), anaesthetize the entry site with 2–3 mL of 1% lidocaine (lignocaine) injected intradermally with a 25 gauge needle. Local anaesthetic cream is an alternative and must be applied at least 1 hour prior to the procedure. Apply a small amount of traction to the skin below the cannulation point to reduce movement of the vein. Hold the cannula with the middle and index finger on either side of the cannula and your thumb on the cap at the end and push the cannula through the skin at an angle of 30–40°. Once the cannula enters the vein, blood will flash back into the cannula. The cannula can then be advanced along the vein while gently withdrawing but not completely removing the trocar. Remove the tourniquet, occlude the tip of the cannula by pressing on the vein immediately above the end of the cannula with your finger. Remove the trocar and flush the cannula with 5–10 mL of 0.9% saline to ensure patency. Attach the plastic cap or giving set and ensure that the fluid is running adequately. A sterile semipermeable film dressing is used to cover the insertion site, and the site inspected twice a day to look for evidence of infection.

Post-procedure care

Intravenous catheters are a source of sepsis, and lines should be removed as soon as possible, e.g. intravenous antibiotics switched to oral when indicated. If prolonged intravenous treatment is required, lines should be changed every 72 hours and the date of insertion documented in the clinical record.

Complications

- 'Tissuing' of drip, i.e. the cannula lies outside of the vein
- Thrombophlebitis.

If you fail...

- Come back and try later.
- Vasodilatation may be achieved by placing the arm in warm water or gently tapping over the vein.
- Ask a colleague for help.
- Consider subcutaneous fluids: glucose and 0.9% saline, but not drugs, can be administered subcutaneously via a butterfly needle.

Arterial sampling

Indications

- Blood gas and acid–base analysis
- Very occasionally if blood cannot be obtained from a vein.

Equipment

- Dedicated blood gas syringe or standard syringe flushed through with 2–3 mL of heparin
- 23 gauge needle
- Cotton wool balls
- Alcohol swab
- Disposable gloves.

Procedure

Note the concentration of any inspired oxygen the patient is breathing, which should be constant for at least 20 minutes

Specific procedures

preceding the test. Decide on the site for arterial puncture: brachial, radial or femoral artery. The radial artery (non-dominant arm preferred) at the wrist is the best site for obtaining an arterial sample because it is near to the surface, relatively easy to palpate and stabilize, and the hand usually has a good collateral supply from the ulnar artery, in case of radial artery damage during the procedure. The collateral supply is assessed by Allen's test in which the patient clenches the fist for 20 seconds, pressure is applied to the ulnar and radial artery for 30 seconds (the open hand should then blanch white), and then the examiner releases the pressure over the ulnar artery. A normal result (hand flushing within 5 seconds) indicates a good collateral circulation. The brachial and femoral arteries do not have a good collateral supply. The femoral artery is more likely to be involved with atheroma, especially in the elderly. Clean the area with the alcohol swab and expel excess heparin from the blood gas syringe. Clean and anaesthetize the skin using local anaesthetic (p. 796). Palpate with three fingers over the course of the artery to determine the area of maximum pulsation. Insert the needle, bevel up, at about 45° to the skin. Once the artery is entered, blood will pulsate into the syringe. If no blood is obtained after the needle has been advanced an appropriate distance, withdraw the needle, exerting gentle traction on the plunger, as blood often enters on removal. If this is not successful the needle must be redirected. Once 1.5–2 mL of blood have been obtained, remove the needle and ask an assistant to apply firm pressure with the cotton wool to the puncture site for 5 minutes. Remove the needle from the syringe and expel any air bubbles. The syringe should be capped and sent for immediate analysis (Table 18.2).

Complications

- Arterial spasm and ischaemia
- Dislodgement of atheroma from femoral artery.

Table 18.2 Normal values for arterial blood gases	
pH	7.35–7.45
$P_a\text{co}_2$	4.3–6.0 kPa
$P_a\text{o}_2$	10.5–14 kPa
Base excess	± 2 mmol/L
HCO_3	22–26 mmol/L
O_2 saturation	95–100%

If you fail...

Do not persist with several attempts but ask a senior colleague for help.

Central venous cannulation

Indications

- Measurement of central venous pressure (CVP)
- Infusion of substances irritant to small veins and tissues, e.g. dopamine
- Difficulty in obtaining peripheral venous access
- Administration of drugs during a cardiac arrest
- Modified central venous lines are used for administration of intravenous feeding, insertion of a Swan–Ganz catheter and temporary transvenous cardiac pacing.

Contraindications

There are no absolute contraindications, but the cannula is placed away from an area of skin sepsis if possible.

Equipment

- Materials for a sterile procedure performed under local anaesthetic (p. 795)
- Scalpel and blade
- Central line pack (e.g. Leader-Cath)
- Infusion fluid already run through a giving set, and a three-way tap
- CVP monitoring set if required.

Method

The aim of central venous cannulation is to place the tip of the cannula in the right atrium or superior vena cava. This is usually achieved by percutaneous puncture of the right internal jugular or subclavian vein. The internal jugular vein is preferred in patients with respiratory disease (the risk of pneumothorax is less than with subclavian vein cannulation) or a bleeding tendency (bleeding can be more easily controlled by direct pressure in the neck if there is inadvertent arterial puncture). Correct placement of a catheter in the vein is more likely if sited under ultrasound guidance, although this expertise in not always available.

Specific procedures

This is a sterile procedure performed under local anaesthetic with the operator wearing a sterile gown and the working area isolated with sterile drapes (p. 795). The patient is placed in a slightly head-down position and a small skin incision (see site, later) made with a scalpel blade in the anaesthetized skin. A needle, used to locate the vein, is attached to a saline-filled syringe and gentle aspiration is maintained as the needle is advanced through the skin and subcutaneous tissues towards the vein. Once in the vein, the syringe is removed and the needle occluded with a finger to prevent air embolism. The flexible end of the guidewire is passed down the needle into the vein and the needle removed leaving the guidewire in place. The cannula is loaded on to the guidewire and slid into the vein before the wire is removed, leaving the cannula in position. The giving set is attached to the cannula, which is secured in position by a stitch and transparent adhesive dressing. A chest X-ray is taken as soon as possible after insertion to demonstrate the correct position of the cannula tip and exclude complications such as a pneumothorax.

When removing a central line, remember to place the patient in the head-down position and after removing the cannula press with a gauze pad for a few minutes to prevent bleeding and air embolus.

Internal jugular vein puncture The internal jugular vein runs behind the sternomastoid lateral to the carotid artery. The line of the carotid artery is located with the fingers of the left hand and the site of cannula insertion is chosen as a point at or just above an imaginary line drawn across the cricoid membrane; this avoids damage to structures in the root of the neck. With the right hand, the needle is advanced just lateral to the fingers of the left hand and passed parallel to the midline at an angle of 45° to the skin.

Subclavian vein puncture The needle is inserted just below the midpoint of the clavicle and advanced along its posterior surface towards the suprasternal notch. The needle and syringe are kept parallel to the coronal plane at all times to avoid puncturing the pleura or subclavian artery.

Complications

- Puncture of major arteries, pleura and thoracic duct
- Air and catheter embolism

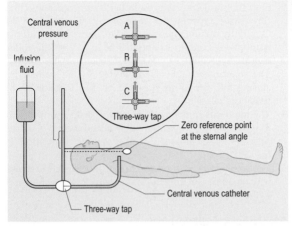

Fig. 18.1 **Measurement of central venous pressure using the mid-axillary line as a reference point.** (After Nicol M (2000) *Essential Nursing Skills*. St Louis, Mosby.)

- Catheter-related sepsis
- Venous thrombosis.

If you fail…

Do not persist with several attempts but ask a senior colleague or anaesthetist for help.

Measurement of central venous pressure

The CVP is the pressure in the right atrium and may be measured continuously using a pressure transducer, or intermittently using a manometer. A constant zero-reference level is essential for accurate measurement; either the mid-axillary line or the sternal angle is usually used. A mark should be made on the skin to indicate the level so that all subsequent readings are made from the same point. The normal value is between 0–4 and 3–7 cmH$_2$O, measured from the sternal angle and mid-axillary line, respectively, as the zero-reference points (Fig. 18.1).

803

1. With the three-way tap in position 'A' allow the 0.9% sodium chloride infusion to run rapidly for a few seconds to check that the line is patent.

2. Stop the infusion using the roller clamp and adjust the three-way tap on the manometer to position 'B'. Gradually open the roller clamp to allow fluid to fill the manometer column to about 5–10 cm. Close the roller clamp.
3. The manometer tube is connected to the patient by closing off the three-way tap to the infusion fluid (position 'C').
4. The meniscus in the manometer will drop steadily until it moves with respiration above and below a mean pressure. The pressure at the end of respiration is the CVP.
5. The infusion is reconnected to the patient via the three-way tap, thus isolating the manometer. Reset the infusion to the prescribed rate.

Electrical cardioversion

Cardioversion is the delivery of energy that is synchronized to the QRS complex, whereas defibrillation is non-synchronized delivery of energy, i.e. the shock is delivered randomly during the cardiac cycle (see below).

Indications

- Elective cardioversion
  - Atrial tachyarrhythmias
- Emergency cardioversion
  - Atrial tachyarrhythmias causing haemodynamic compromise, e.g. hypotension, pulmonary oedema
  - Ventricular tachycardia (VT)
  - Ventricular fibrillation (VF).

Contraindications

- Digitalis toxicity (relative contraindication) – induction of ventricular arrhythmias by cardioversion is more likely
- Atrial fibrillation with onset more than 24 hours previously (due to risk of embolism) unless patient has high-risk symptoms and signs (p. 408).

Equipment

- Defibrillator
- Self-adhesive monitor–defibrillator pad electrodes
- Intravenous cannula in situ.

Table 18.3 Energy levels for monophasic defibrillators

Arrhythmia	Initial shock energy (J)	Subsequent shocks (J)
Supraventricular tachycardia	100	200, 360
Atrial flutter	50	100, 200, 300
Atrial fibrillation	100	200, 360
Ventricular arrhythmias	100	200, 360
Ventricular fibrillation	200	200, 360

Method

General anaesthesia is necessary in a conscious patient to induce amnesia and avoid the pain of the tetanic muscular contraction induced by the electric current through the thorax. Lay the patient flat. If in bed, remove pillows and the head of the bed. The two electrodes are placed in a position that will maximize transmyocardial current flow, and this is usually achieved by placing one at the apex of the heart and the other over the right second intercostal space. For all arrhythmias except VF the defibrillator should be enabled to deliver a synchronized shock, i.e. the shock is delivered on the R wave of the QRS complex. Failure to deliver a synchronized shock may induce VF. Energy selection in cardioversion is arrhythmia dependent (Table 18.3). Energy levels are lower when using a biphasic compared to a monophasic device. Before delivering the shock the operator must make sure that no one, including him- or herself, has any contact with the patient either directly or indirectly, e.g. by touching the bed on which the patient is lying. The operator usually calls 'stand back' before delivering the shock.

Complications

■ Superficial burns to the skin
■ Induction of arrhythmias
■ Systemic embolization. This complication is more likely to occur in patients with AF who have not been anti-coagulated prior to cardioversion (p. 415)
■ Myocardial damage from excessive energy.

If it fails...

Ensure the electrodes have been correctly placed. A change of electrode position, e.g. anterior and posterior chest walls, should be tried. Stop the procedure after a maximum of seven shocks in elective cardioversion. Chemical cardioversion with antiarrhythmic drugs is an alternative.

In the patient who has had a cardiac arrest and is not responding, a difficult decision is when to stop resuscitation and defibrillation efforts. This depends on the patient, the circumstances of the arrest and how long the patient has had a non-perfusing cardiac rhythm. In general, if a patient arrests in hospital and resuscitation has not resulted in a perfusing cardiac rhythm after 30 minutes then further attempts are unlikely to be successful. The prognosis is poorer in patients who arrest outside hospital. There are exceptions: resuscitation is continued for longer in a hypothermic patient.

Pleural aspiration

Indications

- Diagnostic
  - To investigate the cause of a pleural effusion. A pleural biopsy is sometimes performed at the same time, as this increases the diagnostic yield
- Therapeutic
  - To drain large effusions for symptom relief
  - To instil therapeutic agents such as sclerosants.

Equipment

- Materials for a sterile procedure performed under local anaesthesia (p. 795)
- Specimen containers
- For diagnostic tap: 20 mL syringe with 21 gauge needle
- For therapeutic tap:
  - 50 mL syringe with Luer-Lock fitting
  - Three-way tap
  - 14 gauge cannula
  - Receiver for fluid.

Method

This is a sterile procedure performed with a local anaesthetic (p. 795). The patient should be sitting up and leaning over a suitably placed bed table with the arms folded in front of the body. The upper limit of the effusion posteriorly is determined from the chest X-ray and by percussion. The skin and subcutaneous tissues overlying the intercostal space at the chosen level are infiltrated with lidocaine (lignocaine) and the area anaesthetized down to the pleura. The needle is passed over the upper border of the rib to avoid damaging the subcostal neurovascular bundle. For a diagnostic tap 20 mL of fluid is aspirated, placed into appropriate containers and sent for microscopy and culture, including TB, cytology, PH, LDH and protein concentration.

If it fails...

If you cannot obtain any fluid try a different space, usually higher up. If fluid cannot be aspirated or only a small amount is obtained (e.g. with a loculated effusion) an ultrasound examination will identify whether fluid is actually present and, if so, the most promising site for aspiration can be marked.

Complications

- Pneumothorax
- Pulmonary oedema; the risk is greatest with the rapid removal of large quantities of fluid (> 1 litre)
- Damage to the neurovascular bundle which lies in the subcostal groove
- Infection
- Seeding of malignant cells along the tract with a malignant effusion.

Chest drain insertion

Indications

- Pneumothorax
  - In any ventilated patient
  - Tension pneumothorax after initial needle relief
  - Persistent or recurrent pneumothorax after simple aspiration
  - Large secondary pneumothorax in patients over 50 years (p. 548)
- Malignant pleural effusion
- Empyema
- Traumatic haemopneumothorax.

Specific procedures

Equipment

- Materials for a sterile procedure performed under local anaesthetic (p. 795)
- Scalpel and blade
- Chest tube
- Closed drainage system with sterile water
- Suture, e.g. '1' silk
- Instrument for blunt dissection (e.g. curved clamp)
- Artery forceps
- Dressings.

Procedure

Premedication with intravenous midazolam (1–5 mg) may be given immediately before the procedure. This is a sterile procedure performed under local anaesthetic with the operator wearing a sterile gown and the working area isolated with sterile drapes (p. 795). The most common position for insertion of the drain is in the mid-axillary line through the 'safe triangle' (a triangle bordered by the anterior border of latissimus dorsi, the lateral border of the pectoralis major muscle, a line superior to the horizontal level of the nipple, and an apex below the axilla). The position for chest drain insertion is with the patient on the bed, slightly rotated, with the arm on the side of the lesion behind the patient's head, or the patient should be sitting up and leaning over a suitably placed bed table, with the arms folded in front of the body. Small-bore tubes (8–14 French (F)) are adequate for air or low-viscosity effusions. Large-bore drains (28–30 F) are used for blood or pus to minimize blockage. The skin, underlying muscle and pleura is infiltrated with 8–10 mL of 1% lidocaine (lignocaine) advancing over the upper border of the rib below to avoid the subcostal neurovascular bundle. Aspiration is applied intermittently until the pleural cavity is entered and the presence of air or fluid confirmed.

Small-bore tubes   are inserted with the aid of a guideline through the hub of the needle and then the tract enlarged using a dilator. A small-bore tube can then be passed into the thoracic cavity along the wire.

Large-bore tubes   are inserted into the pleural space following blunt dissection of the subcutaneous tissue and muscle into the pleural cavity. A skin incision slightly bigger than the operator's finger and tube, is made just above and parallel to the upper border of the rib below the chosen intercostal space. A simple suture across the incision (wound closure suture for after drain removal) is inserted before blunt dissection. Using a Spencer-Wells clamp or similar, a path is made through the chest wall to open the muscle fibres, and the track widened to allow the passage of a finger ('blunt dissection'). The length of tube required is measured and inserted by holding the tip of the catheter with a curved artery clamp and advancing into the pleural space. The central trocar must not be used to advance the tube.

For both large- and small-bore tubes the tip of the tube should be aimed apically to drain air and basally for fluid. The drain is connected to the underwater drainage system. A stay suture through skin and subcutaneous tissue is inserted to secure the chest drain. With a correctly placed tube, there is drainage of fluid if present, and bubbling of water and respiratory swing in the underwater seal bottle. The position of the tube and expansion of the lung are checked with a chest X-ray. A chest drain should not be clamped other than under the supervision of a respiratory physician or thoracic surgeon. The underwater seal bottle should be kept below the chest drain insertion site. The air outlet of the underwater seal may be connected to moderate suction (-20 cmH$_2$O) to assist in lung re-expansion. This is more often necessary in the presence of an air leak. Large pleural effusions should be drained slowly (< 500 mL per hour) to prevent re-expansion pulmonary oedema. To remove a chest drain, ask the patient to exhale, remove the drain, and tighten the previously placed suture to close the incision.

Complications

- Injury to the neurovascular bundle
- Re-expansion pulmonary oedema
- Infection
- Pneumothorax and surgical emphysema.

If you fail...

Insertion can be carried out under ultrasound control by a senior colleague.

Nasogastric tube insertion

Indications

- To drain gastric secretions, e.g. prior to surgery, acute pancreatitis or for bowel obstruction
- For enteral feeding (using a fine-bore tube) or drug administration.

Equipment

- Nasogastric tube of appropriate size and type, e.g. large-bore (Ryles tube) for drainage of secretions
- 50 mL syringe
- pH indicator strips (0.5 gradation)
- Drainage bag
- Receiver or vomit bowl
- Adhesive tape.

Procedure

Ask the patient to sit up if possible and protect the patient's clothing with a towel. Estimate the length of tube to be inserted by measuring the distance from the patient's nose to the tip of the ear lobe and then to the xiphisternum and mark this distance on the tube. When inserted to the estimated measurement the tip should lie in the patient's stomach. Ask the patient to clear the nasal passages by blowing the nose and select the best nostril. Lubricate the distal end of the tube with water and place into the nostril, advancing slowly along the floor of the nostril to the naso-pharynx. As the tube enters the pharynx, ask the patient to take a sip of water and to swallow as you advance the tube into the oesophagus. Once the tube has reached the measured distance and is thought to be in the stomach, gently insufflate 10–20 mL of air down the enteral tube to clear the tube of any substance that may alter the pH result. Aspirate fluid with the syringe and test for acid with graded pH paper (*not* blue litmus paper). A pH < 5.5 (unless patient on antacids, H_2-receptor antagonists or proton pump inhibitors) indicates that the tube is in the stomach. The pH is higher (pH 6–7) in the lung and small intestine. If no aspirate is obtained repeat the aspiration after each of the following manoeuvres: turn the tube a quarter circle; turn the patient onto the left side; turn the patient onto the right side; and hold syringe below level of stomach. If no aspirate is obtained or the pH is >5.5 an X-ray will be needed to confirm tube placement in the stomach. Secure the tube in position with adhesive tape and record the measurable part of the tube on the observation chart. Tube placement with gastric pH testing should be checked on each occasion:

- Before administration of feed
- Before giving medication
- Following an episode of vomiting or retching
- Following evidence of tube displacement.

Complications

- Aspiration
- Gastro-oesophageal reflux
- Local trauma to nose.

If you fail…

- Try the other nostril.
- Put tube in the refrigerator, which usually causes it to stiffen.

Digital examination of the rectum

Place the patient in the left lateral position with the buttocks at the edge of the couch and ask the patient to curl up with the knees towards the chest. Wear a disposable glove on the right hand and separate the patient's buttocks with both hands. Examine the perineum and anus for inflammation, skin tags, external piles, fissures, fistulae and sinuses. If a prolapse is suspected ask the patient to bear down, and look for the rectal mucosa or bowel appearing through the anus.

Put some lubricant on the index finger of the right hand and place the pulp of the finger flat on the anus. Introduce the finger into the anal canal by pushing gently in a slightly backwards direction. Extreme pain and spasm of the anal sphincter at this stage suggest an anal fissure, which may make further examination impossible. The lower end of the fissure, which is usually situated posteriorly, may be visible if the buttocks are gently separated. To examine the rectum, the finger is advanced and rotated through 180° so that the pulp of the finger lies anteriorly. The walls of the rectum are normally smooth and soft, and any deviation, e.g. polyps, carcinoma, should be noted. Posteriorly the coccyx and sacrum can be felt through the rectal wall, and anteriorly the prostate gland in men and the cervix in women. The normal prostate gland is smooth and firm with a shallow midline groove separating two lateral lobes. A hard, irregular gland with loss of the median groove is characteristic of carcinoma.

After withdrawal, the examining finger should be inspected for blood and the colour of the faeces noted.

Abdominal paracentesis

Indications

- To investigate the cause of ascites
- Rapid relief of large-volume ascites.

Equipment

- Materials for a sterile procedure performed under local anaesthetic (p. 795)
- For diagnostic tap: 20 mL syringe with 21 gauge needle
- For therapeutic tap
  - Large-bore (14 gauge) cannula with three-way tap
  - Collecting system and specimen containers
  - Intravenous giving set and plasma expander.

Procedure

This is a sterile procedure performed under local anaesthesia (p. 795). Ask the patient to empty their bladder before the procedure. Place the patient in a semi-recumbent position and confirm the presence of ascites clinically.

Clean and anaesthetize the skin over the right or left iliac fossa. For a diagnostic tap, a standard 21 gauge (green) needle attached to a 20 mL syringe is introduced along the anaesthetized track in the left or right iliac fossa to the peritoneal cavity, and fluid aspirated and sent for white cell count, microscopy and culture (after inoculation into blood culture bottles), cytology and measurement of protein, albumin (to determine serum–ascitic albumin gradient) and amylase. If indicated, fluid is also sent for measurement of lipids and examination for acid-fast bacillus. For therapeutic paracentesis a large-bore cannula or dedicated paracentesis cannula is introduced in a similar fashion until fluid is aspirated. The stylet is then removed and a 50 mL syringe way tap. Aspiration is continued either via aspiration or free bag drainage until the desired volume of fluid is removed. If large-volume paracentesis is planned (> 3–4 L) in a patient with ascites due to portal hypertension, an intravenous drip should be set up and albumin infused at a concentration of 8 g per litre of ascitic fluid removed. Following the procedure a simple dry dressing is applied.

Complications

- Infection
- Ascitic fluid leak
- Puncture of intra-abdominal viscus
- Renal impairment and encephalopathy after large-volume paracentesis in patients with cirrhosis.

If it fails…

Ask the radiologist to perform the procedure under ultrasound control.

Sengstaken tube insertion

Indications

Variceal bleeding not controlled pharmacologically or by endoscopic therapy.

Equipment

- Sengstaken tube
- 50 mL syringe
- Radio-opaque contrast material (e.g. Omnipaque)
- Length of string
- 0.5 litre bag of saline or glucose
- Large collection bowl.

Procedure

Insertion of a Sengstaken tube is best performed with an endotracheal tube in situ to protect the patient's airway and reduce the risk of aspiration. Familiarize yourself with the construction of the tube and identify the four ports: two for aspiration of the oesophagus and stomach, and two for inflation of the oesophageal and gastric balloons (Fig. 18.2). Check the capacity of both the gastric and the oesophageal

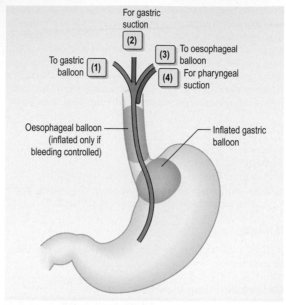

Fig. 18.2 **Diagram of a Sengstaken tube in situ.**

balloon. With the patient on the left lateral side, insert the tube into the mouth and guide into the pharynx with the fingers. The tube should pass easily down the oesophagus. On entry into the stomach, blood is usually readily aspirated through the gastric aspiration port. Insert the tube as far as possible and inflate the gastric balloon with the appropriate volume of fluid (150–250 mL). Using a mixture of water and contrast material aids radiological confirmation of correct placement. The tube is then withdrawn until resistance at the gastro-oesophageal junction is felt, usually at about 35 cm. At this stage the 0.5 L bag of fluid is attached with string to the end of the tube and allowed to hang over the side of the bed, so that constant traction is applied to the balloon. An X-ray is performed to check correct tube placement. It is not normally necessary to inflate the oesophageal balloon. The balloon should be left in place inflated for no longer than 24 hours to minimize the risk of pressure necrosis of the oesophagus. Aspirate every 15 min from the gastric and oesophageal aspiration ports, and if there is continued bleeding inflate the oesophageal balloon to 40 mmHg. The oesophageal balloon should only be inflated if the gastric balloon is inflated.

Complications

- Oesophageal rupture
- Pressure necrosis leading to oesophageal ulceration and stricture
- Aspiration leading to pneumonia.

Urine collection and testing

Urine passed into a clean dry vessel is suitable for chemical tests. A mid-stream specimen of urine (MSU) collected into a sterile specimen pot is necessary for microscopy and culture. The urine should be analysed immediately or stored in a refrigerator to reduce the growth of contaminants.

Urine testing

Commercially prepared paper strips are available to test for urine specific gravity, pH, protein, glucose, ketones, bilirubin, urobilinogen and blood. Usually one strip is impregnated with dyes specific for each test. It is important that the strips are kept in sealed, dry containers and the test areas not handled. The manufacturer's instructions must be followed exactly. The strip is dipped briefly into the urine and its edge then run against the rim of the container to remove excess fluid. The strip is held horizontally (to prevent urine running down the strip and mixing the dyes) and the colour changes read at exactly the times specified by the manufacturer. The colour changes are compared with the colour charts supplied on the outside of the strip containers.

Bladder catheterization (urethral)

Indications

- Relief of urinary retention
- To monitor urinary output in the critically ill
- Urinary incontinence
- Collection of an uncontaminated urine specimen for bacteriological analysis – rarely.

Equipment

- Sterile catheter pack (usually prepacked, containing kidney dish, dressing towels, gallipot for sterile saline and gauze swabs)
- Sterile lidocaine (lignocaine) gel with nozzle
- Sterile 0.9% sodium chloride for cleaning
- 12–14 gauge catheter (usually Foley type)
- Sterile gloves
- 20 mL syringe with sterile water
- Catheter bag with stand/holder
- Disposable waterproof absorbent pad.

Procedure

Place the patient in a supine, slightly reclining position. Women should have their knees flexed and the thighs apart. Remove the bedclothes to expose the genital area and place the disposable pad beneath the buttocks. Wash your hands and open the catheter pack, ensuring that principles of asepsis are maintained throughout. Open the catheter, but do not remove it from its internal wrapping, and place it on the sterile receiver on the trolley. Wash your hands and put on the sterile gloves. Place sterile dressing towels onto the bed area between the patient's legs and over the thighs. In men tear a hole in the centre of the towel and allow the penis to protrude through. In the female use one gloved hand to cleanse the urethral meatus with saline while holding the labia apart with the other. Use a new gauze swab for each stroke and clean from the front towards the anus. In the male the foreskin, if present, should be retracted in order to cleanse the meatus. Apply sterile lidocaine gel to the tip of the catheter and into the urethra in men. Place a kidney dish between the legs in readiness. Insert the catheter into the urethra, holding the penis perpendicular to the body. Gradually advance the catheter out of its wrapper and into the urethra. Gentle pressure is required to advance the catheter into the bladder, at which point urine should flow into the kidney dish. Any resistance should prompt withdrawal and reinsertion. The catheter should be inserted almost to the side arm before inflating the balloon with the volume of sterile water indicated on the catheter. The catheter is then withdrawn to lie at the bladder neck and connected to the catheter drainage bag. Reposition the foreskin in uncircumcised men, and record the volume of urine drained.

Complications

- Infection
- Urethral trauma and stricture formation.

If you fail...

Do not make repeated attempts in the male, as damage to the longer urethra can occur. Ask advice of surgeons/ urologists for consideration of a suprapubic approach through the abdominal wall, directly into the bladder.

Lumbar puncture

Indications

- To obtain a sample of CSF for detection of infection, blood, malignant cells or abnormal proteins
- Administration of chemotherapeutic drugs
- Therapeutic, e.g. removal of CSF in the treatment of benign intracranial hypertension.

A brain CT or MRI scan should be performed before LP in patients who have clinical features that increase the likelihood of having intracranial mass lesions or increase in CSF pressure which would preclude LP: immunosuppression, bleeding tendency, focal neurological signs, papilloedema, loss of consciousness or seizure.

Equipment

- Materials for a sterile procedure performed under local anaesthetic (p. 795)
- 23–24 gauge spinal needle
- Manometer
- Three separate numbered sterile collection bottles.

Procedure

This is a sterile procedure performed under local anaesthetic. Position the patient on the left side on the edge of the bed with the knees curled up to the chest. Identify the L3–L4 interspace by palpating the anterior superior iliac spine and marking the interspace perpendicularly below it. Having cleansed and anaesthetized the skin, insert the spinal needle in the interspace with the stylet in place, aiming for the umbilicus. Resistance is usually felt at the spinal ligaments and again at the dura. The stylet can then be removed, at which stage clear colourless fluid should emerge. The manometer is then attached to measure CSF pressure (normally 80–180 mmH$_2$O with small visible excursions related to pulse and respiration). Fluid is collected into the three separate numbered bottles. A decreasing concentration of red blood cells from bottles 1 to 3 indicates a traumatic tap, rather than blood in the CSF. Fluid should be sent for microscopy and culture, protein, and glucose concentration with a simultaneous plasma glucose sample. Additional investigations may be appropriate depending on the suspected diagnosis. The patient should lie flat for 12 hours after the procedure to avoid a headache that may develop.

Complications

- Post-procedure headache
- Infection
- Herniation of the brainstem through the foramen magnum ('coning').

If you fail...

Try with the patient sitting upright on the edge of the bed (CSF pressure cannot be measured in this position).

PROCEDURES AFTER DEATH

Diagnosis of death

When asked to confirm a patient's death it is important to see the body and to confirm the identity of the patient with the nursing staff.

Confirmation of death involves the demonstration of:

- Fixed and dilated pupils
- Absent carotid pulse
- No breath sounds over 1 minute
- No heart sounds over 1 minute
- No response to painful stimuli, e.g. pressing firmly on the sternum.

Record these details in the notes, giving the time and date of confirmation of death, and sign your name clearly.

Death certification and referral to the Coroner

A death certificate is usually completed on the day following death. It is signed by a doctor who attended the deceased in his or her last illness, and that doctor must have seen the patient both within 14 days before death and after death. Although there is no legal requirement for a doctor to inform the Coroner of a death (this is the legal responsibility of the Registrar of Deaths), it is usual to inform the Coroner of a death under particular circumstances. These include:

- Uncertain cause of death
- The patient has not been seen by the doctor within 14 days before death
- The death was suspicious
- Death occurred within 24 hours of admission to hospital without a firm diagnosis being made
- Deaths due to accidents, injuries, suicide, neglect, poisoning or drug or alcohol overdose
- Death of persons in legal custody
- Death related to medical treatment or within 24 hours of an anaesthetic.

Cremation forms

If the patient is to be cremated you will be asked to complete form B, the Certificate of Medical Attendance, on the cremation form. You must have attended the patient within 14 days prior to death and you must see the patient after death (ensuring that there are no pacemaker implants in the body); make certain that the cause of death on the cremation form is identical to that on the death certificate.

Therapeutics 19

Medicines should be prescribed only when they are necessary; and in all cases the benefit of administering the medicine should be considered in relation to the risk involved. This is particularly important during pregnancy when the risk to both the mother and fetus must be considered. Titles of drugs and preparations should be written in full. Where non-proprietary ('generic') drugs are available they should be used in prescribing other than rare exceptions where stated. Names followed by the symbol ® are or have been used as proprietary names in the UK. Prescriptions should be written legibly in ink or otherwise so as to be indelible, should be dated, should state the full name and address of the prescriber, and the name, address and date of birth or age of the patient.

Any drug may produce unwanted or unexpected adverse reactions. Doctors, dentists, coroners, pharmacists and nurses are encouraged to report suspected adverse reactions to the relevant regulatory agency. The elderly are more susceptible to adverse drug reactions and drug interactions because of co-morbidity, polypharmacy, changes in drug distribution associated with a reduction in body mass and relatively more of the stroke volume reaching the brain (which explains why the elderly are more vulnerable to the effects of drugs acting centrally). Impairment of renal and liver function may necessitate a reduction in drug dosage or contraindicate prescribing of some drugs.

This chapter has listed some of the drugs commonly prescribed, particularly by junior doctors. The doses given are for adults. A full list of drug interactions and dosage adjustment in renal and liver failure is beyond the scope of this chapter and readers should refer to the *National Formulary*.

INFECTIOUS DISEASES

Antimicrobial agents are natural or synthetic chemical substances that suppress the growth of, or destroy, micro-organisms including bacteria, fungi and viruses.

Antibacterials

The choice of antibacterial is based on patient factors and the known or likely causative organism. Factors related to the patient which must be considered include history of drug allergy (e.g. penicillin), renal and hepatic function, susceptibility to infection (e.g. immunosuppressed), severity of illness, age, ability to take drugs by mouth, and in women use of the contraceptive pill, pregnancy or breast-feeding. Antibacterials can be either bacteriostatic (inhibit bacterial growth but do not destroy it, infection is eliminated by the native immune system) or bacteriocidal (kill the micro-organism). Antibacterials are also grouped according to their mechanism of action.

β-Lactam antibacterials

Mechanism of action
Inhibit synthesis of the peptidoglycan layer of the cell wall, which surrounds certain bacteria and is essential for their survival.

Indications
Benzylpenicillin (penicillin G) is effective for many streptococcal and meningococcal infections, leptospirosis and treatment of Lyme disease. *Phenoxymethylpenicillin* (penicillin V) has a similar antibacterial spectrum to benzylpenicillin but it should not be used for serious infections because gut absorption is unpredictable. *Flucloxacillin* is effective for infections due to beta-lactamase-producing staphylococci (most staphylococci are resistant to benzylpenicillin because they produce penicillinases). *Ampicillin* is principally indicated for the treatment of exacerbations of chronic bronchitis and middle ear infections. *Amoxicillin* is a derivative of ampicillin and has a similar antibacterial spectrum. It is better absorbed than ampicillin when given by mouth. Co-amoxiclav consists of amoxicillin with the beta-lactamase inhibitor clavulanic acid which extends the spectrum of activity of amoxicillin.

Preparations and dose

Benzylpenicillin   *Injection: 600 mg vial.*
IM/IV   (slow injection or infusion): 2.4–4.8 g daily in four divided doses. Higher doses may be needed in serious infections.

Phenoxymethylpenicillin   *Tablets: 250 mg; Solution: 125 mg/ 5 mL, 250 mg/mL.*
Oral   500 mg every 6 hours increased up to 1 g every 6 hours in severe infections.

Flucloxacillin   *Capsules: 250 mg, 500 mg; Solution: 125 mg/ 5 mL, 250 mg/5 mL; Injection: 250 mg vial.*
Oral   250–500 mg every 6 hours, at least 30 minutes before food.
IM   250–500 mg every 6 hours.
IV   (slow injection or infusion): 0.25–2 g every 6 hours.

Amoxicillin   *Capsules: 250 mg, 500 mg; Suspension: 125 mg/ 5 mL, 250 mg/5 mL; Injection: 250 mg vial.*
Oral   250–500 mg depending on infection.
IM/IV   (slow injection or infusion): 500 mg every 8 hours increased to 1 g every 6 hours in severe infections.

Ampicillin   *Capsules: 250 mg, 500 mg; Suspension: 125 mg/ 5 mL, 250 mg/5 mL; Injection: 500 mg vial.*
Oral   0.25–1 g every 6 hours 30 minutes before food.
IM/IV   (slow injection or infusion): 500 mg every 4–6 hours increased to 2 g every 6 hours in endocarditis and 2 g every 4 hours in *Listeria* meningitis.

Side-effects

Hypersensitivity reactions include urticaria, fever, rashes, and anaphylaxis. Individuals with a history of anaphylaxis, urticaria or rash immediately after penicillin administration are at risk of immediate hypersensitivity to a penicillin and should not receive a penicillin or cephalosporin (10% of penicillin-allergic patients are also allergic to cephalosporins). Encephalopathy with fits results from excessively high doses or in patients with severe renal failure. Diarrhoea can occur as a result of disturbance of the normal colonic flora. Other effects are interstitial nephritis, and reversible neutropenia and eosinophilia. Aminopenicillins (e.g. amoxicillin) frequently produce a non-allergic maculopapular rash in patients with glandular fever.

823

Cautions/contraindications
Contraindicated in penicillin hypersensitivity (see above); macrolides are an alternative in these patients.

Cephalosporins

Mechanism of action
Inhibit bacterial wall synthesis in a manner similar to the penicillins.

Indications
Broad-spectrum antibiotics which are used for the treatment of septicaemia, pneumonia, meningitis, biliary-tract infections, peritonitis and urinary tract infections.

Preparations and dose
Cephalosporins are often classified by 'generations'. The members within each generation share similar antibacterial activity. Succeeding generations tend to have increased activity against Gram-negative bacilli, usually at the expense of Gram-positive activity, and increased ability to cross the blood–brain barrier.

First-generation
Cefalexin *Capsules: 250 mg, 500 mg; Suspension: 125 mg/5 mL, 250 mg/5 mL.*
Oral 250 mg every 8 hours, doubled for severe infections; maximum 4 g daily.

Cefradine *Capsules: 250 mg, 500 mg; Syrup: 250 mg/5 mL; Injection: 500 mg, 1 g vial.*
Oral 250–500 mg every 6 hours; up to 1 g every 6 hours in severe infections.
IM/IV (over 3–5 min or infusion): 0.5–1 g every 6 hours, increased to 8 g daily in severe infections.

Second generation
Cefaclor *Capsules: 250 mg, 500 mg; Suspension: 125 mg/5 mL, 250 mg/5 mL.*
Oral 250 mg every 8 hours, doubled for severe infections; maximum 4 g daily.

Cefuroxime *Tablets: 125 mg, 250 mg; Suspension: 125 mg/mL; Injection: 250 mg, 750 mg, 1.5 g vial.*
Oral 250 mg twice daily in most infections; double dose for pneumonia. Gonorrhoea: 1 g as a single dose; Lyme disease: 500 mg twice daily for 20 days.

IM/IV 750 mg every 6–8 hours; 1.5 g every 6–8 hours in severe infections. Single injected doses over 750 mg by intravenous route only. Gonorrhoea: 1.5 g in a single dose i.m. (divided between two sites); surgical prophylaxis: 1.5 g by i.v. injection at induction, up to three further doses of 750 mg i.m./i.v. for high-risk procedures.

Third generation

Cefotaxime *Injection: 500 mg, 1 g, 2 g.*
IM/IV (injection or infusion): 1 g every 12 hours increased in severe infections (e.g. meningitis) to 8 g daily in four divided doses.

Ceftazidime *Injection: 250 mg, 500 mg, 1 g, 2 g.*
IM/IV (injection or infusion): 1 g every 8 hours or 2 g every 12 hours; 2 g every 8 hours or 3 g every 12 hours in severe infections. Single doses over 1 g by intravenous route only.

Side-effects
Skin rashes, nausea and vomiting, diarrhoea (including *Clostridium difficile* colitis), hypersensitivity reactions (see penicillin).

Cautions/contraindications
Penicillin hypersensitivity.

Aminoglycosides

Mechanism of action
Inhibit protein synthesis in bacteria by binding irreversibly to the 30S ribosomal unit. This inhibits translation from mRNA to protein. Aminoglycosides are bactericidal.

Indications
Active against many Gram-negative bacteria (including *Pseudomonas* species) and some Gram-positive bacteria but are inactive against anaerobes. Often used for serious Gram-negative infections when they have a complementary and synergistic action with agents that disrupt cell wall synthesis (e.g. penicillins).

Preparations and dose
Examples: gentamicin (the most widely used), amikacin, neomycin, netilmicin, streptomycin, tobramycin.

Gentamicin *Injection: 40 mg/mL.*
IM/IV (slow injection over 3 min or infusion): 3–5 mg/kg in divided doses every 8 hours.

825

Side-effects

Most unwanted effects are dose related and are probably related to high trough concentrations of the drug. Ototoxicity can lead to both vestibular and auditory dysfunction resulting in often irreversible disturbances of balance or deafness. Renal toxicity, acute neuromuscular blockade, nausea, vomiting, rash and antibiotic-associated colitis.

Cautions/contraindications

Contraindicated in myasthenia gravis. Monitor serum concentrations in all patients and reduce dose in renal impairment. In patients with normal renal function serum aminoglycoside concentrations should be measured after three to four doses (earlier and more frequent measurements in patients with renal failure), 1 hour after i.m. or i.v. administration ('peak' concentration to ensure bactericidal efficacy) and also just before the next dose ('trough' concentration to minimize the risk of toxic effects).

Macrolides

Mechanism of action

Interfere with bacterial protein synthesis by binding reversibly to the 50S subunit of the bacterial ribosome. The action is primarily bacteriostatic unless at high concentrations.

Indications

Erythromycin has an antibacterial spectrum that is similar to that of penicillin; it is thus an alternative in penicillin-allergic patients. Indications for erythromycin include respiratory infections, whooping cough, Legionnaires' disease, *Chlamydia* infections and campylobacter enteritis. Erythromycin has poor activity against *H. influenzae*. Clarithromycin is a derivative of erythromycin with slightly greater activity. Azithromycin has slightly less activity than erythromycin against Gram-positive bacteria but enhanced activity against Gram-negative bacteria.

Preparations and dose

Examples: erythromycin, azithromycin, clarithromycin.

Erythromycin *Capsules and tablets: 250 mg; Suspension: 125 mg/5 mL, 250 mg/5 mL, 500 mg/5 mL; Injection: 1 g vial.*
Oral 0.5–1 g daily in two or four divided doses; up to 4 g daily in severe infections. Early syphilis: 500 mg four times daily for 14 days. Uncomplicated genital chlamydia and non-gonococcal urethritis: 500 mg twice daily for 14 days.

IV infusion 25 mg/kg by continuous infusion or in divided doses every 6 hours; 50 mg/kg in severe infections.

Clarithromycin *Tablets: 250 mg, 500 mg; Injection: 500 mg vial.*
Oral 250 mg every 12 hours; increased in severe infections to 500 mg every 12 hours.
IV infusion into larger proximal vein: 500 mg twice daily.

Side-effects

GI upset (epigastric discomfort, nausea, vomiting and diarrhoea) are common with the oral preparation of erythromycin; azithromycin and clarithromycin are better tolerated. Skin rashes, cholestatic jaundice (with erythromycin), prolongation of the QT interval on the ECG, with a predisposition to ventricular arrhythmias. Erythromycin and clarithromycin inhibit P450 drug-metabolizing enzymes and can elevate levels of drugs (e.g. carbamazepine and ciclosporin), requiring these enzymes for metabolism (see National Formulary for list).

Sulphonamides and trimethoprim

Mechanism of action

Inhibit the enzyme dihydrofolate reductase in the synthetic pathway to folic acid. Bacteria cannot utilize external folic acid, a nutrient that is essential for cell growth.

Indications

The importance of the sulphonamides has decreased as a result of increasing bacterial resistance and their replacement by antibacterials that are generally more active and less toxic. Sulfamethoxazole and trimethoprim are used in combination (as co-trimoxazole) because of their synergistic activity. However, co-trimoxazole is associated with rare but serious side-effects (e.g. Stevens–Johnson syndrome, bone marrow suppression) and its use is limited to the treatment of *Pneumocystis carinii* pneumonia, toxoplasmosis and nocardiasis. In other infections it is only used when there is evidence of sensitivity and good reason to prefer this combination to a single drug. Trimethoprim is used in urinary tract infections and acute and chronic bronchitis.

827

Trimethoprim *Tablets: 100 mg, 200 mg; Suspension: 50 mg/5 mL.*
Oral 200 mg every 12 hours.

Side-effects

Nausea, vomiting and diarrhoea, skin rashes. Rarely bone marrow suppression, folate deficiency (in patients with depleted folate stores), photosensitivity and allergic reactions including anaphylaxis.

Cautions/contraindications

Contraindicated in blood dyscrasias.

Metronidazole and tinidazole

Mechanism of action

A toxic metabolite inhibits bacterial DNA synthesis and breaks down existing DNA. Only some anaerobes and some protozoa contain the enzyme (nitroreductase) that converts metronidazole to its toxic metabolite. It is bactericidal.

Indications

Anaerobic infections, protozoal infections, *Helicobacter pylori* eradication, *C. difficile* colitis. Metronidazole is more commonly used than tinidazole.

Preparations and dose

Metronidazole   *Tablets: 200 mg, 400 mg; Suspension: 200 mg/ 5 mL; Intravenous infusion: 5 mg/5 mL; Flagyl® suppositories.*
Oral   400 mg every 8 hours; for surgical prophylaxis, 400 mg before surgery and three further doses of 400 mg every 8 hours for high-risk procedures.
IV infusion   over 20 minutes: 500 mg every 8 hours; for surgical prophylaxis, 500 mg at induction and up to three further doses of 500 mg every 8 hours for high-risk procedures.
By rectum   500 mg every 8 hours; for surgical prophylaxis, 1 g 2 hours before surgery and up to three further doses of 1 g every 8 hours for high-risk procedures.

Side-effects

Nausea, vomiting, metallic taste, disulfiram-like reaction (unpleasant hangover symptoms) with alcohol, skin rashes, and abnormal liver biochemistry. On prolonged therapy, peripheral neuropathy, transient epileptiform seizures and leucopenia.

Cautions/contraindications

Caution with alcohol ingestion; reduce dose in severe liver disease and avoid in porphyria.

Quinolones

Mechanism of action
Inhibit replication of bacterial DNA. The effect is bactericidal.

Indications
Ciprofloxacin has a broad spectrum of activity and is particularly active against Gram-negative bacteria. It has only weak activity against streptococci, staphylococci and anaerobes.

Preparations and dose
Examples: ciprofloxacin, norfloxacin, levofloxacin.

Ciprofloxacin *Tablets: 100 mg, 250 mg, 500 mg, 750 mg; Suspension: 250 mg/5 mL; Intravenous infusion: 2 mg/mL.*
Oral 250–750 mg twice daily depending on infection.
IV infusion (over 30–60 minutes): 200–400 mg twice daily.

Side-effects
Gastrointestinal upset (nausea, vomiting, diarrhoea), CNS effects (dizziness, headache, tremors, rarely convulsions), photosensitive skin rashes, tendon damage (pain, inflammation, rupture).

Cautions/contraindications
Contraindicated in patients with a history of tendon disorders related to quinolone use; risk of tendon rupture is increased by corticosteroids. If tendonitis is suspected, stop quinolone immediately.

GASTROINTESTINAL SYSTEM

Drugs for dyspepsia and peptic ulceration

Antacids

Mechanism of action
Neutralize gastric acid. Other actions may include increased binding of growth factors to ulcers, promotion of angiogenesis and inhibition of pepsin activity. Alginate-containing antacids form a 'raft' that floats on the surface of the stomach contents to reduce reflux and protect the gastro-oesophageal mucosa.

Indications
Symptomatic relief in dyspepsia, gastro-oesophageal reflux and peptic ulceration. Healing of peptic ulcers is much less

Gastrointestinal system

than with antisecretory drugs (see below) and antacids should not be used for this indication.

Preparations and dose

Aluminium hydroxide *Tablets: 500 mg; Oral suspension: 4% w/w in water.*

1–2 tablets chewed or 5–10 mL four times daily and at bedtime, or as required.

Magnesium trisilicate *Mixture.*

10–20 mL three to four times daily.

Co-magaldrox (Mucogel®) *Suspension.* Mixture of aluminium hydroxide 220 mg, and magnesium hydroxide 195 mg/5 mL.

10–20 mL 20 minutes to 1 hour after meals and at bedtime, or as required.

Alginate-containing antacid *Tablets, liquid.* Gaviscon® contains sodium bicarbonate, sodium alginate, calcium bicarbonate.

1–2 tablets chewed or 10–20 mL four times daily after meals and at bedtime.

Side-effects

Magnesium-containing antacids tend to be laxative, whereas aluminium-containing antacids may be constipating; antacids containing both aluminium and magnesium may reduce these colonic side-effects.

Cautions/contraindications

Antacids may interfere with the absorption of other drugs and in general other drugs should be given at least 1 hour before or after each dose of antacid. Antacids and compound alginate preparations with a high sodium content, e.g. magnesium trisilicate mixture (6.3 mmol/10 mL) and Gaviscon® (6.2 mmol/10 mL; 2.0 mmol/tablet) should be avoided in cardiac, renal or hepatic disease. Aluminium hydroxide is contraindicated in hypophosphataemia. Constipating antacids (i.e. those containing aluminium) should be avoided in liver disease.

H$_2$-receptor antagonists

Mechanism of action

These reduce gastric acid secretion as a result of histamine H$_2$-receptor blockade.

Indications

Gastro-oesophageal reflux disease (GORD), prevention of gastroduodenal damage in patients requiring intensive care, prevention of NSAID-induced duodenal ulcers, and in high doses prevention of gastric ulcers (PPI usually preferred).

Preparations and dose

Ranitidine *Tablets: 150 mg, 300 mg; Syrup 75 mg/5 mL; Injection 50 mg/2 mL.*
Oral

- GORD: 150 mg twice daily or 300 mg at night, 150 mg four times daily in severe cases for 4–8 weeks. Reduce to lowest dose possible to relieve symptoms in maintenance treatment.
- NSAID-associated ulceration: 150 mg twice daily or 300 mg at night.

IV   50 mg diluted to 20 mL and given over at least 2 minutes every 6–8 hours.

Cimetidine *Tablets 200 mg, 400 mg; Syrup 200 mg/5 mL.*
Oral

- GORD: 400 mg four times daily for 4–8 weeks; reduce down to lowest dose possible for maintenance treatment.
- NSAID-associated ulceration: 400 mg twice daily or 800 mg at night.

Side-effects

Diarrhoea, altered liver biochemistry, headache dizziness, rash. Rarely other side-effects (see *National Formulary*).

Cautions/contraindications

Cimetidine retards oxidative hepatic drug metabolism by binding to microsomal cytochrome P450. It should be avoided in patients stabilized on warfarin, phenytoin, and theophylline (or aminophylline) but other interactions (see *National Formulary*) may be of less clinical relevance.

Proton pump inhibitors

Mechanism of action

Inhibit gastric acid secretion by blocking the hydrogen/potassium-adenosine triphosphate enzyme system (the 'proton pump') of the gastric parietal cell.

Indications

GORD; healing of peptic ulcers; prevention of NSAID-induced peptic ulcers; in combination with antibacterials for eradication of *Helicobacter pylori*; intravenously and after endoscopic therapy to reduce rebleeding rates in patients with bleeding peptic ulcers; inhibition of gastric acid in pathological hypersecretory conditions, e.g. gastrinoma; prevention of peptic ulcers in critically ill patients; prophylaxis of acid aspiration during general anaesthesia.

Preparations and dose
Omeprazole *Capsules and tablets: 10 mg, 20 mg, 40 mg; Dispersible tablets (Losec® MUPS); Intravenous infusion (Losec®): vial.*

- GORD: 20–40 mg once daily for 4–8 weeks, maintenance 10–20 mg once daily.
- Healing of peptic ulcers: 20 mg daily for 4 weeks.
- Prevention of NSAID-induced ulcers: 20 mg daily.
- Eradication of *H. pylori* (in combination with anti-bacterials): 20 mg twice daily.
- By intravenous injection in bleeding peptic ulcers: 80 mg over 5 minutes and then 8 mg per minute (vial diluted in 100 mL 0.9% sodium chloride or 5% dextrose).
- Gastrinoma: 60 mg once daily, usual range 20–120 mg daily.
- Gastric acid reduction during general anaesthesia: 40 mg on preceding evening then 40 mg 2–6 hours before surgery.

Lansoprazole *Zoton® capsules: 15 mg, 30 mg (also in suspension); Zoton Fastab® (orodispersible tablet): 15 mg, 30 mg.*

- GORD: 30 mg once daily for 4–8 weeks, maintenance 15–30 mg once daily.
- Healing of peptic ulcers: 30 mg daily for 4 weeks.
- Prevention of NSAID-induced ulcers: 15 mg daily.
- Eradication of *H. pylori* (in combination with anti-bacterials): 20 mg twice daily.
- Gastrinoma: 60 mg once daily, usual range 30–120 mg daily.

Side-effects
Gastrointestinal disturbance (diarrhoea, nausea, vomiting), liver dysfunction, hypersensitivity reactions, headache, skin reactions, increased risk of gastrointestinal infections (due to reduced gastric acidity).

Cautions/contraindications
Omeprazole may decrease the effect of warfarin, phenytoin and diazepam. Lansoprazole may increase the effect of warfarin, phenytoin and theophylline. Reduce dose in severe liver disease.

Constipation

Treatment of constipation is initially with lifestyle changes and drugs are reserved for use as second-line treatment. It may be necessary to use a combination of two different types of laxative, e.g. stimulant plus faecal softener. All laxatives are contraindicated in intestinal obstruction or perforation, paralytic ileus, and severe inflammatory conditions of the gut such as Crohn's disease and ulcerative colitis.

Bulk-forming laxatives

Mechanism of action
Absorb water and increase faecal mass, which stimulates peristalsis.

Indications
Treatment of slow-transit constipation and bulking of stool in colostomy, diverticular disease and irritable bowel syndrome.

Preparations and dose
Wheat bran is one of the most effective fibre laxatives, and patients can add it to meals, e.g. cereal (2–6 tablespoons per day).

Ispaghula husk   *Fybogel® granules: 3.5 g sachet or 150 g granules.*
   1 sachet or 2 level 5-mL spoonfuls of granules in water twice daily after meals.

Methycellulose   *Celevac® tablets: 500 mg.*
   3–6 tablets twice daily with at least 300 mL of liquid.

Sterculia   *Normacol® granules: 7 g sachets or 500 g granules.*
   1–2 sachets or 1–2 heaped 5-mL spoonfuls washed down with plenty of liquid once or twice daily after meals.

Side-effects
Flatulence, abdominal distension.

Cautions/contraindications
Maintain adequate fluid intake to prevent faecal impaction; contraindications (see above).

Stimulant laxatives

Mechanism of action
Increase colonic motor activity.

Indications
Short-term treatment of constipation.

Preparations and dose
Bisacodyl *Tablets: 5 mg; Suppositories: 10 mg.*
Oral 5–10 mg at night, occasionally increase to 15–20 mg.
By rectum 10 mg in the morning.

Docusate sodium *Dioctyl® capsules: 100 mg; Docusol® solution: 50 mg/5 mL; Norgalax® Micro-enema: 120 mg in 10 g single-dose pack.*
Oral 500 mg daily in two to three divided doses.
By rectum 10 g unit daily.

Glycerol (glycerin) *Suppositories: glycerol 700 mg.*
  1 suppository moistened with water before use.

Senna *Tablets: 7.5 mg; Senokot® granules: 5.5 mg/g; Senokot® syrup: 7.5 mg/5 mL.*
  2–4 tablets, 1–2 level 5-mL spoonfuls of granules with water, 10–20 mL of syrup at night.

Side-effects
Abdominal cramps, hypokalaemia, prolonged use may precipitate the onset of an atonic non-functioning colon.

Cautions/contraindications
Contraindications (see above).

Osmotic laxatives

Mechanism of action
Draw fluid from the body into the bowel.

Indications
Treatment of constipation. Lactulose is used in the treatment of encephalopathy. Phosphate enemas are used to evacuate the bowel before radiological procedures, flexible sigmoidoscopy and surgery.

Preparations and dose
Lactulose *Solution: 3.1–3.7 g/5 mL.*
  Initially 15 mL twice daily; hepatic encephalopathy: 30–50 mL three times daily adjusted to produce two to three soft stools daily.

Macrogols (polyethylene glycol) *Movicol® (polyethylene glycol '3350' with electrolytes).*

1–3 sachets daily in divided doses; each sachet dissolved in 125 mL of water. For smaller dosing, Movicol-Half® is also available.

Magnesium salts *Magnesium hydroxide mixture; Magnesium sulphate (Epsom salts).*

25–50 mL when required of magnesium hydroxide; 5–10 g of magnesium sulphate in a glass of water before breakfast.

Phosphates (rectal) *Fleet® Ready-to-use Enema: 118 mL.*

One enema inserted 30 minutes before evacuation required.

Sodium citrate (rectal) *Micralax Micro-enema®: 5 mL..*

One enema as required.

Side-effects
Abdominal distension, colic, nausea, local irritation after phosphate enema.

Cautions/contraindications
Contraindications (see above). May also cause electrolyte disturbance. Use with caution in hepatic and renal impairment.

Bowel-cleansing solutions

Indications
Used before colonic surgery, colonoscopy or radiological examination to ensure the bowel is free of solid contents. They are not treatments for constipation. Bowel-cleansing agents are coupled with a low-residue diet for at least 2 days before the procedure, copious intake of water or other clear fluids and cessation of all solid foods on the day before the procedure.

Mechanism of action
This is variable depending on drug.

Preparations and dose
Citramag® *Magnesium carbonate 11.57 g and citric acid 17.79 g/sachet.*

1 sachet at 8.00 a.m. and 1 sachet between 2 and 4 p.m. on day before procedure.

Fleet Phospho-soda® *Sodium dihydrogen phosphate dehydrate 24.4 g, disodium phosphate dodecahydrate 10.8 g/45 mL.*

45 mL diluted with 120 mL of water (half glass), followed by one full glass of water. For morning procedures, the first

dose should be taken at 7 a.m. and the second dose at 7 p.m. the day before the procedure. For afternoon procedures, the first dose should be taken at 7 p.m. on the day before and the second dose at 7 a.m. on the day of the procedure.

Klean-prep®   *Macrogol '3350'.*

2 sachets diluted with water to 2 litres, and 250 mL drunk rapidly every 10–15 minutes. 2 sachets on evening before examination, and 2 sachets on morning of examination.

Picolax®   *Sodium picosulfate 10 mg/sachet with magnesium citrate.*

Dosing as for Citramag®.

Side-effects
Nausea, vomiting, abdominal cramps. Occasionally dehydration and hypotension, electrolyte disturbance.

Cautions/contraindications
See under treatment of constipation.

Diarrhoea

Most cases of acute diarrhoea are infective and will settle without treatment. Oral rehydration salts (Dioralyte®), 1 sachet after every loose motion, are often used especially in the elderly and children. Antidiarrhoeal agents relieve symptoms of acute diarrhoea and can be given in uncomplicated cases. Antidiarrhoeal agents, e.g. loperamide, are also used in the management of chronic diarrhoea.

Loperamide   *Capsules: 2 mg.*

Mechanism of action
Antimotility agent.

Indications
Symptomatic treatment of acute diarrhoea; chronic diarrhoea in adults.

Side-effects
Constipation, abdominal cramps, dizziness.

Cautions/contraindications
Active ulcerative colitis or infective diarrhoea associated with bloody stools.

Nausea and vomiting

Antiemetics should be prescribed only when the cause of vomiting is known (e.g. drugs particularly cytotoxic chemotherapy, postoperative, motion sickness, pregnancy, and migraine) because otherwise they may delay diagnosis. If antiemetic drug treatment is indicated, the drug is chosen according to the aetiology of vomiting. Dexamethasone (p. 880) has antiemetic effects and is used in vomiting associated with cancer chemotherapy. It has additive effects when given with high-dose metoclopramide or with a 5-HT$_3$-receptor antagonist such as ondansetron. The mechanism of action of dexamethasone as an antiemetic is unknown but may involve reduction of prostaglandin synthesis.

Antihistamines

Indications
Motion sickness, drug-induced vomiting, vestibular disorders, such as vertigo and tinnitus.

Mechanism of action
Competitive antagonist at the histamine H$_1$ receptor.

Preparations and dose
Cyclizine *Tablets: 50 mg; Injection 50 mg/mL.*
Oral 50 mg up to three times daily.
IM/IV injection 50 mg three times daily.

Promethazine *Phenergan® tablets: 10 mg, 25 mg; Elixir: 5 mg/mL; Injection: 25 mg/mL.*
Oral 20–25 mg (at bedtime the night before travel).
IM/IV 25–50 mg.

Side-effects
Drowsiness, antimuscarinic effects (urinary retention, dry mouth, blurred vision), palpitations, arrhythmias and rashes.

Cautions/contraindications
Caution in prostatic hypertrophy, urinary retention, glaucoma and pyloroduodenal obstruction (due to antimuscarinic effects). Drug interactions – see *National Formulary*.

Phenothiazines

Mechanism of action
Dopamine antagonists. Act centrally by blocking the chemoreceptor trigger zone (CTZ) in the fourth ventricle. Many drugs produce vomiting by an action on the CTZ.

Indications

Prochlorperazine is used in nausea and vomiting in the postoperative period and in drug-induced, including cytotoxic drug-induced, vomiting. Chlorpromazine is usually reserved for nausea and vomiting of terminal illness.

Preparations and dose

Chlorpromazine hydrochloride See antipsychotics (p. 885).
Oral 10–25 mg every 4–6 hours.
IM 25 mg then 25–50 mg every 3–4 hours.
By rectum In suppositories: 100 mg every 6–8 hours.

Prochlorperazine *Stemetil® tablets and suppositories: 5 mg, 25 mg; Syrup: 5 mg/mL; Injection: 12.5 mg/mL.*
Oral 20 mg initially, then 10 mg after 2 hours; prevention: 5–10 mg two to three times daily.
IM 12.5 mg followed if necessary after 6 hours by an oral dose.
By rectum 25 mg followed if necessary after 6 hours by an oral dose.

Side-effects
See antipsychotics (p. 886).

Cautions/contraindications
See antipsychotics (p. 886).

Domperidone and metoclopramide

Mechanism of action
Block dopamine receptors and inhibit dopaminergic stimulation of the CTZ.

Indications
Domperidone is used particularly in postoperative nausea and vomiting and also gastro-oesophageal reflux disease and dyspepsia. Metoclopramide is particularly used in nausea and vomiting associated with cytotoxics or radiotherapy.

Preparations and dose
Metoclopramide *Tablets: 10 mg; Syrup: 5 mg/mL; Injection: 5 mg/mL.*
Oral/IM/IV (over 1–2 min): 10 mg three times daily.

Domperidone *Tablets: 10 mg; Suspension: 5 mg/mL; Suppositories: 30 mg.*
Oral 10–20 mg three to four times daily; maximum 80 mg.
By rectum 60 mg twice daily.

Side-effects
Central nervous system effects are produced by meto-clopramide and to a lesser extent by domperidone (due to limited passage across the blood–brain barrier). Extrapyramidal effects include acute dystonias (treated by drug cessation and procyclidine 5–10 mg i.m./i.v.), akathisia and a parkinsonism-like syndrome. Drowsiness with high doses of metoclopramide. Galactorrhoea is caused by hyperprolactinaemia as a result of dopamine receptor blockade.

Cautions/contraindications
Contraindicated in gastrointestinal obstruction, 3–4 days after GI surgery where increased motility may be harmful, and phaeochromocytoma.

5-HT3-receptor antagonists

Mechanism of action
Block the 5-HT_3-receptors in the chemoreceptor trigger zone (see phenothiazines) and in the gut.

Indications
Particularly effective against vomiting induced by highly emetogenic chemotherapeutic agents and radiotherapy used for treating malignancy and postoperative vomiting that is resistant to other agents.

Preparations and dose
Examples: dolasetron, granisetron, ondansetron, tropisetron.

Ondansetron *Tablets: 4 mg; Syrup: 4 mg/5 mL; Injection: 2 mg/mL; Suppositories: 16 mg.*

- Chemotherapy: 8 mg by mouth, or 16 mg by rectum 1–2 hours before treatment; or by i.m./i.v. injection, 8 mg immediately before treatment, then by mouth, 8 mg every 12 hours; or by rectum, 16 mg daily. With severely emetogenic chemotherapy, treatment is given i.m./i.v. and continued by infusion 1 mg/h for up to 24 hours.
- Prevention of postoperative nausea and vomiting: by mouth, 16 mg 1 hour before anaesthesia; or by i.m./i.v. injection, 4 mg at induction of anaesthesia, followed by 8 mg at intervals of 8 hours for two further doses.

Side-effects
Headache, constipation, hypersensitivity reactions. Following i.v. administration: seizures, chest pain, arrhythmias, hypotension and bradycardia.

Cautions/contraindications
Caution with prolonged QT interval and cardiac conduction disorders.

NUTRITION AND BLOOD

Anaemia

Oral iron

Mechanism of action
Reference nutrient intake is 8.7 mg for men, 14.8 mg for women.

Indications
Treatment of iron deficiency, prophylaxis in patients with risk factors for iron deficiency, e.g. malabsorption, menorrhagia, pregnancy and post-gastrectomy. Adding a 250 mg ascorbic acid tablet at the time of iron administration enhances the degree of iron absorption (iron is best absorbed as the ferrous (Fe^{2+}) ion in a mildly acidic environment). Iron and folic acid combination preparations are used in pregnancy for women who are at risk of developing iron and folic acid deficiency.

Preparations and dose
Ferrous sulphate   *Tablets: 200 mg (65 mg iron).*
   Treatment: 1 tablet three times daily – continue for 3 months following normal haemoglobin result (the total duration of therapy should be for 6 months); prophylactic: 1 tablet daily.

Ferrous fumarate   *Fersamal® tablets: 210 g (68 mg iron); Syrup 140 mg (45 mg iron)/5 mL.*
   Treatment: 1–2 tablets three times daily or 10–20 mL syrup twice daily; prophylactic: 1 tablet daily.

Ferrous glycine sulphate   *Plesmet® syrup: 25 mg Fe/5 mL.*
   5–10 mL three times daily.

Side-effects
Constipation and diarrhoea. Nausea and epigastric pain are related to the amount of elemental iron ingested and are lower with preparations containing a low elemental iron content.

Cautions/contraindications
Avoid long-term use unless indicated; excretion of iron is fixed at 1–2 mg of iron per day through gastrointestinal loss, and prolonged use may result in iron overload.

Parenteral iron

Indications
Parenteral iron can be given to patients who are iron deficient and when there is intolerance or non-compliance with oral preparations. Intravenous iron sucrose is reasonably well tolerated with a low incidence of serious adverse reactions. Intravenous iron dextran has a greater incidence of serious adverse reactions than iron sucrose but it can be given via the intramuscular route if intravenous access is difficult.

Preparations and dose
Iron sucrose   *Venofer® injection: 20 mg/mL.*
IV   Bolus intravenous dosing (200 mg) over 10 minutes is more convenient than a 2-hour infusion.

Iron dextran   *CosmoFer® injection: 50 mg/mL.*
IV/IM   By deep i.m. injection into the gluteal muscle, or by i.v. infusion. Dose calculated according to bodyweight and iron deficit; consult product literature.

Side-effects
Gastrointestinal side-effects, injection-site reactions, anaphylactoid reactions (fever, urticaria, bronchospasm, pruritus, hypotension).

Cautions/contraindications
Facilities for cardiopulmonary resuscitation must be at hand. Contraindicated in patients with a history of allergic disorders including asthma, eczema and anaphylaxis.

Folic acid

Mechanism of action
Reference nutrient intake 200 μg/day.

Indications
In folate-deficient megaloblastic anaemia, prevention of folic acid deficiency in chronic haemolytic states, renal dialysis and pregnancy, prevention of neural tube defects.

Preparations and dose
Folic acid   *Tablets: 400 μg, 5 mg; Syrup: 400 μg/mL, 2.5 mg/mL; Injection: 15 mg/mL.*

- Folate deficiency: 5 mg daily for 6 months, maintenance 5 mg daily.

- Prevention of first neural tube defect: 400 µg daily before conception and first 12 weeks of pregnancy.
- To prevent recurrence of neural tube defect: 5 mg daily, before conception and first 12 weeks of pregnancy.

Side-effects
Very rarely allergic reactions.

Cautions/contraindications
Folic acid should not be used in undiagnosed megaloblastic anaemia unless vitamin B_{12} is administered concurrently, otherwise neuropathy may be precipitated.

Vitamin B_{12}

Mechanism of action
Reference nutrient intake 1.5 µg/day.

Indications
Vitamin B_{12} deficiency.

Preparations and dose
Hydroxycobalamin *Injection: 1 mg/mL.*

- Vitamin B_{12} deficiency without neurological involvement: 1 mg intramuscularly three times a week for 2 weeks then 1 mg every 3 months life-long.
- Vitamin B_{12} deficiency with neurological involvement: 1 mg intramuscularly daily for 6 days then 1 mg every 2 months.

Cyanocobalamin *Tablets: 50 µg; Liquid: 35 µg/5 mL.*
Vitamin B_{12} deficiency of dietary origin: 50–150 µg or more daily taken between meals.

Side-effects
Itching, fever, nausea, dizziness, anaphylaxis after injection. Hypokalaemia, sometimes fatal, due to intracellular potassium shift upon anaemia resolution after treatment of severe vitamin B_{12} deficiency.

Cautions/contraindications
Contraindicated if hypersensitivity to hydroxycobalamin or any component of preparation.

Fluid and electrolytes

Potassium

Indications
Potassium replacement, particularly in patients taking digoxin or anti-arrhythmic drugs, in patients in whom

secondary hyperaldosteronism occurs (cirrhosis of the liver, severe heart failure), with excessive loss of potassium in the faeces (diarrhoea, laxative abuse, malabsorption) or gastro-intestinal losses (approx. 5–15 mmol/L in gastric, biliary, pancreatic and small bowel secretions).

Preparations and dose

Oral potassium chloride *Effervescent tablets (Sando-K®): 12 mmol of K+; Syrup (Kay-Cee-L®): 1 mmol/mL.*

- Prevention of hypokalaemia: 25–50 mmol in divided doses.
- Treatment of hypokalaemia: 40–100 mmol daily depending on serum potassium and severity of any continuing loss.

Intravenous potassium *Injection: 20 mmol/10 mL; Infusions 10–40 mmol/L.*

A variety of infusion fluids with concentrations of potassium between 10 and 40 mmol/L are available in 500 mL and 1 L size bags. Concentrations over 60 mmol/L must be infused into a large (e.g. femoral) or central vein, as high concentrations are irritant to smaller veins. Maximum rate of i.v. potassium is usually 10–20 mmol/h, although 40–100 mmol/h have been given to selected patients with paralysis or arrhythmias (with ECG monitoring).

Side-effects

Nausea and vomiting, oesophageal and small bowel ulceration with oral preparations; where appropriate, potassium-sparing diuretics are preferable. Cardiac arrhythmias and vein irritation with i.v. administration.

Cautions/contraindications

Use smaller doses in renal impairment, otherwise there is a danger of hyperkalaemia. Oral liquid preparations should be used in preference to tablets when there is any cause for delay in transit through the GI tract.

Ion exchange resins for potassium removal

Mechanism of action

The resin takes up potassium in the gut.

Indications

Hyperkalaemia.

Preparations and dose

Calcium polystyrene sulphonate *Calcium resonium powder.*

Oral 15 g three to four times daily in water or as a paste.
By rectum as an enema: 30 g in methycellulose solution
retained for 9 hours followed by irrigation to remove resin
from the colon.

Side-effects
GI disturbance (anorexia, nausea, constipation, diarrhoea),
hypercalcaemia, hypomagnesaemia, rectal ulceration and
colonic necrosis following rectal administration.

Cautions/contraindications
Avoid in hypercalcaemia from any cause, caution in heart
failure, hypertension, renal failure and oedema (due to salt
loading).

Oral sodium

Indications
In chronic conditions associated with sodium depletion,
e.g. in salt-losing bowel or renal disease. Sodium bicarbonate is used for chronic acidotic states associated with salt
depletion, e.g. renal tubular acidosis. A spot urine sodium
concentration < 20 mmol/L indicates sodium depletion
irrespective of serum sodium.

Preparations and dose
Sodium chloride *Slow sodium® tablets: 600 mg (approx.
10 mmol each of Na^+ and Cl^-).*
   4–8 tablets daily with water; in severe depletion up to a
maximum of 20 tablets daily.

Sodium bicarbonate *Capsules: sodium bicarbonate 500 mg
(approx. 6 mmol each of Na^+ and HCO_3^-).*
   1–4 capsules three times daily.

Side-effects
Excess leads to hypernatraemia, fluid overload and pulmonary oedema.

Cautions/contraindications
Hypernatraemia, fluid retention.

Minerals

Calcium

Mechanism of action
Reference nutrient intake 700 mg.

Indications
Hypocalcaemia, osteomalacia, when dietary calcium intake (with or without vitamin D) is deficient in the prevention and treatment of osteoporosis.

Preparations and dose
Calcium carbonate   *Calcichew® chewable tablets (calcium 500 mg or Ca²⁺ 12.6 mmol); Sandocal® dispersible tablets: 400 (calcium 400 mg or Ca²⁺ 10 mmol), 1000 (calcium 1 g or Ca²⁺ 25 mmol); Calcium-Sandoz® syrup (calcium 108.3 mg or Ca²⁺ 2.7 mmol/5 mL).*

- Osteoporosis and calcium deficiency: 1 g daily, syrup 55–75 mL daily.
- Osteomalacia: 1–3 g daily, syrup 55–155 mL daily.

Calcium gluconate   *Injection: 10% (calcium 89 mg or Ca²⁺ 2.2 mmol/10 mL).*
  10–20 mL over 10 minutes for acute hypocalcaemia.

Side-effects
Gastrointestinal disturbances; with injection, peripheral vasodilatation, fall in blood pressure, injection-site reactions.

Cautions/contraindications
Conditions associated with hypercalcaemia and hypercalciuria.

Magnesium

Mechanism of action
Magnesium is an essential constituent of many enzyme systems.

Indications
Treatment of deficiency states; magnesium is secreted in large amounts in gastrointestinal fluid and excessive losses occur in diarrhoea, stoma or fistulas. Intravenous magnesium is used in the treatment of acute severe asthma, life-threatening cardiac arrhythmias and pre-eclampsia.

Preparations and dose
Magnesium oxide   *Capsules: 160 mg (4 mmol Mg²⁺).*
  2 capsules three times daily, adjusted according to magnesium levels.

Magnesium sulphate   *Injection.*
  See asthma.

Side-effects
Hypermagnesaemia causing muscle weakness and arrythmias.

Cautions/contraindications
Increased plasma levels may occur with renal failure.

Zinc

Mechanism of action
Involved in many metabolic pathways, essential for the synthesis of RNA and DNA. Reference nutrient intake is 9.5 mg (145 µmol) for men, 7 mg (110 µmol) for women.

Indications
Treatment of zinc deficiency as a result of malabsorption or skin disease, and in the inherited disorder of zinc absorption, acrodermatitis enteropathica.

Preparations and dose
Zinc *Effervescent tablets: 125 mg (45 mg zinc).*

Side-effects
Abdominal pain, dyspepsia, nausea, vomiting, diarrhoea, gastric irritation.

Cautions/contraindications
Caution in acute renal failure – zinc may accumulate.

Vitamins

Vitamin B

Mechanism of action
Water-soluble vitamins: thiamine (B_1) is an essential cofactor in carbohydrate metabolism, reference nutrient intake 0.4 mg per 1000 kcal; pyridoxine (B_6) is a cofactor in the metabolism of many amino acids, reference nutrient intake 15 µg/g of dietary protein.

Indications
Deficiency of the B vitamins is uncommon other than deficiency of vitamin B_{12} (see above). The severe deficiency states Wernicke's encephalopathy and Korsakoff's psychosis are best treated initially by the parenteral administration of B vitamins (Pabrinex®) followed by oral administration of thiamine in the long term.

Preparations and dose
Pyridoxine *Vitamin B_6 tablets: 20 mg, 50 mg.*

- Deficiency states: 20–50 mg up to three times daily.
- Isoniazid neuropathy prophylaxis: 10 mg daily.
- Idiopathic sideroblastic anaemia: 100–400 mg daily in divided doses.

Thiamine   *Vitamin B₁ tablets: 50 mg, 100 mg; Pabrinex®: i.v. high-potency vitamins B and C.*

Oral   50 mg three times daily.

IV   Each pair of ampoules must be given over 10 minutes, or in 50–100 mL sodium chloride 0.9% or glucose 5% infused over 15–30 minutes. In alcohol withdrawal, give 1 ampoule pair/day. In Wernicke–Korsakoff's syndrome give two pairs every 8 hours for 48 hours until oral thiamine can be introduced.

Vitamin B complex   *Vitamin B tablets: Compound Strong tablets (nicotinamide 20 mg, pyridoxine 2 mg, riboflavin 2 mg, thiamine 5 mg).*

1–2 tablets three times daily for treatment of vitamin B deficiency.

Vitamin C (ascorbic acid)

Mechanism of action

Water-soluble vitamin necessary for the formation of collagen; reference nutrient intake 40 mg/day.

Indications

Treatment of scurvy, and less florid manifestations of vitamin C deficiency commonly found especially in the elderly. Also used in iron deficiency to increase iron absorption (see p. 839).

Preparations and dose

Ascorbic acid   *Tablets: 50 mg, 100 mg, 200 mg, 500 mg.*

- Prophylaxis: 25–75 mg daily.
- Therapeutic: at least 100 mg three times daily.

Vitamin D

Mechanism of action

Fat-soluble vitamin whose main action is to promote intestinal absorption of calcium. An oral supplement of 10 μg (400 units) prevents deficiency.

847

Indications

- Prevention of vitamin D deficiency in those at risk, e.g. Asians consuming unleavened bread and in elderly patients, particularly those who are housebound or live in residential or nursing homes.

- As an adjunct in the prevention and treatment of osteoporosis where dietary intake of vitamin D (and calcium) is suboptimal.
- Vitamin D deficiency caused by intestinal malabsorption, chronic liver disease and severe renal impairment.
- Hypocalcaemia of hypoparathyroidism.

Preparations and dose

Ergocalciferol   *Calciferol (vitamin D₂) tablets: 250 μg (10 000 units); Calcium (97 mg) and ergocalciferol (10 μg, 400 units) tablets.*

- Prevention of vitamin D deficiency: calcium and ergocalciferol tablets 1–2 daily.
- Adjunct in treatment of osteoporosis: calcium and ergocalciferol tablets 1–2 daily.
- Deficiency caused by malabsorption or chronic liver disease: up to 1 mg (40 000 units) calciferol.
- Hypocalcaemia of hypoparathyroidism: up to 2.5 mg (100 000 units) calciferol.

Alfacalcidol   *1α-Hydroxycolecalciferol capsules: 250 ng, 500 ng, 1 μg.*
Vitamin D treatment in patients with severe renal impairment: 0.25–1 μg daily.

Calcitriol   *1,25-Dihydroxycolecalciferol: 250 ng, 500 ng.*
Vitamin D treatment in patients with severe renal impairment: 250–1000 ng daily.

Side-effects

Symptoms of overdosage include anorexia, lassitude, nausea and vomiting, polyuria, thirst, headache and raised concentrations of calcium and phosphate in plasma and urine. All patients on pharmacological doses of vitamin D should have plasma calcium concentration checked at intervals (initially weekly) and if nausea and vomiting are present.

Cautions/contraindications

Contraindicated in hypercalcaemia and metastatic calcification.

Vitamin K

Mechanism of action

Fat-soluble vitamin necessary for the production of blood clotting factors and proteins necessary for the normal calcification of bone; reference nutrient intake 1 µg/kg bodyweight.

Indications

Water-soluble form to prevent deficiency in patients with fat malabsorption (especially biliary obstruction or hepatic disease); intravenously for excessive anticoagulation with warfarin and in patients with prolonged INR (due to fat malabsorption) prior to invasive procedures (e.g. ERCP or liver biopsy) or in whom there is bleeding.

Preparations and dose

Phytomenadione *Vitamin K₁ tablets: 10 mg; Injection: 10 mg/mL.*

Oral Excessive anticoagulation (INR > 8.0): 0.5–2.5 mg.

IV Excessive anticoagulation and major bleeding (any INR value): 5 mg over 10 minutes together with FFP (15 mL/kg).

Menadiol sodium phosphate *Water-soluble tablets: 10 mg.* For prevention of vitamin K deficiency in patients with fat malabsorption: 10 mg daily.

Side-effects

Anaphylaxis with i.v. preparation.

Cautions/contraindications

Caution with menadiol in G6PD deficiency and vitamin E deficiency (risk of haemolysis).

Multivitamin preparations

Multivitamins BP *Tablets.*

Abidec *Drops.*

1 tablet or 0.6 mL daily contains lower reference nutrient intake for vitamins A, B, group C, and D.

Pabrinex IVHP *Injection*, vitamins B and C, see page 845.

Multivitamin and mineral supplements

Forceval® *Capsules.*

1 capsule daily contains all vitamins, minerals and trace elements as an adjunct in synthetic diets.

849

RHEUMATOLOGY

Anti-inflammatories and pain relief

Aspirin is indicated for transient musculoskeletal pain and pyrexia. In inflammatory conditions non-steroidal anti-inflammatory agents are usually given. Paracetamol is similar in efficacy to aspirin, but has no demonstrable anti-inflammatory activity. It should always be considered for first-line use in pain relief where anti-inflammatories are not routinely indicated. Codeine may be added when paracetamol alone is insufficient.

Non-steroidal anti-inflammatory drugs (NSAIDs)

Mechanism of action

Inhibition of cyclo-oxygenase, the enzyme which catalyzes the synthesis of cyclic endoperoxidases from arachidonic acid to form prostaglandins. Inhibition of the COX-1 isoform in the gastrointestinal tract leads to a reduction in protective prostaglandins and predisposes to gastroduodenal damage.

Indications

- Chronic disease accompanied by pain and inflammation.
- Transient musculoskeletal pain.
- Pain in dysmenorrhoea.
- Pain caused by secondary bone tumours.

Preparations and dose

Ibuprofen *Tablets: 200 mg, 400 mg, 600 mg, 800 mg; Syrup: 100 mg/5 mL.*
Oral Initially 1.2–1.8 g daily in three to four divided doses after food, increased to a maximum of 2.4 g daily if necessary. Maintenance 0.6–1.2 g daily in divided doses.

Diclofenac *Tablets: 25 mg, 50 mg; Suppositories: 25 mg, 50 mg, 100 mg; Injection: 75 mg/3 mL.*
Oral/rectal 75–150 mg daily in two to three divided doses.
IM 75 mg once or twice daily for up to 2 days.

Indometacin *Capsules: 25 mg, 50 mg; Suppositories: 100 mg.*
Oral 50–200 mg daily in divided doses with food.
Rectal 100 mg once or twice daily.

Mefenamic acid *Capsules: 250 mg; Tablets: 500 mg.*
Oral 500 mg three times daily, after food.

Side-effects

All NSAIDs are associated with serious gastrointestinal toxicity; the risk is higher in the elderly. Inflammation and ulceration can occur throughout the gut but are clinically most apparent in the stomach and duodenum (dyspepsia, erosions, ulceration, bleeding). Ibuprofen is associated with the lowest risk, and piroxicam, indometacin and diclofenac with intermediate risk. NSAIDs associated with the risk are generally preferred, and the lowest NSAID compatible with symptom relief should be prescribed. Other side-effects include hypersensitivity reactions (particularly rashes, bronchospasm, angio-oedema), blood disorders, fluid retention (may precipitate cardiac failure in the elderly), acute renal failure, hepatitis, pancreatitis and exacerbation of colitis.

Cautions/contraindications

NSAIDs are best avoided in patients taking anticoagulants or corticosteroids. The combination of NSAID and aspirin may increase the risk of gastrointestinal side-effects, and this combination should be used only if absolutely necessary. It is preferable to avoid NSAIDs in patients with active or previous gastrointestinal ulceration or bleeding but this may not be possible in patients with serious rheumatic diseases. In this case gastroprotection (usually with a proton pump inhibitor) should be offered to patients at high risk of developing peptic ulceration or patients who might not withstand an ulcer complication (previous peptic ulceration, warfarin users, elderly, associated co-morbidity, e.g. severe heart failure). NSAIDs are contraindicated in patients with a history of hypersensitivity to aspirin or any other NSAID – which includes those in whom attacks of asthma, angio-oedema, urticaria or rhinitis have been precipitated by aspirin or any other NSAID. In patients with renal, cardiac or hepatic impairment, caution is required since NSAIDs may impair renal function. Use with caution in inflammatory bowel disease – may cause flares. For interactions of NSAIDs, see the *National Formulary*.

Selective COX-2 inhibitors (Coxibs)

Mechanism of action
Selective inhibition of the COX-2 isoform.

Indications
Where NSAIDs are indicated but where there is a particularly high risk of developing gastroduodenal ulceration, perforation or bleeding.

851

Preparations and dose
Etoricoxib *Arcoxia® tablets: 60 mg, 90 mg, 120 mg.*
Oral Osteoarthritis: 60 mg once daily; rheumatoid arthritis: 90 mg daily; acute gout: 120 mg daily.

Celecoxib   *Celebrex® tablets: 100 mg, 200 mg.*
Oral   Osteoarthritis: 200 mg daily in one to two divided doses, increased if necessary to 200 mg twice daily; rheumatoid arthritis: 200–400 mg daily in two divided doses.

Side-effects
Dry mouth, dyspepsia, cough.

Cautions/contraindications
Increased risk of myocardial infarction and stroke with selective COX-2 inhibitors compared with placebo. Coxibs are contraindicated in patients with established ischaemic heart disease and cerebrovascular disease. Caution in inflammatory bowel disease (see above). Contraindicated in active peptic ulceration.

Drugs affecting bone metabolism

Bisphosphonates

Mechanism of action
Adsorbed onto hydroxyapatite crystals in bone, slowing both their rate of growth and dissolution, and thereby reducing the rate of bone turnover.

Indications
Prophylaxis and treatment of osteoporosis in combination with calcium (800 mg daily) and vitamin D (800 IU/day if dietary intake inadequate), treatment of Paget's disease and hypercalcaemia of malignancy, treatment of osteolytic lesions and bone pain in bone metastases associated with breast cancer or multiple myeloma.

Preparations and dose
Disodium etidronate   *Didronel® tablets: 200 mg.*
Oral   For Paget's disease: 5 mg/kg daily for up to 6 months. May be repeated after interval of 3 months.
  Didronel PMO®: Pack consisting of 400 mg tablets and calcium carbonate (Cacit®) 1.25 g tablets.
Oral   For treatment and prevention of osteoporosis: given in 90-day cycles, 1 Didronel® tablet daily for 14 days, then 1 Cacit® tablet daily for 76 days.
  Advise patients to avoid food 2 hours before and after taking tablets.

Alendronic acid   *Fosamax® tablets: 5 mg, 10 mg; Fosamax® Once Weekly: 70 mg.*

Oral

■ Treatment and prevention of glucocorticoid osteoporosis: 10 mg daily at least 30 min before breakfast or 70 mg once weekly.
■ Prevention of osteoporosis in postmenopausal women. 5 mg daily.

Because of severe oesophageal reactions (oesophagitis, oesophageal ulcers and strictures), patients should be advised to take the tablets with a full glass of water on rising, to take them on an empty stomach at least 30 minutes before the first food or drink of the day and to stand or sit for at least 30 minutes. Also advise patients to stop the tablets and seek medical attention if symptoms of oesophageal irritation develop.

Risedronate   *Actonel® tablets: 5 mg, 30 mg; Actonel® Once a Week: 35 mg.*
Oral

■ Prevention and treatment of osteoporosis: 5 mg daily or 35 mg weekly.
■ Paget's disease: 30 mg daily for 2 months; may be repeated if necessary after at least 2 months.

Precautions for taking risedronate are as for alendronate (above). No food or drink for 2 hours after risedronate.

Disodium pamidronate   *Injection: 15 mg, 30 mg, 60 mg, 90 mg.*
IV   Patients should be hydrated first.

■ Hypercalcaemia of malignancy: according to serum calcium concentration 15–90 mg in single infusion or in multiple infusions over 2–4 consecutive days. Each 60 mg must be diluted with at least 250 mL sodium chloride and given over at least 1 hour. Serum calcium < 3.0 mmol/L, give 15–30 mg; serum calcium > 4.0 mmol/L, give 90 mg.
■ Osteolytic lesions and bone pain in bone metastases associated with breast cancer or multiple myeloma: 90 mg every 4 weeks (or every 3 weeks to coincide with chemotherapy in breast cancer).
■ Paget's disease: 30 mg once a week for 6 weeks; may be repeated every 6 months.

Side-effects
Gastrointestinal side-effects (dyspepsia, nausea, vomiting, abdominal pain, diarrhoea, constipation), influenza-like symptoms, oesophageal reactions (see above), musculoskeletal pain.

Cautions/contraindications
Correct vitamin D deficiency and hypocalcaemia before starting, caution with risedronate and alendronate in symptomatic oesophageal disorders, caution in severe renal impairment.

CARDIOVASCULAR SYSTEM

Diuretics

Diuretics reduce sodium and chloride reabsorption at different sites in the nephron and thus increase urinary sodium and water loss.

Thiazide diuretics

Mechanism of action
Inhibition of sodium reabsorption at beginning of distal convoluted tubule.

Indications
To relieve oedema due to chronic heart failure and, in lower doses to reduce blood pressure.

Preparations and dose
Bendroflumethiazide (bendrofluazide)   *Tablets: 2.5 mg, 5 mg.*
Oral
- Hypertension: 2.5 mg each morning – higher doses rarely necessary.
- Oedema: initially 5–10 mg each morning.

Metolazone   *Tablets: 5 mg.*
Oral   Oedema resistant to other diuretics: start at 5 mg each morning and gradually increase if necessary to 20 mg daily in resistant oedema.

Side-effects
Postural hypotension, hypokalaemia, hyponatraemia, anorexia, diarrhoea, aggravates diabetes mellitus and gout. Profound diuresis with metolazone, particularly when combined with loop diuretics.

Cautions/contraindications
Symptomatic hyperuricaemia, severe renal and hepatic impairment, hyponatraemia, hypercalcaemia, untreated hypokalaemia.

Loop diuretics

Mechanism of action
Inhibit sodium reabsorption from the ascending limb of the loop of Henle.

Indications
Heart failure, intravenously in patients with acute pulmonary oedema, oedema associated with renal disease, oedema associated with liver disease in combination with potassium-sparing diuretics. High doses may be needed with impaired renal function.

Preparations and dose
Furosemide (frusemide) *Tablets: 20 mg, 40 mg, 500 mg; Syrup containing: 1, 4, 8 or 10 mg/mL; Injection: 20 mg/2 mL.*
Oral For oedema, usually 20–80 mg daily.
IV Initially 20–80 mg; if multiple dose, rate not to exceed 4 mg per minute.

Bumetanide *Tablets: 1 mg, 5 mg; Injection 1 mg/2 mL; Liquid 1 mg/5 mL.*
   (1 mg bumetanide = 40 mg furosemide (frusemide) at low doses.)
Oral Initially 1 mg (0.5 mg in the elderly) daily, increased according to response.
IV 1–2 mg repeated after 20 minutes if necessary. Higher doses usually given as infusion over 30–60 minutes.

Side-effects
Hypokalaemia, hypomagnesaemia, hyponatraemia, GI disturbance, hyperuricaemia, hyperglycaemia, tinnitus and deafness with rapid i.v. administration or high doses, myalgia (bumetanide at high doses).

Cautions/contraindications
Untreated severe electrolyte disturbance, coma due to liver failure.

Potassium-sparing diuretics

Mechanism of action
Inhibition of sodium reabsorption in the cortical collecting tubule. Amiloride and triamterene directly decrease sodium channel activity; spironolactone inhibits aldosterone. They have weak natriuretic activity.

Indications
Spironolactone is used in oedema in chronic liver disease

and in low doses to improve survival in severe heart failure. Amiloride and triamterene in combination with loop diuretics are used as an alternative to giving potassium supplements and in resistant oedema.

Preparations and dose

Amiloride   *Tablets: 5 mg; Syrup 5 mg/5 mL.*
Oral   5–10 mg daily. Maximum 20 mg daily if used alone.

Spironolactone   *Tablets: 25 mg, 50 mg, 100 mg; Suspension: 5 mg, 10 mg, 25 mg, 50 mg, 100 mg/5 mL.*
Oral
- Heart failure: initially 25 mg daily increased to 50 mg if necessary.
- Ascites in chronic liver disease: 100 mg in combination with 40 mg of furosemide (frusemide), increasing gradually to a maximum of 400 mg and 160 mg respectively.

Side-effects

Hyperkalaemia, gynaecomastia (spironolactone).

Cautions/contraindications

Avoid in renal impairment; co-administration with ACE inhibitors may cause hyperkalaemia.

It is preferable to prescribe thiazides and potassium-sparing diuretics separately. The use of fixed drug combinations (e.g. co-amilozide 2.5/25; amiloride hydrochloride 2.5 mg, hydrochlorothiazide 25 mg) may be justified if compliance is a problem.

Beta-blockers

Mechanism of action

Block the β-adrenoceptors in the heart, peripheral vasculature, bronchi, pancreas and liver. They decrease heart rate, reduce the force of cardiac contraction, lower blood pressure. These effects reduce myocardial oxygen demand and give more time for coronary perfusion.

Indications

Hypertension, angina, myocardial infarction, arrhythmias, stable heart failure, to alleviate symptoms of anxiety, prophylaxis of migraine, prevention of variceal bleeding and symptomatic treatment of thyrotoxicosis (no effect on thyroid function tests).

Preparations and dose

Most β-blockers are equally effective but there are

differences between them which may affect choice in particular diseases or individual patients, e.g. sotalol is used for the management of supraventricular and ventricular arrhythmias, propranolol in the treatment of thyrotoxicosis, prevention of variceal bleeding and prophylaxis of migraine (usually), bisoprolol and carvedilol in the management of heart failure (usually specialist initiated).

Propranolol *Tablets: 10 mg, 40 mg, 80 mg, 160 mg; Oral solution: 5 mg/mL; Injection 1 mg/mL.*
Oral
- Hypertension: initially 80 mg twice daily, increased at weekly intervals as required; maintenance 160–320 mg daily.
- Portal hypertension: initially 40 mg twice daily, increased according to heart rate; maximum 160 mg twice daily.
- Angina: initially 40 mg two to three times daily; maintenance 120–240 mg daily.
- Arrhythmias: anxiety, thyrotoxicosis, migraine prophylaxis, essential tremor, 10–40 mg three times daily.

IV Arrhythmias and thyrotoxic crisis: 1 mg over 1 minute; if necessary repeat at 2-minute intervals; maximum 10 mg.

Atenolol *Tablets: 25 mg, 50 mg, 100 mg.*
Oral
- Hypertension: 25–50 mg daily.
- Angina: 25–100 mg daily in one or two doses.
- After MI: 25–100 mg daily.

IV For arrhythmias: 2.5 mg at a rate of 1 mg/min, repeated at 5-min intervals to a maximum of 10 mg, or by infusion 150 μg/kg over 20 minutes, repeated every 12 hours if required.

Metoprolol *Tablets: 50 mg, 100 mg; Injection: 1 mg/mL.*
Oral
- Hypertension: 50–100 mg twice daily.
- After MI: 100 mg twice daily.
- Angina, arrhythmias, anxiety, thyrotoxicosis, migraine prophylaxis, essential tremor: 50–100 mg two to three times daily.

IV For arrhythmias: up to 5 mg at a rate of 1–2 mg/min, repeated after 5 min to a maximum of 10–15 mg.

Sotalol *Tablets: 40 mg, 80 mg, 160 mg; Injection: 10 mg/mL.*
Oral 80 mg daily in one to two divided doses, increased

gradually at intervals of 2–3 days to usual dose of 160–320 mg daily.

IV Over 10 minutes: 20–120 mg with ECG monitoring repeated at 6-hour intervals if necessary.

Side-effects

Bradycardia, exacerbation of intermittent claudication, lethargy, nightmares, hallucinations, deterioration of glucose tolerance and interference with metabolic and autonomic responses to hypoglycaemia in diabetics.

Cautions/contraindications

Contraindicated in asthma, COPD, diabetics with frequent episodes of hypoglycaemia, severe peripheral arterial disease, second- or third-degree heart block, uncontrolled heart block, phaeochromocytoma (apart from specific use with alpha-blockers).

Drugs affecting the renin–angiotensin system

Renin produced by the kidney in response to glomerular hypoperfusion catalyzes cleavage of angiotensinogen (produced by the liver) to angiotensin (AT), which in turn is cleaved by angiotensin-converting enzyme (ACE) to angiotensin II, which acts on two receptors. The AT_1 receptor mediates the vasoconstrictor effects of AT. The actions of the AT_2 receptor are less well defined.

Angiotensin-converting enzyme inhibitors

Mechanism of action

Inhibit the conversion of angiotensin I to angiotensin II and reduce angiotensin II mediated vasoconstriction.

Indications

Heart failure, hypertension, diabetic nephropathy, ischaemic heart disease.

Preparations and dose

Perindopril *Coversyl® tablets: 2 mg, 4 mg, 8 mg.*

- Hypertension: initially 2 mg daily, usual maintenance 4 mg daily, maximum 8 mg daily.
- Heart failure: initially 2 mg daily, maintenance usually 4 mg daily.

Lisinopril *Tablets: 2.5 mg, 5 mg, 10 mg, 20 mg.*

- Hypertension: initially 5 mg daily, maintenance 10–20 mg daily, maximum 40 mg daily.

- Heart failure: initially 2.5 mg daily, maintenance 5–20 mg daily.
- After MI: maintenance 5–10 mg daily.

Ramipril *Tritace® tablets: 1.25 mg, 2.5 mg, 5 mg, 10 mg.*

- Hypertension: initially 1.25 mg daily, maintenance 2.5–5 mg daily, maximum 10 mg once daily.
- Heart failure: initially 1.25 mg daily, increased if necessary to maximum 10 mg daily.
- After MI: 2.5 mg twice daily, maintenance 2.5–5 mg daily.

Side-effects
First-dose hypotension (use small initial doses) in heart failure and patients taking diuretics, dry cough, hyperkalaemia, sudden deterioration in renal function in patients with renal artery stenosis and in patients taking NSAIDs (check urea and electrolytes 1–2 weeks after starting treatment), loss of taste, rashes, hypersensitivity reactions.

Cautions/contraindications
Bilateral renal artery stenosis, pregnancy, angio-oedema, severe renal failure, severe or symptomatic mitral or aortic stenosis and hypertrophic obstructive cardiomyopathy (risk of hypotension).

Angiotensin II receptor antagonists

Mechanism of action
Antagonist of the type 1 subtype of the angiotensin II receptor (AT_1 receptor).

Indications
Hypertension, heart failure or diabetic nephropathy in patients intolerant to ACE inhibitors because of cough.

Preparations and dose
Candesartan *Amias® tablets: 2 mg, 4 mg, 8 mg, 16 mg.*

Hypertension: initially 4 mg daily, increased as necessary to 16 mg daily.

Valsartan *Diovan® capsules: 40 mg, 80 mg, 160 mg.*

Hypertension: 80 mg once daily (40 mg in caution groups) and increased if necessary after 4 weeks to 160 mg daily.

Side-effects
Postural hypotension, rash, abnormalities in liver biochemistry, hyperkalaemia.

Caution/contraindications

Lower dose in liver and renal impairment, patients taking high-dose diuretics, elderly over 75 years. Caution in renal artery stenosis, aortic or mitral valve stenosis and in obstructive hypertrophic cardiomyopathy.

Nitrates, calcium-channel blockers and potassium-channel activators

Nitrates, calcium-channel blockers and potassium-channel activators have a vasodilating effect leading to a reduction in venous return, which reduces left ventricular work and dilatation of the coronary circulation.

Nitrates

Mechanism of action

Increase in cyclic guanosine monophosphate (cGMP) in vascular smooth muscle cells causes a decrease in intracellular calcium levels and smooth muscle relaxation with dilatation of veins and arteries, including the coronary circulation.

Indications

Prophylaxis and treatment of angina, adjunct in congestive heart failure, intravenously in the treatment of acute left ventricular failure and unstable angina.

Preparations and dose

Glyceryl trinitrate *Sublingual tablets: 300 μg, 500 μg, 600 μg – expire after 8 weeks once bottle opened; Spray 400 μg/dose.*

Angina: one or two tablets or sprays under the tongue (sublingual use avoids hepatic first-pass metabolism) repeated as required. More effective if taken before exertion known to precipitate angina. Advantage of tablets over spray is that they can be spat out if side-effects occur (headache, hypotension).

Glyceryl trinitrate *Transiderm-Nitro® patches: 5 mg, 10 mg, 15 mg/24 h.*

Angina: apply patch to chest or outer arm and replace at different site every 24 hours. If tolerance (with reduced therapeutic effect) is suspected, the patch should be left off for 4–8 consecutive hours – usually at night as this is the least symptomatic period.

Glyceryl trinitrate buccal   *Suscard® tablets: 2 mg, 3 mg, 5 mg.*
- Angina: 1–5 mg three times daily.
- Heart failure: 5 mg (increased to 10 mg in severe cases) three times daily.

Glyceryl trinitrate injection   *5 mg/mL (to be diluted before use).*

0.6–0.9 mg/h i.v., then increase dose cautiously until response is achieved, keeping systolic BP > 100 mmHg. Usual range 2–10 mg/h.

Isosorbide mononitrate   *Tablets: 10 mg, 20 mg, 40 mg.*

10–40 mg twice daily, 8 hours apart rather than 12 to prevent nitrate tolerance.

Isosorbide mononitrate (modified release)   *Isotard® 25XL (25 mg), to Isotard 60XL (60 mg).*

25–60 mg once daily. Reserve for patients where twice-daily dosing (above) has proved unacceptable. Build up dose gradually to avoid headaches, Up to 120 mg daily may be required.

Side-effects
These are mainly due to vasodilating properties and are minimized by initiating therapy with a low dose. Flushing, headache, postural hypotension; methaemoglobinaemia (p. 959) with excessive dosage.

Cautions/contraindications
Hypertrophic obstructive cardiomyopathy, aortic stenosis, mitral stenosis, cardiac tamponade, marked anaemia, closed-angle glaucoma. Nitrates potentiate the effect of other vasodilators and hypotensive drugs. Sildenafil is contraindicated in patients taking nitrates.

Calcium-channel blockers

Different modified-release preparations of calcium antagonists have different bioavailabilities and so the brand should be stated on the prescription.

Mechanism of action
Block calcium channels and modify calcium uptake into myocardium and vascular smooth muscle cells. The dihydropyridine calcium-channel blockers (e.g. amlodipine, nifedipine, nimodipine) are potent vasodilators with little effect on cardiac contractility or conduction. In contrast,

verapamil and to a lesser extent diltiazem are weak vaso-dilators but depress cardiac conduction and contractility.

Indications

Hypertension, prophylaxis of angina. Verapamil in the treatment of some arrhythmias. Nimodipine for the prevention of ischaemic neurological deficits following aneurysmal subarachnoid haemorrhage.

Preparations and dose

Amlodipine   *Istin®: 5 mg, 10 mg.*
   5–10 mg once daily.

Verapamil   *Tablets: 40 mg, 80 mg, 120 mg, 160 mg; Oral solution: 40 mg/5 mL; Securon SR® modified-release (slow-release) tablets: 120 mg, 240 mg; Securon® injection: 2.5 mg/mL.*

- Angina: 80–120 mg three times daily. SR 240 mg once or twice daily.
- Hypertension: 240–480 mg daily in two to three divided doses. SR 120–240 mg once or twice daily.
- Supraventricular arrhythmias: oral 40–120 mg three times daily, i.v. 5–10 mg over 10 minutes, further 5 mg after 5–10 minutes if required.

Nifedipine modified release   *Adalat® LA tablets: 20 mg, 30 mg, 60 mg.*

- Angina: initially 30 mg once daily, increased if necessary to 90 mg once daily.
- Hypertension: initially 20 mg once daily, increased if necessary.

Diltiazem   *Tablets: 60 mg.*
   Angina: 60 mg three times daily.

Diltiazem slow release   *Adizem-SR® capsules: 90 mg, 120 mg, 180 mg; Adizem-XL® capsules: 120 mg, 180 mg, 240 mg, 300 mg.*

- *Adizem SR:* hypertension, 120 mg twice daily; angina, 90 mg twice daily increased to 180 mg twice daily if required.
- *Adizem XL:* angina and hypertension, 240 mg once daily increased to 300 mg once daily.

Side-effects

Mainly due to vasodilator properties: flushing, dizziness, tachycardia, hypotension, ankle swelling, headache. Side-effects are minimized by starting with a low dose and increasing slowly. Constipation with verapamil. Worsening heart failure with verapamil and diltiazem.

Cautions/contraindications
Aortic stenosis. Verapamil and diltiazem diminish cardiac contractility and slow cardiac conduction; thus they are relatively contraindicated in patients taking beta-blockers, left ventricular failure, sick sinus syndrome, heart failure. Verapamil is contraindicated for treatment of arrhythmias complicating Wolff–Parkinson–White syndrome. Short-acting calcium antagonists increase mortality and are contraindicated immediately after myocardial infarction.

Potassium-channel activators

Mechanism of action
Hybrid action of nitrates (p. 858) and potassium channel activator. The latter causes an increase in potassium flow into the cell and indirectly leads to calcium-channel blockade and arterial dilatation.

Indications
Refractory angina in patients who are uncontrolled on standard regimens of aspirin, beta-blockers, nitrates, calcium antagonists and statins.

Preparations and dose
Nicorandil   *Ikorel® tablets: 10 mg, 20 mg.*
  5–30 mg twice daily.

Side-effects
Headache (often temporary), flushing, nausea, vomiting, dizziness, hypotension, tachycardia.

Cautions/contraindications
Contraindicated in left ventricular failure and cardiogenic shock. Sildenafil is contraindicated in patients taking nicorandil.

Cardiac glycosides

Digoxin is the most commonly used cardiac glycoside.

Mechanism of action
Inhibition of myocardial cell Na^+/K^+-ATPase results in an increase in intracellular sodium and, indirectly by reducing activity of the Na–Ca cotransporter, an increase in intracellular calcium. There is an increase in the force of myocardial contraction and reduced conductivity at the AV node.

Indications

■ Heart failure with atrial fibrillation; its main role is for controlling the heart rate.

■ Supraventricular arrhythmias, particularly atrial fibrillation.

Preparations and dose

Digoxin *Tablets: 62.5 μg, 125 μg, 250 μg; Injection: 250 μg/mL; Lanoxin-PG® elixir: 50 μg/mL.*

Oral loading   250–500 μg daily. For urgent digitalization: 1–1.5 mg in divided doses over 24 hours.

Oral maintenance   62.5–500 μg daily according to renal function and heart rate.

IV loading   0.75–1 mg total dose as an infusion over 2 hours. Half the dose given over 10–20 minutes followed by a further fraction of the dose every 4–8 hours according to response. Oral maintenance dose after that time.

Side-effects

Usually associated with excessive dosage; they include anorexia, nausea, vomiting, diarrhoea, visual disturbances, drowsiness, confusion, delirium, hallucinations, heart block. Digoxin has a narrow therapeutic index and serum digoxin levels are measured in suspected toxicity at least 6 hours after the last oral dose.

Cautions/contraindications

Complete heart block, second-degree AV block, supra-ventricular arrhythmias caused by Wolff–Parkinson–White syndrome, hypertrophic obstructive cardiomyopathy. Avoid hypokalaemia as it predisposes to toxicity. Check renal function and electrolytes before starting therapy; reduce dose in the elderly and in renal impairment. Digoxin is potentiated by amiodarone, diltiazem, nicardipine, verapamil, quinidine, quinine and itraconazole. Reduced absorption may occur with antacids or colestyramine. Tetracycline, erythromycin and possibly other macrolides enhance the effect of digoxin. Rifampicin reduces serum concentrations.

Digoxin-specific antibody fragment (Fab) Digibind® is indicated for suspected toxicity where measures beyond withdrawal of digoxin and correction of any serum electrolyte abnormalities are felt to be necessary.

Drugs for arrhythmias

SUPRAVENTRICULAR ARRHYTHMIAS

Adenosine

Mechanism of action
Adenosine is a purine nucleotide. It acts on adenosine receptors and enhances the flow of potassium out of myocardial cells and produces hyperpolarization of the cell membrane and stabilizes the cell membrane. It has potent effects on the SA node, producing sinus bradycardia, and slows impulse conduction through the AV node.

Indications
Reversion to sinus rhythm of paroxysmal supraventricular tachycardia, including those associated with accessory pathways, e.g. Wolff–Parkinson–White syndrome.

Preparations and dose
Adenosine   *Adenocor®: 3 mg/mL.*
IV   By rapid intravenous injection into a central or large peripheral vein, 3 mg over 2 seconds with cardiac monitoring and resuscitation equipment available; if necessary followed by 6 mg after 1–2 minutes, and then 12 mg after a further 1–2 minutes; increments should not be given if high-level AV block develops at any dose.

Side-effects
Unwanted effects are common; however, they are usually transient. Patients should be warned before drug administration of side-effects usually lasting less than 1 minute.

- Bradycardia and AV block
- Facial flushing, headache, chest pain or tightness
- Bronchospasm.

Cautions/contraindications
Contraindicated in second- or third-degree AV block and sick sinus syndrome (unless pacemaker fitted), asthma.

SUPRAVENTRICULAR AND VENTRICULAR ARRHYTHMIAS

865

Amiodarone hydrochloride

Mechanism of action
Class III drug action (p. 415) which prolongs the duration of the action potential, thus increasing the absolute refractory

period. Inhibits the potassium channels involved in repolarization. Also has b-adrenoceptor antagonist activity.

Indications

Intravenous injection of amiodarone may be used in cardiopulmonary resuscitation for ventricular fibrillation or pulseless tachycardia unresponsive to other interventions. Oral and intravenous amiodarone is used in the treatment of arrhythmias (supraventricular and ventricular tachycardia, atrial fibrillation and flutter) particularly when other drugs are ineffective or contraindicated. In the non-emergency setting it should only be initiated under specialist supervision. Unlike many other antiarrhythmic drugs, amiodarone causes little or no myocardial depression.

Preparations and dose

Amiodarone   *Tablets: 100 mg, 200 mg; Injection: 30 mg/mL or concentrate 50 mg/mL.*

Oral   200 mg three times daily for 1 week reduced to 200 mg twice daily for a further week; maintenance, usually 200 mg daily or the minimum required to control the arrhythmia.

IV   Via central line catheter (in an emergency, e.g. ventricular tachycardia, can be given via a large peripheral line, but is a vesicant drug and therefore requires caution), initially 5 mg/kg in 250 mL glucose 5% (drug incompatible with sodium chloride) over 20–120 minutes with ECG monitoring. This may be repeated if necessary to a maximum of 1.2 g in 24 hours in 500 mL. As soon as an adequate response has been obtained, oral therapy should be initiated and the i.v. therapy phased out.

Side-effects

Amiodarone contains iodine and can cause both hypothyroidism and hyperthyroidism. Thyroid function tests including T_3 should be measured before treatment and then every 6 months of treatment. Amiodarone is also associated with liver toxicity, and liver biochemistry should be measured before and then every 6 months of treatment. Other side-effects are reversible corneal microdeposits (drivers may be dazzled by headlights at night), phototoxic skin reactions (advise patients to use total sunblock creams), pneumonitis and peripheral neuropathy.

Cautions/contraindications

Contraindicated in sinus bradycardia or sinoatrial heart block, unless pacemaker fitted.

Many drugs interact with amiodarone including warfarin and digoxin (check *National Formulary* for full list). It has a very long half-life (extending to several weeks) and many months may be required to achieve steady-state concentrations, this is also important when drug interactions are considered.

Disopyramide

Mechanism of action
Class Ia antiarrhythmic drug (p. 415). Produces Na^+ channel blockade and increases refractoriness of the cell.

Indications
Ventricular and supraventricular arrhythmias.

Preparations and dose
Disopyramide   *Capsules: 100 mg, 150 mg; Injection: 10 mg/mL.*
Disopyramide SR   *Tablets: 150 mg, 250 mg.*
Oral   300–800 mg daily in divided doses. SR preparation: 250–375 mg every 12 hours.
IV   By slow intravenous injection: 2 mg/kg over at least 5 minutes to a maximum of 150 mg with ECG monitoring, followed immediately by *either* 200 mg by mouth, then 200 mg every 8 hours for 24 hours *or* 400 µg/kg/h by intravenous infusion; maximum 300 mg in first hour and 800 mg daily.

Side-effects
Gastrointestinal disturbances, powerful negative inotropic effect, avoid in heart failure. Antimuscarinic effects, especially dry mouth, urinary retention and blurred vision.

Cautions/contraindications
Contraindicated in second- and third-degree heart block and sinus node dysfunction (unless pacemaker fitted), cardiogenic shock, severe uncompensated heart failure. Interactions with other drugs including astemizole, terfenadine and amiodarone (check *National Formulary* for full list).

VENTRICULAR ARRHYTHMIAS

867

Lidocaine (lignocaine) hydrochloride

Mechanism of action
Class 1b antiarrhythmic. Na^+-channel blockade and increases duration of the action potential.

Indications
Ventricular arrhythmias, especially after myocardial infarction.

Preparations and dose
Lidocaine *Injection: 2%, 20 mg/mL; Infusion 0.1% (1 mg/mL), 0.2% (2 mg/mL).*
IV injection 100 mg as a bolus over a few minutes (50 mg in lighter patients or those whose circulation is severely impaired) followed immediately by infusion of 4 mg/min for 30 minutes, 2 mg/min for 2 hours, then 1 mg/min; reduce concentration further if infusion continued beyond 24 hours.

Side-effects
Dizziness, paraesthesias, drowsiness, confusion particularly if injection too rapid. Other side-effects are convulsions, hypotension, bradycardia, and hypersensitivity.

Cautions/contraindications
Contraindicated in sinoatrial disorders, all grades of AV block, severe myocardial depression, porphyria.

Anticoagulants

Low-molecular-weight heparins

Mechanism of action
Mainly anti-Xa activity.

Indications
Prevention and treatment of deep venous thrombosis (DVT) and pulmonary embolism, myocardial infarction, acute coronary syndromes. Low-molecular-weight heparin is almost always used for these indications. For patients at high risk of bleeding, heparin (unfractionated) is more suitable than low-molecular-weight heparin because its effect can be terminated rapidly by stopping the infusion. Refer to the *National Formulary* for dosing for heparin.

Preparations and dose
Low-molecular-weight heparin *Enoxaparin – Clexane® injection: 20 mg, 40 mg, 60 mg, 80 mg, 100 mg, 120 mg, 150 mg.*

■ Prophylaxis of DVT by subcutaneous injection:
Surgical patients: moderate risk 20 mg once every 24 hours for 7–10 days with first dose 2 hours before surgery; high risk (e.g. orthopaedic patients) 40 mg every 24 hours for 7–10 days with first dose 12 hours before surgery.
Medical patients: 40 mg every 24 hours.

- Treatment of DVT and pulmonary embolism: 1.5 mg/kg (150 units/kg) by subcutaneous injection every 24 hours, usually for at least 5 days and until oral anticoagulation is established.
- Unstable angina and non ST-elevation myocardial infarction: 1 mg/kg (100 units/kg) by subcutaneous injection every 12 hours usually for 2–8 days.

Side-effects
- Haemorrhage.
- Thrombocytopenia, which is immune mediated and does not usually develop until after 6–10 days; it may be complicated by thrombosis. Platelet counts are recommended for patients receiving heparin for more than 5 days. Heparin should be stopped immediately and not repeated in those who develop thrombocytopenia or a 50% reduction of platelet count.
- Hyperkalaemia due to aldosterone secretion.
- Osteoporosis after prolonged use.

Cautions/contraindications
Contraindicated with bleeding disorders, thrombocytopenia, recent cerebral haemorrhage, severe liver disease, severe untreated hypertension, recent surgery to eye or nervous system.

Oral anticoagulants

Mechanism of action
Their anticoagulant effect is mediated by inhibition of vitamin K-dependent gamma carboxylation of coagulation factors II, VII, IX and X, thus leading to biologically inactive forms.

Indications
Prophylaxis of embolization in atrial fibrillation, cardioversion and dilated cardiomyopathy (target INR 2.5); prophylaxis of embolization after insertion of mechanical prosthetic heart valve (target INR 3.5); prophylaxis and treatment of venous thrombosis and pulmonary embolism (target INR 2.5). Warfarin takes at least 48–72 hours for the anticoagulant effect to develop fully.

Preparations and dose
Warfarin *Tablets: 1 mg, 3 mg, 5 mg.*

Maintenance dose usually 3–9 mg daily taken at the same time each day. Daily monitoring of the INR in the early days of treatment, then at longer intervals depending on response.

Side-effects

Haemorrhage (see *National Formulary* for management of bleeding in patients receiving warfarin), skin necrosis in patients with protein C or protein S deficiency, soon after starting treatment.

Cautions/contraindications

Contraindicated if underlying abnormalities of haemostasis (e.g. haemophilia, thrombocytopenia), severe uncontrolled hypertension, active peptic ulceration and severe liver disease.

Many drugs interact with warfarin (check *National Formulary* for full list) and the patient's INR should be measured frequently whenever any drug is added to, or withdrawn from, the patient's therapeutic regimen. Warfarin activity is particularly *increased* by alcohol, amiodarone, aspirin and other NSAIDs, cimetidine, ciprofloxacin, clofibrate, co-trimoxazole, dipyridamole, macrolide antibiotics such as erythromycin, metronidazole, statins, tamoxifen, levothyroxine (thyroxine). Warfarin activity is particularly *decreased* by carbamazepine, rifampicin, rifabutin, griseofulvin, and some herbal remedies, e.g. St John's wort. Warfarin activity may be *increased* or *decreased* by phenytoin, corticosteroids, colestyramine.

Antiplatelet agents

Mechanism of action

Antiplatelet agents decrease platelet aggregation and inhibit thrombus formation in the arterial circulation, where anticoagulants have little effect. Aspirin inhibits the enzyme cyclo-oxygenase, reducing production of thromboxane A_2, a stimulator of platelet aggregation. Dipyridamole inhibits phosphodiesterase-mediated breakdown of cyclic AMP, which leads to impaired platelet activation by multiple mechanisms. Clopidogrel blocks binding of ADP to platelet receptors and thus inhibits activation of the GP IIb/IIIa complex and platelet activation.

Preparations and dose

Aspirin   *Tablets: 75 mg, 300 mg, also as a dispersible form.*

- Secondary prevention of thrombotic cerebrovascular or cardiovascular disease: 300 mg chewed followed by maintenance dose of 75 mg.
- Primary prevention of vascular disease when the estimated 10-year coronary heart disease risk $\geq 15\%$, and

provided that blood pressure is controlled.

■ After coronary artery bypass grafting: 75 mg daily.

■ In combination with clopidogrel – see below.

■ Atrial fibrillation (selected cases): 75 mg daily.

■ Transient musculoskeletal pain and pyrexia (see rheumatology).

Dipyridamole   *Tablets: 100 mg; Oral suspension: 50 mg/mL; Persantin® Retard (modified release) capsules: 200 mg.*

Secondary prevention of ischaemic stroke and transient ischaemic attacks: 300–600 mg daily in three to four divided doses before food. MR preparation, 200 mg twice daily.

Clopidogrel   *Plavix® tablets: 75 mg.*

■ Where aspirin is contraindicated for the prevention of atherosclerotic events in patients with history of ischaemic stroke, myocardial infarction, or established peripheral artery disease: 75 mg daily.

■ Following coronary artery stent insertion: 300 mg daily, then 75 mg daily with aspirin 75 mg daily. Continue clopidogrel for 1 month – 9 months if a drug-eluting stent.

■ Acute coronary syndrome: 300 mg, then 75 mg daily in addition to aspirin and other treatments. Continue clopidogrel for 9 months.

Side-effects
Haemorrhage. Aspirin causes peptic ulceration. Patients with a past history of ulceration must be co-prescribed proton pump inhibitors (PPI) while taking aspirin, to prevent recurrent ulceration. In patients with a history of peptic ulcer bleeding while taking aspirin, co-administration of a PPI is associated with a reduced rate of re-bleeding compared to administration of clopidogrel.

Cautions/contraindications
Active bleeding, haemophilia and other bleeding disorders. Aspirin also causes bronchospasm and must be prescribed with caution to patients with asthma. Aspirin interacts with a number of other drugs, and its interaction with warfarin is a special hazard (refer to *National Formulary* for details).

Fibrinolytic drugs

Mechanism of action
Hydrolyse a peptide bond in plasminogen to yield the active enzyme, plasmin, which promotes clot lysis.

Preparations and dose

Tenecteplase   *Metalyse® injection: 40 mg (8000 units) and 50 mg (10 000 units) vials.*

For acute myocardial infarction: by intravenous injection over 10 seconds 30–50 mg according to bodyweight (500–600 µg/kg) to a maximum of 50 mg. Tenecteplase must be administered within 6 hours of the first onset of symptoms. After 6 hours an alternative agent is used, e.g. streptokinase. Heparin should be administered concurrently with tenecteplase, e.g. enoxaparin 1 mg/kg subcutaneously every 12 hours up to a maximum of 7 days.

Streptokinase   *Injection: 1.5 million international units.*
- Myocardial infarction: 1.5 million units over 60 minutes.
- In selected cases of DVT, pulmonary embolism, acute arterial thromboembolism, central retinal venous or arterial thrombosis: by intravenous infusion 250 000 units over 30 minutes, then according to clinical condition.

Side-effects

Haemorrhage, cardiac arrhythmias during reperfusion of the myocardium, hypotension and allergic reactions (bronchospasm, urticaria) with streptokinase.

Cautions/contraindications

Gastrointestinal bleeding, aortic dissection, severe uncontrolled hypertension, intracranial aneurysm, recent major surgery or invasive diagnostic procedure (within last 7–10 days), recent stroke or head injury, proliferative diabetic retinopathy, bleeding disorders, recent obstetric delivery, recent trauma including vigorous cardiopulmonary resuscitation.

Lipid-regulating drugs

Statins

Mechanism of action

Inhibition of 3-hydroxy-3-methylglutaryl coenzyme A (HMG-CoA) reductase, an enzyme involved in cholesterol synthesis, especially in the liver. More effective at lowering LDL-cholesterol than other classes of drugs but less effective than the fibrates in reducing triglycerides.

Indications

Secondary prevention of coronary and cardiovascular events in patients with history of angina or myocardial infarction, peripheral artery disease, non-haemorrhagic stroke, transient ischaemic attack. *Primary prevention* of coronary events in patients at increased risk of coronary heart disease such as inherited dyslipidaemias or a 10-year risk of 15% calculated using tables such as the Joint British Societies Coronary Risk Prediction Chart in the *British National Formulary*.

Preparations and dose
Atorvastatin   *Lipitor® tablets: 10 mg, 20 mg, 40 mg, 80 mg.* 10 mg once daily at night increased at intervals of at least 4 weeks to 40 mg once daily. Maximum 80 mg daily.

Simvastatin   *Tablets: 10 mg, 20 mg, 40 mg, 80 mg.* 10 mg at night, increased at intervals of at least 4 weeks up to 40 mg at night. For secondary prevention, initially 20 mg at night, increased up to 80 mg at intervals.

Side-effects
Reversible myositis/myopathy – ask patients to report unexplained muscle pain, measure serum creatine kinase (CK) and stop statin if CK $> 5 \times$ upper limit of normal. Altered liver biochemistry – liver biochemistry should be measured before and within 1–3 months of starting treatment, and thereafter at intervals of 6 months for 1 year, unless indicated sooner by signs or symptoms suggestive of hepatotoxicity. Stop treatment if serum transaminase concentration rises to, and persists at, three times the upper limit of the reference range. Gastrointestinal effects including abdominal pain, diarrhoea, flatulence and vomiting.

Cautions/contraindications
Contraindicated in most types of active liver disease, pregnancy (adequate contraception during treatment and for 1 month afterwards) and myositis. Increased risk of myositis and rhabdomyolysis if statins are given with a fibrate, ciclosporin, digoxin, warfarin, erythromycin, and ketoconazole.

RESPIRATORY SYSTEM

Most drugs described in this section are used in the management of asthma and COPD. Drug inhalation delivers the drug directly to the airways; the dose is smaller than that for the drugs given by mouth, and side-effects are reduced. *Metered-dose inhalers* (MDI) are the method of first choice for drug delivery. An *MDI with a spacer device* (e.g. AeroChamber plus spacer device) removes the need to coordinate actuation of an MDI and inhalation, and may

873

improve drug delivery for patients who have difficulty using a pressurized MDI. They increase airway drug deposition and reduce oropharyngeal deposition. Local adverse effects from inhaled corticosteroids, e.g. oropharyngeal candidiasis, are reduced and a spacer device should be co-prescribed with inhaled corticosteroids for children, patients on high doses and those with poor inhaler technique. *Breath-activated inhalers* or *dry powder inhalers* are also available. A *nebulizer* converts a solution of a drug into an aerosol for inhalation and delivers a higher dose of drug than is usual with standard inhalers. Nebulizers are used in the management of acute severe asthma, chronic persistent asthma and brittle asthma.

Bronchodilators

Short-acting selective β_2-adrenoceptor stimulants

Mechanism of action

β-agonists interact with β-receptors on the surface of a variety of cells and lead to bronchial smooth muscle relaxation, decrease release of mediators from mast cells, inhibit neutrophil and eosinophil functional responses and increase mucociliary transport.

Indications

Inhalers used as required (on a p.r.n. basis) for relief of symptoms in asthma and on an as needed (p.r.n.) or regular basis in COPD. Prophylactic treatment should be considered for asthma patients using an inhaler more than once daily. Oral preparations are used by patients who cannot manage the inhaled route, and the intravenous route is used for acute severe asthma.

Preparations and dose

Salbutamol *Metered dose inhaler(MDI): 100 μg/puff; Breath-actuated inhaler (Easi-Breathe)®: 100 μg/puff; Tablets: 2 mg, 4 mg; Oral solution: 2 mg/5 mL; Nebules: 2.5 mg/2.5 mL, 5 mg/2.5 mL; For infusion: 5 mg/5 mL.*

Inhaled MDI or breath-actuated inhaler: one to two puffs inhaled when required up to three to four times daily.

Oral 4 mg three to four times daily. Elderly and sensitive patients 2 mg initially.

Nebules 2.5–5 mg inhaled, repeated according to clinical need.

IV infusion Add 5 mg in 5 mL to a 500 mL bag of sodium chloride 0.9% or glucose 5%, to give a 10 μg/mL solution.

Infuse at a rate of 5 µg per minute and adjust according to response. Usual maintenance: 3–20 µg/min.

Salbutamol SR *Ventmax SR capsules: 4 mg, 8 mg.*
Oral 8 mg twice daily.

Terbutaline *Bricanyl® metered-dose inhaler (MDI): 250 µg/ puff; Dry powder inhaler (Turbohaler®): 500 µg/inhalation; Injection (Bricanyl®): 500 µg/mL.*

Inhaled

■ One to two puffs of MDI inhaled when required up to three to four times daily.

■ One inhalation of dry powder inhaler when required up to four times daily.

IV 250–500 µg up to four times daily. Give i.v. over 1–2 minutes or dilute 1.5–2.5 mg in 500 mL glucose 5% and give as a continuous infusion at a rate of 1.5–5 µg/min for 8–10 hours.

Side-effects
Fine tremor, tachycardia, palpitations, headache, disturbances of sleep. Hypokalaemia with high doses (monitor plasma potassium in severe asthma).

Cautions/contraindications
Caution in untreated/poorly controlled hyperthyroidism, arrhythmias.

Long-acting selective inhaled b2-adrenoceptor stimulants

Mechanism of action
As above for short-acting selective β_2-adrenoceptor stimulants.

Indications
Long-acting inhaled β_2 agonists are added to existing inhaled corticosteroid therapy to prevent asthma attacks. They are not used for an acute asthma attack. They are also used in COPD without inhaled corticosteroids.

Preparations and dose
Salmeterol (Serevent®) *Metered-dose inhaler: 25 µg/puff.*
Two puffs inhaled twice daily.
Accuhaler (dry powder for inhalation): 50 µg/blister.
1 blister twice daily.
Diskhaler (dry powder for inhalation): 50 µg/blister.
1 blister twice daily.

Formoterol (eformoterol)   *Foradis® Turbohaler (dry powder): 6 and 12 μg/inhalation.*
6–24 μg inhaled twice daily.

Side-effects
As above.

Cautions/contraindications
As above.

Antimuscarinic bronchodilators

Mechanism of action
Antagonize the actions of acetylcholine by competition at the type 3 muscarinic receptor (M_3) site located on airway smooth muscle. Antagonism of acetylcholine results in airway smooth muscle relaxation and bronchodilatation.

Indications
In combination with β-agonists for the emergency treatment of acute severe asthma. They are not usually used as first-line bronchodilators to treat chronic asthma but are often used in the management of COPD.

Preparations and dose
Ipatropium bromide   *Atrovent® metered-dose inhaler: 20 and 40 μg/puff.*
20–80 μg inhaled three to four times daily.
Atrovent® Aerocaps (dry powder for inhalation): 40 μg.
20–80 μg inhaled three to four times daily.
Nebules: 250 μg/mL.
100–500 μg inhaled up to four times daily.

Side-effects
Dry mouth, nausea, constipation, headache, acute angle-closure glaucoma.

Cautions/contraindications
Use with caution in patients with myasthenia gravis, narrow-angle glaucoma (protect patient's eyes from nebulized drug), benign prostatic hypertrophy, bladder neck obstruction.

Theophylline

Mechanism of action
Increases the intracellular concentration of cyclic nucleotides in airway smooth muscle and inflammatory cells by

inhibiting phosphodiesterase-mediated hydrolysis, in turn leads to smooth muscle relaxation and bronchodila tation. Theophylline also has anti-inflammatory/immuno-modulatory and bronchoprotective effects that may be mediated by other molecular mechanisms.

Indications

- Intravenously in acute severe asthma.
- In patients with chronic asthma whose asthma is not adequately controlled with inhaled corticosteroids. A single dose at night can help control nocturnal asthma and early morning wheezing.

Preparations and dose

Aminophylline is a mixture of theophylline and ethylene-diamine; the ethylenediamine confers greater solubility in water.

Theophylline *Slo-Phyllin® SR capsules: 60 mg, 125 mg, 250 mg.*

250–500 mg every 12 hours.

Uniphyllin Continus® SR tablets: 200 mg, 300 mg, 400 mg.

200 mg every 12 hours, increased after 1 week to 300 mg every 12 hours. Patients over 70 kg: 200–300 mg every 12 hours, increased after 1 week to 400 mg every 12 hours.

Aminophylline *Tablets: 100 mg; SR (Phyllocontin Continus®) tablets: 225 mg; Injection: 250 mg/10 mL.*

Oral 100–300 mg three to four times daily, or SR 225–450 mg twice daily.

IV loading 5 mg/kg (250–500 mg) over 20 minutes.

IV maintenance Add 500 mg to 250–500 mL sodium chloride 0.9% or glucose 5%, and give 500 μg/kg/h, adjusted according to plasma theophylline concentration.

Side-effects

Tachycardia, palpitations, nausea and other gastrointestinal disturbances, headache, CNS stimulation, insomnia, arrhythmias and convulsions especially if given rapidly by intravenous infusion. There is a narrow margin between therapeutic and toxic dose.

877

Cautions/contraindications

All modified-release theophylline preparations should be prescribed by brand name as the bioavailability between different brands may vary. Plasma theophylline concentration should be monitored in patients on oral therapy (8–12 hours after the last dose) and on intravenous treatment for longer than 24 hours (stop infusion for 15 minutes before taking the blood sample). Plasma theophylline concentration for optimum response 10–20 mg/L (55–110 μmol/L).

Theophylline is metabolized in the liver; there is considerable variation in plasma-theophylline concentration particularly in smokers, in patients with hepatic impairment or heart failure, or if certain drugs are taken concurrently – check *National Formulary* for details.

Intravenous magnesium sulphate

Mechanism of action
Relaxation of bronchial smooth muscle leading to bronchodilatation.

Indications
A single dose of i.v. magnesium sulphate is given to patients with:

- Acute severe asthma who have not had a good initial response to inhaled bronchodilator therapy
- Life-threatening or near fatal asthma.

Preparations and dose
Magnesium sulphate *50% (Mg^{2+} approx. 2 mmol/mL): 2 mL (1 g), 5 mL (2.5 g), 10 mL (5 g) ampoule.*
IV (Magnesium sulphate concentration should not exceed 20%; dilute 1 part of magnesium sulphate injection 50% with at least 1.5 parts of water for injection.) 1.2–2 g i.v. infusion over 20 minutes.

Side-effects
Nausea, vomiting, flushing, hypotension, arrhythmias, drowsiness, muscle weakness.

Cautions/contraindications
Profound hypotension reported with concomitant use of calcium-channel blockers.

Corticosteroids

878

Mechanism of action
The precise mechanisms for benefits in asthma are not known. Corticosteroids induce the synthesis of inhibitory factor kappa B (IκB), a protein that traps and thereby inactivates nuclear factor kappa B. The latter protein

activates cytokine genes, and thus steroids inhibit the synthesis of most cytokines. Steroids reduce airway inflammation and hence reduce oedema and secretion of mucus into the airway.

Indications

Inhaled For prophylactic treatment of asthma when patients are using a β_2-agonist more than once daily. In patients with COPD who have an improvement in lung function after a trial of oral corticosteroids.

Oral Acute severe asthma and in patients with chronic asthma when the response to other anti-asthma drugs is small.

Parenteral Acute severe asthma.

Preparations and dose

Inhaled

Beclometasone *Metered-dose inhaler: 50, 100, 200, 250 μg/ puff.*

200 μg inhaled twice daily, or for more severe cases up to 800 μg daily may be used.

Breath-activated inhaler: 50, 100, 250 μg/puff.

200 μg inhaled twice daily, or for more severe cases up to 800 μg daily may be used.

Dry powder for inhalation: 100, 200, 400 μg/puff.

400 μg inhaled twice daily.

Budesonide *Pulmicort® metered-dose inhaler: 50, 200 μg/puff.*

50 μg inhaled twice daily, or for more severe cases up to 400 μg twice daily.

Turbohaler® (dry powder): 100, 200, 400 μg/inhalation.

100–800 μg inhaled twice daily.

Fluticasone *Seretide® metered-dose inhaler: 50, 125, 250 μg/ puff.*

100–200 μg inhaled twice daily, increased up to 1 mg twice daily when necessary. Higher doses initiated by a specialist.

Seretide® dry powder for inhalation: 50, 100, 250, 500 μg/ blister.

100–200 μg inhaled twice daily, increased up to 1 mg twice daily when necessary. Higher doses initiated by a specialist.

Oral preparations

See page 880.

Intravenous preparations
See page 880.

Side-effects

The adverse effects of oral corticosteroids are listed on page 625. Inhaled corticosteroids have many fewer side-effects than oral corticosteroids but adverse effects are reported. Hoarseness and oropharyngeal candidiasis are reduced by rinsing the mouth with water after inhalation of a dose and/or by using a spacer device. Higher doses of inhaled corticosteroids have the potential to induce adrenal suppression, and patients on high doses should be given a 'steroid card' and may also need corticosteroid cover during an operation or illness. High doses may also reduce bone mineral density and the dose should be reduced when asthma control is good. There is a small increased risk of glaucoma.

Cautions/contraindications

Caution with inhaled corticosteroids in active or quiescent tuberculosis. Paradoxical bronchospasm may be prevented (if mild) by inhalation of a β_2-agonist before corticosteroid treatment.

ENDOCRINE SYSTEM

Thyroid and antithyroid drugs

Thyroid hormones

Mechanism of action
Synthetic thyroxine.

Indications
Hypothyroidism, diffuse non-toxic goitre, thyroid carcinoma.

Preparations and dose
Levothyroxine sodium (thyroxine)   *Tablets: 25 μg, 50 μg, 100 μg.*

50 μg daily (25 μg in elderly patients or those with cardiac disease) increased in steps of 25–50 μg every 3–4 weeks until the high serum TSH values return to the reference range. Usual maintenance dose to relieve hypothyroidism 100–200 μg daily.

Side-effects
These usually occur at excessive dosage but may do so at start of therapy with rapid increase in metabolism.

Arrhythmias, palpitations, skeletal muscle cramps and weakness, vomiting, diarrhoea, tremors, restlessness, headache, flushing, sweating, fever, excessive loss of weight and sometimes anginal pain where there is latent myocardial ischaemia.

Cautions/contraindications
Panhypopituitarism or predisposition to adrenal insufficiency from other causes (initiate corticosteroid therapy before starting levothyroxine), lower dose in the elderly or cardiovascular disease, diabetes mellitus (dosage increase may be needed for antidiabetic drugs including insulin). Contraindicated in thyrotoxicosis.

Antithyroid drugs

Mechanism of action
Interfere with synthesis of thyroid hormones.

Indications
Long-term management of thyrotoxicosis and to prepare patients for thyroidectomy. Antithyroid drugs may be given with propranolol, 40 mg three times daily, for initial symptom control.

Preparations and dose
Carbimazole   *Tablets: 5 mg, 20 mg.*

Most commonly used drug for thyrotoxicosis in the UK. Initial treatment 15–40 mg daily; occasionally a larger dose is required. This dose is continued until the patient becomes euthyroid, usually after 4–8 weeks, and the dose is then gradually reduced to a maintenance dose of 5–15 mg. Treatment is usually given for 12–18 months. A combination of carbimazole, 40–60 mg daily, with levothyroxine (thyroxine), 50–150 µg daily, is used in a *blocking–replacement regimen* (not in pregnancy).

Propylthiouracil   *Tablets: 50 mg.*

Dosing schedule is as for carbimazole but initial treatment is 200–400 mg daily and maintenance dose 50–150 mg daily.

Side-effects
Bone marrow suppression particularly with carbimazole; patients should be asked to report symptoms and signs suggestive of infection, especially sore throat. A white cell count should be performed if there is any clinical evidence

of infection, and treatment should be stopped immediately if there is clinical or laboratory evidence of neutropenia. Nausea, gastrointestinal disturbance, headache, rashes and pruritus with carbimazole. Cutaneous vasculitis, hepatic necrosis, nephritis and lupus-like syndrome with propylthiouracil.

Cautions/contraindications
Liver disorders; overtreatment can result in rapid development of hypothyroidism.

Corticosteroids

Mechanism of action
Replacement therapy The adrenal cortex normally secretes hydrocortisone (cortisol) which has glucocorticoid activity and weak mineralocorticoid activity. It also secretes the mineralocorticoid aldosterone. In *primary adrenal insufficiency* physiological replacement is best achieved with a combination of hydrocortisone and the mineralocorticoid fludrocortisone; hydrocortisone alone does not usually provide sufficient mineralocorticoid activity for complete replacement. In *hypopituitarism* glucocorticoids are given but aldosterone is not necessary as production is regulated by the renin–angiotensin system.
Anti-inflammatory actions include induction of the synthesis of IκB, an inhibitory protein which binds NF-Kappa B.

Indications
■ A wide variety of inflammatory conditions of the joints, lungs, skin and bowel, acute transplant rejection, auto-immune conditions, nephritic syndrome (particularly in children), septic shock, cerebral oedema, acute hyper-sensitivity reactions such as angio-oedema of the upper respiratory tract and anaphylactic shock.
■ For replacement therapy in adrenal insufficiency and hypopituitarism.

The type of steroid preparation used depends on the indication, e.g. dexamethasone is a very potent steroid with insignificant mineralocorticoid activity (see below) and this makes it particularly suitable for high-dose therapy in conditions where fluid retention (mineralocorticoid side-effect) would be a disadvantage, e.g. cerebral oedema. Prednisolone has predominantly glucocorticoid activity and is the corticosteroid most commonly used by mouth for long-term disease suppression. The relatively high mineralocorticoid activity of cortisone and hydrocortisone, and the resulting fluid retention, make them unsuitable for disease suppression on a long-term basis. Hydrocortisone is used for adrenal replacement therapy and intravenously in the emergency management of some conditions, e.g. severe ulcerative colitis, anaphylactic shock. Corticosteroids are also used by inhalation in asthma, by rectal administration in inflammatory bowel disease, and topically in the treatment of inflammatory conditions of the skin. These preparations are not discussed in this section.

Preparations and dose

The equivalent anti-inflammatory doses of corticosteroids and their mineralocorticoid activity are shown in Table 19.1.

Prednisolone *Tablets: 1 mg, 5 mg, 25 mg; Soluble tablets: 5 mg; Enteric-coated tablets: 2.5 mg, 5 mg.*
Oral Initially 10–40 mg daily, up to 60 mg in severe disease as a single dose after breakfast. Maintenance usually 2.5–15 mg.

Hydrocortisone *Tablets (Hydrocortone®): 10 mg, 20 mg; Injection (Solu-Cortef®): 100 mg powder for reconstitution.*
Oral Replacement therapy: 20–30 mg daily in divided doses.
IV/IM 100–500 mg, three to four times daily or as required, by a slow bolus or as an infusion in sodium chloride 0.9% or glucose 5%.

Dexamethasone *Tablets: 500 μg, 2 mg; Oral solution: 2 mg/ 5 mL; Injection: 4 mg/mL, 24 mg/5 mL.*

Table 19.1 Equivalent anti-inflammatory doses of corticosteroids	
	Mineralocorticoid activity
Prednisolone 5 mg	Slight
= Betamethasone 750 μg	Negligible
= Cortisone acetate 25 mg	High
= Deflazacort 6 mg	Slight
= Dexamethasone 750 μg	Negligible
= Hydrocortisone 20 mg	High
= Methylprednisolone 4 mg	Slight
= Triamcinolone 4 mg	Slight

Oral   0.5–10 mg daily in divided doses.

IV/IM   Initially 0.5–20 mg daily in divided doses; i.v. injection must be given over at least 3–5 minutes or as an infusion in sodium chloride 0.9% or glucose 5%.

Methylprednisolone   *Tablets (Medrone®): 2 mg, 4 mg, 16 mg, 100 mg; Injection (Solu-Medrone®): 40 mg, 125 mg, 500 mg, 1 g, 2 g vial.*

Oral   Usual range 2–40 mg daily.

IV/IM   Initially 10–500 mg daily, dose depends on condition. Slow i.v. injection or infusion.

Side-effects

Glucocorticoid side-effects include diabetes and osteoporosis (p. 625). Precautions for patients taking prolonged therapy with corticosteroids are discussed on page 624. *Mineralocorticoid* side-effects include hypertension, sodium and water retention and potassium loss.

Cautions/contraindications

Untreated systemic infection, avoid live virus vaccines in those receiving immunosuppressive doses.

DRUGS USED IN DIABETES

Oral antidiabetic drugs

Oral antidiabetic drugs are used for the treatment of type 2 diabetes mellitus. They are usually only prescribed if the patient fails to respond to at least 3 months' restriction of energy and carbohydrate intake, and an increase in physical activity.

Sulphonylureas

Mechanism of action
Augment insulin secretion.

Indications
Patients with type 2 diabetes mellitus who are not overweight, or in whom metformin is contraindicated or not tolerated.

Preparations and dose
Several sulphonylureas are available and choice is determined by side-effects and the duration of action as well as the patient's age and renal function. Glibenclamide is long acting and associated with a greater risk of hypoglycaemia and should be avoided in the elderly.

Gliclazide and tolbutamide are shorter acting and are a better choice.

Glibenclamide   *Tablets: 2.5 mg, 5 mg.*

Initially 5 mg daily with or immediately after breakfast, adjusted according to response; maximum 15 mg daily.

Tolbutamide   *Tablets: 500 mg.*

0.5–1.5 g (max. 2 g) daily in divided doses with or immediately after breakfast.

Gliclazide   *Tablets: 80 mg.*

Initially 40–80 mg daily, adjusted according to response up to 160 mg as a single dose or 320 mg daily in divided doses.

Side-effects

Generally mild and infrequent and include gastrointestinal disturbances such as nausea, vomiting, diarrhoea and constipation. May encourage weight gain. Sulphonylurea-induced hypoglycaemia may persist for many hours and must always be treated in hospital. Occasionally cholestatic jaundice, hepatitis, allergic skin reactions and blood disorders.

Cautions/contraindications

Use short-acting form in renal impairment. Avoid sulphonylureas in severe renal and hepatic impairment, and in porphyria. Contraindicated in breast-feeding, and substitute insulin during pregnancy.

Biguanides

Mechanism of action

Decrease gluconeogenesis and increase peripheral utilization of insulin.

Indications

Drug of first choice in overweight patients in whom strict dieting has failed to control diabetes. Also used in combination with sulphonylureas, pioglitazone, rosiglitazone, repaglinide, nateglinide or insulin if diabetes is inadequately controlled with metformin alone. Also used in polycystic ovary syndrome.

Preparations and dose

Metformin   *Tablets: 500 mg, 850 mg.*

500 mg once daily initially, then titrate upwards to every 8 hours or 850 mg every 12 hours; maximum 3 g daily in divided doses.

Side-effects
Anorexia, nausea, vomiting, diarrhoea (usually transient), abdominal pain, metallic taste, rarely lactic acidosis (withdraw treatment). Hypoglycaemia does not usually occur with metformin.

Cautions/contraindications
Contraindicated in even mild renal impairment (increased risk of lactic acidosis). Measure serum creatinine before treatment and once or twice annually during treatment. Withdraw if tissue hypoxia likely (e.g. sepsis, respiratory failure, recent myocardial infarction, hepatic impairment), use of iodine-containing X-ray contrast media (do not restart until renal function returns to normal) and use of general anaesthesia (suspend metformin 2 days before surgery and restart when renal function returns to normal). Contraindicated in pregnancy and breast-feeding.

Treatment of hypoglycaemia

Initially glucose 10–20 g (2–4 teaspoons sugar, 3–6 sugar lumps) is given by mouth. If sugar cannot be given by mouth (e.g. unconscious patient), glucose or glucagon can be given by injection.

Mechanism of action
Glucagon mobilizes glycogen stored in the liver.

Indications
Acute hypoglycaemia where glucose cannot be given either by mouth or intravenously.

Preparations and dose
Glucagon   *GlucaGen® Hypokit: 1 mg vial with prefilled syringe containing water for injection.*
   By subcutaneous, intramuscular, or intravenous injection 1 mg.

Side-effects
Nausea, vomiting, abdominal pain, hypokalaemia, hypotension, hypersensitivity reactions.

Cautions/contraindications
Phaeochromocytoma.

NEUROLOGY

Hypnotics and anxiolytics

Hypnotics and anxiolytics should be reserved for short courses (because dependence and tolerance may occur with long-term use) to alleviate acute conditions after causal factors have been established. Benzodiazepines are the most commonly used anxiolytics and hypnotics.

Hypnotics

Mechanism of action

Benzodiazepines bind to specific receptor sites that are closely linked to the $GABA_A$ receptor, inducing a conformational change that enhances the action of the inhibitory neurotransmitter GABA. Zopiclone is not a benzodiazepine but binds to the same receptor.

Indications

Transient or short-term insomnia due to extraneous factors such as shift work or an emotional problem or serious medical illness. Short-term use only – up to 4 weeks.

Preparations and dose

Temazepam   *Tablets: 10 mg, 20 mg; Oral solution: 10 mg/5 mL.*
Oral   10–20 mg at bedtime.

Zopiclone   *Tablets: 3.75 mg, 7.5 mg.*
Oral   7.5 mg at bedtime; elderly, initially 3.75 mg.

Side-effects

Drowsiness and lightheadedness, confusion and ataxia, especially in the elderly (avoid if possible). Hangover effects of a night-time dose may impair driving the following day. Paradoxical increase in anxiety and aggression; adjustment of the dose up or down usually improves the problem. Tolerance may develop within 3–14 days.

Cautions/contraindications

Contraindicated in respiratory depression, acute breathlessness, severe liver disease, myasthenia gravis, sleep apnoea syndrome. Withdrawal symptoms (may be delayed for 3 weeks with long-acting preparation) if drug stopped abruptly after long-term use, consisting of anxiety, insomnia, depression, psychosis and convulsions.

Anxiolytics

Mechanism of action
As above.

Indications
- Short-term relief in severe anxiety.
- In panic disorders resistant to antidepressant treatment.
- Intravenously for short-term sedation with medical procedures, e.g. colonoscopy.
- Prevention of the alcohol withdrawal syndrome.
- Benzodiazepines also used in the acute management of status epilepticus.

Preparations and dose
Diazepam *Tablets: 2 mg, 5 mg, 10 mg; Oral solution: 2 mg/ 5 mL, 5 mg/5 mL; Emulsion injection: 10 mg/2 mL; Rectal solution: 2.5 mg/1.25 mL, 5 mg/2.5 mL, 10 mg/2.5 mL.*
Oral Anxiety: 2 mg three times daily, increasing if necessary to 15–30 mg daily in divided doses. Elderly: half adult dose. Insomnia associated with anxiety: 5–15 mg at bedtime.
IM/IV (into a large vein at a rate not more than 5 mg/min) for severe acute anxiety and control of panic attacks: 10 mg repeated if necessary after not less than 4 hours.
  In status epilepticus:
IV 10–20 mg repeated if necessary after 30–60 minutes; may be followed by infusion to maximum 3 mg/kg over 24 hours.
By rectum 500 μg/kg up to maximum 30 mg (elderly, half dose) repeated after 12 hours if necessary.

Lorazepam *Tablets: 1 mg, 2.5 mg; Injection 4 mg/mL.*
Oral Anxiety: 1–4 mg daily in divided doses (elderly, half dose). Insomnia associated with anxiety: 1–2 mg at bedtime.
IM/IV (into a large vein by slow injection) for severe acute anxiety and control of panic attacks: 25–30 μg/kg, repeated if necessary every 6 hours.
  In status epilepticus: by intravenous injection into a large vein: 4 mg.

Chlordiazepoxide *Capsules: 5 mg, 10 mg; Tablets: 5 mg, 10 mg.*
Oral Anxiety: 10 mg three times daily in anxiety, increased if necessary to 60–100 mg daily. In alcohol withdrawal: 10–50 mg four times daily (under supervision) and reduced gradually over 7–14 days.

Oxazepam   *Tablets: 10 mg, 15 mg, 30 mg.*
Oral   Anxiety: 15–30 mg three to four times daily (half dose in elderly). Insomnia associated with anxiety: 15–25 mg (max. 50 mg) at bedtime.

Short acting and used as an alternative to chlordiazepoxide in alcohol withdrawal for patients with severe liver dysfunction, 15–30 mg four times daily (under supervision) and reduced gradually over 7–14 days.

Antipsychotics ('neuroleptics')

Mechanism of action
Blockade of CNS dopamine (D_2) receptors.

Indications
In the short term to quieten disturbed patients whatever the underlying psychopathology, e.g. schizophrenia, mania, toxic delirium. Used in the long-term management of schizophrenia. Also used in intractable hiccup and nausea and vomiting.

Preparations and dose
Chlorpromazine   *Tablets: 10 mg, 25 mg, 50 mg, 100 mg; Oral solution: 25 mg/5 mL, 100 mg/5 mL; Suppositories: 100 mg.*

Initially 25–50 mg three times daily or 75 mg at night; adjust according to response.

Haloperidol   *Capsules: 500 µg; Tablets: 500 µg, 1.5 mg, 5 mg, 10 mg, 20 mg; Oral liquid: 5 mg/5 mL, 10 mg/5 mL; Injection: 5 mg/mL, 20 mg/mL.*
Oral   Psychoses: initially 1.5–3 mg (3–5 mg in severe cases) two to three times daily, may be increased to maximum 30 mg daily in divided doses and then reduced to maintenance dose when control achieved. Hiccup and vomiting: 1–1.5 mg three times daily.
IM/IV   2–10 mg repeated every 4–8 hours according to response to a maximum of 18 mg daily.

Side-effects
Acute drowsiness, hypotension, tachycardia, convulsions, antimuscarinic symptoms (dry mouth, constipation, difficulty with micturition, blurred vision), neuroleptic malignant syndrome (hyperthermia, fluctuating conscious level, muscular rigidity, autonomic dysfunction). Extrapyramidal, haematological and endocrine side-effects with longer-term use (see *National Formulary*).

Cautions/contraindications

Use with caution in liver disease, renal impairment, cardio-vascular disease, Parkinson's disease, epilepsy, myasthenia gravis, glaucoma. Contraindicated in coma and phaeochromocytoma. Many drug interactions (check *National Formulary*).

Antiepileptics

Drug of choice for seizure type in adults. The newer antiepileptic drugs are not described here and should be initiated by a specialist.

Carbamazepine

Mechanism of action

Inhibition of repetitive neuronal firing is produced by reduction of transmembrane Na^+ influx, by use-dependent blockade of Na^+ channels.

Indications

Drug of choice for simple and complex partial seizures, and for tonic–clonic seizures secondary to a focal discharge.

Preparations and dose

Carbamazepine *Tablets: 100 mg, 200 mg, 400 mg; Tegretol® liquid: 100 mg/5 mL; Tegretol® suppositories: 100 mg; Modified-release tablets (Tegretol® Retard): 200 mg, 400 mg.*

Initially 100 mg once or twice daily increased slowly to usual dose of 0.8–1.2 g daily (epilepsy) or 200 mg three to four times daily (trigeminal neuralgia). Total daily doses are the same for Tegretol Retard but given twice daily (may provide better steady-state levels).

Side-effects

Nausea and vomiting, especially early in treatment. Central nervous system toxicity leads to double vision, dizziness, drowsiness and ataxia. Transient leucopenia is common, especially early in treatment – severe bone marrow depression is rare. Hyponatraemia caused by potentiation of antidiuretic hormone.

Cautions/contraindications

Contraindicated in AV conduction abnormalities (unless paced), history of bone marrow depression, porphyria. Hepatic enzyme induction leading to accelerated metabolism of the oral contraceptive pill (dose of oestrogen should be increased to avoid failure of contraception), warfarin (reduced anticoagulant effect), ciclosporin and others (see *National Formulary*). Interactions also with other antiepileptic drugs.

Valproate

Mechanism of action
Blockade of transmembrane Na^+ channels, thus stabilizing neuronal membranes.

Indications
Effective for all forms of epilepsy.

Preparations and dose
Sodium valproate *Tablets: 100 mg, 200 mg; Solution: 200 mg/5 mL; Injection powder for reconstitution: 400 mg.*

600 mg daily in two divided doses, increasing by 200 mg/day at 3-day intervals to usual dose of 1–2 g daily in divided doses.

Side-effects
Gastrointestinal upset (nausea, vomiting, anorexia, abdominal pain, acute pancreatitis), increased appetite and weight gain, transient hair loss, dose-related tremor, thrombocytopenia, rarely severe hepatotoxicity. Drug concentration in plasma does not correlate with therapeutic effect and monitoring is only necessary to assess complications of suspected toxicity.

Cautions/contraindications
Acute liver disease, porphyria. Monitor liver biochemistry 6-monthly in those most at risk of severe liver damage (see *National Formulary*). Many drug interactions with antiepileptics and other drugs (see *National Formulary*).

Phenytoin and fosphenytoin

Mechanism of action
Inhibit sodium influx across the cell membrane, reduce cell excitability.

Indications
All forms of epilepsy except absence seizures. Also used in management of status epilepticus and in trigeminal neuralgia.

Preparations and dose
Phenytoin *Capsules: 25 mg, 50 mg, 100 mg, 300 mg; Suspension: 30 mg/5 mL; Injection: 50 mg/mL.*

Oral 150–300 mg daily (single dose or two divided doses) increased gradually as necessary (with plasma-phenytoin concentration monitoring); usual dose 200–500 mg. Reference range for concentration 40–80 µmol/L (10–20 mg/L) immediately before the next dose.

IV By slow i.v. injection or infusion (with blood pressure and ECG monitoring), status epilepticus: 15 mg/kg at a rate not exceeding 50 mg per minute, as a loading dose; maintenance doses of about 100 mg should be given thereafter at intervals of every 6–8 hours, monitored by measurement of plasma concentrations; rate and dose reduced according to weight.

Fosphenytoin   *Pro-Epanutin® for injection: 75 mg/mL.*

Pro-drug of phenytoin which can be given more rapidly and causes fewer infusion site reactions. Dose expressed as phenytoin sodium equivalent (PE) (fosphenytoin 1.5 mg = phenytoin sodium 1 mg).

Status epilepticus: initially 15 mg PE/kg by i.v. infusion (with blood pressure, ECG and respiratory rate monitoring during and for at least 30 minutes after infusion) at a rate of 100–150 mg PE/min. Maintenance 4–5 mg PE/kg daily (in one to four divided doses) by i.v. infusion at a rate of 50–100 mg PE/min.

Side-effects

Intravenous injection may cause CNS, cardiovascular (hypotension, heart block, arrhythmias) and respiratory depression. If hypotension occurs, reduce infusion rate or discontinue. Other side-effects are dose related and include impaired brainstem and cerebellar function (nystagmus, double vision, vertigo, ataxia, dysarthria), chronic connective tissue effects (gum hyperplasia, coarsening of facial features, hirsutism), skin rashes (withdraw treatment), folate deficiency, increased vitamin D metabolism and deficiency, blood dyscrasias, lymphadenopathy and teratogenic effects.

Cautions/contraindications

Contraindicated in sinus bradycardia, heart block and porphyria. Many drug interactions (see *National Formulary*). Highly protein bound and can be displaced by valproate and salicylates, which therefore enhance the effect. Induction of hepatic drug-metabolizing enzymes and metabolism of warfarin and ciclosporin increased (see *National Formulary* for full list).

ETHICS

1. You are covering for your colleague in the GP practice who is unwell and likely to be off work for at least 2 weeks. A patient of his has asked to see you urgently in order to find out the result of the HIV test which your colleague had arranged last week. The patient is extremely anxious. He is a 31-year-old journalist who is happily married and healthy. Five years previously he had spent several months in Zambia and had unprotected sex with a girlfriend he met there. He has read in the newspapers of the high rates of HIV infection in Africa and has become increasingly worried that he has AIDS. He and his wife are planning to start a family and he requested the HIV test. His test result is positive. What points would you bring out in your consultation with the patient?

2. You have been asked to see the wife of a 67-year-old male inpatient with advanced metastatic gastric cancer. He had been admitted after returning from holiday in Australia where he initially became unwell. The medical notes, radiology and histology have been sent with the patient. He is cachectic, and treatment is obviously palliative. His wife is aware of the diagnosis and prognosis and she has requested that you promise her that you will not tell her husband the diagnosis. She tells you that she has always been the 'decision-maker' and her husband would go along with whatever she thought best. She tells you that he would not cope with the diagnosis, would give up immediately, and she wants his remaining life to be as good as it can be. What points would you bring out in the discussion with the patient's wife?

3. Which of the following are true in relation to the consent process?

(a) A 39-year-old severely mentally disabled man is admitted with haematemesis to a London teaching hospital. His mother who is his main carer accompanies him to the hospital and provides the history. On admission, his pulse is 104/min, BP 90/60 mmHg and Hb 8.4 g/dL. He needs an upper gastrointestinal endoscopy after appropriate resuscitation to determine the source of bleeding and if necessary control bleeding with endoscopic therapy. The endoscopy cannot go ahead without the written consent of his mother.

(b) A 15-year-old boy admitted with appendicitis wants to sign the consent form for appendicectomy. This is legally binding.

(c) A 56-year-old woman is admitted with massive haematemesis. She has been taking indometacin for arthritis and you suspect a bleeding peptic ulcer. She is pale, sweaty, and has a poor-volume pulse of 140/min. Her BP is 70/40 mmHg. You explain the likely diagnosis to her and say that you would like to take some blood for a variety of tests to further assess her condition and also to crossmatch her for blood transfusion. She tells you that she is a Jehovah's Witness and will not have a blood transfusion or any blood products. She can refuse a blood transfusion even if it will save her life.

(d) A 36-year-old man is admitted after a road traffic accident. He has a Glasgow Coma Score of 4 and an obvious external head injury. CT scan shows a massive extradural haematoma. The neurosurgeons are called and want to take him to theatre that afternoon to evacuate the haematoma. He is unable to provide consent. The surgeons are allowed to proceed with surgery.

(e) You are a third-year medical student and have attended the cardiology clinic to sit in with the consultant. It is unnecessary for the consultant to seek each patient's consent for you to be present at the consultation.

Answers

1. After explaining to the patient that your colleague is absent and unable to be present himself today you

should check if your colleague discussed the details of the tests and the patient's understanding of the implications of a positive test. The patient may require you to go over this information again. The patient should be reassured that the test result is confidential and will only be available to those staff involved with his care. Explain that the natural history of HIV infection is variable and there is nothing to suggest that he has AIDS. You should also explain to the patient that his wife has a right to know about the test result and the implications of a positive test. He should be encouraged to tell his wife and you should offer to facilitate this. His wife could be HIV positive and should also be tested. He should also be advised that he should not have unprotected sex with his wife or other partners to prevent disease transmission. Finally the patient should be offered a follow-up visit in the near future.

2. First, clarify why she does not want her husband to know the diagnosis. Explain that he is very unwell and he himself must be aware that something is seriously wrong. Explain to her that her husband may ask you directly about the diagnosis and that you must tell him and provide him with information about the disease. Explain that you will answer his questions honestly and give a guide to the prognosis. Also explain that this can be a gradual process and does not need to be done in one consultation. However, you cannot promise not to tell her husband and you should explain that you cannot lie and you have a responsibility to the patient. He may, for example, want to put his affairs in order if he knows that he has a terminal disease. Also explain to the patient's wife that if she does not tell her husband, he may lose trust in his carers if the diagnosis becomes apparent.

3. (a) False. Legally in England, Wales and Northern Ireland, no person can give consent to treatment on behalf of another adult, even if that person has Enduring Power of Attorney. The view of people close to the patient has no legal status in terms of decision making. Doctors may treat a patient who lacks capacity to consent to treatment, without consent, providing the treatment is necessary and in the patient's best interests. However, it is good practice for the healthcare team to consult with

895

people who are close to the patient, particularly when assessing the patient's best interests. Any such discussions should take into consideration the duty of confidentiality owed to the patient. In this case it would be in the patient's best interests to have an upper gastrointestinal endoscopy. In Scotland the law allows people over 16 to appoint a proxy decision maker who has the power to give consent to medical treatment when the patient loses capacity. The courts may also appoint a proxy decision maker on behalf of an incapacitated adult.

(b) True. A young person of any age can give a valid consent to treatment or examination provided he or she is considered to be competent to make the decision. At the age of 16 there is a presumption that the patient is competent to give a valid consent. Up to the age of 18, where the person lacks capacity, a person or local authority with parental responsibility (mother, father if the parents have ever been married, legally appointed guardian) can give consent on behalf of the patient.

(c) True. Competent adult patients are entitled to refuse consent to treatment even when doing so may result in permanent physical injury or death. A Jehovah's Witness can refuse a blood transfusion even where this is essential for survival. Where the consequences of refusal are grave, it is essential that patients understand this.

(d) True. In an emergency, where consent cannot be obtained, doctors should provide medical treatment that is in the patient's best interests and is immediately necessary to save life or avoid significant deterioration in the patient's health. If, however, the patient is an adult and there is clear evidence of a valid advance refusal of a particular treatment (such as a refusal of blood by a Jehovah's Witness) that treatment should not be given.

(e) False. The consultant should explain to each patient that you are a medical student and that you would like to sit in on the consultation and observe the clinic. He should also explain that you are doing this as a part of your medical training. Patients should feel able to refuse consent to the presence of students or other observers during their consultation and/or examination. They should be reassured that their decision will in no way affect their treatment. Wherever possible, patients should be given the option of considering this request prior to the arrival of the observers.

INFECTIOUS DISEASES AND TROPICAL MEDICINE

1. Describe briefly the intestinal infections produced by:
   (a) *Campylobacter* sp.
   (b) *Yersinia* sp.
   (c) *Clostridium difficile*.

2. A 1-year-old boy has been unwell for 6 hours, temperature 40.5°C with eight petechial spots on the trunk and legs. He is drowsy, with systolic blood pressure of 45 mmHg.
   (a) What is the probable diagnosis?
   (b) What immediate treatment would you give?
   (c) What treatment would you give the rest of the family?
   (d) Can the disease be prevented in this age group?
   (e) What complications would you examine for at an outpatient visit 6 weeks later?

3. A 35-year-old man with AIDS presents with headache, fever, confusion and fits. His CD4 count is 73/mL. A brain CT scan shows multiple ring-enhancing lesions. Which of the following is the most likely cause?
   (a) Tuberculosis
   (b) *Cryptosporidium parvum*
   (c) *Toxoplasma gondii*
   (d) Meningioma
   (e) Kaposi's sarcoma.

4. A 47-year-old man returns from a week's holiday in Kenya. He presents 18 days later to Accident and Emergency with headache and fever of 38.9°C. There are no abnormal findings other than a fever on examination. What is the most likely cause of his illness?
   (a) *Plasmodium falciparum*
   (b) *Plasmodium ovale*
   (c) Typhoid fever
   (d) Dengue fever
   (e) Viral haemorrhagic fever.

5. A 64-year-old man with heart failure presents with a fever and a red macular area over his shin. The margins are not well demarcated and you note that the involved skin is swollen, warm to touch and tender. In relation to the presenting problem, which of the following are true?
   (a) The most likely cause is beta-haemolytic streptococci.
   (b) The pathogen responsible is likely to be identified on blood cultures.
   (c) The site of involvement is atypical.
   (d) Leg oedema is a risk factor.
   (e) Clindamycin would be a suitable treatment.

Answers

1. (a) The only campylobacter producing intestinal infection is *Campylobacter jejuni*. *Campylobacter* and *Salmonella* species account for most cases of food poisoning (poultry is the main source of infection in both). Campylobacter infection produces a prodromal febrile infection lasting 1–4 days, followed by a diarrhoeal phase which may last 1–2 weeks. Severe abdominal pains often accompany the diarrhoea, which may be blood-stained. Septicaemia may occur, but rarely death. Sigmoidoscopy may show an acute colitis resembling ulcerative colitis. Diagnosis is made by microscopy (seen as motile rods) and culture of faeces. Infection is usually self-limiting; antibiotic treatment with erythromycin is given to those with systemic symptoms. Complications include cholecystitis, pancreatitis, reactive arthritis and Guillain-Barré syndrome.
   (b) There are three main *Yersinia* species in humans, all of which are uncommon in Britain. *Y. pseudotuberculosis* and *Y. enterocolitica* cause diarrhoea, terminal ileitis and mesenteric adenitis (may be confused with appendicitis). Diagnosis is usually by serology, demonstrating a rise in antibody titre on paired samples. The illness is usually self-limiting, but tetracycline may be helpful for treating a severe infection. The third species, *Y. pestis*, causes plague.
   (c) *Clostridium difficile* produces pseudomembranous colitis, which is an uncommon complication of antibiotic therapy. *C. difficile* is present in the colon

of some healthy individuals, and colitis has been attributed to the selection of drug-resistant *C. difficile* that proliferates in the colon and produces a necrotizing toxin. Diagnosis is by demonstration of the toxin in stool and by typical sigmoidoscopic appearances (pseudomembranous on an erythematous background). Treatment is with oral metronidazole 400 mg three times daily or oral vancomycin 250 mg four times daily for up to 10 days.

2. (a) The temperature and hypotension indicate septicaemic shock. The petechial spots suggest this is caused by infection with *Neisseria meningitidis* (not all of these infections produce meningitis). Fulminant meningococcaemia is a severe life-threatening illness with a rapidly progressive downhill course.

(b) The initial treatment is intravenous benzylpenicillin (cefotaxime or chloramphenicol if penicillin allergic), which must be started immediately the diagnosis is clinically suspected. The management of suspected bacterial meningitis is outlined in Emergency Box 16.3.

(c) Household contacts of a patient with meningococcal disease should be prescribed prophylaxis with rifampicin (600 mg twice daily for 2 days), ciprofloxacin or, for pregnant contacts, ceftriaxone. The purpose of chemoprophylaxis is to eliminate carriage in the contact group. It does not prevent illness in those already infected so contacts should continue to be alert to the symptoms of meningococcal disease.

(d) A vaccine for meningococcal group C and *Haemophilus influenzae* is available and is part of routine childhood immunization in the UK. Contacts of a case should be treated as above.

(e) A small number of patients develop chronic complications, e.g. arthritis, vasculitis and pericarditis, which may be due to immune complex disease.

3. (c) This patient is severely immunosuppressed (CD4 count < 200/μL) and in these patients the most likely cause of a CNS mass lesion is opportunistic infection and AIDS-associated tumours. The typical findings of cerebral toxoplasmosis in an AIDS patient are multiple

ring-enhancing lesions on CT or MRI (p. 53). Toxoplasma and lymphoma are the most common causes of brain lesions in AIDS patients but other infections including cryptococcosis, histoplasmosis, aspergillosis, and tuberculosis may also cause brain abscesses in AIDS patients. In AIDS patients, latent toxoplasma can reactivate and cause disease, particularly when the CD4 count is < 100/mL. *Cryptosporidium parvum* causes gastrointestinal disease, usually diarrhoea. In AIDS patients this can be prolonged and severe and there may also be biliary tract involvement (cholangitis, cholecystitis). Kaposi's sarcoma is a low-grade vascular tumour predominantly affecting the skin, oral cavity, gastrointestinal tract and lungs.

4. (a) Malaria is the most likely cause of a fever in a traveller from Kenya (p. 25). The majority of imported malaria infection is caused by either *P. falciparum* (about 70%) or *P. vivax* and most malaria deaths are due to *P. falciparum*. The usual incubation period for *P. falciparum* is 12–14 days but may be longer if malaria prophylaxis was taken. A febrile illness unrelated to foreign travel would be almost as common as malaria as a cause of fever in a returning traveller. Typhoid and paratyphoid fever are much less common than malaria. Dengue fever (much less common than malaria) is almost excluded as the cause if patients develop symptoms more than 14 days after their return, and most would have a rash.

5. (a) True; (b) False; (c) False; (d) True; (e) True.
The description is consistent with cellulitis (p. 21). The lower limbs are preferentially involved and the diagnosis is clinical. In the majority of patients no organism is cultured from blood, skin aspirates or skin biopsy specimens and routine culturing is not necessary. For most patients empiric antibiotic therapy is reasonable.

GASTROENTEROLOGY

1. A 30-year-old man presents with a 1-week history of bloody diarrhoea.
   (a) What questions would you ask to help determine the cause?
   (b) What are the most common infectious causes and what are the most useful initial investigations?

2. A 30-year-old man presents with a 10-week history of discomfort in the right iliac fossa. He has also noticed some weight loss. The ESR is raised (50 mm/h).
   (a) What are the likely causes?
   (b) What imaging tests might be appropriate?

3. A 23-year-old beautician, who is otherwise well, gives a 5-year history of alternating morning diarrhoea, constipation, flatulence and left lower quadrant abdominal pain.
   (a) What is the most likely diagnosis?
   (b) How would you manage the problem?

4. A man of 30 presents with a 3-month history of difficulty in swallowing. What features of the history would help in making a diagnosis?

5. A 45-year-old man presents with a 6-month history of loose, pale, bulky offensive stools that are difficult to flush away and associated with mild abdominal discomfort.
   (a) Discuss the differential diagnosis.
   (b) What features in the history would you particularly focus on to help determine the cause?

6. A 20-year old woman who is 3 months pregnant presents with a 2-year history of chronic bloody diarrhoea and weight loss. Her stool frequency is eight times per day, serum albumin 28 g/L, Hb 9.0 g/dL and ESR 45 mm/h. One year ago a colonoscopy showed pancolonic inflammation, and colonic biopsies showed a chronic inflammatory infiltrate in the mucosa and lamina propria, crypt distortion and crypt abscesses. Select the best medication for this patient.
   (a) Oral prednisolone
   (b) Oral aminosalicylates
   (c) Rectal aminosalicylates
   (d) Intravenous hydrocortisone
   (e) Antibiotics.

7. A 55-year-old man presents with an episode of massive haematemesis.
   (a) Discuss the likely causes of this.
   (b) Outline your plan of management.

Answers

1. (a) Bloody diarrhoea suggests colonic disease. The common causes are inflammatory bowel disease (IBD) and infections, although colon cancer (usually

blood mixed in with the stools, not frank diarrhoea) and acute intestinal ischaemia should be borne in mind. This patient should be asked about his previous medical history, family history of colorectal disease, and drug ingestion (prescribed, illicit and over-the-counter). The diagnosis of colorectal cancer would be unlikely in a young man with no family history. Cocaine and other vasoconstricting drugs have been associated with mesenteric ischaemia and a careful drug history should be taken. Recent antibiotic use supports a diagnosis of *Clostridium difficile* infection and pseudomembranous colitis, although watery diarrhoea is a more common presentation. He should be asked about previous similar episodes of diarrhoea, with or without blood, and a family history of IBD. Recent travel abroad and other family members similarly affected would suggest an infectious cause.

(b) A short history (< 2 weeks) in the absence of previous episodes is most suggestive of an infectious cause. The infectious causes of bloody diarrhoea include *Campylobacter jejuni, Shigella* sp. (bacillary dysentery), *Entamoeba histolytica* (amoebic dysentery, occurring in the tropics), some types of *Escherichia coli* and, rarely, *Salmonella* sp. and *Clostridium difficile*. The most useful initial investigations are stool microscopy and culture, and a sigmoidoscopy and colonic biopsy.

2. (a) In a young person, right iliac fossa discomfort associated with weight loss and a raised ESR strongly suggests Crohn's disease (p. 97). An appendix mass must be considered, although the history is long. In immigrants, ileocaecal tuberculosis should be considered (p. 523). Amoebiasis may sometimes cause right iliac fossa pain, usually with the formation of an 'amoeboma', and this should be considered in people resident in tropical areas or travellers from the tropics.

(b) Imaging is with abdominal ultrasonography and small-bowel barium follow-through. Colonoscopy with direct visualization of the ileum may also be indicated.

3. (a) These features, particularly in a young, otherwise healthy female, are very suggestive of irritable bowel syndrome.

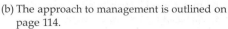
    (b) The approach to management is outlined on
       page 114.

4. The causes of dysphagia are listed on page 61.
   Progressive dysphagia associated with weight loss is
   suggestive of malignancy, although this would be
   unusual in a young man. A preceding history of
   heartburn suggests reflux with a complicating peptic
   stricture. Chest pain, regurgitation and dysphagia for
   liquids points to a motility disorder such as achalasia.
   Oesophageal candidiasis or cytomegalovirus infection
   may cause dysphagia in patients with AIDS.

5. (a) These features are strongly suggestive of
      malabsorption leading to steatorrhoea, which
      usually results from chronic pancreatic insufficiency
      or disease of the small intestine.
   (b) He should be asked about a history of intestinal
      resection, pancreatic resection or chronic pancreatitis.
      Intestinal resection can lead to steatorrhoea through
      three mechanisms: massive small gut resection and
      reduced area for absorption; resection of the terminal
      ileum (usually > 100 cm leading to bile salt
      malabsorption and deficiency); or small bowel
      bacterial overgrowth and bile salt deconjugation. A
      history of heavy alcohol consumption would support
      a diagnosis of chronic pancreatitis. He should be
      asked about a family history of coeliac disease and
      Crohn's disease. Chronic giardia infection causes
      steatorrhoea and, although the disease is acquired
      world-wide, attack rates are particularly high after
      travel to parts of Eastern Europe and Russia.

6. (d) The diagnosis suggests ulcerative colitis affecting
      the whole colon. The current presentation is consistent
      with acute severe colitis (Table 3.8) and the treatment is
      intravenous steroids (p. 101). Steroids are not
      contraindicated in pregnancy and it is essential for the
      health of the baby that her disease is rapidly brought
      under control.

7. (a) The causes of haematemesis are outlined on
      page 83, though massive haematemesis is usually
      the result of bleeding from varices (usually
      oesophageal, can be gastric) or large peptic ulcers.
   (b) Patients are usually shocked on presentation and
      must be aggressively resuscitated, initially with
      plasma expanders (p. 556) and subsequently with

whole blood. After adequate resuscitation, the source of bleeding is localized at gastroscopy; further management depends on the cause. A stepwise approach to management is outlined in Emergency Box 3.1.

LIVER, BILIARY TRACT AND PANCREATIC DISEASE

1. A 50-year-old woman complains of itching, passing dark urine and pale stools, and is deeply jaundiced.
   (a) What specific questions would you want to ask in the history to help you determine the cause?
   (b) What is the most useful initial investigation?

2. A 36-year-old woman presents with a 4-day history of painless jaundice. There is no previous history of medical illness and on examination she is deeply jaundiced with palmar erythema and multiple spider naevi. Initial investigations show:
   - Hb 11.5 g/dL, WCC 36×10^9/L, MCV 106 fL, platelets 41×10^9/L
   - Serum sodium 129 mmol/L, potassium 2 mmol/L, urea 1.4 mmol/L
   - Serum bilirubin 190 µmol/L, alkaline phosphatase 350 U/L, AST 260 U/L, ALT 104 U/L, γ-GT 250 U/L.
   Hepatitis B and A antibody titres are not elevated. Serum vitamin B_{12} and folate are normal.
   (a) What is the probable diagnosis?
   (b) What further tests would be useful?
   (c) What is the initial management?

3. You have been asked to see a 40-year-old woman in Accident and Emergency with a 4-day history of epigastric pain with radiation to the back. She has been vomiting, and on examination there is tenderness with guarding in the epigastrium. There have been no previous similar attacks. The serum amylase is 798 U/L (normal range < 125 U/L).
   (a) What is the most likely diagnosis?
   (b) What further specific questions would you ask to determine the aetiology?

4. A 42-year-old man presents with tiredness, lethargy and arthralgia. His blood tests show abnormal serum liver biochemistry (ALT 63 U/L, alkaline phosphatase 90 U/L, bilirubin 17 µmol/L) and a random blood

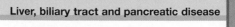
glucose of 15 mmol/L. Which of the following is the most likely diagnosis?

(a) Primary biliary cirrhosis
(b) Hepatitis B infection
(c) Haemochromatosis
(d) Chronic pancreatitis
(e) Alcoholic liver disease.

5. (a) A 29-year-old man who at a routine medical examination is found to have a serum bilirubin of 47 µmol/L with otherwise normal liver biochemistry. Full blood count and reticulocyte count are normal. He is fit and well and takes no medication.

(b) A 60-year-old woman with itching and xanthomas. Serum alkaline phosphatase 350 U/L, bilirubin 25 µmol/L, aspartate aminotransferase 47 U/L.

(c) An 80-year-old man who has hypertension and is otherwise fit and well. Serum alkaline phosphatase 749 U/L, gamma glutamyl transpeptidase 24 U/L.

(d) A 40-year-old intravenous drug abuser with AST 3639 U/L, INR 1.3, alkaline phosphatase 341 U/L.

(e) A 19-year-old man with tremor, dysarthria and abnormal liver biochemistry.

Select the best match for each of the above:

A. Paget's disease
B. Wilson's disease
C. Primary biliary cirrhosis
D. Gilbert's syndrome
E. Acute hepatitis B infection.

Answers

1. (a) The jaundice is associated with pruritus, dark urine and pale stools, and is therefore cholestatic. The next step is to establish whether this is intrahepatic or extrahepatic. The causes are listed in Figure 4.2. You would want to know how long she had been jaundiced and if there had been any previous episodes. Previous episodes may suggest bile duct stones. The patient should be asked about episodes of biliary pain. Risk factors for hepatitis A (ingestion of shell fish, recent travel) and hepatitis B and C should be sought (intravenous drug use, previous blood transfusions or operations, unprotected sex

with a person at risk for hepatitis B or C). Hepatitis E infection (HEV) would be unlikely unless the patient had travelled to an area of the world that is endemic for HEV (North Africa, Asia, Middle East) within the incubation period (2–7 weeks). A history of prodromal symptoms (nausea, vomiting, malaise, abdominal discomfort) in the weeks preceding the onset of jaundice would support a diagnosis of viral hepatitis.

A detailed alcohol and drug history should be taken including medicines bought over the counter.

She should be asked about weight loss and abdominal pain which in the presence of cholestatic jaundice suggests a malignant cause for biliary obstruction.

(b) The most useful initial investigation is an ultrasound of the gall bladder, biliary tree and pancreas to determine if there are dilated bile ducts suggesting extrahepatic cholestasis. In some cases ultrasound will also show the cause of obstruction if the ducts are dilated.

2. (a) The most probable diagnosis is alcoholic hepatitis superimposed on a background of chronic alcoholic liver disease. The raised MCV (with a normal vitamin B_{12} and folate), very high γ-GT and thrombocytopenia all suggest alcohol abuse. The very high WCC and AST : ALT ratio > 2 is typical of alcoholic hepatitis (p. 163). The sodium is probably low because of inability to excrete a free water load and dilutional hyponatraemia (p. 317).

(b) and (c) Further investigations and initial management are discussed on page 133. In addition, thiamine must be given to prevent Wernicke's encephalopathy (p. 584).

3. (a) The serum amylase is greater than six times the upper limit of normal and together with the clinical history suggests a diagnosis of acute pancreatitis (p. 175). An elevated serum amylase level is a non-specific finding because it occurs in a number of conditions other than acute pancreatitis but a level more than three times the upper limit of normal is strongly suggestive of acute pancreatitis.

(b) The causes of acute pancreatitis are listed in Table 4.11. A prior history of biliary pain (p. 170) suggests a diagnosis of gallstone pancreatitis. Excess alcohol ingestion causes acute and chronic pancreatitis, and a careful alcohol history should be taken. Many drugs have been associated with pancreatitis due to either an idiosyncratic effect or direct toxic effect. Trauma (blunt or penetrating), ERCP and major surgery are other causes of acute pancreatitis, and it is likely these causes would be immediately apparent from a brief history. High serum triglyceride concentrations can precipitate attacks of acute pancreatitis, and the patient should be asked about a personal and family history of lipid disorders and acquired causes of hypertriglyceridaemia (e.g. diabetes mellitus, hypothyroidism). Premature activation of pancreatic enzymes within the pancreas is the proposed pathogenic mechanism for acute pancreatitis seen in patients with hereditary pancreatitis. Affected patients usually present with a family history and at a young age and the condition is therefore unlikely to be presenting for the first time in this patient.

4. (c) The combination of symptoms, a mildly raised ALT and probable diabetes mellitus suggests haemochromatosis. Chronic pancreatitis causes diabetes but does not explain the arthralgia and abnormal liver biochemistry. Primary biliary cirrhosis is commoner in women and typically presents with a rise in alkaline phosphatase. Acute hepatitis B infection can present with a polyarthritis but does not explain the rise in blood glucose.

5. (a) D
   (b) C
   (c) A
   (d) E
   (e) B

DISEASES OF THE BLOOD AND HAEMATOLOGICAL MALIGNANCIES

1. You are asked to assess a 25-year-old woman who is found to have a low haemoglobin at her first antenatal booking clinic. There are no physical abnormalities. The values are as follows: Hb 10.7 g/dL, MCV 64 fL, WBC 7.2×10^9/L, platelets 202×10^9/L.

(a) What diagnoses do you consider?

(b) What simple investigations would you request in the first instance?

2. A 36-year-old woman complains of being easily tired over 6 months, and her stools have become more frequent. An FBC shows an Hb of 8 g/dL, MCV 110 fL.

(a) What are the most likely causes of the raised MCV?

(b) List three investigations that you would perform in the first instance to determine the diagnosis?

3. A 65-year-old woman comes to see you complaining of severe headaches for several weeks, and of now having lost vision in one eye. Initial investigations show: Hb 10.5 g/dL, WBC 8.0×10^9/L, ESR 90 mm/h.

(a) What is the probable diagnosis?

(b) What features would you pay attention to in the physical examination?

(c) What further diagnostic investigation would you arrange?

(d) What treatment would you give?

(e) What possible complications of this treatment would concern you in a patient of this age?

4. A 60-year-old woman with repeated sore throats has a blood count carried out by her general practitioner who seeks your advice. Investigations reveal: Hb 9.1 g/dL, WBC 2.0×10^9/L, platelets 80×10^9/L.

(a) What does the blood count show?

(b) What causes should you consider?

5. A 40-year-old man, resident in the UK, is found to have an Hb 18.9 g/dL and a haematocrit 55% on routine blood testing. What specific points in the history would help you to determine the cause?

6. What are the causes of persistent enlargement of the cervical lymph nodes in a man aged 25 years?

7. (a) A 35-year-old woman with a history of systemic lupus erythematosus presents with epistaxis and purpura.

(b) A 21-year-old man with a history of spontaneous bleeding into the joints.

(c) A 40-year-old woman with a history of nose bleeds presents with prolonged bleeding after a tooth extraction. Her father suffered with a similar problem.

(d) A 69-year-old man admitted to ITU with cholangitis and septicaemia, now bleeding spontaneously from venepuncture sites and the mouth.

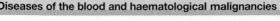

Select the best match for each of the above:

A. Prolonged APTT; normal platelet count; normal bleeding time and prothrombin time; plasma factor VIII:C reduced; and von Willebrand factor level normal

B. Severe thrombocytopenia; prolonged prothrombin time, APTT, and thrombin time; reduced plasma fibrinogen; and elevated fibrin degradation products and D-dimer

C. Bleeding time is prolonged; prothrombin time and APTT are normal

D. Bleeding time is prolonged; prolonged APTT; and normal PT. Levels of plasma factor VIII:C and von Willebrand factor reduced.

8. A 65-year-old man has a routine full blood count after presenting to his GP for a 'general check-up'. He is asymptomatic and previously fit and well. The total white cell count is raised (45.4×10^9/L) with a predominant lymphocytosis. The haemoglobin and platelet count are normal. What is the most likely diagnosis?

   (a) Infectious mononucleosis
   (b) Chronic myeloid leukaemia
   (c) Chronic lymphocytic leukaemia
   (d) Acute myeloid leukaemia
   (e) Myeloma.

Answers

1. (a) This patient has a mild microcytic anaemia. The most probable causes are thalassaemia trait (particularly with the very low MCV) and iron deficiency anaemia (Table 5.2). Iron requirements increase during pregnancy (2 mg/day) as a result of transfer of iron to the fetus and an increased red cell mass. These processes occur largely in the second trimester, and therefore it is likely that she was iron deficient before pregnancy (if this is the cause of the anaemia). In a young woman the most probable cause of iron deficiency is heavy menstrual blood loss (suggested by frequent periods, the passage of clots and frequent changes of pads/tampons).

   (b) Investigations are Hb electrophoresis and iron studies (p. 187).

2. (a) Anaemia with an MCV > 100 fL is most probably the result of vitamin B_{12} or folate deficiency (Table 5.2). The frequent stools suggest gastrointestinal disease. Taking these two together, the most likely diagnosis is small bowel disease, either Crohn's or coeliac disease (pp. 96 and 88).

   (b) The investigations are measurement of serum vitamin B_{12}, red cell folate, anti-endomysial and tissue transglutaminase antibodies, small bowel barium follow-through and distal duodenal biopsies. There may also be malabsorption of iron, and iron deficiency must be excluded (p. 186). Treatment is that of the underlying disease and the replacement of haematinics (pp. 840 and 841).

3. (a) The most probable diagnosis is giant cell arteritis (p. 762) causing central retinal artery occlusion and anaemia of chronic disease.

   (b) Examine the temporal arteries (tender and thickened), the eyes (milky-white fundus as a result of oedema) and look for systemic features of disease (fever, weight loss). In patients who also have polymyalgia rheumatica the range of motion of the shoulders and hips may be limited due to pain and the muscles may be tender to palpation.

   (c) and (d) The diagnosis and treatment of giant cell arteritis are discussed on page 763.

   (e) Complications of steroid treatment are osteoporosis and fractures, diabetes mellitus, hypertension, depression, and psychosis.

4. (a) This elderly woman has pancytopenia.

   (b) The causes of pancytopenia are listed in Table 5.6. The probable cause may be suggested by a detailed history (particularly drugs) and physical examination. A bone marrow trephine biopsy is the key investigation.

5. This is polycythaemia and the causes are listed on page 211. The most common cause of polycythaemia is hypoxia secondary to pulmonary disease. Shortness of breath, chronic cough, a history of sleep apnoea, or a history of cardiorespiratory disease may point to chronic hypoxia as the cause of polycythaemia. A detailed smoking and drug history should be obtained. Anabolic steroids and self-injection of erythropoietin (in athletes to improve performance) results in an increased red

cell mass. A history of thrombosis, haemorrhage or pruritus are suspicious for polycythaemia vera. Primary renal and hepatocellular cancers produce erythropoietin, and the patient should be asked about symptoms suggestive of these, although they are likely to be non-specific. Extended periods of time at high altitude results in polycythaemia but is not a consideration in this patient.

6. Persistent enlargement of a group of nodes makes most infections unlikely. In a young man this is most probably the result of Hodgkin's lymphoma, leukaemia, or possibly TB. Non-Hodgkin's lymphoma is uncommon in a young person. If there are risk factors, HIV infection (usually generalized lymphadenopathy) must be considered. Initial investigations include FBC and blood film, ESR, and lymph node biopsy for histological examination. Further investigation, which includes chest X-ray, CT scan of chest and abdomen, bone marrow examination and HIV test, would depend partly on initial results.

7. (a) C. The history and clotting abnormalities suggest autoimmune thrombocytopenia associated with SLE.
   (b) A. The history of bleeding into joints suggests a deficiency of clotting factors. A deficiency or functional abnormality of platelets is characterized by bleeding into skin and from mucous membranes.
   (c) D. This is von Willebrand's disease. The clinical features suggest a mild form with autosomal dominant inheritance.
   (d) B. This is the typical clinical and haematological picture of disseminated intravascular coagulation.

8. (c) About 25% of patients with CLL are diagnosed after a routine blood count reveals an absolute lymphocytosis. They feel well and are asymptomatic. The commonest presentation in other patients is painless swelling of lymph nodes. The commonest age for presentation is in the 60s. Viral infections may present with a lymphocytosis, although not usually this high and this patient has no symptoms. In addition, most older adults are not susceptible to infection because of prior exposure.

RHEUMATOLOGY

1. A 50-year-old man presents with acute arthritis of his left ankle.
   (a) What are the likely causes?
   (b) What is the most useful initial investigation?

2. A 45-year-old woman with a long-standing history of rheumatoid arthritis presents with a 6-month history of increasing dyspnoea. She does not experience orthopnoea. The venous pressure is not elevated and her heart sounds are normal. Her electrocardiogram is normal. Blood gases on air show an arterial Po_2 7.7 kPa, venous Pco_2 4.9 kPa, pH 7.45.
   (a) What is the probable diagnosis?
   (b) What other physical signs would you look for?
   (c) What other investigations would be helpful and what would you expect the results to show?

3. You are asked to see a 23-year-old woman in Accident and Emergency with tetany.
   (a) What is the most likely cause?
   (b) What other causes would you consider?

4. A woman of 55 presents with backache which proves to be osteoporotic in origin.
   (a) What investigations would lead to this diagnosis?
   (b) What are the predisposing factors?
   (c) How would you treat her?

5. A 60-year-old woman with a long history of alcohol abuse presents because she can no longer climb stairs or rise from chairs. She has recently begun treatment with NSAIDs given by her general practitioner for presumed osteoarthritis of both hips. Biochemical investigations reveal the following data: serum sodium 142 mmol/L, potassium 4.2 mmol/L, chloride 102 mmol/L, urea 8 mmol/L, creatinine 60 μmol/L, corrected calcium 2.2 mmol/L, phosphate 0.5 mmol/L, alkaline phosphatase 1000 U/L.
   (a) What do you consider to be the most likely diagnosis?
   (b) Describe appropriate investigations to support your diagnosis.
   (c) What is the best treatment?

6. (a) A 60-year-old man with severe pain and swelling at the base of the big toe.

(b) A 25-year-old woman with polyarthralgia and vesiculopustular skin lesions.

(c) A 34-year-old with arthralgia, an erythematous skin rash and generalized lymphadenopathy 4 weeks after trekking in a forest in Connecticut.

(d) A 40-year-old woman with rheumatoid arthritis treated with infliximab develops a scaling erythematous rash on the face and arms, arthralgias and positive antinuclear antibodies.

(e) A 29-year-old man with ulcerative colitis develops low back pain and stiffness that is particularly bad in the mornings.

Select the best match for each of the above:
A. Drug-induced systemic lupus erythematosus
B. Ankylosing spondylitis
C. Acute gout
D. Disseminated gonococcal infection
E. Lyme disease.

7. In a 34-year-old female with active rheumatoid arthritis, which of the following is the drug of first choice to delay disease progression?
(a) Indometacin
(b) Oral prednisolone
(c) Methotrexate
(d) Paracetamol
(e) Infliximab.

Answers

1. (a) The causes of a large joint monoarthritis are discussed on pages 255 and 278.

   (b) The most useful initial investigation is joint aspiration and synovial fluid analysis (Emergency Box 6.1). Subsequent tests would depend on the findings on joint aspiration, and may include X-ray of the joint and the measurement of serum uric acid concentration.

2. (a) The probable diagnosis is fibrosing alveolitis, a rare complication of rheumatoid arthritis. Less probably it is drug induced (rare side-effects of gold and methotrexate). She has type I respiratory failure (p. 563).

   (b) Physical signs to look for are central cyanosis, clubbing, reduced chest expansion and end-expiratory crackles at the lung bases.

(c) Investigations to confirm the diagnosis are listed on page 534.

3. (a) In a 23-year-old, presumably otherwise healthy, woman the most probable cause is respiratory alkalosis secondary to hyperventilation. Alkalosis causes tetany by reducing ionization of calcium salts (ionized calcium is physiologically active).

    (b) Other causes of tetany – hypocalcaemia (p. 636), hypokalaemia (p. 322) and hypomagnesaemia (p. 326) – are much less likely, but must be considered.

4. (a) Backache occurs in osteoporosis as a result of vertebral collapse or a crush fracture (not osteoporosis per se), which is seen on a plain X-ray. Bone densitometry (DXA) is used to confirm the diagnosis of osteoporosis and measure the response to treatment.

    (b) The predisposing factors are listed on page 300; of these, the most likely is early menopause.

    (c) The treatment is analgesia in the short term and, in the long term, elimination of risk factors where possible, maintenance of calcium intake, and bisphosphonates (p. 301).

5. (a) There is a borderline low serum calcium, a very low serum phosphate and markedly raised alkaline phosphatase. The diagnosis is probably osteomalacia (resulting from vitamin D deficiency), causing a proximal myopathy. Against this is the very high alkaline phosphatase, which is usually only moderately raised in osteomalacia. The myopathy may be the result of alcohol, but this does not explain the very high alkaline phosphatase. The serum urea is raised and the creatinine is at the lower end of the normal range. This picture is seen with dehydration or a gastrointestinal bleed (possibly related to ingestion of NSAIDs).
    Vitamin D deficiency is most likely to be a result of liver disease and poor diet but coeliac disease should be excluded with appropriate serology (p. 88).

    (b) Measurement of serum 25-OH-vitamin D will confirm the low levels.

    (c) Treatment is with ergocalciferol (10 000 units per day) and calcium (1000 mg/day). The aim is to normalize serum and urinary calcium levels and

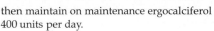
then maintain on maintenance ergocalciferol
400 units per day.

6. (a) C
   (b) D
   (c) E
   (d) A
   (e) B

7. (c) Corticosteroids are used as a bridge between the
   initiation and therapeutic effects of disease-modifying
   agents and/or in the treatment of acute synovitis. They
   are not used to slow disease progression, as the
   evidence is conflicting and there are major side-effects
   of chronic steroid use (p. 625). NSAIDs and paracetamol
   have no effect on disease progression. Biological
   agents, such as the anti-TNF agent infliximab, are
   not used in the UK as first-line treatment in RA.
   Methotrexate is one of the disease-modifying drugs
   and is used to slow disease progression in RA.
   Methotrexate is teratogenic. It is contraindicated in
   pregnancy, and following administration to a woman
   or man, they should avoid conception for 3 months
   after stopping.

WATER AND ELECTROLYTES

1. A 39-year-old woman is admitted to a hospital with a
   3-week history of nausea, vomiting and weakness
   following a chest infection. She has a past history of
   depression and hypothyroidism, for which she was
   taking thyroxine. On examination she is dehydrated,
   drowsy and pigmented, with a blood pressure of
   70/40 mmHg. She is oliguric, and investigation shows:
   haemoglobin 14.9 g/dL, white blood cells 7.4×10^9/L,
   urea 22.8 mmol/L, creatinine 290 µmol/L, sodium
   118 mmol/L, potassium 5.7 mmol/L, bicarbonate
   23 mmol/L, thyroxine 29.6 mmol/L, free T_4 4.5 pmol/L,
   TSH > 50 mU/L.
   (a) What are the probable diagnoses and their cause?
   (b) What further investigations are indicated?
   (c) What is the initial treatment?

2. (a) A 74-year-old man with congestive heart failure is
       brought to Accident and Emergency by his
       daughter, having 'gone off his legs' and 'hardly
       eaten or drunk' for 2 days. On examination, his JVP

is raised by 4 cm and he has ankle and peripheral oedema. Serum Na^+ 126 mmol/L, K^+ 5.5 mmol/L, urea 9 mmol/L, creatinine 159 μmol/L.

(b) A 40-year-old man with severe diarrhoea, heart rate 114/min and blood pressure 100/60 mmHg with a postural drop of 20 mmHg.

(c) An 80-year-old woman who is brought to Accident and Emergency with a history of increasing confusion over 2 weeks and found by a neighbour on the floor of her flat unable to get up. Serum Na^+ 150 mmol/L, K^+ 5.0 mmol/L, urea 24 mmol/L, creatinine 160 μmol/L.

(d) A 30-year-old man who is 2 days post-appendicectomy. He is completely well and receiving a 5% dextrose drip. His serum Na^+ is 99 mmol/L.

(e) A 60-year-old man with small cell lung cancer presenting with seizures and a serum Na^+ 114 mmol/L and osmolality 240 mmol/L.

Select the best option for each of the above:
A. Glucose 5%
B. Sodium chloride 0.9%
C. Sodium chloride 3% (hypertonic)
D. Water restriction 500 mL/day
E. Repeat the blood test.

3. A 40-year-old chronic homeless alcoholic was admitted to hospital 4 days ago. His electrolytes are as follows: serum Na^+ 135 mmol/L, K^+ 3.2 mmol/L, Mg^{2+} 0.4 mmol/L, phosphate 0.32 mmol/L. The most likely intervention that has precipitated this electrolyte imbalance is:
(a) Spironolactone
(b) Vitamin D
(c) Enteral nutrition
(d) Thiamine
(e) Furosemide (frusemide).

Answers

1. (a) This presentation is typical of an Addisonian crisis precipitated by the chest infection. The patient is markedly hypotensive and dehydrated on clinical examination. The raised urea and creatinine are compatible with dehydration and prerenal acute

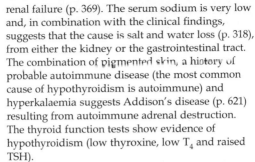

renal failure (p. 369). The serum sodium is very low and, in combination with the clinical findings, suggests that the cause is salt and water loss (p. 318), from either the kidney or the gastrointestinal tract. The combination of pigmented skin, a history of probable autoimmune disease (the most common cause of hypothyroidism is autoimmune) and hyperkalaemia suggests Addison's disease (p. 621) resulting from autoimmune adrenal destruction. The thyroid function tests show evidence of hypothyroidism (low thyroxine, low T_4 and raised TSH).

(b) Blood glucose (to look for hypoglycaemia), random plasma cortisol and ACTH, chest X-ray, blood cultures, serum adrenal autoantibodies.

(c) The immediate and subsequent management of an Addisonian crisis is given in Emergency Box 13.3.

2. (a) D. This man has evidence of fluid overload on examination and has a low serum sodium which is dilutional secondary to a relative water excess.

(b) B. He has evidence of decreased extracellular volume (p. 312) suggesting depletion of both sodium and water.

(c) A. Hypernatraemia is usually the result of reduced water intake. The history suggests that this patient has been unable to get access to water.

(d) E. The very low serum sodium is inconsistent with a well patient. It is likely the blood has been taken from the drip arm and should be repeated in the first instance.

(e) C. The history and blood results are suggestive of syndrome of inappropriate ADH secondary to small cell lung cancer. He has seizures as a result of severe hyponatraemia and the immediate treatment is hypertonic saline.

3. (c) The electrolyte picture with a low serum phosphate, potassium and magnesium is typical of the refeeding syndrome (p. 123). Alcoholics are frequently underweight and are at risk of the refeeding syndrome. Spironolactone is a potassium-sparing diuretic and is not associated with hypokalaemia. Alcoholic patients are at risk of thiamine deficiency and should be given thiamine immediately on admission to hospital and certainly before administration of nutritional

supplements which may precipitate deficiency. Vitamin D deficiency causes secondary hyperparathyroidism and hypophosphataemia.

RENAL DISEASE

1. (a) What clinical and other evidence would lead you to suspect the diagnosis of chronic renal failure in a 50-year-old man?
   (b) How would you determine the cause of chronic renal failure?

2. In a patient presenting with a plasma creatinine of 500 μmol/L, which of the following features would suggest that the renal failure is chronic, rather than acute?
   (a) Reduced renal size detected by ultrasonography
   (b) A urine sodium concentration of less than 10 mmol/L
   (c) Elevated serum alkaline phosphatase and subperiosteal erosions on X-ray of the hands
   (d) A haemoglobin of 14 g/L
   (e) The presence of ureteric obstruction on renal ultrasonography
   (f) Evidence of polyneuropathy.

3. A previously healthy 20-year-old male has developed acute renal failure following a road traffic accident where he has sustained multiple injuries.
   (a) What are the factors contributing to the development of the renal failure?
   (b) What are the initial steps in management?

4. A 50-year-old man presents with bilateral ankle swelling and is found to have a serum albumin of 28 g/L. He has otherwise developed no new symptoms.
   (a) What particular points in the history and physical examination would help you to determine the cause?
   (b) What further investigations are indicated?

5. A 45-year-old man presents through Accident and Emergency. He is non-specifically unwell and feeling sick. His investigations show a serum creatinine of 900 μmol/L and serum potassium 7.1 mmol/L. The ECG is abnormal with absent P waves and a widened QRS complex. His electrolytes and ECG were normal 2 weeks ago. The immediate treatment indicated is:
   (a) Urgent check on the electrolytes

(b) Calcium gluconate intravenously
    (c) Insulin and dextrose intravenously
    (d) Salbutamol nebulizer
    (e) Calcium resonium.

6. A 66-year-old man is admitted with acute renal failure.
   The physical examination and ultrasound examination
   of the kidneys, ureters and bladder exclude
   hypovolaemia and urinary obstruction. Which of the
   following are indications for haemodialysis?
       (a) Pulmonary oedema refractory to furosemide
           (frusemide) infusion
       (b) Urea 35 mmol/L
       (c) Pericarditis
       (d) Creatinine of 750 μmol/L, serum potassium of
           7.0 mmol/L after insulin and dextrose
       (e) Urine output 20 mL/h.

7.   (a) Renal cell carcinoma
       (b) Prostate cancer
       (c) Ovarian cancer
       (d) Non-seminoma germ cell tumour of the testes
       (e) Colorectal cancer

   Select the best match for tumour with tumour marker:
       A. Alpha-fetoprotein
       B. Ca-125
       C. Erythropoietin
       D. Prostate-specific antigen
       E. CEA.

Answers

1.   (a) A patient presenting with any of the complications
   discussed on page 378 would lead you to suspect
   chronic renal failure (CRF), but the usual ways in
   which patients present are with hypertension,
   nocturia and polyuria, or with symptoms of anaemia.
     (b) The investigations for renal failure are discussed on
   page 377. A renal biopsy is performed in patients
   with normal-sized kidneys. Small kidneys are
   technically difficult to biopsy, histological
   investigations are hard to interpret, and at this late
   stage the prognosis would not be influenced by
   treatment of the underlying condition.

2. (a), (c) and (f) suggest chronic renal failure. The urine
   sodium concentration is very low, and this may occur

919

with prerenal acute renal failure (when the kidney is conserving sodium) and with chronic renal failure when the concentrating ability of the kidney is lost and large amounts of dilute urine are produced. The normal Hb is in favour of acute renal failure.

3. (a) The most probable cause is poor renal perfusion secondary to hypovolaemia from blood loss. Other causes include rhabdomyolysis (extensive crush injury to muscle leads to the release of myoglobin, which is directly toxic to renal tubular cells), ruptured urethra (suspect with severe pelvic fractures and anuria) and later septicaemia and drugs (e.g. gentamicin).

   (b) Initial management is to correct hypovolaemia with whole blood (measurement of central venous pressure will guide replacement) followed by a bolus of furosemide (frusemide) (p. 372) if the patient remains oliguric. If urine output does not increase and urethral rupture is excluded as the cause of oliguria, then treatment is as for established acute tubular necrosis (p. 375). The investigations must include measurement of the muscle enzyme creatinine phosphokinase.

4. (a) Hypoalbuminaemia is caused by decreased synthesis (liver disease or systemic illness) or increased loss from the kidneys or, rarely, the gut (protein-losing enteropathy). The main differential in this case is between liver disease and nephrotic syndrome. Important points in the history are risk factors for chronic liver disease (e.g. alcohol, intravenous drug abuse) and diseases that may be associated with nephrotic syndrome (e.g. diabetes, chronic infections and amyloidosis, drugs). Signs of chronic liver disease must be looked for on physical examination.

   (b) Initial investigations are liver biochemistry and measurement of urinary protein excretion (p. 337).

5. (b) He has acute renal failure complicated by severe hyperkalaemia with ECG changes. This is a medical emergency. Immediate treatment (p. 325) with intravenous calcium is indicated, which directly antagonizes the membrane actions of hyperkalaemia. Beta$_2$-adrenergic agonists (salbutamol) and insulin drive potassium into cells by increasing Na/K-ATPase activity but take 30 minutes to act. The anion-exchange

resin, calcium resonium, takes up potassium and increases excretion but is slow to lower potassium.

6. (a), (c), and (d) Indications for dialysis in acute renal failure are hyperkalaemia, refractory fluid overload, profound acidosis, rapidly rising urea (> 50 mmol/L) and signs of uraemia such as pericarditis.

7. (a) C. Renal cell carcinoma produces a host of hormones. The commonest are erythropoietin (causing polycythaemia) and parathyroid hormone-related protein (causing hypercalcaemia).

   (b) D. PSA is produced by prostate epithelial cells. The major causes of an elevated serum level are benign prostatic hyperplasia, prostate cancer, prostatic inflammation and perineal trauma. Higher levels are more predictive of prostate cancer.

   (c) B. Serum Ca-125 is elevated in about 80% of women with ovarian cancer. Like all tumour markers it is not specific. It is also increased in patients with other malignancies and with pleural and peritoneal disease.

   (d) A. Serum concentrations of the beta subunit of human chorionic gonadotrophin (β-HCG) and alpha-fetoprotein (AFP) are elevated in most men with non-seminomatous germ cell tumours of the testes. β-HCG, but not AFP, is elevated in about 20% of patients with seminomas. These tumour markers are not sensitive or specific for testicular cancer but can be useful in the assessment of prognosis and response to treatment.

   (e) E. CEA is not specific for colon cancer; raised serum levels may occurs in other malignancies and benign conditions, and normal levels may occur in early-stage disease. It is most useful in disease follow-up after treatment.

CARDIOVASCULAR DISEASE

1. A 55-year-old man presents with a 3-day history of retrosternal chest pain radiating to the left arm and jaw and occasionally occurring at rest. The character of the pain is suggestive of myocardial ischaemia.

   (a) What additional features in the clinical history would suggest that the pain is angina rather than myocardial infarction?

(b) What features in the history would suggest that this is unstable angina?

2. (a) How would you differentiate acute pericarditis from acute myocardial infarction clinically?
   (b) Pericarditis may be a complication of myocardial infarction. When after the infarction does it typically occur?
   (c) What are the most common causes of acute pericarditis in the UK?

3. A 60-year-old woman presents with a 2-month history of breathlessness and clinical features of mild heart failure. She is found to have atrial fibrillation with an uncontrolled ventricular response (130 beats/min).
   (a) Give four possible causes for the atrial fibrillation.
   (b) Name three drugs that may be used to control the ventricular response.
   (c) What investigations would you order?

4. A 44-year-old woman is admitted to hospital with malaise and fever. She has felt unwell for 6 months. Examination shows pallor, an apical pansystolic murmur and splenomegaly. A blood count sent by the general practitioner shows a haemoglobin of 8.4 g/dL, WBC 7.2×10^9/L and platelets 394×10^9/L.
   (a) What investigations are required?
   (b) How might treatment be monitored?

5. (a) Describe the clinical features of an acute attack of left ventricular failure.
   (b) Name three physical findings that would be of most value in distinguishing it from other causes of severe shortness of breath.
   (c) What are the key points to the management of acute pulmonary oedema?

6. A 50-year-old man complains of a painful red swollen calf.
   (a) What are the likely causes?
   (b) How would you discriminate between the causes?

7. A 61-year-old man is admitted following a year's history of dizziness on exertion, culminating in a black-out while cutting the lawn. On admission he has a slow rising pulse and a systolic ejection murmur. There is no history of angina.
   (a) What is the likely diagnosis?
   (b) How would you estimate its clinical severity?

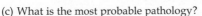
Answers

(c) What is the most probable pathology?

(d) What is the treatment?

8. A 68-year-old man with known ischaemic heart disease is admitted with three prolonged episodes of typical anginal pain over the last 24 hours. He usually takes aspirin, nitrates, a statin, metformin and atenolol. He has a history of hypertension, type II diabetes mellitus and hypercholesterolaemia. His admission ECG is normal and 12-hour serum troponin is raised. Which of the following is the most appropriate intervention after appropriate medical treatment in this case?

(a) Exercise ECG

(b) Coronary angiography

(c) Stress echocardiogram

(d) Further investigation only if recurrent chest pain.

Answers

1. (a) The pain of angina is usually less severe than that of myocardial infarction. Classic angina comes on with exercise and is relieved by rest, and the pain is usually not accompanied by other symptoms such as sweating, nausea or vomiting. The pain of myocardial infarction may come on at rest, is persistent and may last several hours, and is often accompanied by sweating, nausea and vomiting.

(b) Unstable angina is angina of recent onset (less than 1 month), worsening angina or angina at rest.

2. (a) Acute pericarditis and myocardial infarction are discussed on pages 474 and 442. They can usually be differentiated on the basis of the nature, the site and radiation of the pain, and the presence of associated symptoms and signs (e.g. nausea, vomiting, breathlessness, pericardial rub on auscultation).

(b) Pericarditis is common in the first few days, particularly in anterior wall infarction. Post-myocardial infarction syndrome (Dressler's syndrome) is much less common. It occurs weeks or months after an acute myocardial infarction and consists of pericarditis, fever and a pericardial effusion. It is caused by an autoimmune response to damaged cardiac tissue.

(c) Coxsackie viral infection and myocardial infarction.

923

3. (a) The causes of atrial fibrillation are listed on page 413.
   In an elderly woman the probable causes are
   ischaemic heart disease, mitral valve disease,
   thyrotoxicosis and cardiomyopathy.
   (b) The drugs usually used to control the ventricular
   rate are those that slow conduction through the AV
   node: digoxin, β-blockers and verapamil.
   (c) Investigations should include an ECG (which will
   show fibrillation and may show evidence of
   ischaemia or mitral valve disease, Fig. 9.10b), a chest
   X-ray (which may confirm the clinical diagnosis of
   heart failure and show evidence of mitral valve
   disease, Fig. 9.2), an echocardiogram, and thyroid
   function tests.

4. (a) This combination of clinical signs suggests infective
   endocarditis affecting the mitral valve.
   Investigations are discussed on page 462.
   (b) Treatment is monitored clinically (patient
   well-being, temperature charts, evidence of heart
   failure) and by regular blood counts, ESR and
   echocardiography. Antibiotic doses are adjusted
   according to bacteriological studies (minimum
   bactericidal concentration) and gentamicin levels (to
   ensure therapeutic levels are obtained but without
   toxic levels likely to cause side-effects).

5. (a) Clinical features of acute left ventricular failure are
   listed on page 432.
   (b) A gallop rhythm, widespread crackles and pulsus
   alternans differentiate pulmonary oedema from
   other causes of acute shortness of breath (listed in
   Table 10.2). In pulsus alternans the arterial pressure
   alternates between high and low systolic peaks. Its
   presence indicates severe left ventricular failure.
   (c) The key points in the management of pulmonary
   oedema are listed in Emergency Box 9.2.

6. (a) The differential diagnosis of a swollen calf includes
   deep venous thrombosis (DVT), cellulitis or a
   ruptured Baker's cyst. Oedema in heart failure or
   hypoalbuminaemia also causes a swollen calf, but
   this is usually bilateral. A Baker's cyst (popliteal
   cyst) is a synovial cyst in the popliteal fossa which
   sometimes occurs in patients with a knee effusion.
   Rupture of the cyst produces sudden and severe
   pain, swelling and tenderness of the upper calf.

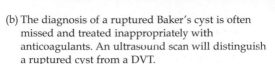
(b) The diagnosis of a ruptured Baker's cyst is often missed and treated inappropriately with anticoagulants. An ultrasound scan will distinguish a ruptured cyst from a DVT.

7. (a) The history and examination are typical of aortic stenosis (p. 457). As in this case, presentation is usually in the sixth decade.

(b) The presence of symptoms indicates at least moderately severe aortic stenosis. A longer ejection systolic murmur, clinical and ECG evidence of left ventricular hypertrophy all indicate more severe stenosis. The severity may be more accurately assessed by Doppler echocardiography.

(c) The most likely pathology is a calcified bicuspid aortic valve.

(d) Treatment in a symptomatic patient is valve replacement.

8. (b) He has a TIMI risk score of at least 5 (we are not told if he has had a previous angiography) and is at high risk (at least 25%) of death, MI or severe recurrent ischaemia. This is an indication for early coronary angiography followed by revascularization by balloon angioplasty or CABG if appropriate.

RESPIRATORY DISEASE

1. A 17-year-old girl presents to Accident and Emergency with an acute exacerbation of asthma.
   (a) What features on clinical examination would indicate a severe attack of asthma?
   (b) What is your immediate treatment of this patient?

2. A 45-year-old woman develops breathlessness and wheezing following a cold. What features in the history would you seek to support a diagnosis of asthma?

3. A 28-year-old previously healthy Caucasian female presents with a persistent dry cough for 4 weeks. She has also recently developed a nodular rash on her legs. She does not smoke and works in an office. Physical examination reveals coarse crackles at both lung bases and a rash on her legs. A chest X-ray shows prominent bilateral hilar lymphadenopathy and reticulonodular infiltrates in both lung fields.
   (a) What is the most likely diagnosis?
   (b) What is the most likely cause of the rash on the legs?

(c) If a lung biopsy were obtained, what would you expect it to show?

4. A 35-year-old woman is admitted as an emergency with acute onset of shortness of breath and central chest pain. She was recently discharged from hospital after a cholecystectomy. On examination she is obese, pale, sweating, pulse 120/min and BP 80/50. The JVP is raised by 4 cm and there is a left parasternal heave. She smokes 30 cigarettes per day and takes the combined oral contraceptive pill.
   (a) What is the most likely diagnosis?
   (b) In this patient, what are the risk factors for the presumed diagnosis?
   (c) What is the immediate treatment of this condition?

5. A 50-year-old ventilation engineer presents with a 3-day history of dry cough, confusion and diarrhoea. His temperature is 39.5°C and investigations show serum Na^+ 129 mmol/L, AST 99 U/L, bilirubin 29 μmol/L, alkaline phosphatase 150 U/L. A chest X-ray shows consolidation in the left lower lobe. What is the most appropriate antibiotic treatment?
   (a) Penicillin
   (b) Gentamicin
   (c) Trimethoprim–sulfamethoxazole
   (d) Erythromycin
   (e) Clarithromycin.

6. A 20-year-old otherwise fit young man develops sudden onset of shortness of breath and left-sided chest pain that is worse on inspiration. He attends Accident and Emergency later that afternoon and on examination he is found to be well with a respiratory rate of 22/min. A chest X-ray shows a 1.5 cm visible rim between the left lung margin and chest wall (i.e. a small left-sided pneumothorax). The correct management is:
   (a) Discharge home
   (b) Chest drain insertion
   (c) Aspirate air with a needle
   (d) Inpatient observation
   (e) Administer diazepam to control the respiratory rate.

7. (a) A 24-year-old woman with wheezing and a night-time cough. She is a non-smoker.
   (b) A 54-year-old man with gradual onset of shortness of breath and a dry cough. Examination reveals clubbing and end-inspiratory crepitations.

(c) A 67-year-old man with a 3-month history of shortness of breath, cough, and recently a hoarse voice.

(d) An 18-year-old man with hypogammaglobulinaemia, shortness of breath, and cough productive of copious amounts of sputum.

(e) A 34-year-old homosexual man with a 3-month history of cough with sputum and haemoptysis, weight loss and night sweats.

Match each of the above with the most likely diagnosis:

A. Tuberculosis
B. Bronchial carcinoma
C. Asthma
D. Idiopathic pulmonary fibrosis
E. Bronchiectasis.

Answers

1. (a) Features of a severe attack of asthma are:
    - Inability to complete a sentence in one breath
    - Pulse > 110 beats/min
    - Respirations ≥ 25 breaths/min
    - PEFR 30–50% of predicted value or 30–50% of patient's best.

    There are additional clinical features which suggest that the attack is *life-threatening*, and these are listed on page 514.

    (b) Acute severe asthma is a medical emergency and an indication for urgent treatment. The management is summarized in Emergency Box 10.1. Immediate treatment is 60% oxygen, salbutamol 5 mg or terbutaline 10 mg via oxygen-driven nebulizer, and hydrocortisone 100 mg intravenously or 60 mg orally.

2. The classic triad of symptoms associated with asthma consists of wheezing, cough, and shortness of breath. However, one or more of these symptoms may be absent and they are not specific for asthma. A history of intermittent, seasonal waxing and waning of symptoms; nocturnal episodes; exacerbation of symptoms on exposure to stimuli such as exercise, cold air, allergens, air pollutants and with upper respiratory tract infections argues for the diagnosis of asthma.

3. (a) There are many causes of hilar lymphadenopathy. However, the clinical history together with the bilateral hilar enlargement suggest sarcoidosis.

   (b) Erythema nodosum.

   (c) Lymphocytes, macrophages and sometimes fibrosis. Non-caseating granulomas are the key histopathological feature of sarcoidosis and are found in lymph nodes and in a lymphatic distribution in the lung.

4. (a) The history and examination findings are suggestive of a massive pulmonary embolism with acute right heart strain. A similar clinical picture may also be seen with a right ventricular infarct, but she has a number of risk factors which are more in favour of pulmonary embolism.

   (b) Recent surgery, smoking, obesity and the combined oral contraceptive pill.

   (c) 100% oxygen and pain relief with diamorphine. This patient has a massive embolism with hypotension and right heart strain (raised JVP and right ventricular heave) and you should give thrombolysis after imaging to confirm the diagnosis. She may also require intravenous fluids to try to raise the filling pressure of the right ventricle, thereby increasing cardiac output. Treatment with heparin and subsequently warfarin should also be given to reduce the chance of further emboli. The management of a pulmonary embolism is summarized in Emergency Box 9.5.

5. (e) He has pneumonia. In a ventilation engineer pneumonia may be the result of any of the causes of community-acquired pneumonia (p. 517), but he is particularly at risk of infection with *Legionella* sp. The clinical clues that are suspicious (but not pathognomonic) for Legionnaire's disease in a patient with pneumonia are: presence of gastrointestinal symptoms especially diarrhoea, neurological complications especially confusion, fever > 39°C, hyponatraemia, hepatic dysfunction and haematuria. The newer macrolides (clarithromycin and azithromycin) and respiratory tract quinolones (especially levofloxacin) are the treatments of choice for *Legionella* infection.

6. (a) This is a small pneumothorax in an otherwise young fit man, i.e. a primary pneumothorax.

Methods to estimate the size of a pneumothorax are controversial and the most accurate is a chest CT scan but this is not practicable in all patients. The most commonly used method to estimate the size of a pneumothorax is to measure the distance from the lateral edge of the lung to the inner wall of the thoracic cage on a chest X-ray (Fig. 10.5). A distance > 2 cm implies that the pneumothorax is at least 50%, and hence large in size. Patients with a small (< 2 cm) primary pneumothorax and minimal symptoms do not require hospital admission, but before discharge they should be instructed to return in the event of developing more severe breathlessness. Air slowly resorbs from the pleural space at a rate of about 1.5% a day. His pneumothorax is about 22% and will resolve in about 15 days. Inhaled oxygen speeds up the process.

7. (a) C
   (b) D
   (c) B
   (d) E
   (e) A

INTENSIVE CARE MEDICINE

1. A man aged 55 years who underwent right hemicolectomy for carcinoma of the caecum 4 days ago has developed acute circulatory failure ('shock'), with an arterial pressure of 65/40 mmHg and heart rate of 120/min.
   (a) List the probable causes of this occurrence.
   (b) Indicate the clinical features that would aid you in distinguishing between them, and outline your initial management of the situation.

2. The following patients all have a blood pressure of 70/40 mmHg:
   (a) A 67-year-old man with anterior myocardial infarction
   (b) A 74-year-old woman 3 days after a total hip replacement
   (c) A 34-year-old man with a pericardial effusion
   (d) A 65-year-old woman taking NSAIDs with epigastric pain and an Hb 8.0 g/dL
   (e) A 34-year-old man who became wheezy after eating peanuts.

Select the most likely cause for shock in each case:
A. Pulmonary embolus
B. Cardiac tamponade
C. Cardiogenic shock
D. Anaphylaxis
E. Hypovolaemia.

3. A 49-year-old man is admitted with cellulitis. He develops severe facial swelling, stridor and shortness of breath shortly after admission to hospital. His blood pressure is 90/50 mmHg. The most appropriate immediate management is:
(a) Penicillin
(b) Intravenous saline
(c) Intramuscular epinephrine (adrenaline)
(d) Intravenous hydrocortisone
(e) Intravenous Haemaccel.

Answers

1. (a) The two most likely causes are sepsis or a massive pulmonary embolism. Less likely are gastrointestinal haemorrhage and a perioperative myocardial infarction complicated by cardiogenic shock.
   (b) The clinical features of each of these conditions are discussed on pages 13, 556 and 466, respectively. Management involves:
   - Emergency resuscitation with 60% oxygen, large-bore intravenous cannulae and administration of colloid.
   - Make a diagnosis: temperature charts and physical examination will often reveal the cause. ECG, blood gases and chest X-ray should be performed.
   - Further treatment depends on the response to fluids and the likely cause.
2. (a) C
   (b) A
   (c) B
   (d) E
   (e) D

3. (c) The clinical description is suggestive of anaphylactoid shock with respiratory distress due to oedema of neck. The most appropriate treatment is intramuscular epinephrine (adrenaline). Hydrocortisone and

intravenous fluids are part of the management but the most immediate treatment is epinephrine.

POISONING, DRUG AND ALCOHOL ABUSE

1. After a disagreement with her boyfriend, a 20-year-old woman was seen to ingest 50 tablets of aspirin (i.e. 15 g total) and was brought to hospital 4 hours later. You find her alert and complaining of mild tinnitus only. The salicylate concentration in a blood sample taken in the Accident and Emergency department is within the therapeutic range. Select the best option for treatment.
   (a) No further treatment necessary
   (b) Single-dose activated charcoal
   (c) Multiple-dose activated charcoal
   (d) Urine alkalinization
   (e) Intravenous fluids.

2. A girl aged 17 is admitted after a suicide attempt with a single drug. Initial blood gases were: P_aO_2 13.7 kPa, P_aCO_2 3.7 kPa, pH 7.49.
   (a) What is the metabolic abnormality?
   (b) What drug has this woman probably taken?
   (c) What acid–base changes may occur later?
   (d) When she has recovered, what features would alert you to the risk of a further life-threatening suicide attempt?

3. (a) A 24-year-old woman who has taken an overdose of paracetamol.
   (b) A 17-year-old patient with respiratory arrest from an overdose of heroin.
   (c) A 30-year-old woman who has taken an overdose of temazepam and has a Glasgow Coma Score of 7.
   (d) A 58-year-old woman who has taken an overdose of atenolol, with a pulse rate of 35/minute.
   (e) A 33-year-old man comatose from carbon monoxide poisoning.

   Select the best treatment of each of the above:
   A. Hyperbaric oxygen
   B. *N*-acetylcysteine
   C. Flumazenil
   D. Naloxone
   E. Atropine.

4. A well-known alcoholic is admitted through Accident and Emergency having been found wandering in the

street by the police. He is agitated, disorientated and says that there are insects on the ward curtains. On examination he is tachycardic. What is the most appropriate treatment?

(a) Chlordiazepoxide
(b) 5% dextrose drip
(c) Carbamezepine
(d) Beta-blockers
(e) Ethanol.

Answers

1. (e) Ingestion of 10–20 g of aspirin may produce severe toxicity. This case represents a very serious overdose and serum levels are within the normal range because intestinal absorption is still taking place (see p. 575). Initial management involves administration of intravenous fluids to correct dehydration and initiate a diuresis; further management depends on the salicylate concentration in a repeat blood sample taken 6 hours after drug ingestion (p. 576). More than one drug is often taken in overdose cases, and this should be sought from the history and measurement of plasma paracetamol levels. Several points suggest that the overdose is not a serious suicide attempt (Table 12.4) and psychiatric referral is probably not necessary.

2. (a) The patient has a respiratory alkalosis.
   (b) Aspirin.
   (c) Respiratory alkalosis is due to direct stimulation of the respiratory centre by salicylates. Initially, renal excretion of bicarbonate will bring the pH towards normal, producing some compensation of the alkalosis. Subsequently, a combined respiratory and metabolic acidosis develops because:
   - Hypotension and dehydration impair renal function with retention of organic acids.
   - Salicylates interfere with carbohydrate, fat and protein metabolism, as well as with oxidative phosphorylation. This gives rise to increased lactate, pyruvate and ketone bodies, all of which contribute to the acidosis.
   - Salicylate and its metabolites are acidic and further enhance the metabolic acidosis.

■ Severe overdose produces depression of the
respiratory centre and a respiratory acidosis.
(d) Risk factors for suicide are listed in Table 12.4.
3. (a) B
    (b) D
    (c) C
    (d) E
    (e) A
4. (a) This is delirium tremens (p. 586). Benzodiazepines
    (chlordiazepoxide, diazepam, oxazepam, lorazepam)
    are used to treat the alcohol withdrawal syndromes.
    Thiamine should be administered prior to any glucose-
    containing solutions in order to decrease the risk of
    precipitating Wernicke's encephalopathy. Alcohol
    withdrawal seizures are usually self-limited and do not
    require specific anticonvulsant medication. Phenytoin
    is used if there is status epilepticus. Carbamezepine
    should not be used in the management of alcohol
    withdrawal seizures.

ENDOCRINOLOGY

1. An otherwise healthy 36-year-old woman presents with
    8 months of feeling anxious and tremulous. On
    examination her pulse is 115 per minute, BP 155/90
    and there is a moderately enlarged, non-tender, non-
    nodular thyroid and hyperreflexia.
    (a) What is your clinical diagnosis?
    (b) What tests would you order?
    (c) What would you expect the results to show?
    (d) What are the main treatment options for this
        patient?
2. A 29-year-old man presents with 5 days of pain and
    tenderness over the thyroid gland. He feels jittery but
    otherwise well. On examination, he is afebrile, pulse
    120 per minute, BP 140/90. His thyroid is enlarged and
    diffusely tender, with no evidence of nodules.
    (a) What is your clinical diagnosis?
    (b) How would you confirm it?
    (c) How would you treat this patient?
    (d) What is his prognosis?
3. An 85-year-old woman is found lying on the floor of
    her unheated flat; hypothermia is suspected.
    (a) How would you confirm the diagnosis?

(b) What abnormality might there be on ECG?

(c) What would be your management?

4. A 72-year-old woman with known breast cancer presents with dehydration, confusion and vomiting. Her corrected serum calcium is 3.8 mmol/L. What are the immediate measures to reduce the serum calcium?

5. (a) Serum TSH 10 mU/L (normal range 0.3–3.5 mU/L), normal serum total T_4, free T_4 and T_3.

   (b) Serum TSH 15 mU/L, low serum total T_4, free T_4 and T_3.

   (c) Serum TSH 0.1 mU/L, low serum total T_4, free T_4 and T_3.

   (d) Serum TSH < 0.01 mU/L, increased serum T_4, free T4 and T_3.

   (e) Serum TSH < 0.01 mU/L, normal serum T_4 and free T_4, increased T_3.

   Select the best matches for each of the above:

   A. T_3 toxicosis

   B. Thyrotoxicosis

   C. Compensated euthyroidism

   D. TSH deficiency

   E. Hypothyroidism.

6. A 49-year-old man presents with a vertebral fracture. He is noted on examination to have hypertension, a proximal muscle weakness and purple striae on his abdomen. You suspect Cushing's syndrome, and a 24-hour urine collection shows a grossly elevated cortisol excretion. Which one of the following clinical and laboratory features suggests ectopic ACTH production?

   (a) Impaired suppression of cortisol secretion during a low-dose dexamethasone suppression test

   (b) Plasma ACTH is high

   (c) Suppression of cortisol secretion during a high-dose dexamethasone suppression test

   (d) Serum potassium of 4.0 mmol/L

   (e) Plasma ACTH levels are unchanged after administration of corticotrophin-releasing hormone.

7. A 60-year-old smoker presents with a serum sodium of 129 mmol/L. Which of the following support a diagnosis of syndrome of inappropriate ADH?

   (a) A history of watery diarrhoea and a postural drop of blood pressure of 20 mmHg

934

(b) Absence of signs of fluid overload or depletion and a serum creatinine of 90 μmol/L

(c) A history of myocardial infarction 3 months earlier, a raised JVP and ankle oedema

(d) Vitiligo, a postural drop in blood pressure and a blood glucose of 2.2 mmol/L

(e) Signs of chronic liver disease and ascites.

Answers

1. (a) Hyperthyroidism which, clinically and epidemiologically, is likely to be Graves' disease.

   (b) and (c) Serum TSH will be low, often undetectable. Serum T_4 and T_3 will be high. Serum microsomal and thyroglobulin antibodies will be present in the serum in most cases of Graves' disease.

   (d) Antithyroid drugs given for about 2 years in the hope that the disease remits on its own. These include:
   - Carbimazole, most often used in the UK
   - Methimazole, the active metabolite of carbimazole, used in the USA
   - Propylthiouracil, occasionally used.

   β-Blockers for symptomatic relief, but they do not alter the course of the disease.

   Radioiodine is more commonly preferred for definitive treatment of Graves' disease; surgery is particularly suited to patients with large goitres which are unlikely to remit after medical treatment.

2. (a) The presence of diffuse swelling and tenderness of the thyroid gland, together with the history of pain, suggests de Quervain's thyroiditis. Inflammation of the gland leads to the release of preformed hormone.

   (b) The serum TSH would be low. A radioactive iodine uptake scan would show reduced uptake by the thyroid because the gland is not actively synthesizing thyroid hormone. This test is not routinely performed, but in other cases of hyperthyroidism there would be increased uptake.

   (c) The disease is generally mild and limited to a few weeks, so definitive therapy is rarely needed. β-Blockers are used for symptomatic relief. Patients may become transiently hypothyroid during recovery.

   (d) Spontaneous remission in a few weeks.

3. (a) The diagnosis and management of hypothermia are discussed on pages 644–645. Hypothermia is diagnosed when the core (rectal) temperature is < 35°C measured with a low-reading rectal thermometer.

   (b) The ECG abnormalities are 'J' waves (pathognomonic of hypothermia), a tachycardia with a bradycardia developing at temperatures < 32°C. At very low temperatures there may be ventricular arrhythmias.

   (c) The treatment is described on page 645.

4. Severe hypercalcaemia such as this is a medical emergency and almost certainly related to malignancy. Management is discussed in Emergency Box 13.4. Other causes of hypercalcaemia are listed in Table 13.16.

5. (a) C
   (b) E
   (c) D
   (d) B
   (e) A

   The interpretation of thyroid function tests is summarized in Table 13.7.

6. (e) Ectopic adrenocorticotrophin (ACTH) syndrome refers to excess ACTH production by a source outside of the pituitary, leading to signs and symptoms of Cushing's syndrome (p. 626). The most common causes are small cell carcinoma of the lung, carcinoid tumours and islet cell tumours of the pancreas. A low-dose dexamethasone suppression test is used to make a diagnosis of Cushing's syndrome; it does not establish the cause. A raised plasma ACTH in a patient with Cushing's syndrome indicates only that secretion is ACTH dependent, i.e. it is due to excess ACTH secretion from the pituitary, or from an ectopic source; or very rarely due to excess secretion of corticotrophin-releasing hormone. Suppression of plasma cortisol during a high-dose dexamethasone suppression test usually indicates pituitary-dependent Cushing's syndrome in a patient with high plasma ACTH levels. Patients with ectopic ACTH secretion often have hypokalaemia, and plasma ACTH levels do not respond to CRH administration.

7. (a) and (d) have evidence of fluid depletion and the low serum sodium is likely to be due to gastrointestinal and renal loss of sodium respectively. There are also

features in (d) which suggest a diagnosis of adrenal insufficiency. (c) and (e) have evidence of fluid overload due to heart failure and chronic liver disease respectively, and the low serum sodium is likely to be due to relative water excess, although total body sodium is increased. (b) is most suggestive of SIADH, i.e. no evidence of fluid overload or depletion in the presence of normal renal function. This patient is a smoker and may have SIADH secondary to lung cancer.

DIABETES MELLITUS AND OTHER DISORDERS OF METABOLISM

1. A 45-year-old West African woman weighing 95 kg and 160 cm (5 feet 4 inches) tall is found, on routine examination, to have glycosuria without ketonuria, and a random blood glucose on two occasions of > 13 mmol/L.
   (a) What is the diagnosis?
   (b) What type do you suspect?
   (c) What is the initial management?
2. An 18-year-old man who is a known diabetic is admitted as an emergency. His parents say that he has become unwell over the last 3 days, with vomiting and confusion. Laboratory investigations reveal a blood glucose 36 mmol/L, serum sodium 147 mmol/L, urea 12 mmol/L, potassium 5.0 mmol/L and arterial blood pH 7.1.
   (a) What is the diagnosis?
   (b) Considering the serum potassium concentration, is his total body potassium high, low or normal?
   (c) Outline your initial treatment of this patient.
3. A 20-year-old woman complains of being very thirsty and passing large quantities of urine.
   (a) What are the likely causes?
   (b) How would you establish the diagnosis?
4. (a) What are the features of an attack of hypoglycaemia? Suggest the mechanism of each manifestation.
   (b) What causes of a series of proven attacks ought to be considered?
5. A man of 56 has been diabetic since the age of 20. He now complains of bilateral ankle swelling.
   (a) What is the differential diagnosis?

(b) How would you investigate and manage this
patient?

6. A 60-year-old man attends his GP because he is
worried that he is diabetic. His wife has recently been
diagnosed and already has complications. He
understands that complications can sometimes be
prevented and would like to 'start early' if he is a
diabetic. He has no symptoms. Which of the following
investigations would confirm a diagnosis of diabetes?
   (a) Positive urinalysis for glucose
   (b) Random plasma glucose of 11.7 mmol/L
   (c) Fasting plasma glucose of 8 mmol/L and 2-hour
       value of 11.7 mmol/L in a standard glucose
       tolerance test
   (d) HbA$_{1c}$ of 6.9%
   (e) Fasting plasma glucose of 8 mmol/L.

7. (a) A 22-year-old man presenting with diabetic
       ketoacidosis.
   (b) A 49-year-old female with a BMI of 35 kg/m^2 found
       at a routine medical examination to have a fasting
       plasma glucose between 12 and 14 mmol/L on two
       occasions.
   (c) A 67-year-old man with type 2 diabetes, BMI
       25 kg/m^2 and moderate renal impairment.
   (d) An 87-year-old man with type 2 diabetes and
       no symptoms, taking tolbutamide. His HbA$_{1c}$
       is 8%.
   (e) A 59-year-old man with type 2 diabetes mellitus
       presenting with an acute anterior myocardial
       infarction.

   Select the best option for each of the above:
   A. Tolbutamide
   B. Metformin
   C. Bolus insulin
   D. Insulin infusion
   E. Gliclazide.

8. A 65-year-old with type 2 diabetes mellitus is admitted
with an anterior myocardial infarction. He is normally
treated with metformin and review of his notes show
that his HbA$_{1c}$ when measured 2 months ago, was
6.7%. His blood sugar on admission is 12.5 mmol/L.
What is the immediate best treatment for his
diabetes?

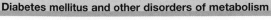
(a) Continue metformin
(b) Continue metformin and add twice-daily intermediate acting insulin
(c) Continue metformin and add a sulphonylurea
(d) Stop metformin and start a sulphonylurea
(e) Stop metformin and start a subcutaneous four-times-daily bolus insulin regimen.

9. A 37-year-old man presents for an evaluation because his brother recently died of coronary disease in his early 40s. The patient's father also has a history of elevated cholesterol and early coronary disease. The patient denies smoking cigarettes and has eliminated high-fat dairy products, most red meat and alcohol from his diet. There is no history of hypertension and physical examination is unremarkable. Measurement of plasma lipids shows a triglyceride of 1.5 mmoL, total cholesterol 9.0 mmol/L, LDL-cholesterol 6.8 mmol/L, HDL-cholesterol 1.5 mmol/L.
    (a) What lipid abnormality do you suspect?
    (b) What other tests would you perform?
    (c) What drug therapy would you prescribe in order to lower the cholesterol?

10. Describe the effects on serum cholesterol of changes in:
    (a) dietary saturated fat
    (b) dietary unsaturated fat
    (c) dietary cholesterol
    (d) sugar.

Answers

1. (a) The random blood sugar confirms the presence of diabetes mellitus.
    (b) Her age, obesity (body mass index > 30) and absence of symptoms or ketosis suggest that this is type 2 diabetes mellitus.
    (c) Initial management involves patient education and weight reduction, achieved with a 1000–1600 kcal diet planned in conjunction with a dietician. Diabetic complications must be sought by physical examination, blood tests and urinalysis (p. 337). Oral hypoglycaemics (p. 653) are necessary if blood glucose remains high in spite of weight loss having been achieved.

939

2. (a) This is diabetic ketoacidosis, as shown by the high blood glucose and acidosis. This is the typical hyperglycaemic emergency of the young diabetic.

    (b) The serum potassium concentration is a poor indicator of total body potassium because most potassium is intracellular. Total body potassium is low with diabetic ketoacidosis because of increased potassium excretion in the urine and loss in the vomit.

    (c) The initial treatment is with intravenous saline, soluble insulin and potassium supplements (p. 660).

3. (a) Frequency of micturition must not be confused with polyuria (usually > 3 L/day); a 24-hour urine output chart is helpful if there is doubt.

    (b) The first and most simple test to perform is a random blood sugar, which will be high if polyuria is secondary to diabetes mellitus. Other causes are primary or hysterical polydipsia (a relatively common cause of polyuria and polydipsia in young women), cranial diabetes insipidus (CDI), nephrogenic DI (p. 630) and chronic renal failure. A full history and examination must include a drug history (e.g. lithium causes nephrogenic DI). Investigations, other than a blood glucose, include serum osmolality, urine osmolality, serum urea, electrolytes and calcium. A water deprivation test may be necessary (p. 632).

4. (a) Symptoms are the result of secretion of counter-regulatory hormones (catecholamines cause hunger, sweating, pallor and tachycardia) and neuroglycopenia (e.g. confusion, drowsiness, fits and eventually coma).

    (b) The causes of hypoglycaemia are listed on page 671. In an otherwise healthy person (e.g. in the absence of cancer, severe liver or renal failure), the most likely causes of recurrent hypoglycaemia are drugs, factitious hypoglycaemia, alcoholic binges and insulinoma. Often the cause will be apparent from the history, physical examination and measurement of blood glucose and plasma insulin during a hypoglycaemic episode. A supervised fast with measurement of glucose, insulin and C-peptide may be needed (p. 672).

5. (a) The most probable causes of leg oedema in this patient are complications resulting from long-standing diabetes, i.e. nephrotic syndrome (p. 665) or heart failure (secondary to ischaemic heart disease).

   (b) These will be distinguished by physical examination, chest X-ray, urine testing for protein and measurement of the serum albumin. Further management depends on the cause and is described on pages 351 and 428.

6. (c) The diagnosis of diabetes is based on plasma glucose, not on measurement of glycosylated haemoglobin or glycosuria (p. 650). In the absence of symptoms (as with this patient) a single high fasting or random plasma glucose is not sufficient to make a diagnosis of diabetes.

7. (a) D

   (b) B

   (c) E

   (d) A

   (e) C

   Diabetic ketoacidosis is treated with an insulin infusion. Acutely ill patients admitted to hospital who are eating should be treated with a bolus insulin regimen. Metformin is useful for patients with type 2 diabetes mellitus who are overweight, but it is contraindicated in renal failure. Gliclazide, which is metabolized by the liver, is a safer option in these patients. Tolbutamide is a safe drug in the elderly because of its short duration of action. The patient in (d) has a HbA_{1c} slightly above the optimum range, but in the very elderly reasonable glucose control and absence of symptoms is the aim.

8. (e) The HbA_{1c} indicates that diabetic control on metformin has been good leading up to this event. However, glucose control in an acutely ill patient is likely to deteriorate, and metformin is contraindicated in severe illness because of the risk of lactic acidosis. Metformin should be stopped. Tight diabetic control will reduce mortality and since he is eating he can be managed with a four-time-daily bolus regimen (p. 670).

9. (a) The patient may have monogenic familial hypercholesterolaemia caused by a defect in the LDL receptor gene (p. 675), or he may have a

polygenic predisposition to elevated LDL-cholesterol. The distinction is not clinically important.

(b) Secondary causes of hyperlipidaemia must be identified. Screening for diabetes mellitus (with a fasting blood glucose) and hypothyroidism (with a serum TSH) should be performed.

(c) Drugs of choice are the HMG-CoA reductase inhibitors and fibrates.

10. Serum cholesterol is mainly derived from endogenous synthesis and thus any dietary modification will have only a small effect. Hypercholesterolaemia is reduced by restricting the intake of cholesterol and saturated fat (both found in animal fat) and replacing with vegetable fat (containing unsaturated fats). Carbohydrate restriction reduces serum triglyceride levels.

NEUROLOGY

1. A woman of 70 wakes one morning with weakness in the right arm and some difficulty in speaking. The symptoms are present the following day and her family bring her to the Accident and Emergency Department.
   (a) What are the likely causes?
   (b) How would you manage this patient?
   (c) What information would you give to the patient and relatives?

2. A man of 65 suddenly develops weakness and numbness of the left arm, which gradually passes off after 15 minutes.
   (a) What are the likely causes?
   (b) How might they be investigated?

3. A 16-year-old girl presents with a 1-day history of severe headache with fever, nausea, vomiting, muscle and joint pains. Over the last 6 hours she had become disorientated and developed a rash. Findings on examination were pulse 125/minute, BP 95/55, temperature 39.5°C. Petechiae and purpura were present on the hands and legs.
   (a) What is your clinical diagnosis?
   (b) What is your immediate management?
   (c) Despite treatment, she deteriorated rapidly and developed a widespread haemorrhagic rash,

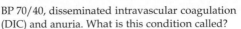
BP 70/40, disseminated intravascular coagulation (DIC) and anuria. What is this condition called?

4. A 40-year-old known alcoholic is brought into Accident and Emergency unconscious and smelling of alcohol.
   (a) What are the most likely causes of coma in this patient?
   (b) Describe your management?

5. (a) List the potentially treatable or reversible causes of apparent dementia.
   (b) What features of the history and clinical findings might arouse your suspicions?

6. A 34-year-old homosexual man with a previous episode of *P. carinii* pneumonia first noted 1 week prior to admission, had poor control of his left hand, and walked to his left. He also noticed difficulty in remembering events, understanding what was read, and dressing apraxia. He had also had early-morning headaches. On examination he was afebrile, he had oral thrush, and fundal examination showed white exudates. He had a left-sided weakness, left homonymous hemianopia and left-sided neglect.
   (a) Do you think this patient has AIDS?
   (b) The history and examination is suggestive of a space-occupying lesion. Where is it situated?
   (c) A brain CT scan shows a ring-enhancing lesion with surrounding oedema and some compression of the adjacent ventricle. What is your differential diagnosis in this patient?

7. A 23-year-old woman was admitted through Accident and Emergency with a 2-day history of symmetrical leg weakness and paraesthesiae. Later she was unable to sit up in bed and reported difficulty in coughing and stiffness of the face. Two weeks previously she had had a short-lived episode of diarrhoea.
   (a) What is the most likely diagnosis?
   (b) What confirmatory tests would you obtain?
   (c) What is the most common antecedent infection to this condition?
   (d) What is the management of this condition?

8. Give three common causes of ptosis and mention the associated features in each case.

9. (a) What are the features of Horner's syndrome?
   (b) Briefly describe the anatomical pathways involved.
   (c) What underlying causes may be responsible?

10. A 30-year-old Asian is admitted with headache and
neck stiffness. CSF findings: pressure 23 mmH$_2$O, red
blood cells 0, white cells 290 × 10^6/L (lymphocytes
82%, monocytes 10%, neutrophils 8%), protein 2 g/L,
glucose 1.8 mmol/L; blood glucose 6 mmol/L.
(a) What are the abnormalities?
(b) What is the diagnosis?

Answers

1. (a) The history is of sudden onset of right-sided
weakness and dysphasia, which is almost certainly
due to a vascular lesion (i.e. stroke). The causes of
stroke are discussed on page 726; in a woman of
this age it is most likely to be due to thrombosis at
the site of atheromatous degeneration in the
middle cerebral artery (p.727).

(b) The investigations and treatment of stroke are
discussed on page 729. A brain CT scan will
differentiate between infarction and haemorrhage.
Aspirin is given to patients with infarction to
reduce the risk of further attacks.

(c) The family must be told that some recovery of
function is expected. Any recovery of speech is
likely to be within the first few days.

2. (a) This is a transient ischaemic attack (TIA), probably
in the territory of the right middle cerebral artery.

(b) The causes and investigation of a TIA are listed on
page 732.

3. (a) Meningitis. The petechial skin rash suggests
meningococcal meningitis.

(b) Immediate intravenous benzylpenicillin should be
given. In the presence of a typical skin rash, lumbar
puncture is not usually necessary and the organism
is found on blood cultures. A CT scan should be
performed if there is any suspicion of an intracranial
mass lesion. Emergency management of suspected
meningitis is outlined in Emergency Box 16.3 on
page 753.

(c) The rapid downhill course is suggestive of
fulminant meningococcaemia
(Waterhouse–Friderichsen syndrome).
Haemorrhage into the adrenal glands may or may
not be present.

4. (a) Coma must never be ascribed to excess alcohol until a thorough history (from relatives, ambulance staff), physical examination and investigation have ruled out other causes. The most likely causes (Table 16.8) in this case are alcohol, drug overdose (with alcohol as a second agent), hypoglycaemia, intracerebral haemorrhage, infarction and Wernicke–Korsakoff syndrome (p. 584).

   (b) The initial management consists of emergency resuscitation to stabilize the patient (p. 724). Intravenous thiamine and glucose (see later) are given. Further assessment (p. 723) and investigations (p. 724) are performed to find the cause of coma. Further management consists of treatment of the underlying cause and care of the unconscious patient (p. 724).

5. (a) The causes of dementia are listed in Table 16.26.

   (b) Treatable causes include hypothyroidism, vitamin B_{12} deficiency, uraemia, hepatic failure, operable cerebral tumour, subdural haematoma and normal pressure hydrocephalus (p. 760). Depression may produce a clinical picture that is indistinguishable from dementia (pseudodementia) and resolves with treatment. Neurosyphilis (p. 755) and Wernicke–Korsakoff syndrome (p. 584) may cause dementia; treatment should always be given, as the disease process may be arrested but rarely reversed. Young age, focal neurological signs, a history of head injury and evidence of anaemia or hypothyroidism should arouse suspicion that this is not Alzheimer's disease (the usual cause of dementia).

6. (a) The history of *P. carinii* pneumonia and oral thrush suggests AIDS.

   (b) Right parietal lobe.

   (c) Ring-enhancing lesions in HIV-infected patients may be caused by *Toxoplasma gondii*, bacteria or lymphoma. Ring enhancement is non-specific and indicates increased vascularity. This patient had a brain abscess caused by infection with *T. gondii* due to reactivation of a previous infection.

7. (a) The distal weakness progressing proximally is the typical picture of Guillain–Barré syndrome (GBS, acute inflammatory polyneuropathy) (p. 774), the

commonest cause of acute generalized muscle weakness.

(b) The diagnosis is made clinically, by nerve conduction studies and examination of the CSF obtained at lumbar puncture.

(c) *Campylobacter jejuni* is a major cause of antecedent infection in GBS patients, and may be associated with a more severe form that tends to be exclusively motor.

(d) The management is:
- *General.* The monitoring and general treatment of these patients is discussed on page 775. In this particular case the difficulty in coughing suggests involvement of the respiratory muscles, and ventilation may well be necessary.
- *Specific.* All patients with any but the mildest deficit should have either plasma exchange or intravenous immune globulin, started as early as possible. Which one is given will often depend on local preference and circumstances.

8. The causes of ptosis are third-nerve lesions (usually complete unilateral ptosis with other eye signs, p. 715), sympathetic paralysis (partial unilateral ptosis with other features of Horner's syndrome, p. 713), myopathy (partial bilateral), congenital (present since birth, usually partial, no other neurological signs) and syphilis (tabes dorsalis, p. 756).

9. The features and causes of Horner's syndrome are described on page 713.

10. (a) There is a CSF lymphocytosis, reduced glucose (in the absence of hypoglycaemia), markedly raised protein and raised CSF pressure. A raised CSF protein occurs with any inflammatory lesion of the CNS. A reduced CSF glucose occurs with bacterial or tuberculous meningitis, and rarely with viral and fungal infections and malignancy. The CSF lymphocytosis is against bacterial meningitis unless it has been partially treated.

(b) The findings are most likely to be due to tuberculous meningitis, which is particularly common in Asians.

DERMATOLOGY

1. A 24-year-old woman complains of a rash on her lower legs.
   (a) What features would lead you to suspect that this is erythema nodosum?
   (b) What are the common causes of erythema nodosum?
   (c) How would you investigate a patient with this condition?

2. Which of the following are true for psoriasis:
   (a) Nail changes are indicators of severe disease.
   (b) Bacterial infections are important triggers of the disease.
   (c) The disease is confined to the skin and not associated with systemic features.
   (d) Granulomas are typically found on skin biopsy.
   (e) Biological therapy (e.g. infliximab) is only indicated in severe disease.

Answers

1. (a) The causes and clinical features of erythema nodosum are listed on page 792.
   (b) Sarcoidosis and inflammatory bowel disease are the most common causes in the UK. A history of recent antibiotic ingestion, oral contraceptives, TB contact or alteration in bowel habit should be sought.
   (c) Basic investigations should include a full blood count, ESR, antistreptolysin O titre (ASOT), throat swab and chest X-ray. Further investigations will depend on the history and associated clinical findings. For instance, in a patient who also has diarrhoea it would be reasonable to perform a small bowel barium follow-through examination to look for Crohn's disease. In a patient who is otherwise well and with a single attack, further investigation may be unnecessary.

2. (a) False. Nail changes may predate the development of skin manifestations and may be present in isolation.
   (b) True. Streptococcal infection of the throat etc. is often associated with a flare-up of the disease, particularly the guttate form.
   (c) False. Systemic features are not uncommon, with arthritis developing in 10% of cases.

947

(d) False. Granulomas are not a feature on skin biopsy.
(e) True. The newer biological therapies are not yet
    licensed for use in the UK and are restricted to
    unresponsive disease.

Dictionary of terms

There are excellent on-line medical dictionaries with definitions for thousands of medical words and conditions. Sites for two of them are:

http://www.medterms.com
http://cancerweb.ncl.ac.uk/omd/

Adenoma A benign epithelial neoplasm in which the cells form recognizable glandular structures or in which they are clearly derived from glandular epithelium.

Adjuvant Term applied to chemotherapy or hormone therapy given after local treatment, in tumours where dissemination is undetectable but can be assumed to have occurred. If effective, it should lead to an increase in cure rate or overall disease-free survival.

Aerobic In microbiology refers to growing, living or occurring in the presence of molecular oxygen. Bacteria that require oxygen to survive (aerobic bacteria).

Afterload The load against which the cardiac muscle exerts its contractile force, i.e. the peripheral vascular tree.

Agonist A drug that has affinity for and in some way activates a receptor when it occupies it.

Alkaptonuria Inborn error of amino acid metabolism resulting from a defect in the enzyme homogentisic acid oxidase and causing an accumulation of homogentisic acid in the urine. The condition is characterized by ochronosis (accumulation of a blue-black pigment in connective tissues) and arthritis. The slate blue-black pigmentation is most apparent in the sclera of the eyes, the external ears, and the tympanic membranes.

Allogeneic transplantation When another individual acts as the donor.

Alopecia   Hair loss from areas where it is normally present.

Alport's syndrome   Hereditary disorder characterized by progressive sensorineural hearing loss, nephritis and renal failure, and, occasionally, ocular defects; transmitted as an autosomal dominant or X-linked trait.

Ambulant (ambulatory)   Able to walk; may be used to describe patients who do not require a wheelchair or are not confined to bed.

Anaerobic   Lacking molecular oxygen. Growing, living or occurring in the absence of molecular oxygen, pertaining to an anaerobe.

Angiography   A radiographic technique where a radio-opaque contrast material is injected into a blood vessel for the purpose of identifying its anatomy on X-ray.

Annular lesions   Lesions occurring in rings.

Antagonist   A drug that binds to a cell receptor and does not activate it.

Antibody   An immunoglobulin molecule that has a specific amino acid sequence by virtue of which it interacts only with the antigen that induced its synthesis in cells of the lymphoid series (especially plasma cells), or with antigen closely related to it.

Antigen   Any substance, organism or foreign material recognized by the immune system as being 'non-self', which will provoke the production of a specific antibody.

Antineutrophil cytoplasmic antibodies (ANCAs)   These are detected on fixed human neutrophils. There are two types:
- Antibodies directed against proteinase 3 (PR3-ANCA), formerly called cytoplasmic or cANCA. Present in 90% of patients with Wegener's granulomatosis.
- Antibodies directed against myeloperoxidase, formerly called perinuclear or pANCA. Present in 60% of some other vasculitides, such as microscopic polyangiitis and Churg–Strauss syndrome. Also found in inflammatory bowel disease and rheumatological disease which is not associated with a vasculitis.

Antinuclear antibodies (ANA)   Represent a wide spectrum of autoantibodies. They are non-specific and may occur at low titre (e.g. 1 : 10) in healthy individuals.

Antioxidant   An enzyme or other organic substance that has the ability to counteract the damaging effects of oxygen in tissues. It has been suggested that antioxidant vitamins such as vitamin E may provide protection against certain diseases, including atherosclerosis.

Aphasia (dysphasia)   A disturbance of the ability to use language, whether in speaking, writing or comprehending. It is caused by left frontoparietal lesions, often a stroke.

- Broca's aphasia (expressive aphasia) is due to a lesion in the left frontal lobe. There is reduced fluency of speech, with comprehension relatively preserved. The patient knows what he/she wants to say but cannot get the words out.
- Wernicke's aphasia (receptive aphasia) is due to a left temporoparietal lesion. The patient speaks fluently but words are put together in the wrong order, and in the most severe forms the patient speaks complete rubbish with the insertion of non-existent words. Comprehension is severely impaired.
- Global aphasia is due to widespread damage to the areas concerned with speech. The patient shows combined expressive and receptive dysphasia.

Apoptosis   Programmed cell death, as signalled by the nuclei in normally functioning cells when age or state of cell health dictates.

Apraxia   Loss of the ability to carry out familiar purposeful movements in the absence of paralysis or other motor or sensory impairment.

Ataxia   Is due to failure of coordination of complex muscular movements despite intact individual movements and sensation.

Atrophy   Thinning (e.g. of the skin).

Autoantibody   An antibody that reacts with an antigen which is a normal component of the body.

Autologous   When the patient acts as his or her own source of cells.

Autosomal dominant   Requires only one affected parent to have the trait to pass it on to offspring.

Autosomal recessive Mutation carried on an autosome (i.e. a chromosome not involved in sex determination) that is deleterious only in homozygotes (identical alleles of the gene are carried). Both affected parents must have the trait to pass it on to their offspring.

Baker's cyst A synovial cyst located in the back of the knee, in the popliteal space, arising from the semimembranous bursa or the knee joint. May rupture and cause calf swelling.

Behçet's disease A rare multisystem chronic recurrent disease characterized by recurrent ulceration in the mouth and genitalia, iritis, uveitis, arthritis, superficial thrombophlebitis and major vascular thrombosis (usually venous). Often treated with immunosuppressive therapy (corticosteroids, chlorambucil).

Benign intracranial hypertension (pseudotumour cerebri) Increased pressure within the brain in the absence of a tumour. Presents with symptoms of raised intracranial pressure. Most common in women between the ages of 20 and 50. The cause is usually not known. May be associated with some drugs. Diagnosis is by brain imaging and lumbar puncture.

Bone marrow Is obtained for examination by aspiration from the anterior iliac crest or sternum. In many cases a trephine biopsy (removal of a core of bone marrow tissue) is also necessary.

Bronchoalveolar lavage At bronchoscopy a lung segment is washed with saline and the fluid retrieved for cell analysis.

Bulla A large vesicle.

Bursa A closed fluid-filled sac lined with synovium that functions to facilitate movement and reduce friction between tissues of the body. Bursitis is inflammation of a bursa.

C1 esterase inhibitor (C1-INH) deficiency (hereditary angio-oedema, hereditary angioneurotic oedema) Presents with recurring attacks of transient oedema suddenly appearing in areas of the skin or mucous membranes and occasionally of the viscera, often associated with dermatographism, urticaria, erythema, and purpura.

Carcinoma   A malignant neoplasm arising from epithelium.

Cardiac catheterization   The passage of a small catheter through a peripheral vein (for study of right-sided heart structures) or artery (for study of left-sided heart structures) into the heart, permitting the securing of blood samples, measurement of intracardiac pressures and determination of cardiac anomalies.

Cardiac nuclear imaging   Uses radiotracers (injected intravenously) which diffuse freely into myocardial tissue or attach to red blood cells.

- Thallium-201 is taken up by cardiac myocytes. Ischaemic areas (produced by exercising the patient) with reduced tracer uptake are seen as 'cold spots' when imaged with a γ camera.
- Technetium-99m is used to label red blood cells and produce images of the left ventricle during systole and diastole.

Caseating   Developing a necrotic centre.

CD (cluster differentiation) antigens   Antigens on the cell surface that can be detected by immune reagents and which are associated with the differentiation of a particular cell type or types. Many cells can be identified by their possession of a unique set of differentiation antigens, e.g. CD4, CD8.

Cheyne–Stokes respiration   An abnormal breathing pattern in which there are periods of rapid breathing alternating with periods of no breathing or slow breathing.

Choledochal cyst   A congenital anatomical malformation of a bile duct, including cystic dilatation of the extra-hepatic bile duct or the large intrahepatic bile duct. Classification is based on the site and type of dilatation. Type I is most common.

Chronic granulomatous disease   A recessive X-linked defect of leucocyte function in which phagocytic cells ingest but fail to digest bacteria, resulting in recurring bacterial infections with granuloma formation.

Chronotropic   Positively chronotropic means to increase the rate of contraction of the heart; negatively chronotropic is the opposite.

Clone   A population of identical cells or organisms that are derived from a single cell or ancestor and contain identical DNA molecules.

Clubbing   Broadening or thickening of the tips of the fingers and toes with increased lengthwise curvature of the nail and a decrease in the angle normally seen between cuticle and finger-nail. Causes include congenital, respiratory (lung cancer, tuberculosis, bronchiectasis, lung abscess or empyema, lung fibrosis), cardiac (bacterial endocarditis, cyanotic congenital heart disease), and rarely gastrointestinal (Crohn's disease, cirrhosis).

Clubfoot (talipes equinovarus)   A deformed foot in which the foot is plantar flexed, inverted and adducted.

Congenital   Something that is present at birth. It may or may not be genetic (inherited).

Constructional apraxia   Inability to copy simple drawings: often seen in hepatic encephalopathy, when the patient is unable to copy a five-pointed star.

Contraindication   Any condition, especially a disease or current treatment, which renders some particular line of treatment undesirable.

C-reactive protein (CRP)   Is synthesized in the liver and produced during the acute-phase response. It is quick and easy to measure and is replacing measurement of the ESR in some centres.

Crust   Dried exudate on the skin.

Cryoglobulins   Immunoglobulins that precipitate when cold or during exercise. They may be monoclonal or polyclonal, e.g. mixed essential cryoglobulinaemia, and result in a cutaneous vasculitis or occasionally a multi-system disorder.

Cryptogenic   A disease of obscure or unknown origin.

CT scan (computed tomography)   CT combines the use of X-rays with computerized analysis of the images to assimilate multiple X-ray images into a two-dimensional cross-sectional image. With helical or spiral CT scanning, computer interpolation allows reconstruction of standard transverse scans or images in any preferred plane. CT angiography uses X-rays to visualize blood flow in arterial vessels throughout the body.

Cytokines Soluble messenger molecules which enable the immune system to communicate through its different compartments. Cytokines are made by many cells, such as lymphocytes (lymphokines) and other white cells (interleukins). Examples of cytokines, other than inter-leukins, include tumour necrosis factor (TNF), interferons and granulocyte colony-stimulating factor (G-CSF).

Dextrocardia The heart is in the right hemithorax, with the apex directed to the right.

DIDMOAD syndrome (Wolfram's syndrome) Hereditary association of diabetes insipidus, diabetes mellitus, optic atrophy and deafness.

Distal A term of comparison meaning farther from a point of reference; it is the opposite of proximal.

Doppler ultrasound A form of ultrasound that can detect and measure blood flow. Doppler ultrasound depends on the Doppler effect, a change in the frequency of a wave resulting from the motion of a reflector, i.e. the red blood cell in the case of Doppler ultrasound.

Down's syndrome Chromosome disorder associated either with a triplication or translocation of chromosome 21. Clinical manifestations include mental retardation, short stature, flat hypoplastic face with short nose, prominent epicanthic skinfolds, small low-set ears with prominent antihelix, fissured and thickened tongue, laxness of joint ligaments, pelvic dysplasia, broad hands and feet, stubby fingers, transverse palmar crease, lenticular opacities and heart disease. Patients with Down's syndrome have an increased risk for leukaemia and early onset of Alzheimer's disease.

Dysarthria Disordered articulation. Any lesion that produces paralysis, slowing or incoordination of the muscles of articulation, or local discomfort, will cause dysarthria. Examples are upper and lower motor lesions of the lower cranial nerves, cerebellar lesions, Parkinson's disease and local lesions in the mouth, larynx, pharynx and tongue.

Dysplasia Abnormal cell growth or maturation of cells.

Ecchymoses   Bruises > 3 mm in diameter.

Echocardiography   Non-invasive method of recording the position and motion of the structures of the heart by echo obtained from beams of ultrasonic waves directed through the chest wall.
  ■ Transoesophageal echo uses miniaturized transducers incorporated into special endoscopes. It allows better visualization of some structures and pathology, e.g. aortic dissection, prosthetic valve endocarditis.
  ■ Doppler echocardiography uses the Doppler principle (in this case, the frequency of ultrasonic waves reflected from blood cells is related to their velocity and direction of flow) to identify and assess the severity of valve lesions.

Ectopic   Located away from its normal position, such as an ectopic pregnancy.

Ejection fraction   The fraction of the ventricular end-diastolic volume that is ejected during cardiac systole. It is usually equal to about 60%.

Electroencephalogram (EEG)   Electrodes applied to the patient's scalp pick up small changes in electrical potential which, after amplification, are recorded on paper or displayed on a video monitor. It is used in the investigation of epilepsy and diffuse brain disorders.

Electromyography (EMG)   A needle electrode is inserted percutaneously into voluntary muscle. Amplified action potentials are recorded on an oscilloscope. Normal resting muscle shows no activity, and during increasing muscle contractions progressively larger numbers of motor units are recruited. EMG is useful in the diagnosis of primary muscle disease (myopathies and dystrophies – individual motor unit potentials are small) and of lower motor neurone lesions (denervation – spontaneous activity appears at rest).

Empirical   Based on experience. Empirical treatment refers to treatment given to an individual that is based on the experience of the physician in treating previous patients with a similar presentation. It is not completely 'scientific' treatment.

End-diastolic volume   The volume of blood in the ventricle at the end of diastole.

Endemic   Present in a community at all times.

Endogenous   Related to or produced by the body.

Enzyme-linked immunosorbent (ELISA) assay   A serologic test used for the detection of particular antibodies or antigens in the blood. ELISA technology links a measurable enzyme to either an antigen or antibody. In this way it can then measure the presence of an antibody or an antigen in the bloodstream.

Eosinophilia   (normal range $0.04–0.44 \times 10^9$/L, 1–6% of total white cells) occurs in asthma and allergic disorders, parasitic infections (e.g. *Ascaris*), skin disorders (urticaria, pemphigus and eczema), malignancy and the hyper-eosinophilic syndrome (restrictive cardiomyopathy, hepatosplenomegaly and very high eosinophil count).

Epidemic   An outbreak of a disease affecting a large number of individuals in a community at the same time. The number of people affected is in excess of the expected.

Epidemiology   The study of the distribution and determinants of health-related states and events in populations.

Epitope   That part of an antigenic molecule to which an antibody or T-cell receptor responds.

ERCP   Endoscopic retrograde cholangiopancreatography. The ampulla of Vater is cannulated, and after injection of radio-opaque contrast medium the pancreatic and common bile ducts (CBD) can be visualized. The sphincter of Oddi may be cut (sphincterotomy) to facilitate the removal of stones and insertion of stents.

Erythema   Redness.

Erythrocyte sedimentation rate (ESR)   The rate of fall of red cells in a column of blood; a measure of the acute-phase response. The speed is mainly determined by the concentration of large proteins, e.g. fibrinogen. The ESR is higher in women and rises with age. It is raised in a wide variety of systemic inflammatory and neoplastic diseases. The highest values (> 100 mm/h) are found in chronic infections (e.g. TB), myeloma, connective tissue disorders and cancer.

Erythroderma   Widespread redness of the skin, with scaling.

Euthanasia   The illegal act of killing someone painlessly, especially to relieve suffering from an incurable disease.

Excoriation   Linear marks caused by scratching.

Excretion urography   (intravenous urography (IVU) or intravenous pyelography (IVP)). Serial radiographs are taken of the kidney and the full length of the abdomen, following intravenous injection of contrast, usually an organic iodine-containing medium.

Exogenous   Developed or originated outside of the body.

Extractable nuclear antigens (ENA)   Nuclear components that are soluble in saline. Examples are Sm, Ro, La and ribonucleoprotein (RNP) antigen. The presence of serum anti-Sm antibodies is highly specific for SLE. Anti-Ro (SS-A) and anti-La (SS-B) occur in patients with Sjögren's syndrome and in some patients with SLE.

Exudate   Fluid rich in protein and cells, which has leaked from blood vessels and been deposited in tissues.

Factitious   Artificial, self-induced.

Familial Mediterranean fever   Inherited disorder more common in those of Mediterranean descent. Recurrent episodes of abdominal pain (due to peritoneal inflammation), fever and arthritis.

Fissure   A cleft, groove or slit, e.g. an anal fissure is an ulcer in the anal canal.

Fistula   A tunnel or abnormal passage connecting two epithelial surfaces, frequently designated according to the organs or parts with which it communicates, e.g. a vesicocolic fistula connects the bladder to the colon.

Fitz-Hugh–Curtis syndrome   Inflammation of the liver capsule associated with genital tract infection – occurs in about 25% of patients with pelvic inflammatory disease. *Neisseria gonorrhoeae* and *Chlamydia trachomatis* are the main causes. Women present with sharp right upper quadrant pain with or without signs of salpingitis. Diagnosis is often clinical and treatment is with appropriate antibiotics.

Gaucher's disease Inherited (autosomal recessive) disorder of lipid metabolism caused by a deficiency of the enzyme β-glucocerebrosidase. Clinical features include hepatosplenomegaly and sometimes neurological dysfunction.

Generic drugs Non-proprietary drugs. They should usually be used when prescribing in preference to proprietary titles.

Glomerular filtration rate (GFR) This is the most widely used test of renal function. In routine clinical practice the most reliable index of GFR is measurement of endogenous creatinine clearance, which is calculated from measurement of a single serum creatinine value.

Hallucinations Perceptions that occur in the absence of external stimuli and while an individual is awake. They may involve any of the senses, including hearing (auditory hallucinations), vision (visual hallucinations), smell (olfactory hallucinations), taste (gustatory hallucinations), and touch (tactile hallucinations). Hallucinations may be drug induced or caused by chronic alcohol excess, temporal lobe epilepsy, psychotic illnesses, or certain organic disorders, such as Huntington's disease.

Histocompatibility antigens Genetically determined isoantigens present on the membranes of nucleated cells. They incite an immune response when grafted on to genetically disparate individuals, and thus determine the compatibility of cells in transplantation.

Howell–Jolly bodies DNA remnants in peripheral RBCs seen post-splenectomy, and in leukaemia and megaloblastic anaemia.

Human leucocyte antigens (HLA) Human histocompatibility antigens determined by a region on chromosome 6. There are several genetic loci, each having multiple alleles, designated HLA-A, HLA-B, HLA-C, HLA-DP, -DQ and -DR. The susceptibility to some diseases is associated with certain HLA alleles (e.g. HLA-B27 in 95% of patients with ankylosing spondylitis), although their exact role in aetiology is unclear.

Hyperplasia The abnormal multiplication or increase in the number of normal cells in normal arrangement in a tissue.

Hypertrophy The enlargement or overgrowth of an organ or part due to an increase in size of its constituent cells.

Iatrogenic Induced inadvertently by medical treatment or procedures, or activity of attending physician.

Idiopathic Of unknown cause.

Idiosyncratic Relates to idiosyncrasy – an abnormal susceptibility to a drug or other agent which is peculiar to the individual.

Incidence An expression of the rate at which a certain event occurs, as the number of new cases of a specific disease occurring during a certain period.

Inotropic Positively inotropic means increasing the force of cardiac muscle contraction.

Insidious Subtle, gradual, or imperceptible development. May be used to refer to the onset of symptoms or signs before the diagnosis of a disorder.

In vitro Outside of the body in an artificial environment such as a test tube.

In vivo Within the body.

Kawasaki's disease An acute febrile illness (lasting more than 5 days) of unknown aetiology that occurs mainly in children. Features include damage to the coronary arteries which is reduced by treatment with aspirin and intravenous γ-globulin.

Left shift Immature white cells appear in the peripheral blood, e.g. with infection.

Leucocytosis An increase in the total circulating white cells ($> 11 \times 10^9$/L).

Leucoerythroblastic reaction Immature red and white cells appearing in the peripheral blood. It occurs in marrow infiltration (e.g. malignancy), myeloid leukaemia and severe anaemia.

Leucopenia A decrease in the total circulating white cells ($< 4.0 \times 10^9$/L).

Leukaemoid reaction A reactive but excessive leucocytosis characterized by the presence of immature cells in the peripheral blood.

Macule A flat circumscribed area of discolouration.

Maculopapule A raised and discoloured circumscribed lesion.

Magnetic resonance imaging (MRI) Uses the body's natural magnetic properties to produce detailed images from any part of the body. It does not involve radiation. Gadolinium is used as an intravenous contrast medium. MRI scanning is potentially life threatening for patients who have had medical or surgical (or accidental) metal implants (e.g. pacemakers, metallic clips, metal valves and joints) because of potential movement within a magnetic field. A metal check (including foreign bodies in the eye) should be done before requesting an MRI. Some implants are MRI safe and some are not. Most MRI departments will have a comprehensive safety check list of such devices and implants.

Marfan's syndrome Autosomal dominant connective tissue disorder associated with mutations in the fibrillin 1 gene on chromosome 15. Up to one-third are new mutations. Clinical features include tall stature, long thin digits (arachnodactyly), high-arched palate, hypermobile joints, lens subluxation, incompetence of aortic and mitral valves, aortic dissection and spontaneous pneumothorax.

Ménétrier's disease (giant hypertrophic gastritis) Gastritis with hypertrophy of the gastric mucosa. Characterized by giant gastric folds, diminished acid secretion, excessive secretion of mucus, and hypoproteinaemia. Symptoms include vomiting, diarrhoea and weight loss.

Metaplasia A change in the type of cells in a tissue to a form which is not normal for that tissue.

Methaemoglobinaemia A condition in which the iron within haemoglobin is oxidized from the ferrous (Fe^{2+}) state to the ferric (Fe^{3+}) state, resulting in the inability to transport oxygen and carbon dioxide. Clinically, there is cyanosis. May be congenital or acquired (after exposure to certain drugs and toxins).

Micturating cystoscopy Used mainly for the evaluation of vesicoureteric reflux in children. Contrast medium is instilled into the bladder via a catheter, and the ureters and kidneys are then screened during micturition.

Miller Fisher syndrome A variant of the Guillain–Barré syndrome characterized by the acute onset of oculomotor dysfunction, ataxia, and loss of deep tendon reflexes with relative sparing of strength in the extremities and trunk. Facial weakness and sensory loss may also occur.

Mirizzi's syndrome Obstructive jaundice caused by compression of the common hepatic duct by a stone in the cystic duct or the neck of the gall bladder.

Monocytosis (normal range $0.04–0.44 \times 10^9$/L, 1–6% of total white cells) occurs in chronic bacterial infections (e.g. TB), myelodysplasia and malignancy, particularly chronic myelomonocytic leukaemia.

Mutation A change in a gene, such as loss, gain, or substitution of genetic material, that alters its function or expression. This change is passed along with subsequent divisions of the affected cell. Gene mutations may occur randomly for unknown reasons or may be inherited.

National Institute for Health and Clinical Excellence (NICE) This is part of the National Health Service (NHS) in the UK and its role is to provide patients, health professionals and the public with authoritative, robust and reliable guidance on current 'best practice'.

nd Notifiable disease.

Necrosis Morphological changes indicative of cell death and caused by the progressive degradative action of enzymes; it may affect groups of cells or part of a structure or an organ.

Neutropenia Decrease in circulating neutrophils in the peripheral blood (normal range $2–7.5 \times 10^9$/L, 40–75% of total white cells). Causes include racial (in black Africans), viral infection, severe bacterial infection, megaloblastic anaemia, pancytopenia and drugs (marrow aplasia or immune destruction).

Neutrophil leucocytosis Occurs in bacterial infection, tissue necrosis, inflammation, corticosteroid therapy, myeloproliferative disease, leukaemoid reaction, leuco-erythroblastic anaemia, acute haemorrhage and haemolysis.

Nodulo A circumscribed large palpable mass > 1 cm in diameter.

Normoblasts Immature nucleated red blood cells (RBCs) seen in the peripheral blood with a leucoerthyroblastic reaction and severe anaemia.

Objective Structured Clinical Examination (OSCE) Examination based on planned clinical encounters in which the candidate (student, doctor or nurse) inter-views, examines, informs, or otherwise interacts with a standardized patient (SP). SPs are individuals who are scripted and rehearsed to portray an actual patient with a specific set of symptoms or clinical findings. SPs may be able-bodied individuals or actual patients with stable findings.

Oligoarticular Affecting a limited number of joints.

Oncogene Gene coding for proteins which are either growth factors, growth factor receptors, secondary messengers or DNA-binding proteins. Mutation of the gene promotes abnormal cell growth.

Osmolality The concentration of osmotically active particles in solution expressed in terms of osmoles of solute per kilogram of solvent.

Osmolarity The concentration of osmotically active particles expressed in terms of osmoles of solute per litre of solution.

Pancytopenia Deficiency of all cell elements of the blood.

Papule A circumscribed raised palpable area.

Pathognomonic A symptom or sign that, when present, points unmistakably to the presence of a certain definite disease.

Persistent vegetative state A condition of life without consciousness or will as a result of brain damage.

Petechiae Bruises < 3 mm in diameter.

Phenotype The appearance and function of an organism as a result of its genotype and its environment.

Plaque   A disc-shaped lesion; can result from coalescence of papules.

Polychromasia   Blue tinge to red blood cells in the blood film caused by the presence of young red cells.

Polymerase chain reaction (PCR)   Technique for rapid detection and analysis of DNA and, by a modification of the method, RNA. Using oligonucleotide primers and DNA polymerase, minute amounts of genomic DNA can be amplified over a million times into measurable quantities.

Positron emission tomography (PET) scanning   Allows the imaging of structures by virtue of their ability to concentrate specific molecules that have been labelled with a positron-emitting isotope, e.g. a glucose analogue (that is not metabolized by the cell) tagged with fluorine (FDG). Metabolically active cells including malignant cells utilize and import more glucose than other tissues and thus take up FDG more avidly. False positives occur with active infections or inflammatory processes.

Prevalence   Total number of cases of a disease in existence at a certain time in a designated area.

Prognosis   A forecast as to the probable outcome of an attack or disease.

Promyelocytes, myelocytes and metamyelocytes   Immature white cells seen in the peripheral blood in leucoerythroblastic anaemia.

Prophylaxis   Prevention of disease.

Proximal   A term of comparison meaning nearer or closer to a point of reference; for example, proximal myopathy is weakness of muscles nearest to the trunk, e.g. quadriceps.

Purpura   Extravasation of blood into the skin; does not blanch on pressure.

Pustule   A pus-filled blister.

Radioimmunoassay (RIA)   Any system for testing antigen–antibody reactions in which use is made of radioactive labelling of antigen or antibody to detect the extent of the reaction.

Refractory Resistant to or not responding readily to treatment.

Retrograde pyelography Following cystoscopy a catheter is placed in the ureteral orifice and contrast injected. It is used to investigate lesions of the lower ureter and to define the lower level of ureteral obstruction shown on ultrasound or antegrade studies.

Rhabdomyolysis The destruction of skeletal muscle cells. May be due to electrical injury, alcoholism, injury, drug side-effects or toxins.

Rheumatoid factors (RhF) Autoantibodies found in the serum, usually of the IgM class, which are directed against the Fc portion of human IgG. They are found in high titre in 70% of patients with rheumatoid arthritis. They may also be detected in other autoimmune rheumatic diseases, autoimmune hepatitis, chronic infections, and in elderly people at low titres.

Scales Dried flakes of dead skin.

Serum The cell-free portion of blood from which fibrinogen has been separated in the process of clotting. Serum is the supernatant obtained by high-speed centrifugation of whole blood collected in a plain tube.

Sinus A blind track opening onto the skin or a mucous surface.

Syndrome A set of signs or a series of events occurring together that point to a single condition as the cause.

Target cells ('Mexican hat cells') Red blood cells with central staining surrounded by a ring of pallor and an outer ring of staining. They occur in thalassaemia, sickle cell disease and liver disease.

Telangiectasia A visible, dilated blood vessel creating small focal red lesions in skin, mucous membranes or gut.

Teratogenic Possessing the ability to disrupt normal fetal development and causing fetal abnormalities.

TNM classification (tumour, node, metastasis) Staging system for many cancers. T is the extent of primary tumour, N is the involvement of lymph nodes and M indicates the presence or absence of metastases. For instance T0–T4 indicates increasing local tumour spread.

Transudate A plasma-derived fluid that accumulates in tissues/cavities as a result of venous and capillary pressure.

Tumour suppressor genes Genes whose protein products induce the repair or self-destruction (apoptosis) of cells containing damaged DNA. Unlike oncogenes, they restrict undue cell proliferation.

Turner's syndrome Females with chromosomes 45X instead of the normal female chromosomes, 46XX. Growth failure, gonadal dysgenesis, widely spaced nipples, webbed neck, cardiac abnormalities, intelligence usually normal.

Vesicle A small, visible, fluid-filled blister.

Von Hippel–Lindau syndrome Autosomal dominant disorder characterized by cerebellar and retinal neoplasms, clear cell renal carcinoma, pheochromocytoma, pancreatic tumours, and inner ear tumours. Associated with germline mutations of the VHL tumour suppressor gene.

Weal A transiently raised reddened area associated with scratching.

Xenotransplantation Transplantation of organs or tissues between different species.

Zoonosis Transmission of a disease from an animal or non-human species to humans. The reservoir for the disease is not human.

Index

Normal values